Magnetic Resonance Imaging: Principles, Techniques and Clinical Applications

Magnetic Resonance Imaging: Principles, Techniques and Clinical Applications

Edited by Zachary Garcia

AMERICAN
MEDICAL PUBLISHERS
www.americanmedicalpublishers.com

American Medical Publishers,
41 Flatbush Avenue,
1st Floor, New York,
NY 11217, USA

Visit us on the World Wide Web at:
www.americanmedicalpublishers.com

ISBN: 978-1-63927-074-3

Cataloging-in-Publication Data

Magnetic resonance imaging : principles, techniques and clinical applications / edited by Zachary Garcia.
p. cm.
Includes bibliographical references and index.
ISBN 978-1-63927-074-3
1. Magnetic resonance imaging. 2. Diagnostic imaging.
3. Imaging systems in medicine. I. Garcia, Zachary.
RC78.7.N83 M34 2022
616.075 48--dc23

Table of Contents

Preface

The technique that is used in radiology to form pictures of the physiological processes and the anatomy of the body is known as magnetic resonance imaging (MRI). Magnetic field gradients, radio waves and strong magnetic fields are used in it to generate images of the organs in the body. Magnetic resonance imaging is different from CT scan and PET scan and does not involve X-rays and the use of ionizing radiation. In hospitals and clinics, magnetic resonance imaging is primarily used for staging of disease, medical diagnosis, and follow-up without getting body exposed to radiation. MRI is widely used in cardiovascular imaging, spinal imaging, neuroimaging, angiography, etc. This book contains some path-breaking studies in the field of magnetic resonance imaging. It strives to provide a fair idea about this discipline and to help develop a better understanding of the latest advances within this field. This book aims to equip students and experts with the advanced topics and upcoming concepts in this area.

The information shared in this book is based on empirical researches made by veterans in this field of study. The elaborative information provided in this book will help the readers further their scope of knowledge leading to advancements in this field.

Finally, I would like to thank my fellow researchers who gave constructive feedback and my family members who supported me at every step of my research.

Editor

Unusual MRI findings in an immunocompetent patient with EBV encephalitis

Paola Di Carlo[1*], Marcello Trizzino[1], Lucina Titone[1], Giuseppina Capra[1], Piero Colletti[2], Giovanni Mazzola[2], Daniela Pistoia[1] and Caterina Sarno[3]

Abstract

Blackground: It is well-known that Epstein-Barr virus (EBV) can affect the central nervous system (CNS).

Case presentation: Herein the authors report unusual timely Magnetic Resonance Imaging (MRI) brain scan findings in an immunocompetent patient with EBV encephalitis.
Diffusion weighted MRI sequence performed during the acute phase of the disease was normal, whereas the Fast Relaxation Fast Spin Echo T2 image showed diffuse signal intensity changes in white matter. The enhancement pattern suggested an inflammatory response restricted to the brain microcirculation. Acyclovir and corticosteroid therapy was administered. After three weeks, all signal intensities returned to normal and the patient showed clinical recovery.

Conclusion: This report demonstrates that EBV in an immunocompetent adult can present with diffuse, reversible brain white matter involvement in the acute phase of mononucleosis. Moreover, our case suggests that a negative DWI sequence is associated with a favorable improvement in severe EBV CNS infection. More extensive studies are needed to assess what other instrumental data can help to distinguish viral lesions from other causes in the acute phase of disease.

Keywords: Epstein-Barr virus encephalitis, MRI, Diffusion-weighted imaging

Background

Epstein-Barr virus (EBV) is the causative agent of infectious mononucleosis (IM) and can lead to various central nervous system (CNS) complications, such as demyelinating disease, acute encephalitis, meningitis and acute cerebellar ataxia [1-3]. The illness usually runs a benign course, though fatal cases have been reported [4].

Neurological involvement has been reported in children during the acute phase of the disease and sequelae occur in a substantial number of patients [4-6]. Neurological manifestations associated with reactivation of EBV infection in immunocompetent adults have recently been reported [7,8]. Furthermore, evidence suggests that EBV plays a role in multiple sclerosis (MS) disease activity and in Acute disseminate encephalomyelitis (ADEM), an immune-mediated inflammatory disorder of the CNS, characterized by a multifocal demyelination that involves the white matter of the brain and spinal cord [9,10].

Magnetic resonance imaging (MRI) shows small or multiple CNS lesions more clearly, allowing rapid diagnosis and the formulation of more effective therapeutic strategies [6,11]. Diffusion-weighted imaging (DWI) sequence identifies CNS lesions earlier than T2W or Fluid Attenuated Inversion Recovery (FLAIR) imaging [11-15].

Herein we report an unusual timely CNS imaging sequence in an immunocompetent patient with acute infectious mononucleosis.

Case presentation

A 19-year-old Italian male student came to the Emergency Department of the "Policlinico Paolo Giaccone" University Hospital in Palermo, Italy, with fever, headache and altered consciousness. The fever started one week before presentation; he had experienced

* Correspondence: pdicarlo@unipa.it
[1]Dipartimento di Scienze per la Promozione della Salute, Università di Palermo, Italy
Full list of author information is available at the end of the article

pharyngitis, lymphadenopathy and asthenia. He had no other history of disease and was immunocompetent. An initial cranial CT scan was normal.

On admission, he had a Glasgow score of 12 and a temperature of 38.6°C; he had visual disorders including blurred vision, impaired accommodation and diplopia.

He presented with cervical lymphadenopathy and hepatosplenomegaly.

Laboratory tests revealed that he had a white blood cell count of 15400 cell mm^{-3}, with 20% neutrophils, 36,2% lymphocytes, 33,1% monocytes and hypertransaminasemia (aspartate aminotransferase level of 78 IU l^{-1} and an alanine aminotransferase level of 271 IU l^{-1}).

Lumbar puncture revealed 81 cells/μL with 27% mononuclear cells and a protein content of 102 mg dl^{-1}.

Real Time quantitative PCR of Cerebrospinal Fluid (CSF) was positive for EBV (2.200 copies/mL). We used the BAMHI-W fragment region of the EBV genome as the target of our PCR screening [16].

PCR of the CSF sample was negative for Herpes Virus 1 And 2, Varicella Zoster Virus, Cytomegalovirus and Enterovirus. Bacterial cultures were negative for *Mycobacterium tuberculosis* and other pathogens which are epidemiologically relevant in our geographic area (e.i. *Rickettsia conorii, Brucella spp*).

On admission, serological tests for HIV, VDRL, CMV, HSV, hepatitis A, hepatitis C, b Borrelia and Brucella were all negative. Serological tests for EBV confirmed primary infection: VCA IgM positive, EA IgG positive, VCA IgG positive, and EBNA IgG negative.

An MRI scan of the brain using gadolinium contrast enhancement was performed 18 hours after the patient was admitted to hospital. Images were taken of the axial, coronal and sagittal sections.

MRI was initially performed with a 1.5-T unit (General Electric, United State) with a single channel receiver coil and body coil for excitation. The examination protocol included FRFSE T2W, FLAIR T2W, DWI and FSE T1W before and after intravenous administration of Gadobutrol. A power injector was used to administer 0,1 mL of Gadovist® (Gadobutrol, 1 M, Bayer Schering Pharma AG, Berlin, Germany) per kg of body weight (equivalent to 0,1 mmol/kg body weight) followed by 20 ml of saline. Injection rate was 2 mL/s. Sequence parameters are reported in Table 1.

The DWI sequence did not show any signal abnormalities (figure 1, A) whereas the T2 Fast relaxation fast spin echo sequence detected demyelinating alteration of the sub- and supra-tentorial white matter, and internal and external capsule and periventricular white matter and semioval center involvement, with scattered, partly confluent white matter changes (figures 1, B)

Fourth ventricle size was reduced, which is consistent with cerebral edema, and we also observed hyperintensity in the ponto-mesencephalic region (cortico spinal tract), on the T2 FLAIR sequence. (figure 1, C).

Contrast agent enhancement pattern suggested an inflammatory response restricted to the brain microcirculation (figure 1, D).

The patient was treated with intravenous acyclovir (10 mg/kg every 8 h) combined with methylprednisolone

Table 1 MRI sequence parameters

	T2WI	DWI	FLAIR	T1WI
TR, ms	4325	7000	9000	500
TE, ms	102	98	118	10,8
b, s/mm²	-	1000	-	-
FOV, mm	220	200	220	220
Matrix	256 × 256	128 × 128	256 × 256	256 × 256
Thickness, mm	5,0	5,0	5,0	5,0
Slices, n	22	44	22	22

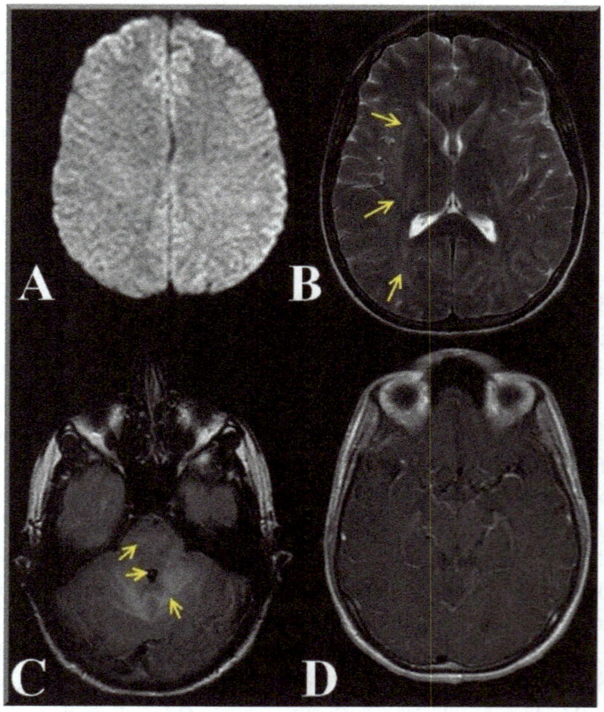

Figure 1 Initial MR imaging of the patient. Magnetic Resonance Imaging of the brain in the acute phase of neurological involvement. Diffusion Weighted MR Imaging of the brain performed in the acute phase of encephalitis (A). Axial T2 FRFSE image shows hyperintensity of white matter with involvement of internal and external capsule (B). Axial T2 FLAIR image demonstrates hyperintensity of white matter; involvement of the ventricular system with reduction in the size of the fourth ventricle is also shown (C). On the T1W Axial FLAIR there is enhancement of cerebral vessels after contrast agent was administered. Hyperintensity of cerebral vessel (D).

(500 mg intravenous bolus for 3 days then 1 mg/kg daily for 21 days).

Neurological improvement was noted at day 10 (Glasgow score of 14) but his diplopia symptoms persisted. PCR on CSF performed three weeks after admission was negative for EBV.

An MRI scan of the brain after three weeks showed markedly decreased hyperintensity on T2W and contrast enhancement had disappeared on post-gadolinium T1-W (figure 2, B,C,D).

Scanner and sequence parameters were identical to those used previously (Table 1).

Six months later, the patient had residual diplopia but was otherwise normal.

Discussion

A brain infection is a medical emergency. Immediate diagnosis and initiation of symptomatic and specific therapy has a dramatic influence upon survival and reduces the extent of permanent brain damage in survivors. In cases of herpes virus encephalitis, EBV has rarely been reported as the cause of CNS lesions, although fatal events and severe sequelae have been described, mostly in cases of acute primary infection [17,18].

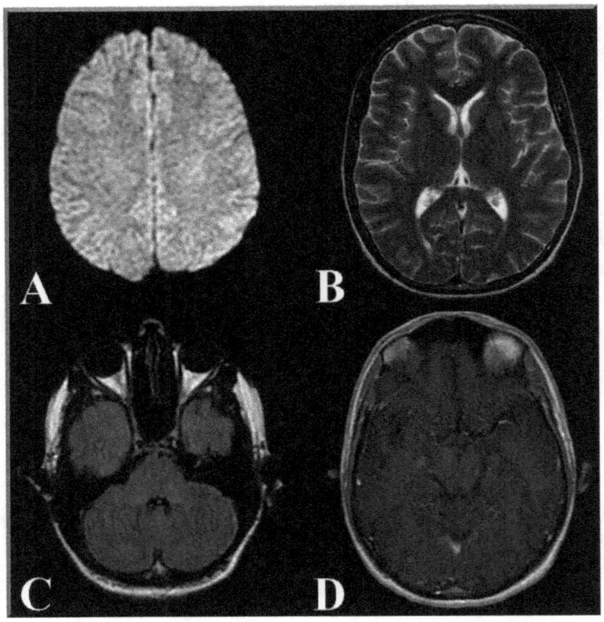

Figure 2 MR imaging of the patient at follow-up 3 weeks later. DWI remains the same, without any signal alteration (A). On the Axial T2 FRFSE image, we can see substantial regression of the previous lesions and no new lesions (B). The Axial T2 FLAIR image shows that the fourth ventricle has returned to its normal size. All signal intensities are normalized (C). On the T1W Axial FLAIR there is no enhancement of cerebral vessels after contrast medium was administered, as described above (D).

DWI sequences provide image contrast that is dependent on the molecular motion of water; this is important in cases of increased or restricted diffusion, such as ischemic stroke, intracranial infections or trauma[6,11-13]. Viral infections of the nervous system are characterized by alterations in water diffusion caused by cytotoxic edema, which can be detected by DWI. Reports have shown that DWI is usually the first sequence that is activated during cytotoxic cortical edema in tissue undergoing necrosis in EBV encephalitis [11-15].

In our case, we did not detect any abnormal signs in the DWI sequence, whereas T2W images showed mainly sub- and supra-tentorial white matter demyelination.

Our young patient's favorable course of CNS EBV infection and clearance suggests that EBV damage may be reversible when no abnormalities are detected on DWI, and appropriate therapy is initiated [14].

Apparent Diffusion Coefficient (ADC) maps can predict outcome in acute encephalitis [15]; we did not calculate this at the time of admission as this feature is not available at our hospital under emergency conditions.

We observed diffuse cerebral micro circular enhancement on T1W images after contrast agent was administered. In the course of inflammatory neurological disorders, adhesion molecule expression on endothelial cells is increased. This amplifies the inflammatory process in viral encephalitis where there is a lymphocytic infiltration of the CNS [19]. Research studies conducted on animals suggest that the herpes virus has an endotheliotropism that may depend on the susceptibility of CNS microvascular endothelial cells [20]. Moreover, EBV infection of human brain microvessel endothelial cells has recently been associated with the onset of multiple sclerosis [21].

Besides other infectious agents are responsible for mononucleosis-like illnesses, such as cytomegalovirus, HIV, cat scratch disease and syphilis, we investigated additional pathogens which are responsible for meningo-encephalitis in our geographic area, such as tuberculosis, rickettsial and brucellosis diseases.

ADEM was one of the non-infective CNS inflammatory diseases which we considered in the differential diagnosis of our patient. ADEM is a monophasic autoimmune demyelinating disease of the CNS that may occur after an infection or vaccination. However, ADEM lesions involve basal ganglia, thalami and the brainstem in particular [10] and this was not the case for our patient. Furthermore, clinical and instrumental resolution does not occur as early as it did in this case.

EBV-specific antiviral therapy does not exist, but acyclovir or gancyclovir have been recommended for the treatment of CNS involvement [6,7]. There is some debate surrounding corticosteroid therapy, but it seems to be a reasonable option when vasculitis is suspected, as our patient's neuroimaging findings suggested.

In conclusion, this report demonstrates that EBV in an immunocompetent adult can present with diffuse, reversible brain white matter involvement in the acute phase of mononucleosis.

Consent

Written informed consent was obtained from the patient for publication of this case report and any accompanying images.

List of abbreviations

ADC: Apparent Diffusion Coefficient; ADEM: Acute Disseminated Encephalomyelitis; CNS: Central Nervous System; CSF: Cerebrospinal Fluid; CT: Computed Tomography; DWI: Diffusion Weighted Imaging; EA: Early Antigen; Ig: Immunoglobulin; EBNA: Epstein-Barr virus nuclear antigen; EBV: Epstein-Barr Virus; FLAIR: Fluid Attenuated Inversion Recovery; FRFSE: Fast Relaxation Fast Spin Echo; FSE: Fast Spin Echo; MRI: Magnetic Resonance Imaging; PCR: Polymerase Chain Reaction; T1W: T1-weighted; T2W: T2-weighted; VCA: Viral Capsid Antigen; VDRL: Venereal Disease Research Laboratory test; CMV: Cytomegalovirus; HIV: Human immunodeficiency virus; HSV: Herpes Simplex Virus.

Author details

[1]Dipartimento di Scienze per la Promozione della Salute, Università di Palermo, Italy. [2]Dipartimento di Medicina Clinica e delle Patologie Emergenti, Azienda Ospedaliera Universitaria Policlinico "Paolo Giaccone" di Palermo, Palermo, Italy. [3]Dipartimento di Scienze Radiologiche, Azienda Ospedaliera Universitaria Policlinico "Paolo Giaccone" di Palermo, Palermo, Italy.

Authors' contributions

PD, MT and CS developed the idea of the study, participated in its design and coordination and helped to draft the manuscript. PC, GM and LT contributed to the acquisition and interpretation of data. DP and GC performed and collected laboratory tests and molecular genetic studies. CS was involved in critically reviewing neuro-imaging data for important intellectual content. All authors read and approved the final manuscript.

Competing interests

The authors declare that they have no competing interests.

References

1. Cohen JI: **Epstein-Barr Virus Infection.** *N Engl J Med* 2000, **343**:481-492.
2. Connelly KP, DeWitt LD: **Neurologic complications of infectious mononucleosis.** *Pediatr Neurol* 1994, **10(3)**:181-4.
3. Phowthongkum P, Phantumchinda K, Jutivorakool K, Suankratay C: **Basal ganglia and brainstem encephalitis, optic neuritis, and radiculomyelitis in Epstein-Barr virus infection.** *J Infect* 2007, **54(3)**:141-4.
4. Biebl A, Webersinke C, Traxler B, Povysil B, Furthner D, Schmitt K, Weis S: **Fatal Epstein-Barr virus encephalitis in a 12-year-old child: an underappreciated neurological complication?** *Nat Clin Pract Neurol* 2009, **5(3)**:171-4.
5. Fujimoto H, Asaoka K, Imaizumi T, Ayabe M, Shoji H, Kaji M: **Epstein-Barr virus infections of the central nervous system.** *Intern Med* 2003, **42(1)**:33-40.
6. Majid A, Galetta SL, Sweeney CJ, Robinson C, Mahalingam R, Smith J, Forghani B, Gilden DH: **Epstein-Barr virus myeloradiculitis and encephalomyeloradiculitis.** *Brain* 2002, **125()**:159-65.
7. Merelli E, Bedin R, Sola P, Gentilini M, Pietrosemoli P, Meacci M, Portolani M: **Encephalomyeloradiculopathy associated with Epstein-Barr virus: primary infection or reactivation?** *Acta Neurol Scand* 1997, **96(6)**:416-20.
8. Minjolle S, Arvieux C, Gautier AL, Jusselin I, Thomas R, Michelet C, Colimon R: **Detection of herpes virus genomes by polymerase chain reaction in cerebrospinal fluid and clinical findings.** *J Clin Virol* 2002, **25(1)**:S59-70.
9. Maghzi AH, Marta M, Bosca I, Etemadifar M, Dobson R, Maggiore C, Giovannoni G, Meier UC: **Viral pathophysiology of multiple sclerosis: A role for Epstein-Barr virus infection?** *Pathophysiology* 2011, **18(1)**:13-20.
10. Menge T, Hemmer B, Nessler S, Wiendl H, Neuhaus O, Hartung HP, Kieseier BC, Stüve O: **Acute disseminated encephalomyelitis: an update.** *Arch Neurol* 2005, **62(11)**:1673-80.
11. Kastrup O, Wanke I, Maschke M: **Neuroimaging of infections.** *NeuroRx* 2005, **2(2)**:324-32.
12. Hagemann G, Mentzel HJ, Weisser H, Kunze A, Terborg C: **Multiple reversible MR signal changes caused by Epstein-Barr virus encephalitis.** *AJNR Am J Neuroradiol* 2006, **27(7)**:1447-9.
13. Schaefer PW, Grant PE, Gonzalez RG: **Diffusion-weighted MR imaging of the brain.** *Radiology* 2000, **217(2)**:331-45.
14. Kuker W, Nagele T, Schmidt F, Heckl S, Herrlinger U: **Diffusion weighted MRI in herpes simplex encephalitis: a report of three cases.** *Neuroradiology* 2004, **46(2)**:122-125.
15. Axer H, Ragoschke-Schumm A, Böttcher J, Fitzek C, Witte OW, Isenmann S: **Initial DWI and ADC imaging may predict outcome in acute disseminated encephalomyelitis: report of two cases of brain stem encephalitis.** *J Neurol Neurosurg Psychiatry* 2005, **76(7)**:996-8.
16. Lo YM, Chan LY, Lo KW, Leung SF, Zhang J, Chan AT, Lee JC, Hjelm NM, Johnson PJ, Huang DP: **Quantitative analysis of cell-free Epstein-Barr virus DNA in plasma of patients with nasopharyngeal carcinoma.** *Cancer Res* 1999, **59(6)**:1188-91.
17. Takei H, Eldin KW, Adesina AM, Bhattacharjee MB: **Fatal Epstein-Barr virus meningitis: an autopsy report.** *Clin Neuropathol* 2006, **25(3)**:115-22.
18. Francisci D, Sensini A, Fratini D, Moretti MV, Luchetta ML, Di Caro A, Stagni G, Baldelli F: **Acute fatal necrotizing hemorrhagic encephalitis caused by Epstein-Barr virus in a young adult immunocompetent man.** *J Neurovirol* 2004, **10(6)**:414-7.
19. Brankin B, Hart MN, Cosby SL, Fabry Z, Allen IV: **Adhesion molecule expression and lymphocyte adhesion to cerebral endothelium: effects of measles virus and herpes simplex 1 virus.** *J Neuroimmunol* 1995, **56(1)**:1-8.
20. Hasebe R, Kimura T, Nakamura K, Ochiai K, Okazaki K, Wada R, Umemura T: **Differential susceptibility of equine and mouse brain microvascular endothelial cells to equine herpesvirus 1 infection.** *Arch Virol* 2006, **151(4)**:775-86.
21. Casiraghi C, Dorovini-Zis K, Horwitz MS: **Epstein-Barr virus infection of human brain microvessel endothelial cells: A novel role in multiple sclerosis.** *J Neuroimmunol* 2011, **230()**:173-7.

2

Tumour size measurement in a mouse model using high resolution MRI

Mikael Montelius[1*], Maria Ljungberg[1,2], Michael Horn[1,3] and Eva Forssell-Aronsson[1,2]

Abstract

Background: Animal models are frequently used to assess new treatment methods in cancer research. MRI offers a non-invasive *in vivo* monitoring of tumour tissue and thus allows longitudinal measurements of treatment effects, without the need for large cohorts of animals. Tumour size is an important biomarker of the disease development, but to our knowledge, MRI based size measurements have not yet been verified for small tumours (10^{-2}–10^{-1} g). The aim of this study was to assess the accuracy of MRI based tumour size measurements of small tumours on mice.

Methods: 2D and 3D T2-weighted RARE images of tumour bearing mice were acquired *in vivo* using a 7 T dedicated animal MR system. For the 3D images the acquired image resolution was varied. The images were exported to a PC workstation where the tumour mass was determined assuming a density of 1 g/cm^3, using an in-house developed tool for segmentation and delineation. The resulting data were compared to the weight of the resected tumours after sacrifice of the animal using regression analysis.

Results: Strong correlations were demonstrated between MRI- and necropsy determined masses. In general, 3D acquisition was not a prerequisite for high accuracy. However, it was slightly more accurate than 2D when small (<0.2 g) tumours were assessed for inter- and intraobserver variation. In 3D images, the voxel sizes could be increased from 160^3 µm^3 to 240^3 µm^3 without affecting the results significantly, thus reducing acquisition time substantially.

Conclusions: 2D MRI was sufficient for accurate tumour size measurement, except for small tumours (<0.2 g) where 3D acquisition was necessary to reduce interobserver variation. Acquisition times between 15 and 50 minutes, depending on tumour size, were sufficient for accurate tumour volume measurement. Hence, it is possible to include further MR investigations of the tumour, such as tissue perfusion, diffusion or metabolic composition in the same MR session.

Keywords: Animal model, Magnetic resonance, Volume determination, Cancer

Background

The efficacy of new tumour treatment methods are usually tested in animal models prior to clinical trials (e.g. [1-3]). The end-point studied is often the change in tumour size using mice with subcutaneous xenografts of human tumour tissue (e.g. [4]). Two or three perpendicular diameters of the tumour are measured and volume is calculated under assumptions of e.g. ellipsoidal tumour shape (e.g. [5]). These methods are fast, inexpensive, and do not require anaesthesia. Studies on orthotopic and metastatic tumour models have increased [6-9]. Generally, such studies exclude external volume measurements and require non-invasive imaging techniques, such as magnetic resonance imaging (MRI), computed tomography (CT), positron emission tomography or single photon emission computed tomography [10, 11].

MicroCT imaging allows accurate measurement of very small tumour volumes (~10^{-2} g) in short acquisition time [12], but the radiation exposure might affect tumour growth and thus confound the interpretation of the treatment results. MRI does not expose the animal

* Correspondence: mikael.montelius@radfys.gu.se
[1]Department of Radiation Physics, Institute of Clinical Sciences, Sahlgrenska Cancer Centre, Sahlgrenska Academy, University of Gothenburg, Sahlgrenska University Hospital, Gothenburg SE-413 45, Sweden
Full list of author information is available at the end of the article

to ionizing radiation and gives no known side effects which opens the possibility to follow the same animal by consecutive non-invasive measurements in longitudinal studies. In addition, MRI has intrinsic contrast abilities which can be used to assess tumour tissue characteristics, e.g. diffusion, perfusion and metabolic properties, parameters reflecting cell proliferation, apoptosis, vascularisation, etc. [11, 13-21].

Multiparametric MR imaging requires optimised MR methods for minimum time consumption. Small tumours require careful attention regarding imaging parameters due to the partial volume effect (PVE). To our knowledge, there is a lack of information on the accuracy and precision of MRI based size measurements on small tumours.

The aim of this study was 1) to develop and assess the accuracy of an MRI based method for *in vivo* measurement of tumour size in a small animal tumour model, and 2) to investigate the possibility to reduce acquisition time by reducing image resolution, without affecting the accuracy.

Methods

Tumour models and experimental setup

The study was performed on 17 tumour bearing female, athymic BALB/c and SCID mice s.c. inoculated in the neck/back region with the human midgut carcinoid cell line, GOT1 (n = 15), or the medullary thyroid carcinoma, GOT2 (n = 2) under anaesthesia using tribromoethanol (Avertin®, Winthrop Laboratories, Surbiton, UK). Animals had free access to water and standard diet.

Within two days after MR imaging, animals were sacrificed by surgical incision of the heart after i.p. injection of sodium pentobarbital (Apoteket Farmaci, Stockholm, Sweden). Gauge block measurements of the length, l, width, w and height, h of the tumours were performed. Assuming ellipsoidal tumours, the volume $V = (\pi/6)\cdot l\cdot w\cdot h$, was determined and converted to mass, m_{GB}, assuming a tumour density of 1.0 g/cm^3. The tumour was then surgically removed and weighed for reference tumour mass, m_T, determination. All procedures were approved by the local Animal ethics committee in Gothenburg.

MR imaging

MRI was performed using a 7 T MR system (Bruker BioSpin MRI GmbH, Ettlingen, Germany; software: ParaVision 5.0) equipped with water cooled gradient coils (maximum gradient strength 400 mT/m). A 72 mm volume coil was used for transmission and an actively decoupled 4 channel array rat brain coil was used for signal receiving (RAPID Biomedical GmbH, Rimpar, Germany). Proper animal positioning was assured using a fast gradient-echo localizer scan. All other imaging experiments were based on a respiration triggered and fat suppressed T2-weighted rapid acquisition with relaxation enhancement (RARE) sequence [22]. A 2D set of axial images was acquired (TR = 3438–4186 ms, TE_{eff} = 30 ms, NSA = 2–5, turbo factor Tf = 4, pixel size: ~150·200 μm^2, slice thickness = 700 μm) prior to a 3D volume acquisition (TR = 3000 ms, TE_{eff} = 35–82 ms, NSA = 1–2, Tf = 4–14). In the 3D acquisition, the matrix size was adjusted to achieve 160^3 μm^3 voxels with minimal field-of-view (FOV) but full tumour coverage. The 3D sequence was repeated twice using voxel sizes of 200^3 μm^3 and 240^3 μm^3 but with maintained FOV. The methods are henceforth designated 3D-160, 3D-200 and 3D-240, respectively. Saturation slices were always used in the phase encoding direction.

During the MRI experiments anaesthesia was maintained using a mixture of air and isoflurane (1.5–2.0 %) (Isoba vet., Schering-Plough Animal-health, Farum, Denmark). Body temperature was maintained with a heating pad on the animal bed and a pressure sensitive pad was used for respiratory triggering.

Image processing and tumour mass estimation

The image series were processed on a PC workstation using an in house developed volume estimation tool implemented in MATLAB (R2008b, The MathWorks, USA). Figure 1 shows the volume determination process. The average signal from a manually outlined region containing approximately equal amounts of tumour and background tissue was used for threshold segmentation (Figure 1b). Successful segmentation was ensured by allowing threshold adjustment on an image by image basis, and a polygon function could be used to manually exclude regions where the segmentation had failed (Figure 1b, c). With the tumour border properly defined, regions of low intra-tumour signal intensity, erroneously assigned to the background compartment, were converted using a growing seed algorithm, and the resulting image was used for volume calculation (Figure 1b, d). The number of tumour voxels, multiplied by the voxel volume, was converted to mass assuming a tumour density of 1.0 g/cm^3. The estimated masses from the 2D and 3D images, denoted m_{2D} and m_{3D} respectively, were compared to m_T using regression analysis.

The operator determining the masses from the repeated scans with increasing voxel sizes ($m_{3D\text{-}160}$, $m_{3D\text{-}200}$, and $m_{3D\text{-}240}$) was blinded to images with higher resolution when such existed.

Intra- and interobserver variability

Repeated (n = 10) segmentation and mass calculation was performed to investigate the intraobserver variability. Five image series including a small tumour (m_T = 0.01, 2D and 3D-160), a medium sized tumour (m_T = 0.10 g,

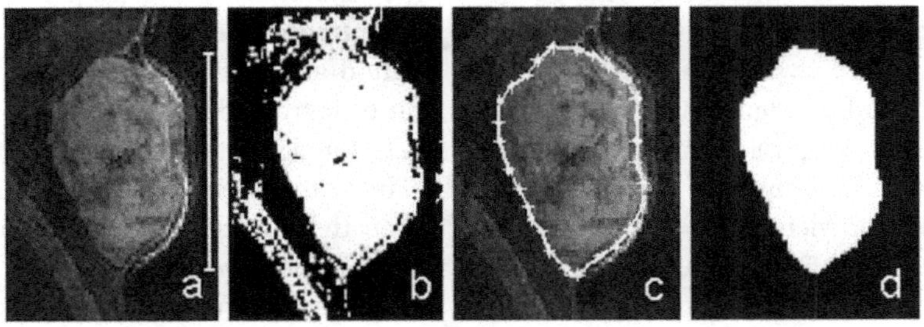

Figure 1 a) 3D-160 MR image of a subcutaneous GOT1 tumour positioned in the neck of the mouse. The tumour is visible as the hyper-intense region central to the image, marked by the 1 cm vertical bar. **b)** The global segmentation threshold is applied and regions of failed segmentation appear outside the tumour. **c)** The manual delineation excludes the areas of failed segmentation, and the final result is shown in **d)** where white pixels represent the region that will be accounted for as tumour volume.

3D-160) and a large tumour ($m_T = 0.87$ g, 2D and 3D-160) were included in the assessment. The operator was blinded to the 3D images when evaluating the 2D images. Learning effects were minimized by presenting the image series in a random order and allowing at least several hours to pass between sessions. The coefficient of variation (CV) was calculated for each image series.

Two additional observers repeated the process on the five image series to investigate interobserver variations. Their results were compared to the corresponding average values obtained by observer 1 in the intraobserver assessment.

Estimation of influence of partial volume effect

A simulation was set up using MATLAB to quantify the maximum influence that PVE could have on volume estimations based on 3D MRI images of a spherically shaped tumour. Tumour diameter and voxel dimensions were used as input parameters. A 3D grid was used to simulate the image matrix, with grid elements acting as image voxels. A sphere, simulating the tumour, was superimposed on the grid with coinciding origins. Grid elements located inside and outside the sphere were defined as tumour and background elements, respectively. Elements intersected by the rim of the sphere were defined as PVE elements. Each one-element thick section of the grid (representing the image slices) was considered for two extreme cases of segmentation, where PVE elements were classified either as tumour elements, or as background elements, thus overestimating or underestimating the true tumour volume, respectively.

The total influence of PVE on the tumour volume estimation was defined as $\frac{\tilde{V}-V}{V} \cdot 100$ %, where $\tilde{V}$ represents the total volume of tumour elements in the simulation and V is the true tumour volume. Voxel sizes of 100^3–250^3 μm^3 and 3–9 mm (diameter) tumours were simulated, and the resulting data were presented as relative volume errors for different number of voxels-per-tumour-diameter ratios.

Statistics

Regression analyses were performed using the Microsoft Excel (2003) statistics toolkit. Pearson's r squared correlation coefficient was used.

Results

Determination of tumour mass

All tumours found at necropsy were well visualized in the MR images. The mass of the resected tumours, m_T, was between 0.01 g and 2.28 g. Tumours with m_T <0.2 g are henceforth classified as small.

A strong correlation was found between the tumour mass estimated from the 3D-160 MR images ($m_{3D\text{-}160}$) and m_T (Figure 2). The correlation was persistent when data only from the small tumours ($m_T < 0.2$ g) were included.

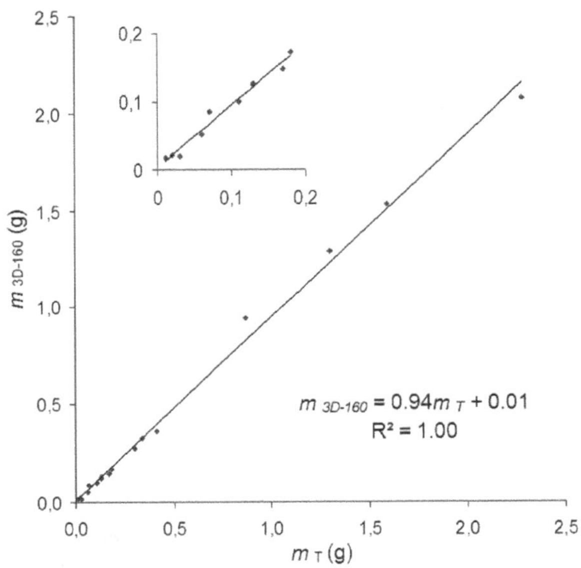

Figure 2 Tumour mass calculated from 3D-160 MR images, $m_{3D\text{-}160}$, vs. tumour mass measured after resection, m_T, n = 17. There is a strong correlation between the parameters. The inserted figure shows the same data when only small tumours (<0.2 g) are included ($m_{3D\text{-}160} = 0.90 m_T + 0.00$, $R^2 = 0.98$, n = 10).

In twelve mice, tumours were measured with gauge blocks in addition to MRI and digital balance. The correlation between m_{GB} and m_T was strong when data from all tumours were included (Figure 3a). When analysing small tumours only, the correlation was markedly reduced ($R^2 = 0.65$). The same subset of tumours analysed with the 3D-160 method yielded $R^2 = 0.97$.

Comparing m_{2D} to m_T (n = 15, one image series was lost, and one did not cover the entire tumour) a strong correlation was obtained ($R^2 = 0.99$) (Figure 3b). Also for small tumours a strong correlation was found ($R^2 = 0.96$), i.e. the 2D method was comparable to the 3D-160 method regarding accuracy.

To exclude the inherent uncertainty of the digital balance, m_{2D} was compared directly to $m_{3D\text{-}160}$. The linear relation in the regression and the correlation approached unity $m_{2D} = 1.01 m_{3D\text{-}160} - 0.00$, $R^2 = 1.00$, n = 15. For small tumours the corresponding relation was $m_{2D} = 1.04\ m_{3D\text{-}160} + 0.00$, $R^2 = 0.99$, n = 9.

The analysis of $m_{3D\text{-}160}$, $m_{3D\text{-}200}$, and $m_{3D\text{-}240}$ vs. m_T did not reveal any obvious voxel size dependence in the range of tumour- and voxel sizes investigated. The acquisition time required for the smallest tumour studied ($m_T = 0.01$ g) was clearly reduced with larger voxels: 55, 34 and 22 minutes for the 160^3, 200^3 and 240^3 μm^3 images, respectively.

Intra- and interobserver variability

The intraobserver variation was in general low for each method and tumour size (CV of 2–3 %), but an indication of increased variability (CV of 7 %) was observed in the 2D image set of the smallest tumour (Table 1).

The interobserver results indicated a difference between the 2D and 3D-160 methods (Table 2). The relative deviation from the average mass was higher when determined from the 2D images compared to the 3D-160 images. The effect was more pronounced for the smallest tumour size.

Computer simulation

Table 3 shows data from the simulations of the maximum possible influence that PVE could have on volume estimation. The largest relative volume error was approximately 40 % for a voxels-per-tumour-diameter ratio of 12, corresponding to, e.g., a tumour of 3 mm diameter (~0.01 g) imaged with the voxel size set to 250^3 μm^3, i.e. the smallest tumour included in this study, in combination with the largest voxel size used in the imaging experiments.

Discussion

The present study evaluated the possibilities and requirements for accurate measurement of small tumour sizes

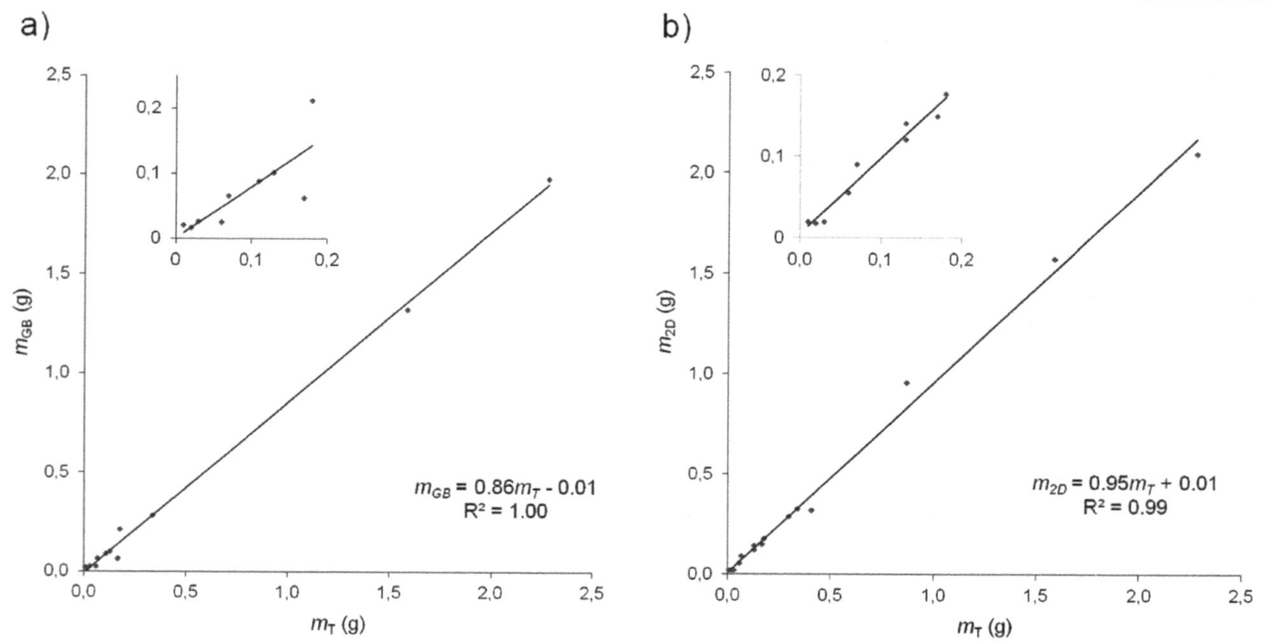

Figure 3 Tumour mass calculated from a) gauge block measurements, m_{GB}, and b) 2D images, m_{2D}, vs. tumour mass measured after resection, m_T. a) m_{GB} vs. m_T (n = 12). The correlation was strong when all tumour sizes were included ($R^2 = 1.0$), but was lower in the assessment of small tumours only (inserted figure; $m_T < 0.2$ g, n = 9, $m_{GB} = 0.78m_T + 0.00$, $R^2 = 0.65$). The corresponding correlation for $m_{3D\text{-}160}$ vs. m_T for the same set of tumours was $m_{3D\text{-}160} = 0.93m_T + 0.00$, $R^2 = 1.00$ ($m_T < 0.2$ g: $m_{3D\text{-}160} = 0.90m_T + 0.00$, $R^2 = 0.97$). **b)** m_{2D} vs. m_T (n = 15). The correlation was strong when all tumour sizes were included ($R^2 = 0.99$), and persisted in the assessment of small tumours only (inserted figure, $m_T < 0.2$ g, n = 9, $m_{2D} = 0.94m_T + 0.00$, $R^2 = 0.96$). The corresponding correlation for $m_{3D\text{-}160}$ vs. m_T for the same set of tumours was $m_{3D\text{-}160} = 0.93m_T + 0.01$, $R^2 = 1.0$ (<0.2 g: $m_{3D\text{-}160} = 0.91m_T + 0.00$, $R^2 = 0.98$).

Table 1 The coefficient of variation (CV) calculated for the five intraobserver variability assessments. The CV is based on 10 volume calculations performed on each of the five image series

m_T (g)	Method	CV (%)
0.01	3D-160	3.1
	2D	6.9
0.10	3D-160	3.1
0.87	3D-160	2.1
	2D	1.9

in mice using MRI. A linear, highly correlated relationship between weighed and MRI measured tumour masses down to 10^{-2} g was found. 3D acquisition should be considered when tumour masses of 10^{-1} gram or less are expected, due to the relative increase of PVE. In very small tumours (10^{-2} g) image acquisition at high resolution (in our setup 160^3 μm^3 voxels) should also be considered. The increased acquisition time using high resolution is compensated for by the smaller FOV needed to cover the tumour. Short acquisition times allow either additional MR investigations on the same animal, such as determining tumour diffusion, perfusion or metabolic parameters within one MR session, or a higher animal throughput.

Initially, the 2D method was included only for anatomical reference since gradient performance limited the minimum slice thickness to 700 μm, resulting in substantial PVE. However, the accuracy of volume estimations based on the 2D images was similar to that based on the 3D images (Figures 2 and 3b). This might be due to the possibility to study adjacent image slices, which probably improves the view of the tumour shape and delineation of the tumour border. However, the 2D method has a higher interobserver variability (Table 2), which supports the use of a 3D method for very small tumours, in order to limit the subjectivity in the evaluation.

Table 2 Interobserver variation. The interobserver variation of tumour mass measurements for three observers given as relative deviation (in per cent) from the average value of the mass (n = 10) obtained by observer 1 for three different tumours and two imaging methods studied

Mean *m* (g)	Method	Interobserver variation (%)		
		Obs1	Obs2	Obs3
0.02	3D-160	–	0.7	−4.7
0.02	2D	–	23	11
0.10	3D-160	–	1.2	−4.3
0.91	3D-160	–	−1.4	0.1
0.99	2D	–	2.2	−9.0

Table 3 Influence of partial volume effect on volume determination. The maximum possible influence of the partial volume effect (PVE) on tumour volume estimations, assuming isotropic voxels and a spherical tumour, determined by simulations

Voxels/diameter (mm^{-1})	Maximum relative volume difference (%)	
	overestimated	underestimated
70	6	−6
45	10	−10
28	16	−14
12	39	−31

The voxels-per-tumour-diameter ratio is listed with the corresponding results from the simulation. The relative difference between over- and underestimated tumour volumes and the analytically calculated volume are given as a percentage of true tumour volume.

In the 3D method, the turbo factor (Tf) was adjusted to reduce acquisition time. An increase in Tf results in an increased point spread function (PSF). Computer simulations assuming similar acquisition parameters as those used, and T2 values common at 7 T [23] showed that the PSF was broadened only by a factor of 1.6 compared to the value for Tf = 1 (data not shown). The minimum TE_{eff} is also affected by the Tf, i.e. the image contrast will vary slightly with Tf. However, tumours were always easily visualized and, altogether, the range of Tfs used in the study might only affect the results to a minor extent.

The most time consuming process in the volume determination was probably when adjusting the threshold value in images where the global segmentation had failed. To reduce the time of analysis one could e.g. calculate an average volume based on two extreme segmentations; one including most of the border, and one excluding it. Such a procedure would, however, overestimate the volume, especially for small voxel-to-diameter ratios, where asymmetry between over- and underestimated volume errors is more pronounced (Table 3). In situations when small tumours require polygon delineation of the tumour border, the decision to assign voxels intersected by the polygon line to the tumour or the background compartment, will require asymmetry consideration since it might have a significant effect on the volume estimation (Table 3).

The tumour density assumption (1.0 g/cm^3) might be an underestimation that would account for the fact that the relations between the determined masses ($m_{3D\text{-}160}$, m_{2D} and m_{GB}) and the weight (m_T) were less than unity. Another contributing factor could be the inherent uncertainty in the digital balance, since errors in the predictor used in regression analysis are typically manifested as a decrease of the slope coefficient towards zero [24]. These two considerations are justified by the fact that the slope was 1.01 when $m_{3D\text{-}160}$ and m_{2D} were compared directly to each other, thus excluding the density effect and predictor uncertainties.

Few studies were found in the literature where the accuracy of MRI based tumour size measurement was verified by e.g. comparison with weight after resection. He et al. found a correlation of $R^2 = 0.96$ ($n = 7$) when comparing volumes of pancreatic tumours in mice from T2-weighted 2D MR images (similar to our 2D method), acquired at 4.7 T, for 0.2–2.0 g tumours [6]. We obtained a similar correlation ($R^2 = 0.96$, $n = 9$) but for smaller tumours (0.01–0.2 g) since we used six times smaller voxel volume, i.e. the influence of PVE might be comparable. Other groups have reported MRI tumour size measurements in mice but without verification with tumour weight, e.g. [7-9]. One group reported MRI measurements of tumours in mouse pancreas down to 0.14 g at 7.0 T using sequence parameters similar to our 2D method (T2-weighted RARE sequence, 0.015 mm^3 voxels), but verified the volume determination by one phantom measurement only [9].

Using high resolution microCT (7 min acquisition time, voxel size of 81^3 μm^3, voxel volume of 0.0005 mm^3) a close correlation was found for 0.02–0.25 g s.c. tumours in mice, verified by weight after resection ($R^2 = 0.97$, $n = 20$) [12]. Thus, microCT is a fast and accurate method, but the absorbed dose delivered to the animal, and especially to the tumour tissue, is a confounding factor in therapy response assessments.

The generally faster T1-weighted sequences have also been used for tumour imaging (e.g. [8]). Often however, the tumour and surrounding tissue have similar T1-values, thus requiring use of contrast agents. T1-weighted sequences without contrast agents may be useful for imaging tumours in e.g. the bladder wall, where fluid constitutes the surrounding tissue, due to widely different T1-values in fluid and solid tissue [7].

Conclusion

This study shows the feasibility of accurate and precise MRI based size measurement of small tumours in mice. Furthermore, short acquisition times that allow additional MR investigations within the same session can be realized by careful selection of MR sequence parameters, e.g. using 2D instead of 3D methods and optimal voxel size.

Competing interests

The authors declare that they have no competing interests.

Authors' contributions

MM designed and carried out the imaging studies, performed the statistical analysis and drafted the manuscript. ML participated in designing and carrying out the imaging study, approved the statistical analysis and helped to draft the manuscript. MH conceived of the study, and participated in its design and coordination. EFA participated in designing the study, performing the statistical analysis and helped to draft the manuscript in addition to supervising the study coordination. All authors read and approved the final manuscript.

Acknowledgements

The authors thank Lilian Karlsson and Ann Wikström for excellent animal handling. This study was supported by grants from the European Commission FP7 Collaborative Project TARCC HEALTH-F2-2007-201962, the Swedish Research Council, the Swedish Cancer Society, BioCARE - a National Strategic Research Program at University of Gothenburg, the King Gustav V Jubilee Clinic Cancer Research Foundation. The work was performed within the EC COST Action BM0607.

Author details

[1]Department of Radiation Physics, Institute of Clinical Sciences, Sahlgrenska Cancer Centre, Sahlgrenska Academy, University of Gothenburg, Sahlgrenska University Hospital, Gothenburg SE-413 45, Sweden. [2]Division of Medical Physics and Medical Engineering, Sahlgrenska University Hospital, Gothenburg SE-413 45, Sweden. [3]Department of Radiology, University of Würzburg, Würzburg, Germany.

References

1. Schmitt A, Bernhardt P, Nilsson O, Ahlman H, Kolby L, Maecke HR, Forssell-Aronsson E: **Radiation Therapy of Small Cell Lung Cancer with 177Lu-DOTA-Tyr3-Octreotate in an Animal Model.** *J Nucl Med* 2004, **45**(9):1542–1548.
2. Masciotti J, Provenzano F, Papa J, Klose A, Hur J, Gu X, Yamashiro D, Kandel J, Hielscher A: **Monitoring Tumor Growth and Treatment in Small Animals with Magnetic Resonance and Optical Tomographic Imaging.** In *Proceedings of SPIE: 21 January 2006; San Jose.* Edited by Fred S. Azar, Dimitris N. Metaxas; 2006:608105-1.
3. Kölby L, Bernhardt P, Johanson V, Schmitt A, Ahlman H, Forssell-Aronsson E, Macke H, Nilsson O: **Successful receptor-mediated radiation therapy of xenografted human midgut carcinoid tumour.** *Br J Cancer* 2005, **93**(10):1144–1151.
4. Tomayko M, Reynolds C: **Determination of subcutaneous tumor size in athymic (nude) mice.** *Cancer chemotherapy and pharmacology* 1989, **24**(3):148–154.
5. Euhus DM, Hudd C, Laregina MC, Johnson FE: **Tumor measurement in the nude mouse.** *J Surg Oncol* 1986, **31**(4):229–234.
6. He Z, Evelhoch JL, Mohammad RM, Adsay NV, Pettit GR, Vaitkevicius VK, Sarkar FH: **Magnetic Resonance Imaging to Measure Therapeutic Response Using an Orthotopic Model of Human Pancreatic Cancer.** *Pancreas* 2000, **21**(1):69–76.
7. Mazurchuk R, Glaves D, Raghavan D: **Magnetic resonance imaging of response to chemotherapy in orthotopic xenografts of human bladder cancer.** *Clin Cancer Res* 1997, **3**(9):1635–1641.
8. Grimm J, Potthast A, Wunder A, Moore A: **Magnetic resonance imaging of the pancreas and pancreatic tumors in a mouse orthotopic model of human cancer.** *Int J Cancer* 2003, **106**(5):806–811.
9. Partecke I, Kaeding A, Sendler M, Albers N, Kuhn J-P, Speerforck S, Roese S, Seubert F, Diedrich S, Kuehn S, *et al*: **In vivo imaging of pancreatic tumours and liver metastases using 7 Tesla MRI in a murine orthotopic pancreatic cancer model and a liver metastases model.** *BMC Cancer* 2011, **11**(1):40.
10. Forssell-Aronsson E, Kjellén E, Mattsson S, Hellström M, Swedish Cancer Society Investigation Group T: **Medical Imaging for Improved Tumour Characterization, Delineation and Treatment Verification.** *Acta Oncologica* 2002, **41**(7):604–614.
11. Weissleder R: **Scaling down imaging: molecular mapping of cancer in mice.** *Nat Rev Cancer* 2002, **2**(1):11–18.
12. Jensen M, Jorgensen J, Binderup T, Kjaer A: **Tumor volume in subcutaneous mouse xenografts measured by microCT is more accurate and reproducible than determined by 18 F-FDG-microPET or external caliper.** *BMC Medical Imaging* 2008, **8**(1):16.
13. Sorensen AG: **Magnetic Resonance As a Cancer Imaging Biomarker.** *J Clin Oncol* 2006, **24**(20):3274–3281.
14. De Schepper AM, De Beuckeleer L, Vandevenne J, Somville J: **Magnetic resonance imaging of soft tissue tumors.** *Eur Radiol* 2000, **10**(2):213–223.
15. Low RN: **Abdominal MRI advances in the detection of liver tumours and characterisation.** *The Lancet Oncology* 2007, **8**(6):525–535.

16. Hakumäki JM, Brindle KM: **Techniques: Visualizing apoptosis using nuclear magnetic resonance.** *Trends Pharmacol Sci* 2003, **24**(3):146–149.
17. Raman V, Pathak AP, Glunde K, Artemov D, Bhujwalla ZM: **Magnetic resonance imaging and spectroscopy of transgenic models of cancer.** *NMR Biomed* 2007, **20**(3):186–199.
18. Kettunen MI, Brindle KM: **Apoptosis detection using magnetic resonance imaging and spectroscopy.** *Prog Nucl Magn Reson Spectrosc* 2005, **47**(3–4):175–185.
19. Barrett T, Brechbiel M, Bernardo M, Choyke PL: **MRI of tumor angiogenesis.** *J Magn Reson Imaging* 2007, **26**(2):235–249.
20. Schmuecking M, Boltze C, Geyer H, Salz H, Schilling B, Wendt TG, Kloetzer K-H, Marx C: **Dynamic MRI and CAD vs. Choline MRS: Where is the detection level for a lesion characterisation in prostate cancer?** *Int J Radiat Biol* 2009, **85**(9):814–824.
21. Pacheco-Torres J, López-Larrubia P, Ballesteros P, Cerdán S: **Imaging tumor hypoxia by magnetic resonance methods.** *NMR Biomed* 2011, **24**(1):1–16.
22. Hennig J, Nauerth A, Friedburg H: **RARE imaging: A fast imaging method for clinical MR.** *Magn Reson Med* 1986, **3**(6):823–833.
23. Crémillieux Y, Ding S, Dunn JF: **High-resolution in vivo measurements of transverse relaxation times in rats at 7 Tesla.** *Magn Reson Med* 1998, **39**(2):285–290.
24. Frost C, Thompson SG: **Correcting for regression dilution bias: comparison of methods for a single predictor variable.** *Journal of the Royal Statistical Society: Series A (Statistics in Society)* 2000, **163**(2):173–189.

3

Quantitative evaluation of an automatic segmentation method for 3D reconstruction of intervertebral scoliotic disks from MR images

Chevrefils Claudia[1,2*], Cheriet Farida[1,2,3], Grimard Guy[2], Miron Marie-Claude[2] and Aubin Carl-Eric[1,2,4]

Abstract

Background: For some scoliotic patients the spinal instrumentation is inevitable. Among these patients, those with stiff curvature will need thoracoscopic disk resection. The removal of the intervertebral disk with only thoracoscopic images is a tedious and challenging task for the surgeon. With computer aided surgery and 3D visualisation of the interverterbral disk during surgery, surgeons will have access to additional information such as the remaining disk tissue or the distance of surgical tools from critical anatomical structures like the aorta or spinal canal. We hypothesized that automatically extracting 3D information of the intervertebral disk from MR images would aid the surgeons to evaluate the remaining disk and would add a security factor to the patient during thoracoscopic disk resection.

Methods: This paper presents a quantitative evaluation of an automatic segmentation method for 3D reconstruction of intervertebral scoliotic disks from MR images. The automatic segmentation method is based on the watershed technique and morphological operators. The 3D Dice Similarity Coefficient (DSC) is the main statistical metric used to validate the automatically detected preoperative disk volumes. The automatic detections of intervertebral disks of real clinical MR images are compared to manual segmentation done by clinicians.

Results: Results show that depending on the type of MR acquisition sequence, the 3D DSC can be as high as 0.79 (±0.04). These 3D results are also supported by a 2D quantitative evaluation as well as by robustness and variability evaluations. The mean discrepancy (in 2D) between the manual and automatic segmentations for regions around the spinal canal is of 1.8 (±0.8) mm. The robustness study shows that among the five factors evaluated, only the type of MRI acquisition sequence can affect the segmentation results. Finally, the variability of the automatic segmentation method is lower than the variability associated with manual segmentation performed by different physicians.

Conclusions: This comprehensive evaluation of the automatic segmentation and 3D reconstruction of intervertebral disks shows that the proposed technique used with specific MRI acquisition protocol can detect intervertebral disk of scoliotic patient. The newly developed technique is promising for clinical context and can eventually help surgeons during thoracoscopic intervertebral disk resection.

* Correspondence: claudia.chevrefils@polymtl.ca
[1]Ecole Polytechnique de Montreal, Biomedical Engineering Institute, Montreal, QC H3C 3A7, Canada
[2]Sainte-Justine University Hospital Center, Montreal, QC H3T 1C5, Canada
Full list of author information is available at the end of the article

Background

Depending on the severity of the curve and the risk of progression, scoliosis can be treated with rigorous observation, bracing or surgery. Several types of surgery can be performed on scoliotic patients to reduce their spinal deformations. Precise positioning of hooks and screws on vertebrae attached to a rod, using anterior or posterior approach, to bring back the normal curvature of the spine is an example [1,2]. For patient with stiff curvature, a disk resection is often required to be able to properly attach instrumentations to the rod and optimise the results of the surgery [3,4]. The disk resection is done with a thoracoscope prior to attach hooks or screws to the rod [5]. The removal of the intervertebral disk with only thoracoscopic images is a tedious and challenging task for the surgeon [6]. Intra-operative thoracoscopic images do not fully describe the actual geometry of the structures of interest due to many factors such as the inherent projection of the imaging modality and the small field of view (which leads to loss of depth perception), the presence of surgical tool in the region of interest and other constraints typically imposed in an operating room. The use of computer assistance in such surgeries could help clinicians to perform their surgical manipulations more precisely by dynamically bringing additional information such as the remaining disk tissue or the distance of surgical tools from critical anatomical structures like the aorta or spinal canal. In this context, multimodal image fusion of a preoperative 3D model of the intervertebral disks with intraoperative thoracoscopic images could be very useful to visualize a 3D spine model including soft tissues and bones in a single view, thus reducing cognitive effort on the part of the surgeon.

A variety of imaging modalities can be used to acquire volumetric information on the patient's anatomy preoperatively. For the current context, MRI is a relevant choice because it is a non invasive imaging modality with the capacity to capture details of soft tissues like intervertebral disks. Manual segmentation of intervertebral disks on every MRI slice is a very time-consuming process and is prone to errors for the radiologist and it is not conceivable in a clinical environment. Time to manually segment one intervertebral disk varies from 15 to 35 minutes depending on the type of MRI sequence, the number of slices covering the volume and the severity of the spinal deformation. Automatic segmentation of intervertebral disks from MRI is an innovative field and it permits reproducible 3D model of the region of interest for an augmented reality system. Towards this goal, we hypothesize that the preoperative 3D geometry of the disk could be extracted from the MRI volume by automatically segmenting the region of interest.

To our knowledge, only one study relates work on segmentation and 3D reconstruction of the intervertebral disk of scoliotic patient [7]. In this study the segmentation of the nucleus pulposus and the annulus fibrosus is done manually. Only few studies relate works on segmentation of MRI spine images from patient with normal spine curvature [8-12]. None of these techniques are useful for our application because of the spinal deformity involved with scoliosis and/or the external constraints namely the unsupervised and closed contours requirements for 3D reconstruction. Indeed, with 3D spine deformation of scoliotic patients, it is impossible to locate the whole spine cord in a single MR image, the intervertebral disks and the verterbrae are often also deformed, bringing an additional challenge to the automatic segmentation method.

Live wire has also been used to segment medical images and it is based on a cost graph principle starting with seeds points given by a user. This technique is a semi automatic segmentation technique that allows the user to select regions of interest by clicking on the images to delineate contour of a specific structure. A graph is built considering pixels as nodes and from each node an edge is created in the four main directions (up,down,left, right). These edges are weighted with features gathered from the sobel filter convolution, so that pixels that stay on the edge are lighter and the ones that go outside the edge are heavier. Several cost function can be used but gradient magnitude is widely used. This type of segmentation is particularly useful to detect complex object contour. Although some work has been done to reduce the problems of the quality of the segmentation and the computational complexity, live wire still necessitates user interaction. Even with the 3D approach [13-16], user has to manually segment the structure of interest on few orthogonal slices or manually delimitate ROI (Region Of Interest) which is a tedious task for the segmentation of more than one intervertebral disk per image.

Watershed has been used in combination with other techniques in cardiology on ultrasound images [17], in neurology on MR images [18,19] and recently we have used this technique on spine MR images [20,21]. The principle of watershed transform is based on the detection of ridges and valleys. The image is viewed as a topological image where intensity represents the altitude of the pixels. The image is flooded from its minimum and it allows the delimitation between the catchment basins and the ridges (watershed lines). Hence the catchment basins represent region of homogeneous intensity representing the region of interest. The results based on the watershed technique showed that the technique is able to cope with variation of topologies and shape and that it was possible to use the algorithm in the sagittal and coronal plane. However, no merging of information (sagittal and coronal plane) was done to encompass the problem of bad boundaries detection in images located at the extreme lateral sides. Also, no 3D quantitative evaluation of this automatic segmentation technique was yet performed.

Segmentation of MR images of patients presenting different degree of scoliotic deformity clearly necessitates the development of a technique able to cope with variations of topology and shape. The purpose of this study is to develop and validate a novel automatic segmentation based on our previous work [20,21]. In these studies only sagittal images or coronal images are used independently. By using only sagittal images, the automatic segmentation had problem to depict interverterbral disk on images located in the lateral side where disks are seen as small structures and are rejected by the automatic segmentation. On the other hand, when the segmentation is done on the coronal images, the same problem occurs on the anterior and posterior side of the intervertebral disk. Hence, using one direction to segment the intervertebral disks on all images covering the volume, in order to have 3D models, is not optimal.

Our first objective is to improve the method developed in [20,21] to take full advantages of MRI by reconstructing coronal images using the sagittal images and merging information from both directions. The second objective is to assess a similarity measure for spatial volumes in order to adequately compare the proposed automatic segmentation results with those of manual segmentation by physicians. Also, because of the 3D spine deformation of scoliotic patients, the intervertebral disks and the verterbrae are often also deformed, bringing an additional challenge to the automatic segmentation method. This clearly motivated the necessity to conduct a robustness evaluation to ascertain the capacity of the proposed technique to cope with different spatial positioning and shape variations of intervertebral disk and surrounding anatomical structures. Hence, the third objective is to evaluate the robustness of the automatic segmentation technique.

Methods

Study data

The MR images were acquired at Sainte-Justine Hospital with a 1.5 Tesla Magnetom Avanto system (Siemens, Erlangen, Germany). The radiofrequency (RF) transmitting and receiving units consisted of a body coil. Three different acquisition protocols were studied on 9 scoliotic patients.

The first acquisition protocol was based on a 3D MEDIC (Multi Echo Data Image Combination) sequence used in the sagittal plane with Repetition Time (TR) = 23 milliseconds (ms), Echo Time (TE) = 12 ms, slice thickness of 1 millimeter (mm) and a matrix of 256 X 256 elements leading to a voxel size of 1 mm^3. The second acquisition used a 3D FISP (Fast Imaging with Steady state Precession) sequence with parameters TR=7.1 ms, TE=2.38 ms, slice thickness of 1 mm and a matrix of 256 X 256 elements leading to a voxel size of 1 mm^3. The third acquisition protocol was a standard 2D Spin Echo used with parameters TR=780 ms and a TE=18 ms, with a slice thickness of 2 mm and 2.4 mm of space between slices using a matrix of 384 mm X 384 mm, leads to a pixel size of 0.67 mm^2 in the sagittal direction. The three acquisition protocols were performed in the sagittal plane because our application calls for high resolution in that plane near the spinal canal and intervertebral disks. The three protocols were acquired in the same session, but since these were lengthy acquisitions we allowed the patient to move between each acquisition. The three MRI acquisition sequences were approved by the ethical committee of Sainte-Justine Hospital, Montreal, Canada and a written consent was obtained from the patients or their relative for publication of study.

The choice of the above acquisition protocols was based on the most commonly used sequence types for segmentation of musculoskeletal images. All three acquisition sequences have relatively short TE's because this makes it possible to see the intervertebral disks without distinguishing between the annulus and the nucleus pulposus, which is what is required in the current study (Figure 1).

Automatic reconstruction of intervertebral disks

The proposed algorithm has three main steps: segmentation, classification and fusion of complementary information coming from coronal and sagittal views, thus taking full advantage of the imaging modality. In brief, this algorithm is an unsupervised segmentation technique able to detect intervertebral disks in short TE MR images of scoliotic patients. As a first step, sagittal images and interpolated coronal images are segmented using the watershed technique applied to modified gradient images as reported by our group [20]. The gradient image is modified using internal and external markers and morphological operators to keep only the most significant and relevant contours for the structures of interest. In the context of the watershed method, internal markers (F^m_{int}) represent sets of connected pixels inside the regions of interest, while the external markers (F^m_{ext}) represent the deepest valley lines surrounding every internal marker. Combined binary markers F^m were imposed as minima on the gradient image and enabled the automatic segmentation of intervertebral disks in MRI of scoliotic patients. This technique resulted in some over-segmentation, thus necessitating a subsequent classification step.

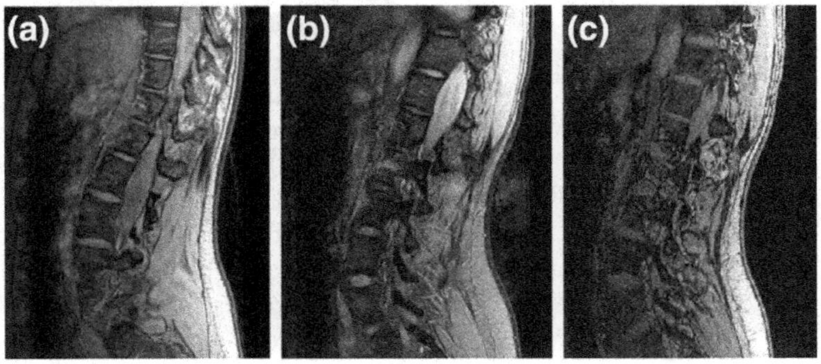

Figure 1 MRI acquisition protocols. Three different acquisition sequences for the same patient from the medium scoliotic severity group: (**a**) 3D MEDIC, (**b**) 2D Spin Echo, (**c**) 3D FISP.

The classification process, as described in [21], is used exclusively in the sagittal images to label the closed contours as either intervertebral disks or background. In short, the classification step allows us to eliminate background regions that are falsely detected as intervertebral disks in the automatic segmentation step. The supervised k-Nearest Neighbours (k-NN) classifier is used with four statistical and four spectral texture features to label each region as either intervertebral disk or background in the sagittal segmented images. The statistical texture features are based on histogram of the closed contour (mean, standard deviation, skewness and entropy). All four spectral texture features are based on the energy Fourier spectrum of the closed region. By using the Fourier spectrum, we have information about the orientation and the frequency of intensity variation of the closed region. To facilitate interpretation, the spectrum is expressed in polar coordinates (r,Θ). Hence, the 4 descriptors of this function used as spectral texture features are the angle θmax at which the spectrum is maximal, the value S(θ)max of the spectrum at θmax, the variance of S(θ) and the difference between S(θ)max and S(θ)mean [21].

The classification step constitutes the second step of the reconstruction process. Being computationally expensive, the classification is limited to the sagittal images because anatomical correspondence can be performed to locate the intervertebral disk regions in the coronal images.

Fusion of disk detection in two plane

The third step of the segmentation process is the fusion of information coming from the sagittal and coronal segmentations and it represents the improvement of the technique proposed in [20,21].

Hence, merging of information is important because, as illustrated in Figure 2 (b), segmentation of intervertebral disks in sagittal images in the lateral regions of the disk is difficult because of the scoliotic deformity (spinal curvature). But, regions where the disks are hard to identify in the sagittal plane, corresponds to regions where disks can easily be segmented in the coronal plane (Figure 2 (c)). The inclusion of the reconstructed coronal image segmentation data thus helped us to delimit more precisely the lateral portions of the disks, corresponding to the shaded elliptical areas in Figure 2 (a). The implementation of this third step addresses the problem of missing sections of the lateral part of the disks as it was pointed out in previous study [20].

Coronal images are reconstructed from the sagittal images without the need of adding another direction of image acquisition during the MRI protocol. From these newly created coronal images, we apply the same segmentation process as for the sagittal images. The fusion of sagittal and coronal segmentation information is achieved as follows: because the slice thickness and the spacing between slices were known, it is possible to join the voxels of the sagittal disk masks and create a reference volume for each disk. The same process is applied to the unlabelled segmented coronal images, creating a set of volumes representing disks and background regions in that case. The centroids of the volumes are calculated and represented the key points for anatomical correspondence between the volumes created from the classified regions in the sagittal plane (reference disk volumes) and the set of volumes created from the segmentation of the coronal planes. Corresponding disk volumes from the two imaging planes are thus superimposed using a union operator. The fusion of the two volumes representing the same disk D is based on the following equation:

$$D = Dref \cup Dcor$$

where *Dref* is the disk volume coming from the sagittal segmentation and *Dcor* is the disk volume coming from the segmentation of coronal images directly. The union of the coronal segmentation with sagittal segmentaion

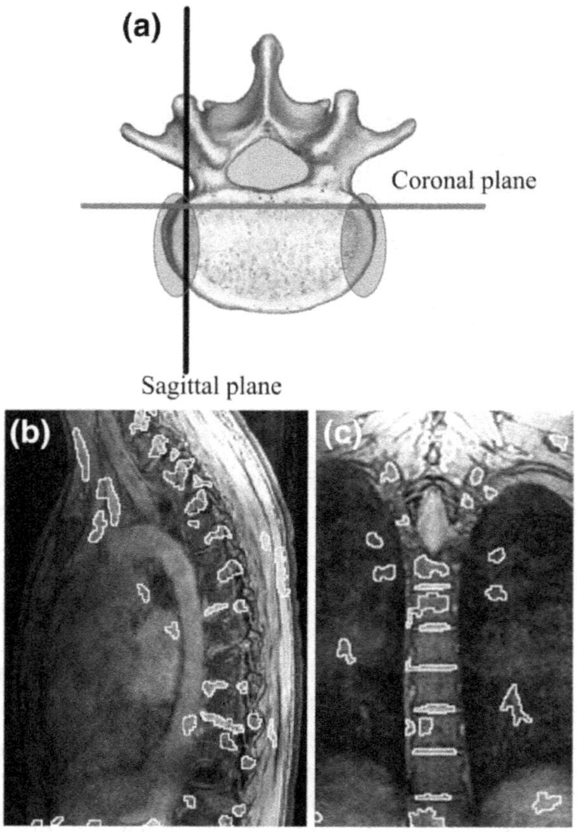

Figure 2 Problematic zone for automatic segmentation. Complementary information is found in different imaging planes. (**a**) Axial view of vertebra showing orientations of sagittal and coronal planes. The shaded ellipses show the regions for which intervertebral disks are hard to segment in sagittal images. (**b**) Segmented sagittal image corresponding to the plane showed in (**a**). None of the intervertebral disks are properly segmented in this sagittal image. (**c**) Segmented coronal image corresponding to the plane showed in (**a**). Several disk contours that the automatic segmentation algorithm is not able to detect in the sagittal plane, are on the other hand, well detected by algorithm in the coronal plane.

allows us to fill empty spaces (created by missing disk detection) encounters in the lateral portion of the disk if only sagittal images where used (figure 2). Moreover, this step enables us to use all the information provided by a volume acquisition modality like MRI and addresses the difficulty of disk segmentation in the lateral regions of the disks when analyzing sagittal images only [21]. A summary of the three steps of the reconstruction process is shown in Figure 3.

Evaluation of the automatic segmentation

To conduct a quantitative evaluation of the automatic segmentation, comparison with gold standard is necessary. The manual segmentations of intervertebral disks performed by 3 clinical experts were considered the gold standard. The validation dataset consists of nine scoliotic patients who underwent magnetic resonance imaging with the three different protocols. Three of the patients have a mild main thoracic curve (Cobb angles from 12° to 24°), three have a moderate curve (Cobb angles from 28° to 35°) and three have a more severe curve requiring surgery (Cobb angles from 43° to 60°). Each user has segmented a total of nine intervertebral disks coming from different patients presenting different curve severities and representing different MRI protocols and different positions relative to the apex of the curve. Experts have carefully indicated the boundaries of the intervertebral disks in every MR slice using the commercially available SliceOmatic™ software (Tomovision, Montreal). While doing the manual segmentation, the experts had access to the orthogonal views, just as in the proposed automatic segmentation approach.

Similarity measure

The Dice Similarity Coefficient (DSC) is used as a statistical metric to evaluate the performance of the novel automatic segmentation method. The DSC has been used in various studies to evaluate the segmentation of many organs in MRI and CT [22-25]. The DSC measures the spatial overlap between two segmentations X and Y. The coefficient is defined as:

$$DSC(X,Y) = \frac{2|X \cap Y|}{|X| + |Y|} \quad (1)$$

where X represents the set of voxels in an intervertebral disk resulting from automatic segmentation and Y the set of voxels contained in the same intervertebral disk resulting from manual segmentation. The values for the DSC range between 0 and 1 where 0 means no overlap and 1 means a perfect overlap between the manual segmentation performed by one of the experts and the corresponding automatic segmentation. A DSC value greater than 0.7 has been reported as indicating good segmentation performance [22,23,25].

The number of voxels contained in the volumes produced by manual and automatic segmentation is also compared to provide an indicator of over- or underestimation of volumes created by the automatic method.

To refine the evaluation of the automatic segmentation, the 2D DSC is also calculated for every sagittal image to locate the intervertebral disk regions that are more prone to produce large errors using automatic segmentation. Moreover, a mean 2D distance in mm between the manually segmented and automatic segmented disk boundaries in the area of the spinal canal is calculated in the sagittal images spanning the canal.

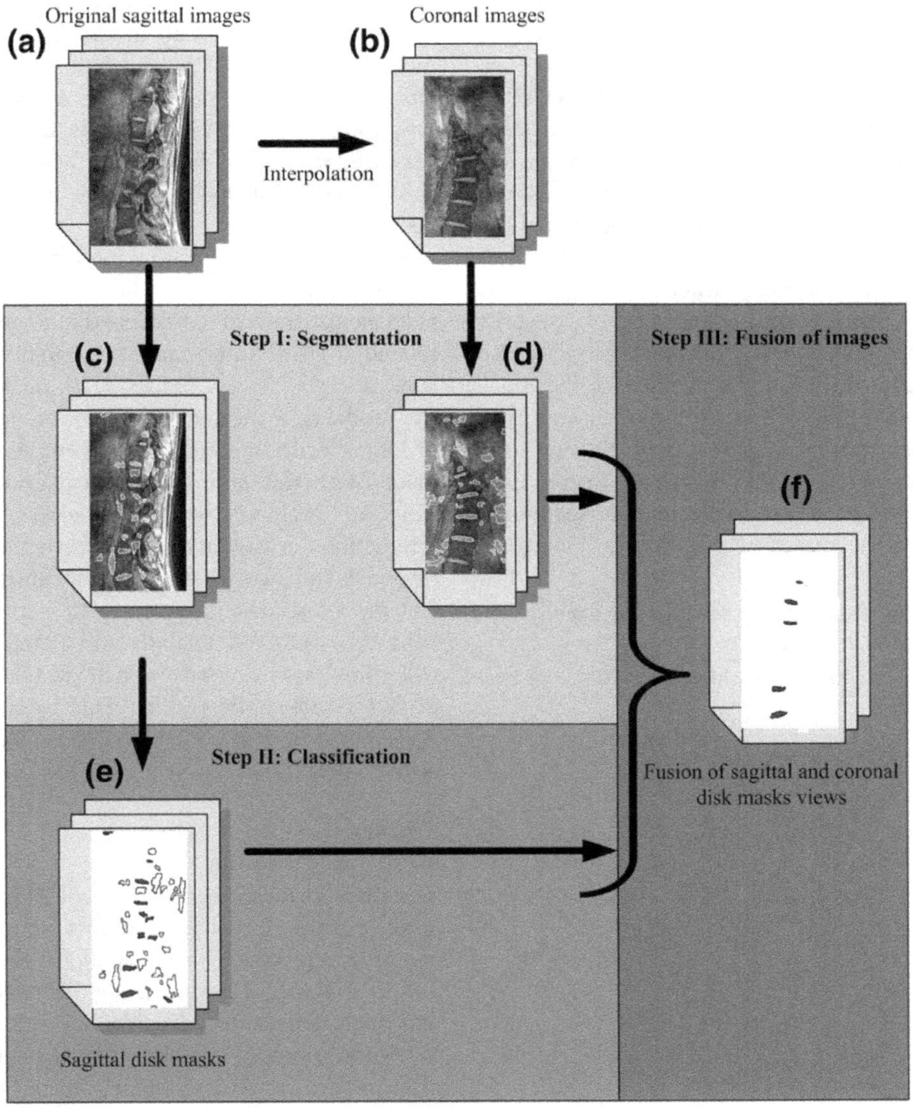

Figure 3 Flowchart of the novel automatic segmentation process. Flow chart of the different steps necessary to obtain the final reconstruction of the intervertebral disks.

Variability

The variance of the results is calculated to compare the variability of the DSC for the proposed segmentation algorithm with the inter-user variability. The inter-user variability represents the degree of concordance between manual segmentations performed by different users. To evaluate the variability, the same three disks are segmented by two clinical experts for each MRI acquisition protocol. The 3D DSC is calculated using (Eq.1) for three different cases: a first case for which manual segmentation of user 1 is compared with the automatic segmentation results, a second case for which manual segmentation of user 2 is compared with the automatic segmentation results and a third case for which manual segmentation of user 1 is compared with manual segmentation of user 2.

Robustness

As the second objective of the paper is to evaluate the robustness of the automatic segmentation algorithm, we have evaluated whether the results of the automatic segmentation are influenced by specific factors characterizing the MR images of scoliotic patients. An experimental factorial design is used to determine the effect of five major characteristics of MR images of scoliotic patients. The studied factors are: 1) the type of MRI acquisition sequence, 2) the position of the intervertebral disk relative to the apex of the curvature, 3) the degree of severity of the curvature, 4) the MRI inter-patient variability for each image acquisition protocol, and finally 5) the user who performed the manual segmentation.

The Table 1 was automatically created with STATISTICA™ from StatSoft Inc. (Oklahoma, U.S.) and it summarizes the setting of the modalities for each factor and each segmentation. Each factor has three modalities represented by 1, 0 and −1 in Table 1. The modalities for the MRI acquisition sequence type are the three acquisition sequences described earlier (3D MEDIC, 3D FISP and 2D Spin Echo). The modalities for the severity of the scoliosis are low severity, moderate severity and high severity deformation. For the position of the intervertebral disk relative to the apex, the modalities corresponds to the disk located at the apex itself, one level superior to the apex and one level inferior to the apex. Three different users have performed manual segmentation and represent the three user modalities. Finally, to verify if the MRI inter-patient variability for a given MRI acquisition sequence can modify the result of the DSC measure, the manual segmentation is divided into three blocks, each block representing a trio of patients with low, moderate and high severity deformations. This is how uncontrollable factor like MRI inter-patient variability can be taken into account in this type of robustness study.

With a factorial design taking into account simple and double interactions of four factors, and with three blocks of patients to also consider the uncontrollable factor related to MRI inter-patient variability, the number of runs is 27: $3^{(4-2)}$ x 3 blocks = 27, or $M^{(k-p)}$ where M is the modality, k the number of factors and p the number of higher order interactions that the user wants to eliminate. With this type of statistical evaluation, it is possible to evaluate whether the simple and double interactions of the factors have an effect on the studied response and also whether the blocking factor has an effect on the studied response with a minimal number of runs. The ANOVA analysis and Pareto chart of effects will allow us to verify which factor or combination of factors affect the results. This part of the evaluation is performed using STATISTICA™ from StatSoft Inc. (Oklahoma, U.S.).

Table 1 Overview of the modality settings for each segmentation created by Statistica

Run	Block	Cobb	Position	MRI	User
1	1	1	0	−1	−1
2	1	0	1	1	0
3	1	−1	−1	1	0
4	1	0	1	−1	−1
5	1	1	0	1	0
6	1	−1	−1	0	1
7	1	1	0	0	1
8	1	−1	−1	−1	−1
9	1	0	1	0	1
10	2	−1	0	0	0
11	2	−1	0	−1	−1
12	2	1	1	1	−1
13	2	0	−1	−1	1
14	2	0	−1	0	0
15	2	0	−1	1	−1
16	2	1	1	0	0
17	2	−1	0	1	−1
18	2	1	1	−1	1
19	3	0	0	1	1
20	3	0	0	−1	0
21	3	−1	1	0	−1
22	3	0	0	0	−1
23	3	1	−1	1	−1
24	3	1	−1	−1	0
25	3	1	−1	0	−1
26	3	−1	1	1	1
27	3	−1	1	−1	0

Results

3D similarity measure

The study included segmentation of 27 intervertebral disks coming from 9 scoliotic patients and 3 different MRI acquisition protocols. Table 2 shows the 3D DSC values and their standard deviation for the three MRI sequences and the number (n) of disks used for the evaluation. Within a group for a given MRI sequence, each of the n disks comes from a different patient. An ANOVA test shows that the 3D DSC of the 3D FISP protocol is statistically lower than the results obtained with the other two protocols. However there is no statistically significant difference between the results obtained for the 3D MEDIC and the Spin Echo sequences. The mean value of the 3D DSC for those two sequences is 0.77 and is higher than the threshold value of 0.70, considered as the minimum for a good segmentation performance.

Table 2 Mean 3D Dice Similarity Coefficient and its standard deviation for the three acquisition sequences, each group composed of *n* disks

MRI Sequences	3D DSC (std dev)	n
3D MEDIC	0.79(0.04)	9
3D FISP	0.64(0.09)	9
Spin Echo	0.75(0.07)	9
All sequences	0.73(0.09)	27
3D MEDIC and Spin Echo	0.77(0.06)	18

To assess the segmentation performance in terms of over- or under-segmentation of the volume of an intervertebral disk, the number of voxels is calculated for the 27 different intervertebral disks. For each type of MRI sequence, there are a total of nine disks, each corresponding to a different patient, and representing different Cobb angles and different positions relative to the apex. Figure 4 shows that for the 3D MEDIC (a) and Spin Echo (b), the majority (all except one) of the automatic segmentations were underestimated compared to manual segmentation (by 25% and 20% respectively). For the 3D FISP (Figure 4 (c)), there is no trend in the over- or under-segmentation of volume for the automatic segmentation compared to the manual segmentation. For this MRI sequence, the automatic volume is either under- or over-estimated by mean 30% compared to manual segmentation.

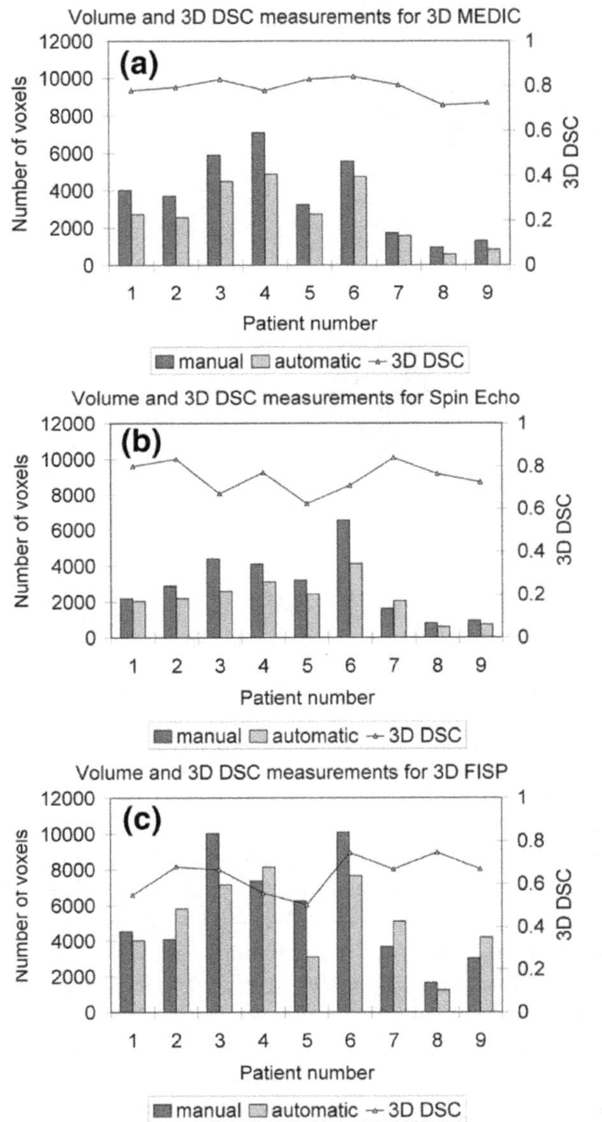

Figure 4 Volume and 3D DSC measurements. The three graphs represent the volumes of the 27 intervertebral disks obtained manually and automatically and the 3D DSC values for each MRI acquisition sequence: (**a**) for the 3D MEDIC, (**b**) for the Spin Echo and (**c**) for the 3D FISP.

Typical results for the 3D reconstruction of intervertebral disks are shown in Figure 5 for the three different MRI acquisitions. By superimposing the volumes and applying transparency (Figure 5 (c) and (f)), it is clear that for the 3D MEDIC and Spin Echo sequences, the error in the spatial overlap between the manual and automatic volumes, as calculated with the 3D DSC, is mainly due to volume underestimation by the automatic process. On the other hand, for the 3D FISP, we can see that the 3D reconstruction of the automatic segmentation (Figure 5 (h)) has more visual discontinuity in the contour than the results obtained for the two other MRI acquisition protocols (Figure 5 (b) and (e)) and than the corresponding manual result (Figure 5 (g)).

2D similarity measure

To complete the performance evaluation of the novel automatic segmentation algorithm, the 2D DSC is calculated on all slices of all the intervertebral disk volumes in this study. Tables 3, 4 and 5 present the mean 2D DSC for the mid-sagittal slices and for the lateral slices for the 3D MEDIC, Spin Echo and 3D FISP MRI sequences respectively. The mid-sagittal slices correspond to 80% of the slices spanning the intervertebral disks, while the remaining 20% are the lateral slices (10% on each side). The number of slices composing each intervertebral disk is also indicated (n). Examination of the results shows that the 2D DSC values for the mid-sagittal slices are always higher than for the lateral slices for every given volume in the case of the 3D MEDIC and Spin Echo images, while this is not the case for the 3D FISP images. Figure 6 shows in detail some typical results for the 2D DSC.

Figure 6 (a), (d) and (g) plot the distribution of the 2D DSC as a function of slice position. These graphs demonstrate that the lower DSC values are found in the lateral slices for the 3D MEDIC and Spin Echo. It is also possible to appreciate visually the under-segmentation by the automatic method in the case of the 3D MEDIC and Spin Echo sequences, which occurs mainly in the lateral slices (lateral portions of the disk) as can be seen in Figure 6 (b) and (e). On the other hand, the mid-sagittal slices (Figure 6 (c) and (f)) show very similar contours for the manual and automatic segmentations. For the 3D FISP case however, the 2D contours show no systematic under-segmentation of the intervertebral disk contours (Figure 6 (h) and (i)) and significant variations of the 2D DSC values are found throughout the volume.

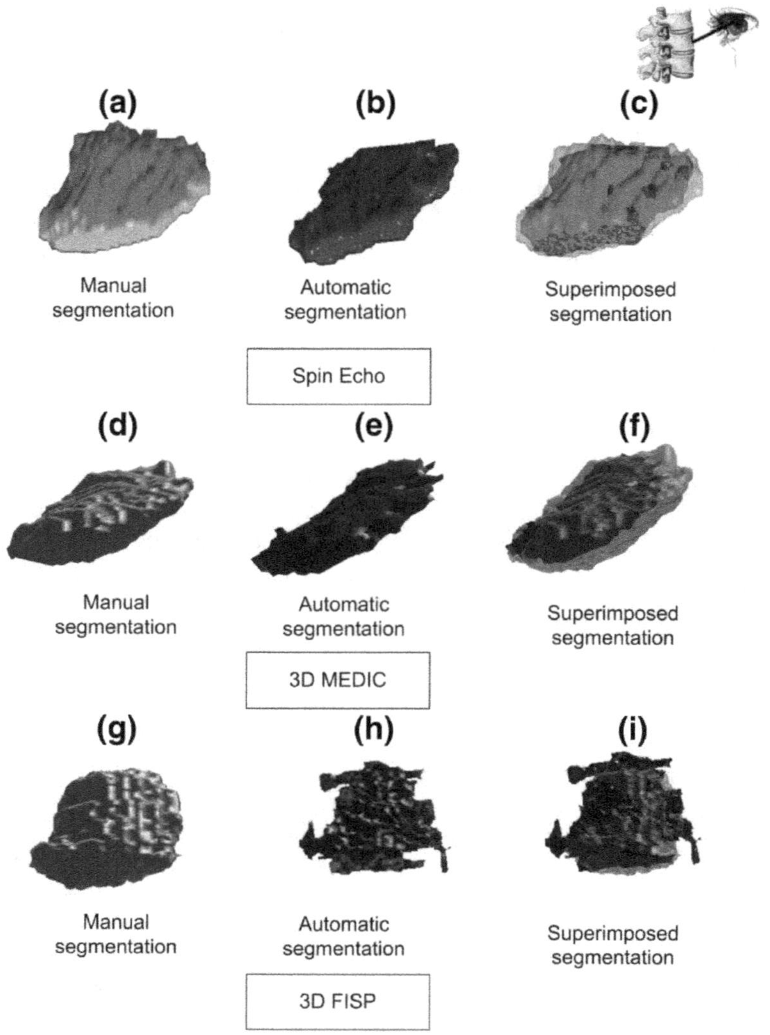

Figure 5 3D reconstruction of intervertebral disks. 3D reconstruction of intervertebral disks obtained with the manual and automatic segmentation procedures. The first column shows a 3D reconstruction in light gray representing the manual segmentation; the second column shows a 3D reconstruction in dark gray representing the automatic segmentation. The third column shows the superimposition of the manual and automatic segmentations. The first row shows the results for the Spin Echo MRI sequence, the second row shows the results for the 3D MEDIC and the third row shows the results for the 3D FISP.

We also sought to quantify the discrepancy between the 2D boundaries of the manual and automatic segmentations in the sagittal imaging slices surrounding the spinal canal, for the Spin Echo and 3D MEDIC sequences. In this evaluation, we find that the automatic segmentation was underestimated (*i.e.* its boundary was farther from the edge of the canal) compared to the manual segmentation by an average distance of 3.4 mm (±1.5mm) and 1.8 mm (±0.8mm) for those two sequences respectively.

Variability of the 3D DSC results

When developing segmentation algorithms for clinical imaging data, an accepted gold standard is the corresponding manual segmentation, but the latter introduces inter-user variability. In our case, a comparison of the variance of the results of the proposed segmentation algorithm with the variance of the manual segmentation results for two users shows that for the 3D MEDIC and Spin Echo sequences, the variability introduced by the automatic segmentation is lower than the inter-user variability for both users. Table 6 is based on a total of 9 intervertebral disks segmented twice by 2 clinical experts.

Table 6 shows that the standard deviations for the inter-user results were 0.07 and 0.05 for the 3D MEDIC and Spin Echo respectively. These values are higher than the variability obtained with the proposed automatic segmentation process. For the 3D FISP, the automatic segmentation leads to a variability of 0.10 when compared to user 2. This variability is higher than the inter-user

Table 3 Mean 2D DSC and standard deviation for the mid-sagittal and lateral slices for 3D MEDIC images of nine patients

3D MEDIC Patients	Mid-sag slices Mean DSC	std dev	n	Lateral slices Mean DSC	std dev	n
p1	0.70	0.29	28	0.52	0.48	8
p2	0.79	0.14	30	0.06	0.12	8
p3	0.86	0.06	32	0.36	0.31	8
p4	0.78	0.17	40	0.05	0.16	10
p5	0.83	0.06	26	0.43	0.46	8
p6	0.83	0.11	33	0.40	0.38	10
p7	0.81	0.09	22	0.65	0.31	6
p8	0.73	0.09	23	0.13	0.24	6
p9	0.66	0.30	25	0.31	0.43	8

Table 5 Mean 2D DSC and standard deviation for the mid-sagittal and lateral slices for 3D FISP images of nine patients

3D MEDIC Patients	Mid-sag slices Mean DSC	std dev	n	Lateral slices Mean DSC	std dev	n
p1	0.43	0.35	29	0.42	0.36	8
p2	0.75	0.09	28	0.50	0.33	8
p3	0.58	0.30	31	0.38	0.41	10
p4	0.41	0.18	36	0.44	0.09	10
p5	0.35	0.34	32	0.11	0.19	10
p6	0.63	0.27	32	0.70	0.16	8
p7	0.66	0.12	26	0.45	0.36	8
p8	0.74	0.22	28	0.20	0.28	8
p9	0.66	0.07	24	0.61	0.27	8

variability of 0.07. Also for the 3D FISP, when comparing user 1 against automatic segmentation, the variability is the same as the inter-user variability.

Robustness

The ANOVA analysis and Pareto chart of effects (Figure 7) reveal that the type of MRI sequence is by far ($p = 0.000285$) the factor that most affects the prediction equation. The user also affects the values of the DSC, but to a lower degree ($p = 0.0418$) than the MRI acquisition sequence. The inter-patient MRI intensity variability (block), the severity of the scoliosis (Cobb angle) and the position of the studied intervertebral disk relative to the apex of the spinal deformity do not influence the response of the system as reported by the 3D DSC measurement. Results also show that interactions between the different factors do not affect the response of the system.

Discussion

Using clinical dataset from real scoliotic patients is important for this study because topology of the spine on MR images varies a lot from normal to scoliotic patient adding important challenge in the segmentation process. In this context, it is commonly accepted to set manual segmentation as gold standard. Aside from the Dice Similarity Coefficient (DSC) used to test the validation criteria, the calculation of volume is also part of the evaluation. The similarity coefficient has the advantage of taking into account the spatial dependency, which is not the case when reporting volumes only. Conversely, although geometrically intuitive, the DSC lacks information about the type of segmentation error, namely whether over- or under-segmentation occurs. By taking into account both metrics (DSC and volume), the current study provides a comprehensive quantitative evaluation of the automatic segmentation applied to a clinical dataset composed of 27 intervertebral disks coming from nine scoliotic patients.

Table 4 Mean 2D DSC and standard deviation for the mid-sagittal and lateral slices for Spin Echo images of nine patients

3D MEDIC Patients	Mid-sag slices Mean DSC	std dev	n	Lateral slices Mean DSC	std dev	n
p1	0.82	0.09	9	0.58	0.25	4
p2	0.83	0.04	9	0.82	0.10	4
p3	0.69	0.08	13	0.26	0.30	4
p4	0.74	0.25	12	0.67	0.21	4
p5	0.56	0.33	11	0.36	0.30	4
p6	0.64	0.30	14	0.58	0.14	4
p7	0.86	0.12	9	0.63	0.43	4
p8	0.74	0.32	8	0.29	0.41	2
p9	0.67	0.28	9	0.28	0.42	4

From the comparison of the automatic segmentation with manual segmentation, we find that the proposed algorithm yields to spatial volumes that are similar to the gold standard, since the average 3D DSC values of 0.79 for the 3D MEDIC and 0.75 for the Spin Echo (Table 2) are higher than the 0.7 threshold for good segmentation performance.

No other study on segmentation based on region detection for 3D reconstruction of intervertebral disk of scoliotic patient exists. However Michopoulou *et al* [12]. have an automatic segmentation for intervertebral disk based on a priori shape information and fuzzy c-mean algorithm. Their segmentation procedure is applied on the mid-sagittal image to evaluate if the disk is degenerated. They have evaluated their segmentation accuracy using a 2D DSC value on the mid-sagittal image. Hence we can partly compare our results with this study. On figure 6 of the current study, the 2D DSC value for the Spin Echo at the mid-sagittal image (image 7) is 0.9 and 0.88 for the 3D MEDIC at the mid-sagittal level. This is

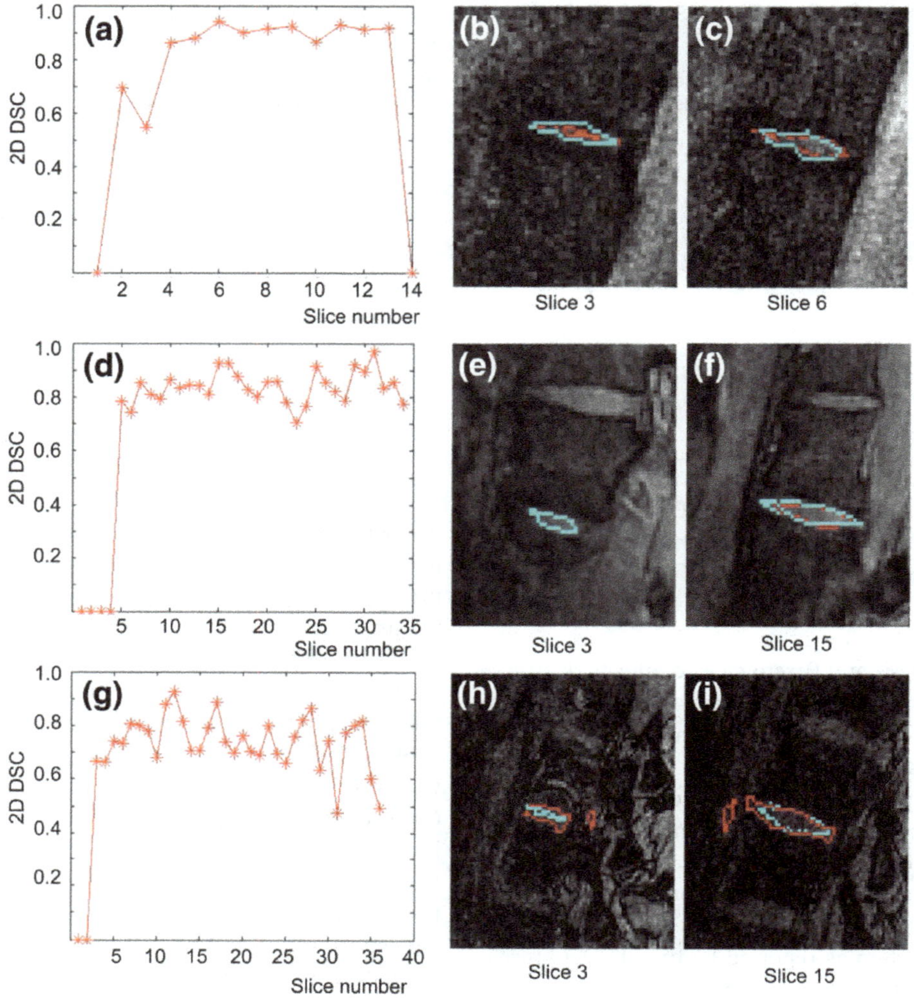

Figure 6 2D measurements. Graphs of the 2D DSC relative to slice number are presented for the (**a**) Spin Echo, (**d**) 3D MEDIC and (**g**) 3D FISP sequences. In the 2D images, cyan represents manual segmentation and red represents automatic segmentation of the intervertebral disk for slices in the lateral and mid-sagittal planes of the disk for the Spin Echo ((**b**) and (**c**)), 3D MEDIC ((**e**) and (**f**)), and 3D FISP (**h**) and (**i**) sequences.

comparable to the results obtained by Michopoulou. Indeed they obtained 0.88 (for the elastic-Atlas-RFCM method), 0.84 (for the Atlas-FCM method) and 0.87 (for the Atlas-RFCM method) on degenerated disk.

Results reveals that the reconstructed 3D volumes of intervertebral disks are systematically underestimated (mean discrepancy of 22.5%) compared to volumes obtained with manual segmentation performed on 3D MEDIC and Spin Echo MR images. For the 3D FISP, there is no trend in over- or under-segmentation but there is a mean discrepancy of 30% between the automatic volumes and the manual volumes. Indeed, there is less consistency from slice to slice for the 3D FISP images because the automatic segmentation algorithm has trouble with the blurred boundaries of intervertebral disks often found in the 3D FISP sequences. The three

Table 6 Mean 3D DSC with standard deviation comparing automatic segmentation against manual segmentation performed by users 1 and 2 and comparing manual segmentation of user 1 against manual segmentation of user 2

Compared volumes	3D MEDIC 3D DSC (std dev)	Spin Echo 3D DSC (std dev)	3D FISP 3D DSC (std dev)	n
User 1 vs automatic	0.77 (0.05)	0.70 (0.05)	0.59 (0.07)	3
User 2 vs automatic	0.72 (0.05)	0.76 (0.04)	0.60 (0.10)	3
User 1 vs User 2	0.81 (0.07)	0.78 (0.05)	0.72 (0.07)	3

The number of disks is specified by n.

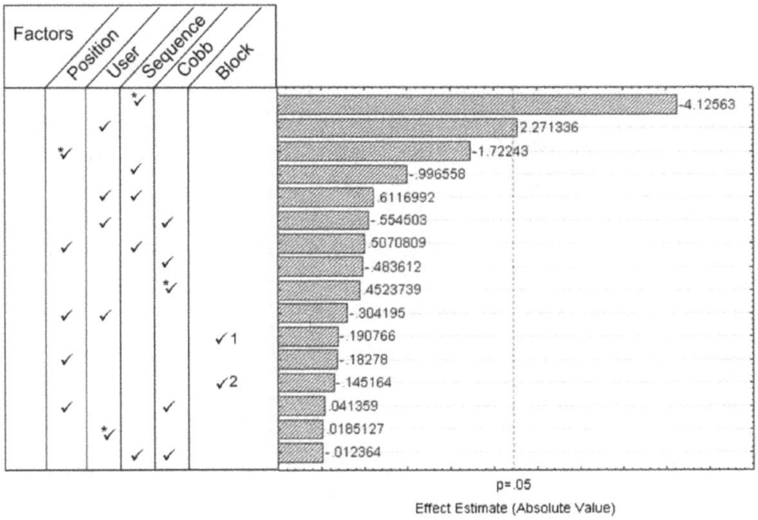

Figure 7 Pareto chart. Pareto Chart of the estimated effects of the 4 controllable factors and 1 uncontrollable factor (Block) on the DSC values. The four controllable factors are the position of the disk relative to the apex of the curvature, the user performing the manual segmentation, the MRI acquisition sequence and the Cobb angle. The uncontrollable factor is the block corresponding to the inter-patient variability. Block 1, Block 2 and Block 3 illustrate the three groups used to create the block. The asterisk * represents the quadratic term and if not specified, the linear term is considered in the equation for the statistical model used to estimate the effect. If more than one factor is specified, this means that the interaction of the 2 specified factors is studied.

clinical experts who performed the manual segmentation all agreed that the intervertebral disks were harder to delimitate in the 3D FISP sequences because of the blurred contours (due to variation of pixel intensities along the boundaries). Hence, even in the manually identified volumes, there is less consistency from slice to slice compared to the two other types of MR images.

The volume underestimation resulting from the automatic segmentation algorithm applied to 3D MEDIC and Spin Echo images occurs more in the lateral slices than in the mid-sagittal slices. Superimposition of volumes in space and 2D evaluation of the DSC (see Tables 3 and 4) show higher 2D DSC results in the mid-sagittal slices than in the lateral slices for all patients, meaning that the differences between the volumes lie mainly in the lateral regions of the disks. For the 3D FISP (Table 5), there is no specific region of volume under- or over-estimation since the results for the 2D DSC vary as much in the mid-sagittal slices as in the lateral slices.

For surgeons, the underestimation of the volume of anatomical structures is viewed as a margin of safety in a computer assistance system. Indeed, by reasonably underestimating the working volume (e.g. the intervertebral disk), surgeons will have more confidence in the 3D model, since they will know that if their surgical tools are inside the 3D model there is no chance to injure critical anatomical structures (e.g. the spinal cord). For example, in spinal release before instrumentation of scoliotic patient, the intervertebral disk must be partially removed and delicate anatomical structures surrounding the disk like the spinal canal and aorta must not be injured during the procedure. These structures are located to the anterior left side of the disk (for the aorta) and to the posterior side (for the spinal canal). The distance in mm between the manual and the automatic segmentations in the sagittal slices spanning the spinal canal is of 3.4 mm (±1.5mm) for the Spin Echo and 1.8 mm (±0.8mm) for the 3D MEDIC. The greater underestimation of the disk for the Spin Echo sequence can be explained by the fact that for half of the patients, the Spin Echo sequence resulted in images with some pixels being brighter in the nucleus compared to the annulus, thus misleading the automatic segmentation process which detected the nucleus boundary as the external disk boundary. A modification of the parameters of the Spin Echo sequence would eliminate this discrepancy between the results in mm of the 3D MEDIC and Spin Echo sequences. Hence, for a disk resection application, a mean underestimation distance of 1.8 mm in the mid-sagittal planes compared to manually segmented contours gives an adequate margin of safety.

The variability associated with the use of automatic segmentation is lower than the variability associated with manual segmentation performed by different users. This is true for both the 3D MEDIC and Spin Echo MR sequences, therefore making the use of the automatic segmentation method clinically feasible. Hence, this study addresses an important issue concerning the use of computer assistance in a clinical environment. Indeed, for an automatic segmentation algorithm to be acceptable, the variability of the 3D model on which the computer assistance system relies should be equal to or lower than the variability of an equivalent 3D model obtained from manual segmentation.

One of the limits of the study is that for the three MRI sequences, the Field Of View (FOV) encompasses only five to seven vertebral levels. It is well known that scoliotic patients often have double curvature (one in the thoracic region and one in the lumbar region of the spine). With such a small FOV it is not possible to image both curvatures at a time. This limitation also entails that in the robustness evaluation, the effect of the position of the disk relative to the spinal region (thoracic or lumbar) has not been considered. Because thoracic disks are smaller than lumbar disks, the behavior of the automatic segmentation algorithm may vary for different vertebral levels. In the current study, the spinal curves included in the MRI were mainly in the lumbar and lower thoracic regions.

However, the robustness study does include an evaluation of the effects of five important factors. Results show that the proposed automatic segmentation algorithm is robust, in light of the fact that the results for the 3D DSC are not affected by the severity of the spinal deformity, the position of the disk relative to the apex or the inter-patient MR intensity variation. On the other hand, the type of MR acquisition sequence is important and could substantially affect the results of the automatic segmentation. Considering that the mean 3D DSC value is significantly lower for the 3D FISP than for the other two sequences (Table 2), the 3D FISP MR acquisition protocol is not recommended for good performance of the proposed automatic segmentation method.

The recommended MR acquisition protocols for the proposed intervertebral disk automatic segmentation method are thus the Spin Echo and 3D MEDIC MR sequences. There is no statistical difference between the 3D DSC results of for these two protocols. The choice between 3D MEDIC and Spin Echo will depend on the clinician. The acquisition time of the 3D MEDIC sequence is 2.5 times longer than for Spin Echo. A longer acquisition time means less reproducible results because patients are more prone to move during the acquisition. Depending on the clinician and on the application, one might decide to use Spin Echo even if some interpolation is required between slices in order to reconstruct in 3D, because an acquisition time of only 12 minutes is more feasible and will have more chance of giving non-blurred images for all patients.

Conclusions

Although the applicability of this method is limited to specific MRI acquisition protocol, the proposed automatic segmentation of intervertebral disks on scoliotic patient is accurate, reliable, and reproducible tool for volume extraction of intervertebral disk of scoliotic patient. The proposed automatic segmentation algorithm is able to cope with patients presenting varying degrees of scoliotic spinal deformity. This work is an important step toward providing reliable pre-operative model updated using intra-operative images to help surgeons to visualize structures of interests during surgeries such as disk resection.

Competing interests

The authors declare that they have no competing interests.

Authors' contributions

CC and FC made substantial conceptual contributions to the design of the study, analysis and interpretation of data, and contributed to drafting of the manuscript. GG and M-CM were involved in manual segmentation and in image data analysis and interpretation of the MRI, and gave their input from a clinical point of view. C-EA gave critical revision of the manuscript regarding important intellectual content. All authors have read and approved the final version of the manuscript.

Acknowledgements

We would like to acknowledge the participation of scoliotic patients. Written consent was obtained from the patient or their relative for publication of study. This project was funded by the Natural Sciences and Engineering Council of Canada (NSERC) and by the Canada Research Chair Program. This work was also supported in part by grants from the Fonds Québécois de la Recherche sur la Nature et les Technologies (FQRNT).

Author details

[1]Ecole Polytechnique de Montreal, Biomedical Engineering Institute, Montreal, QC H3C 3A7, Canada. [2]Sainte-Justine University Hospital Center, Montreal, QC H3T 1C5, Canada. [3]Department of Computer Engineering and Software, Ecole Polytechnique de Montreal, Montreal, QC H3C 3A7, Canada. [4]Department of Mechanical Engineering, Ecole Polytechnique de Montreal, Montreal, QC H3C 3A7, Canada.

References

1. Feng B, Qiu G, Shen J, Zhang J, Tian Y, Li S, Zhao H, Zhao Y: **Impact of Multimodal Intraoperative Monitoring During Surgery for Spine Deformity and Potential Risk Factors for Neurological Monitoring Changes.** *J Spinal Disord Tech* 2012, **25**:e108.
2. Sugarman E, Sarwahi V, Amaral T, Wollowick A, Gambassi M, Seimon L: **Comparative Analysis of Perioperative Differences Between Hybrid Versus Pedicle Screw Instrumentation in Adolescent Idiopathic Scoliosis.** *J Spinal Disord Tech* 2012.
3. Schwab FJ, Smith V, Farcy JP: **Endoscopic thoracoplasty and anterior spinal release in scoliotic deformity.** *Bull Hosp Jt Dis* 2000, **59**(1):27–32.
4. Waisman M, Saute M: **Thoracoscopic spine release before posterior instrumentation in scoliosis.** *Clin Orthop Relat Res* 1997, **336**:130–136.
5. Lieberman IH, Salo PT, Orr RD, Kraetschmer B: **Prone position endoscopic transthoracic release with simultaneous posterior instrumentation for spinal deformity: a description of the technique.** *Spine* 2000, **25**(17):2251–2257.
6. Newton PO, Shea KG, Granlund KF: **Defining the pediatric spinal thoracoscopy learning curve: sixty-five consecutive cases.** *Spine* 2000, **25**(8):1028–1035.
7. Violas P, Estivalezes E, Briot J, Salesde Gauzy J, Swider P: **Objective quantification of intervertebral disc volume properties using MRI in idiopathic scoliosis surgery.** *Magn Reson Imaging* 2007, **25**(3):386–391.
8. Coulon O, Hickman SJ, Parker GJ, Barker GJ, Miller DH, Arridge SR: **Quantification of spinal cord atrophy from magnetic resonance images via a B-spline active surface model.** *Magn Reson Med* 2002, **47**(6):1176–1185.

9. Hoad CL, Martel AL: **Segmentation of MR images for computer-assisted surgery of the lumbar spine.** *Phys Med Biol* 2002, **47**(19):3503–3517.
10. Peng Z, Zhong J, Wee W, Lee JH: **Automated Vertebra Detection and Segmentation from the Whole Spine MR Images.** *Conf Proc IEEE Eng Med Biol Soc* 2005, **3**:2527–2530.
11. Carballido-Gamio J, Belongie SJ, Majumdar S: **Normalized Cuts in 3-D for Spinal MRI Segmentation.** *IEEE Transactions on Medical Imaging* 2004, **23**(1):36–44.
12. Michopoulou SK, Costaridou L, Panagiotopoulos E, Speller R, Panayiotakis G, Todd-Pokropek A: **Atlas-based segmentation of degenerated lumbar intervertebral discs from MR images of the spine.** *IEEE Transactions on Biomedical Engineering* 2009, **56**(9):2225–2231.
13. Udupa JK FAF, Udupa JK: **A 3D generalization of user-steered live-wire segmentation.** *Medical Image Analysis* 2000, **4**(4):389–402.
14. Wieclawek W, Pietka E: **Live-Wire-Based 3D Segmentation Method.** In *Engineering in Medicine and Biology Society.*: EMBS; 2007:5645–5648. *2007 29th Annual International Conference of the IEEE: 22–26 Aug.* 2007.
15. Lu K, Higgins WE: **Improved 3D live-wire method with application to 3D CT chest image analysis.** In *Medical Imaging.* San Diego, CA, United states: SPIE; 2006. Image Processing, Febrary 13, 2006 - Febrary 16, 2006.
16. Farber M, Ehrhardt J, Handels H: **Live-wire-based segmentation using similarities between corresponding image structures.** *Computerized Medical Imaging and Graphics* 2007, **31**:549–560.
17. Cheng J, Foo SW, Krishnan SM: **Watershed-presegmented snake for boundary detection and tracking of left ventricle in echocardiographic images.** *IEEE Transactions on Information Technology in Biomedicine* 2006, **10**(2):414–416.
18. Dokladal P, Bloch I, Couprie M, Ruijters D, Urtasun R, Garnero L: **Topologically controlled segmentation of 3D magnetic resonance images of the head by using morphological operators.** *Pattern Recognition* 2003, **36**(10):2463–2478.
19. Grau V, Alcaniz Raya M, Monserrat C, Juan MC, Marti-Bonmati L: **Hierarchical image segmentation using a correspondence with a tree model.** 2004, **37**(1):47–59.
20. Chevrefils C, Cheriet F, Grimard G, Aubin C-E: **Watershed segmentation of intervertebral disk and spinal canal from MRI images.** In *Image Analysis and Recognition.*: ; 007:1017–1027. th International Conference, ICIAR 2007, 22–24 Aug 2007.
21. Chevrefils C, Cheriet F, Aubin C, Grimard G: **Texture Analysis for Automatic Segmentation of Intervertebral Disks of Scoliotic Spines From MR Images.** *Information Technology in Biomedicine, IEEE Transactions on* 2009, **13**(4):608–620.
22. Zou KH, Warfield SK, Bharatha A, Tempany CM, Kaus MR, Haker SJ, Wells WM, Jolesz FA, Kikinis R: **Statistical validation of image segmentation quality based on a spatial overlap index.** *Acad Radiol* 2004, **11**(2):178–189.
23. Lin D-T, Lei C-C, Hung S-W: **Computer-aided kidney segmentation on abdominal CT images.** *IEEE Transactions on Information Technology in Biomedicine* 2006, **10**(1):59–65.
24. Ibrahim M, John N, Kabuka M, Younis A: **Hidden Markov models-based 3D MRI brain segmentation.** *pt?>Image and Vision Computing* 2006, **24**(10):1065–1079.
25. Zijdenbos AP, Dawant BM, Margolin RA, Palmer AC: **Morphometric analysis of white matter lesions in MR images: method and validation.** *IEEE Transactions on Medical Imaging* 1994, **13**(4):716–724.

4

Quantitative and qualitative assessment of structural magnetic resonance imaging data

Sima Chalavi[1,2*], Andrew Simmons[3,4,5], Hildebrand Dijkstra[6], Gareth J Barker[3,5†] and A A T Simone Reinders[1,2†]

Abstract

Background: Multi-center magnetic resonance imaging (MRI) studies present an opportunity to advance research by pooling data. However, brain measurements derived from MR-images are susceptible to differences in MR-sequence parameters. It is therefore necessary to determine whether there is an interaction between the sequence parameters and the effect of interest, and to minimise any such interaction by careful choice of acquisition parameters. As an exemplar of the issues involved in multi-center studies, we present data from a study in which we aimed to optimize a set of volumetric MRI-protocols to define a protocol giving data that are consistent and reproducible across two centers and over time.

Methods: Optimization was achieved based on data quality and quantitative measures, in our case using FreeSurfer and Voxel Based Morphometry approaches. Our approach consisted of a series of five comparisons. Firstly, a single-center dataset was collected, using a range of candidate pulse-sequences and parameters chosen on the basis of previous literature. Based on initial results, a number of minor changes were implemented to optimize the pulse-sequences, and a second single-center dataset was collected. FreeSurfer data quality measures were compared between datasets in order to determine the best performing sequence(s), which were taken forward to the next stage of testing. We subsequently acquired short-term and long-term two-center reproducibility data, and quantitative measures were again assessed to determine the protocol with the highest reproducibility across centers. Effects of a scanner software and hardware upgrade on the reproducibility of the protocols at one of the centers were also evaluated.

Results: Assessing the quality measures from the first two datasets allowed us to define artefact-free protocols, all with high image quality as assessed by FreeSurfer. Comparing the quantitative test and retest measures, we found high within-center reproducibility for all protocols, but lower *between*-center reproducibility for some protocols than others. The upgrade showed no important effects.

* Correspondence: sima.chalavi@gmail.com
†Equal contributors
[1]Department of Neuroscience, University Medical Center Groningen, and BCN Neuroimaging Center, University of Groningen, Groningen, The Netherlands
[2]King's College London, Institute of Psychiatry, Department of Psychosis Studies, London, UK
Full list of author information is available at the end of the article

Conclusions: We were able to determine (for the scanners used in this study) an optimised protocol, which gave the highest within- and between-center reproducibility of those assessed, and give details of this protocol here. More generally, we discuss some of the issues raised by multi-center studies and describe a methodical approach to take towards optimization and standardization, and recommend performing this kind of procedure to other investigators.

Keywords: Multi-center, Structural MRI, Freesurfer, SPM, Voxel based morphometry, Cortical thickness, Subcortical volumes, Reproducibility, Test-retest, Variability, Relative mean difference

Background

Assessment of brain tissue morphometry is becoming an important biomarker for diagnosis and treatment of a variety of neurological diseases [1-4]. High resolution structural magnetic resonance imaging (sMRI) facilitates quantitative insight into the normal human brain and to changes that occur due to pathology, e.g. in neuro-psychiatric or neurological diseases. Changes in cortical thickness are manifested in normal aging [5] and with the progression of neuro-degenerative diseases such as Alzheimer's disease [6,7], multiple sclerosis [8,9] and schizophrenia [10,11], while alterations in subcortical brain volumes have been reported in normal aging [12,13], Alzheimer's disease [14], Huntington's disease [15,16], and schizophrenia [10,17].

Recently, multi-center MRI studies have increased in popularity. They provide the opportunity to increase subject numbers by pooling data from different centers, which is particularly important for maximising recruitment rates and for studying rare diseases [18-21].

Although manually measuring the brain's volume (using manual tracing techniques) by experienced and trained tracers is often considered as a 'gold standard' [22,23], in large multi-center studies this approach becomes problematic because of the time required; automatic brain measurements are therefore often preferred. There are two types of measurements that can be made by automatic brain analysis tools: quantitative measures, which provide outputs such as brain volumetric and morphometric measures, intended for further analysis, and data quality measures, which give information about the quality of the images, intended to help assess the success of the data analysis approach. One important confound of combining images from different scanners and analysing them with automatic tools is that the volumetric and surface-based brain measurements derived from MR images can be dependent on the scanner manufacturer [24-28], field strength [24-26,28], MRI protocol [25,26,29,30], scanner drift over time [31] and data analysis tool employed [25,32,33], as well as the impact of a scanner upgrade [24,25]. Slight differences in these factors can have a considerable impact on the reliability and reproducibility of the results [20]. It is therefore important to determine whether there is an interaction between the acquisition protocol involved and the effect of interest, and to minimise any such interaction by careful choice of acquisition and analysis methods. Thus, the main aim of the present paper is to report a methodical approach to the choice of MRI protocol for multi-center studies, illustrating the approach using the results from a recent two center study. For our study, we optimized standard vendor derived brain structural MR protocols (with candidate sequences and parameters chosen on the basis of previous reports in the literature) based on their performance with respect to two commonly employed data analysis methodologies. We assessed suitability for the FreeSurfer surface- and volume-based image analysis tool and investigated the reproducibility within and between centers of quantitative measures extracted from FreeSurfer, along with measures from the SPM5 version of Voxel Based Morphometry [34-36].

In this study we collected datasets from two centers equipped with MR scanners with the same field strength and from the same manufacturer. By assessing summary measures of data quality provided by the FreeSurfer program from within-subject within-center datasets, we first aimed to determine the protocols with the highest data quality. Then, by assessing quantitative measures from both FreeSurfer and VBM, we aimed to assess the reproducibility of the MR images 1) within-center, 2) between-center and 3) after scanner upgrade. We report the protocol with the highest reproducibility, which is now in use in a study of Dissociative Identity Disorder (DID) (http://www.neuroimaging-did.com).

Methods

Data acquisition and subjects

In this two-center study, subjects were imaged at two different centers in the Netherlands (Groningen and Amsterdam) which were both equipped with Philips 3 T Intera MR scanners (Philips Medical Systems, Best, NL), referred to here as Center 1 and Center 2. Both centers used the manufacturer's standard 8-channel head coil and software version 2.6.3. We acquired and analyzed five datasets in order to evaluate the quality of images and the reproducibility of different MRI protocols within and between centers. All participants were healthy volunteers with no history of major psychiatric or neurological disease, and provided written informed consent for a study approved by the local ethics committee (Medisch Ethische Toetsingsingscommissie (METc) of the University Medical Center Groningen (UMCG) and Academisch Medisch Centrum (AMC)). For the time period of this study, Periodic Image Quality Tests (PIQT) data, which were collected by the manufacturer as a part of a standard Quality Assurance (QA) protocol, were obtained from both centers and the signal to noise ratio, artefact level and uniformity measurements were investigated.

Comparing T1-weighted volume protocols

As a first step we recommend comparing a range of candidate T1-weighted volume protocols. In our case a single 27-year old healthy female was scanned using six candidate MRI protocols recommended by the vendor and MR physicists at the two centers. While FreeSurfer provided specific protocol recommendations for Siemens scanners, it is difficult to directly translate these to other manufacturer's platforms. We therefore investigated an MPRAGE (Magnetization Prepared RApid Gradient Echo) pulse sequence with similar parameters, along with a number of other pulse sequences and parameters capable of giving whole brain high resolution scans with isotropic or near isotropic voxels, in acceptable imaging times. The protocols included FFE (Fast Field Echo), equivalent to Fast Low Angle SHot (FLASH) on Siemens scanners, and 3D TFE (Turbo Field Echo), equivalent to MPRAGE on Siemens scanners, with 5 different voxel sizes (1.0, 1.05, 1.1, 1.2 and 2.0 mm), two phase encoding directions (right-left and anterior-posterior) and a variety of TR and TE settings (Table 1). This dataset was assessed using quality measures from FreeSurfer's cortical reconstruction process. As these measures are likely to be affected by small changes in the subject position between, or motion during, scans, a thorough visual inspection was made of all data, such that any datasets showing visible bulk motion or artefact likely to be subject-motion related could be excluded from further processing.

Improving T1-weighted volume protocols

The next step is to improve the quality of the images based on the results of the first stage comparison. The details of this stage may vary significantly depending on the results of the first stage. In our case, visual inspection of the images from the first comparison revealed a number of artefacts, in particular a pulsation artefact apparently arising from the carotids. Inconsistencies in phase and amplitude can lead to this kind of artefact, in which ghost images of the vessels or vessel walls are seen along the phase encoding direction. Pulsation artefact can be reduced by adding flow compensation which applies an additional gradient to eliminate phase differences for both stationary and moving spins at the echo time and/or by changing the orientation of phase encoding.. In this study seven variants of the most promising protocols used in the first step were tested (on the same 27-year old healthy female subject) in order to determine protocols which minimized these artefacts while retaining high quality as assessed by FreeSurfer's cortical reconstruction process. Parameter changes included changing the phase encoding direction, adding flow compensation or adding saturation bands using the manufacturer's default settings (Table 1). As previously, a thorough visual inspection was made of all data, such that any datasets showing visible bulk motion or artefact likely to be subject-motion related could excluded from further processing.

Short-term two-center reproducibility

Good short-term multi-center reproducibility is a key minimum requirement for any longitudinal study. In our case the 27 year old healthy female subject was rescanned with two additional young healthy females (26 ± 1.73 years) at both centers with a one day interval, using the three best performing protocols in order to assess the reproducibility of the candidate protocols across centers. This dataset, which was acquired two weeks before a scanner upgrade at Center 1, was also used as part of a scanner upgrade assessment (see below).

Long-term two-center reproducibility

In order to assess the long-term reproducibility of the protocols, the same three participants (27.83 ± 2.31 years) were re-scanned at both centers using the same three protocols 1.5 years later. Long-term reproducibility is also key to longitudinal studies, which normally take place over timescales of months to years. Scanner servicing, replacement of components and long-term scanner drift can all potentially impact on long-term reproducibility.

Assessment of scanner upgrade

To investigate the effect of scanner upgrade the three participants were re-scanned one week after a scanner upgrade at Center 1, when the number of receive channels was changed from 8 to 32 and the scanner operating software was upgraded from 2.6.3 to 3.2.10, again using the same three candidate MR protocols. (Note that although this upgrade provided a 32 channel capability, for the current study the same 8-channel head coil was used before and after the upgrade). Generally it is best to avoid scanner upgrades part way through longitudinal studies, of course, though this will often not be possible due to other operational requirements.

Table 1 Pulse sequence parameters used in the study

Dataset	Protocol name	Protocol type	TR (ms)	TE (ms)	Flip angle	No. Slices	Scan time (sec)	in-plane resolution (mm2)	Phase encoding direction	Slice thickness (mm)	Slice gap (mm)	FC[a]	SB[D]
Initial comparing T1-weighted protocols	A	FLASH	25	4.6	30	160	408	1.0x1.0	Right-left	2.0	−1	-	-
	B	MPRAGE	9.8	4.6	8	120	279	1.16x1.1	Right-left	1.2	0	-	-
	C	MPRAGE	7.6	3.5	8	160	614	1.0x1.0	Anterior-posterior	1.0	0	-	-
	D	MPRAGE	7.6	3.5	8	160	614	1.0x1.0	Anterior-posterior	1.05	0	-	-
	E	MPRAGE	9.8	4.6	8	120	279	1.16x1.1	Right-left	1.2	0	-	-
	F	MPRAGE	7.1	3.3	8	145	557	1.0x1.0	Anterior-posterior	1.1	0	-	-
Optimizing T1-weighted protocols	F	MPRAGE	7.1	3.3	8	145	557	1.0x1.0	Anterior-posterior	1.1	0	-	-
	F1	MPRAGE	7.1	3.3	8	145	557	1.0x1.0	Anterior-posterior	1.1	0	-	✓
	F2	MPRAGE	7.1	3.3	8	145	557	1.0x1.0	Right-left	1.1	0	-	-
	F3	MPRAGE	7.1	3.3	8	145	557	1.0x1.0	Right-left	1.1	0	-	✓
	C1	MPRAGE	9.5	5.3	8	160	614	1.0x1.0	Anterior-posterior	1.0	0	✓	-
	C2	MPRAGE	7.6	3.5	8	160	614	1.0x1.0	Anterior-posterior	1.0	0	-	✓
	C3	MPRAGE	10	5.6	8	160	614	1.0x1.0	Right-left	1.0	0	✓	-

FC[a]: Flow Compensation, manufacturer's default settings.
SB[D]: Saturation band, manufacturer's default settings.

Data analysis

The main interest in our Dissociative Identity Disorder study is volumetric and cortical thickness comparison of different psychiatric groups, so in this study we concentrated on the results from two fully automated brain analysis segmentation tools: FreeSurfer version 4.5 (http://surfer.nmr.mgh.harvard.edu) and Voxel Based Morphometry (VBM) (as implemented within SPM5 (www.fil.ion.ucl.ac.uk/spm)). A brief description of segmentation procedures follows, with further details provided in previous publications [36,37].

The FreeSurfer processing pipeline includes both surface-based [38] and volume-based [37,39] streams. In brief, after preprocessing including motion correction, affine registration to Talairach space, bias field correction, intensity normalization and skull stripping, each voxel is classified as either white matter (WM) or non-WM based on intensity values and neighbor constraints. Hemispheres are separated from each other and an initial WM surface tessellation is generated for each hemisphere and smoothed on the basis of intensity gradients between WM and grey matter (GM) voxels. The white surface is then "nudged" to follow the intensity gradients between the gray matter and cerebrospinal fluid (CSF); this defines the pial surface, and cortical thickness is measured as the average of the shortest distance from the WM surface to the pial surface and from the pial surface to the WM surface [40]. For subcortical segmentation, FreeSurfer combines information about voxel intensity relative to a probability distribution for tissue classes with information about the spatial comparisons to neighboring voxel labels and spatial comparisons to a probabilistic training atlas; structures are determined by assigning each voxel to one of approximately 40 possible labels.

Structural images were also processed using VBM, implemented with Statistical Parametric Mapping software (SPM5) running under Matlab 7.0 (MathWorks, Natick, MA). First, structural images were segmented to determine GM and WM, and normalized to an asymmetric T1-weighted template in Montreal Neurological Institute (MNI) stereotactic space, in a recursive manner [36]. Then images were corrected for volume changes induced by spatial normalization (modulation) [35]. This "modulation" step involves multiplying the spatially normalized gray matter by its relative volume before and after spatial normalization. The resulting gray matter images were finally smoothed with an 8 mm isotropic Gaussian kernel (the default setting for VBM).

We performed two types of measurements:

i. Data quality measures: To determine the MR protocols with the highest performance, we extracted and analyzed summary measures of data quality (described below) from the FreeSurfer analysis of the first two stages and used these as proxies for general image quality.
ii. Quantitative volume and cortical thickness measures: In order to determine which protocols had the best reproducibility within and between centers, and also

after scanner upgrade, we extracted quantitative measures (also described below) from FreeSurfer and VBM analyzed data from the short-term multi-center reproducibility, long-term multi-center reproducibility and scanner upgrade comparisons.

Data quality measures

Artefacts can have an important negative impact both on the visually assessed quality of images, as well as on the performance of automated analysis techniques. Such artefacts include blurring and ghosting artefacts caused by motion or flow which can also influence the scan quality in subtle ways that can often only be assessed qualitatively. In this study all images were therefore visually inspected for artefacts, but in addition we also assessed "summary data quality" measures that, though not specific, are likely to be affected by many types of commonly occurring image artefacts. The FreeSurfer summary data quality measures we used are the "Euler number" and "Contrast to Noise ratio (CNR)" as suggested by Dr Bruce Fischl (http://www.mail-archive.com/freesurfer@nmr.mgh.harvard.edu/msg11456.html) and briefly described here. An examplar dataset from FreeSurfer (known as "Bert"), was also analyzed for comparison purposes. The summary data quality measures from each protocol were compared to the performance of the other protocols, and the protocols with the highest total score were selected for further investigation. In the current study we chose to weight all scores equally, but such a choice needs to be considered on a case by case basis, and for other studies it may be appropriate to give different weights to the factors.

Contrast-to-noise ratio (CNR)

CNR is the ratio of the difference in signal intensity between regions of different tissue types and background (noise) signal. The contrast must be sufficient to obtain robust brain measurements as many automated techniques rely on high contrast boundaries between brain and CSF, or between different tissues (e.g. GM and WM). Selecting an appropriate protocol and also increasing field strength can increase the CNR. CNR information is automatically computed by FreeSurfer [38]. For our purposes we assumed that the higher the CNR the higher the data quality, and the better the assumed performance for FreeSurfer and other segmentations techniques on such data.

Euler Number

It is very important that cortical reconstruction procedures can create a cortical surface model which is geometrically and topologically representative of the cerebral cortex. Lee et al. [41] note that "since the cerebral cortex has the topology of a 2-D sheet, a topologically correct surface model should have no holes and handles and the Euler number should be '2'." For a surface which contains holes or handles, the Euler number is 2-2 g, where g is the number of defects. The Euler number is also automatically computed by the FreeSurfer pipeline [38], and we used this as a metric of cortical surface reconstruction quality: the higher the Euler number, the higher the data quality for FreeSurfer cortical reconstruction.

Quantitative volume and cortical thickness measures

The quantitative volume and cortical thickness measures which were extracted in this paper are: cortical thickness and subcortical volume measurements from FreeSurfer, and total gray matter volume, total white matter volume and whole brain volume (WBV) from VBM-SPM5.

FreeSurfer quantitative measures

In our study, a *global* mean cortical thickness measurement for each subject was computed over the whole cortical surface, combining left and right hemispheres, while *regional* cortical thickness was assessed by limiting cortical thickness measures to one of five major cortical regions: frontal, parietal, temporal, occipital and cingulate.

Volumetric measurements were collected for six subcortical structures which are of particular interest in neuro-degenerative diseases - thalamus (T), caudate (C), putamen (PU), pallidum (PA), hippocampus (H) and amygdala (A). For each of these, the right and left hemisphere volumes were evaluated separately.

Depending on the nature of the multi-center study the most appropriate quantitative measures to assess will, of course, vary.

VBM-SPM quantitative measures

After the smoothing step in VBM, each voxel represents the local average amount of gray or white matter. In this study we report only the total WM and total GM volume results, as the CSF compartment is poorly defined by SPM5 and includes other tissue in non-negligible quantity (areas of skull bone and dura, scalp musculature, fat, upper cervical vertebrae, etc.). Whole brain volume (WBV) was defined in this case as the sum of WM and GM volumes.

Statistical analysis

The reproducibility of each quantitative measure was assessed by calculating the relative mean difference (as a percentage) as described in equation (1) in which Q_{tp1} and Q_{tp2} indicate the quantitative measure extracted at time-point 1 and time-point 2, respectively. Reproducibility and relative mean difference are inversely related i.e. the lower the relative mean difference the higher the reproducibility and vice versa.

Relative mean difference (%) = 100*ABS(Q_{tp1} -Q_{tp2})/ mean(Q_{tp1},Q_{tp2}) (1)

Reproducibility of the protocols was then evaluated within-center, between-center and after scanner upgrade by calculating the relative mean difference in each of the following comparisons:

1) Within-center reproducibility: Center 1 test vs Center 1 retest and Center 2 test vs Center 2 retest.
2) Between-center reproducibility: Center 1 test vs Center 2 test and Center 1 retest vs Center 2 retest.
3) Post scanner upgrade reproducibility: Center 1 retest vs Center 1 upgrade.

Results

Data quality measures

Comparing T1-weighted volume protocols

Visual assessment revealed no datasets that needed to be excluded due to subject motion. Results of the initial FreeSurfer summary data quality measures of the comparing T1-weighted volume protocols (Table 1) are shown in Table 2. In this table each of the protocols was scored according to its rank relative to the other protocols.

The results indicate that FLASH protocol (A) showed lower image quality than both the FreeSurfer example dataset (*"Bert"*) and all the other protocols, so this protocol was excluded from further analysis. Of the remaining protocols, the MPRAGE scans with the highest total score, i.e. protocols C and F were taken forward to the next stage. However, there were a number of artefacts present in the images acquired with these protocols, mostly pulsation artefacts as can be seen as ghost images of the vessels or vessel walls along the phase encoding direction in Figure 1, and as described above, a number of changes were therefore made to the protocols before the second dataset was collected.

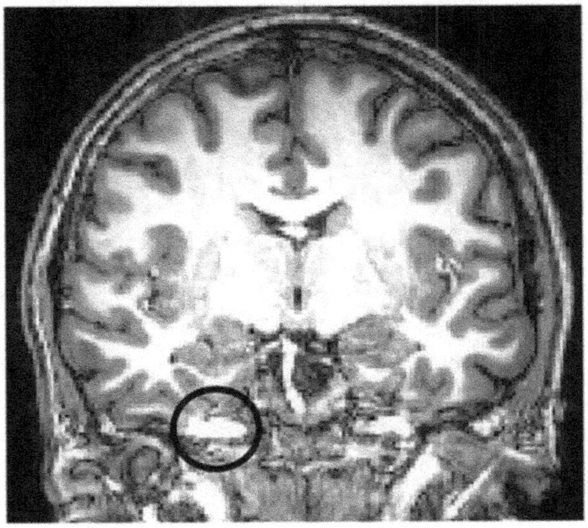

Figure 1 Pulsation artefact detected in the acquired images of initial T1-weighted volume protocols dataset with selected protocols C and F. Inconsistencies in phase and amplitude can result in this kind of artefact, which can be reduced by adding flow compensation and/or changing the phase encoding direction.

Optimization of T1-weighted volume protocols

Table 3 shows the results of the summary data quality measure comparisons for seven protocols from the optimization step. Again, visual assessment revealed no datasets that needed to be excluded due to subject motion. All the protocols gave acceptable results, performing as well as or better than both the protocols in the initial comparisons (Table 2) and the FreeSurfer example dataset *"Bert"*. Visual inspection of images by two independent observers (SC and SR) suggested three artefact-free protocols (F2, F3 and C3), which were selected for further tests.

Quantitative volume and cortical thickness measures

No significant differences were found comparing the signal to noise ratio, artifact level and uniformity

Table 2 Freesurfer summary data quality measures of the initial T1-weighted volume protocols and their ranking relative to the other protocols in parentheses

		Bert	A	B	C*	D	E	F*
Euler No.	**Right**	−40	−396 (1)	−62 (5)	−66 (4)	−78 (3)	−94 (2)	−40 (6)
	Left	−58	−510 (1)	−88 (2)	−72 (4)	−62 (5)	−74 (3)	−52 (6)
CNR	**Grey/white**	2.02	1.50 (1)	2.21 (2)	2.5 (4)	2.59 (5)	2.26 (3)	2.86 (6)
	Grey/CSF	1.09	0.51 (1)	0.69 (2)	0.78 (5)	0.73 (3)	0.75 (4)	0.94 (6)
sum of scores			4	11	17	16	12	24

Protocols with better summary data quality measures are given higher scores.
Criteria:
Euler No : the less negative the better,
Grey/white CNR: the bigger the better,
Grey/CSF CNR : the bigger the better,
Total CNR : the bigger the better.
* The MRI protocols taken forward to the next step.

Table 3 Freesurfer data quality measures of optimized T1-weighted volume protocols

		Bert	F	F1	F2*	F3*	C1	C2	C3*
Euler No	Right	−40	−38	−32	−38	−34	−74	−52	−42
	Left	−58	−46	−42	−28	−44	−66	−72	−48
CNR	Grey/white	2.02	2.92	2.94	2.82	2.89	2.6	2.71	2.67
	Grey/CSF	1.09	1.004	1.004	0.99	1.024	0.92	0.84	0.99

* All the protocols show acceptable image quality results compare to the previous dataset and standard Freesurfer exemplar Bert. However, protocols F2, F3 and C3 were identified as artefact-free and selected for further tests.

measurements of the PIQT data of the two centers (data not shown).

1) Within-center reproducibility

a) Cortical thickness measurements

Figure 2(a) illustrates the average relative mean difference of the cortical thickness measurements from the within-center comparisons. As can be seen, all the protocols showed high reproducibility

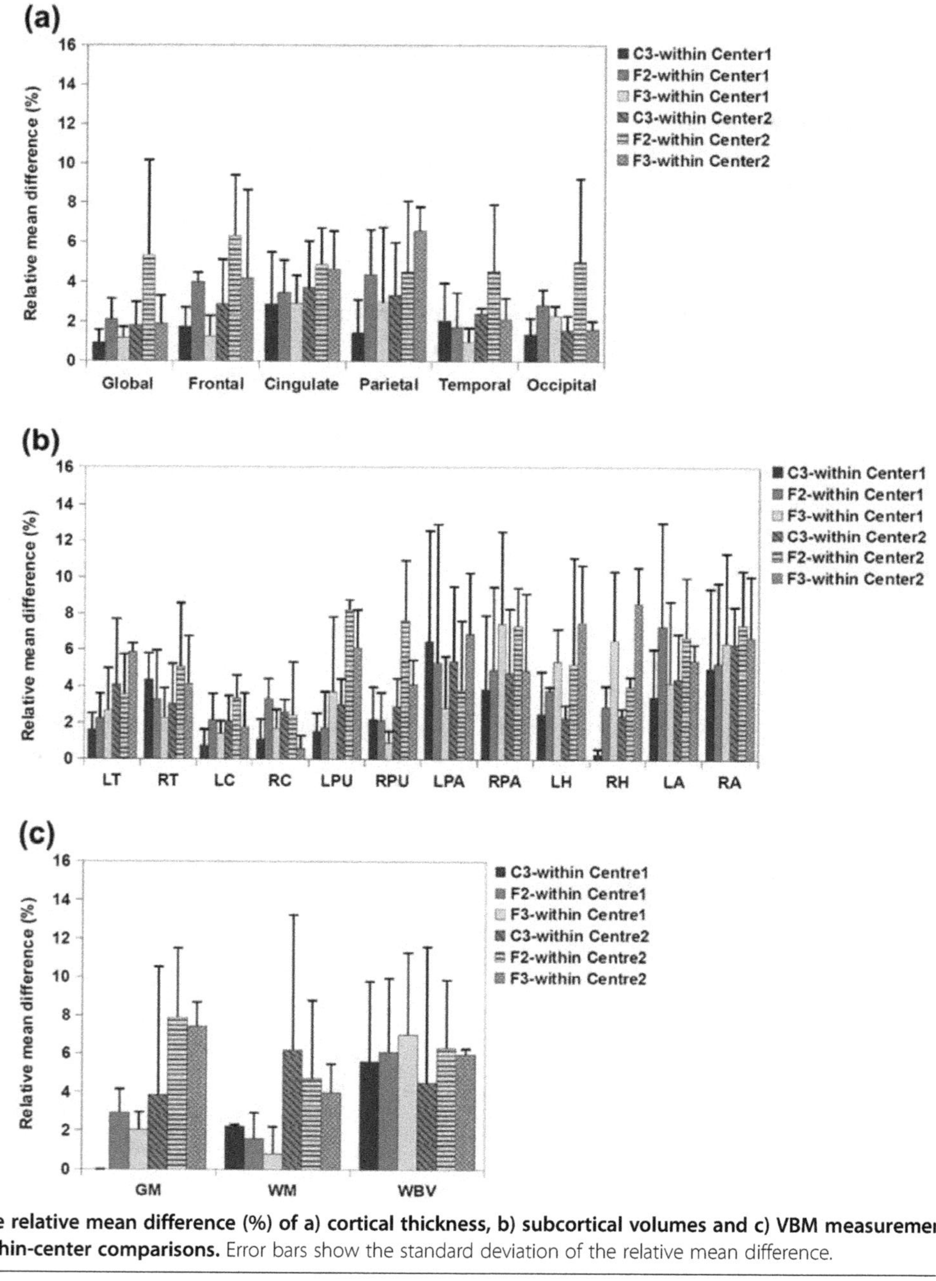

Figure 2 Average relative mean difference (%) of a) cortical thickness, b) subcortical volumes and c) VBM measurements for Center 1 and Center 2 within-center comparisons. Error bars show the standard deviation of the relative mean difference.

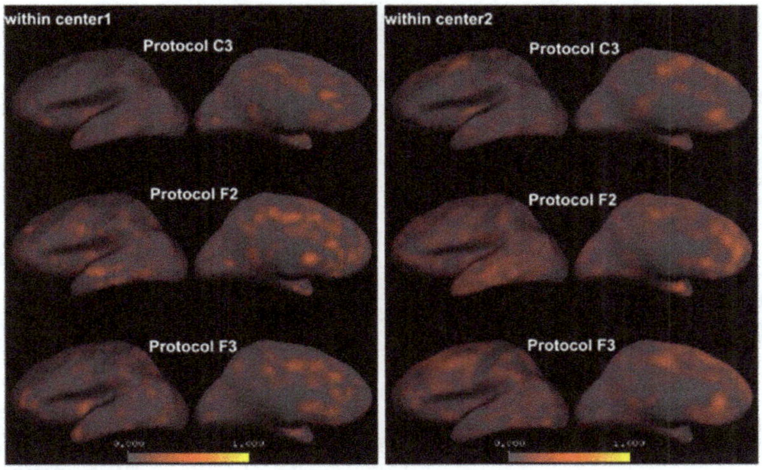

Figure 3 Within-center average absolute cortical thickness differences calculated for each vertex on the left cortical surface (right hemisphere is similar). Comparison between the two centers reveal that while all the protocols are highly reproducible in Center1, in Center2 only protocol C3 shows high reproducibility (less red areas) and the other two protocols show high cortical thickness differences especially in frontal and parietal regions.

in Center 1, with low average relative mean difference (less than 5%) in all cases; However, the reproducibility (for Center 2) of protocols F2 and F3 was not as high as protocol C3 for global, frontal and parietal measurements. Voxel-wise maps of average absolute cortical thickness differences in Figure 3 show that Protocol C3 was highly reproducible at both centers, while protocols F2 and F3 showed lower reproducibility in the frontal and parietal regions, especially at Center 2.

b) Subcortical volume measurements
The average relative mean difference of the subcortical volumes shown in Figure 2(b) illustrate that for Center 1 the volumetric results of most of the structures were highly reproducible for all the protocols (relative mean difference less than 5%). Exceptions were the hippocampal volume acquired using protocols F3 and pallidum and amygdala volumes from all protocols (although the amygdala differences were lowest using protocol C3). However for Center 2, protocols F2 and F3 showed low reproducibility, especially for the putamen, pallidum, hippocampus and amygdala. Protocol C3 showed low reproducibility for pallidum and amygdala (relative mean difference greater than 5%), but again, amygdala differences were the lowest using protocol C3

c) VBM total volume measurements
Figure 2(c) shows the average relative mean difference of the VBM measurements (WM, GM, WBV) of the within-center comparisons. GM and WM measurements acquired using all the protocols were highly reproducible for Center 1 within-center scans, However, for Center2 within-center scans, average relative mean difference for GM measurements acquired using protocol F2 and F3, and WM measurements acquired using C3 and F2 were larger than 5%. Average relative mean difference for WBV measurements from both centers were in the same range for all protocols although protocol C3 was found to have the highest reproducibility for both centers.

2) Between-center reproducibility

a) Cortical thickness measurements
Figure 4(a) illustrates the average relative mean difference of between-center comparisons for the test and retest scans. As can be seen in this figure, for the baseline (test) scans, protocols F2 and F3 show lower reproducibility, especially in cingulate and parietal regions, in which they have average relative mean difference higher than 5%. Vertex-wise maps of average absolute cortical thickness differences (Figure 5) demonstrate that for both centers, while protocol C3 showed low global cortical thickness differences, protocol F2 and F3 showed high cortical thickness differences especially in the aforementioned regions. For the between center retest scans however all the protocols showed high reproducibility (average relative mean difference less than 5%).

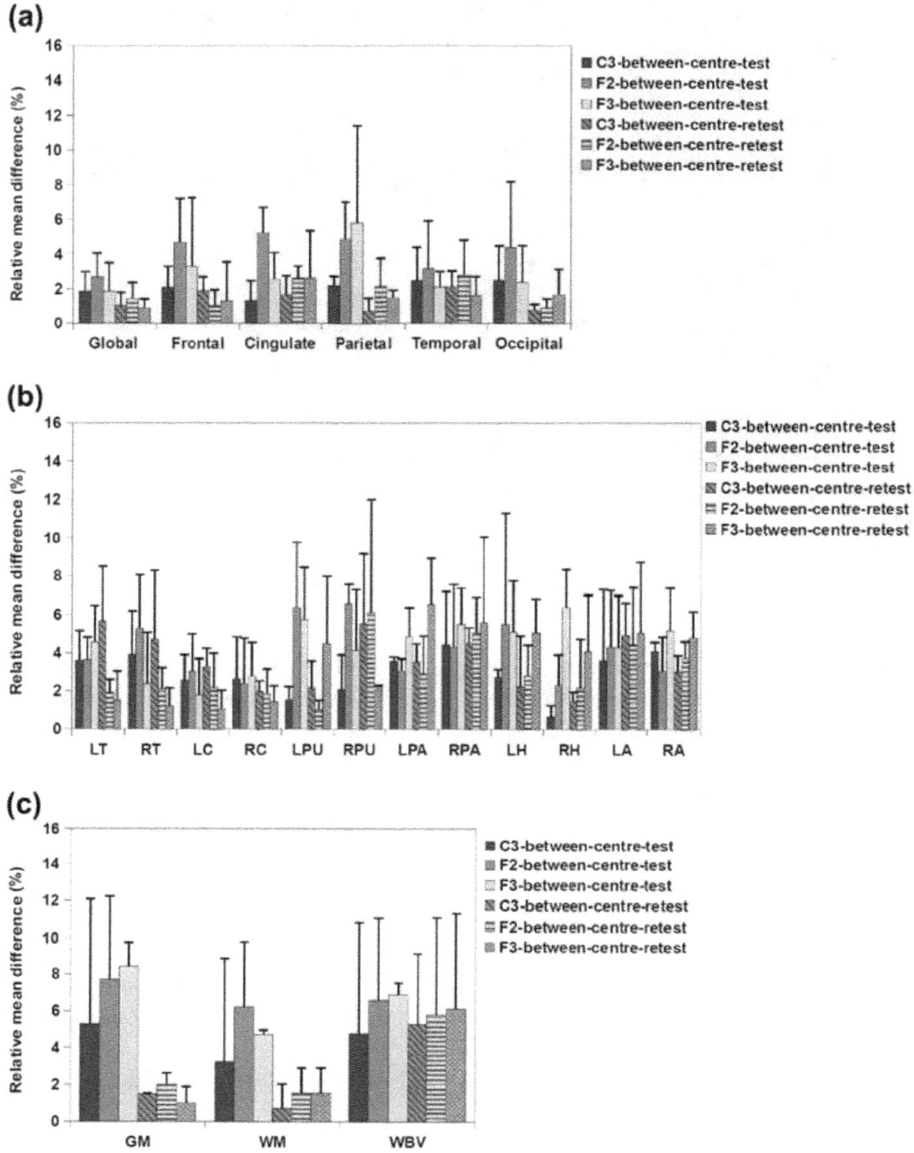

Figure 4 Average relative mean difference (%) of a) cortical thickness, b) subcortical volumes and c) VBM measurements for between-center comparisons of the test and retest scans. Error bars show the standard deviation of the relative mean difference.

b) Subcortical volume measurements
Average relative mean difference of subcortical volumes for the between-center studies shown in Figure 4(b) illustrate that for the baseline scans protocols F2 and F3 were not as reproducible as protocols C3, especially for putamen, pallidum, hippocampus and amygdala. For the retest scans, however, protocol C3 showed low reproducibility for thalamus, putamen and amygdala and protocols F2 and F3 showed low reproducibility for putamen, pallidum, hippocampus and amygdala, protocol F2 showed high average relative mean differences in the putamen, and protocol F3 showed low reproducibility in the pallidum, hippocampus and amygdala.

c) VBM volume measurements
Average relative mean difference of the VBM measurements for between-center comparisons, shown in Figure 4(c), demonstrates that for both baseline (test) and retest scans, protocol C3 is the highest reproducible protocol, with the average relative mean difference always less than 6% whereas protocols F2 and F3 showed higher average relative mean difference for GM and WBV measurements especially for the test comparisons.

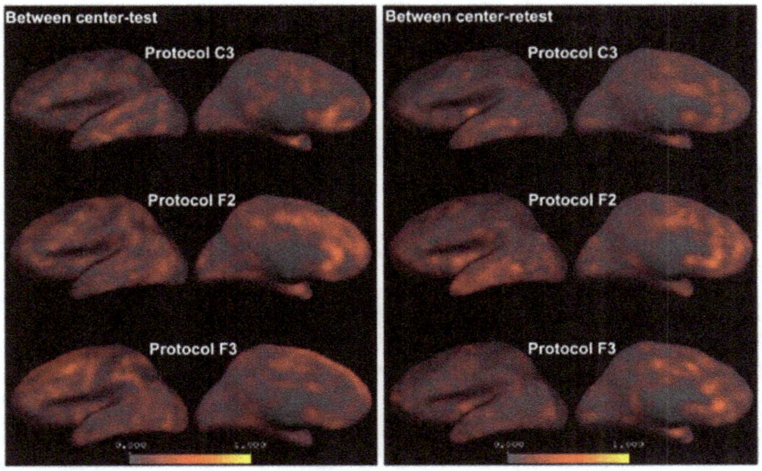

Figure 5 Between-center average absolute cortical thickness differences calculated for each vertex on the left cortical surface (right hemisphere is similar). While protocol C3 shows low average absolute global cortical thickness differences for both test and retest scans, protocol F2 shows high cortical thickness differences especially in frontal, parietal and cingulate regions of the test scans and protocol F3 reveals high cortical thickness differences in cingulate and parietal regions of the test scans.

3) Post scanner upgrade reproducibility

a) Cortical thickness measurements
All the protocols showed low average relative mean difference measures (less than 5%) and therefore high reproducibility results comparing cortical thickness measurements from Center 1 data before and after the upgrade (Figure 6(a), within-center, Center 1 results were also added to this graph for comparison purposes). Voxel-wise average absolute cortical thickness differences illustrating this are shown (for the left hemisphere) in Figure 7.

b) Subcortical volume measurements
Average relative mean difference results of the subcortical volumes illustrated in Figure 6(b) show that the volumetric results of all the structures were highly reproducible using all the protocols except for the pallidum acquired using protocol C3 and putamen, hippocampus and amygdala acquired using protocols F2 and F3.

c) VBM total volume measurements
All the protocols showed low average relative mean difference (less than 5%) when the VBM total volume measurements before and after the scanner upgrade in Center 1 were compared (Figure 6(c)). The standard deviation of the average relative mean difference was also low.

Discussion

Although combining structural MRI scans from different centers provides an opportunity to increase the statistical power of brain morphometric analyses in neurological and neuropsychiatric disorders, one important confound is the potential for scanner and MRI protocol effects to introduce systematic errors, thus making the interpretation of results difficult. In this study, we describe a methodical approach to choosing a T1-weighted volume, based on five steps. We demonstrated our approach for a two-center study, but believe that it can be generalized to larger multi-center studies. We acquired five datasets at two different centers (equipped with scanners from the same manufacturer with the same field strength): two within-subject within-center datasets for an initial comparison of T1-weighted volumes and subsequent optimization of the best performing of these protocols, two between-subject between-center datasets (short-term and long-term comparisons), and one between-subject, within-center dataset after a scanner upgrade in one of the centers. By analysing the summary data quality and quantitative measures extracted from FreeSurfer and VBM (as implemented within SPM5) we aimed to determine an optimised MRI protocol which gave high contrast to noise ratio/image quality (as evidenced by FreeSurfer measures), had minimal image artefacts and was reproducible across centers and over time.

For our initial assessment of image quality, after visual inspection for artefacts we extracted and examined the data quality measures (Euler number and contrast to noise ratio) and used these to compare the scans within the initial T1-weighted volume comparison with each other and with the examplar dataset from FreeSurfer. These quality measures were suggested by Dr. Fischl (http://www.mail-archive.com/freesurfer@nmr.mgh.harvard.edu/msg11456.html) and, while they are inherently interrelated (as the quality of the segmentation of the cortical

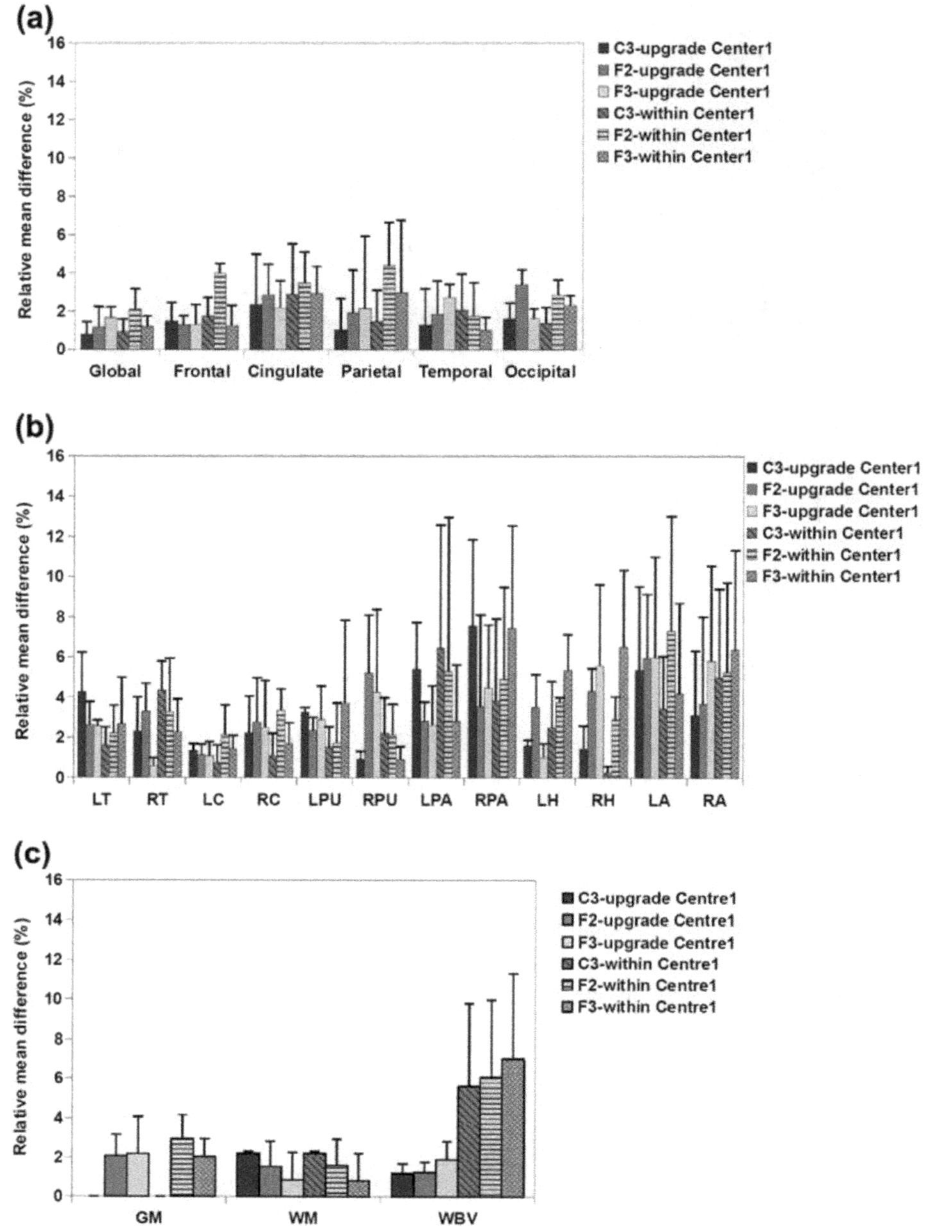

Figure 6 Average relative mean difference (%) of a) cortical thickness, b) subcortical volumes and c) VBM measurements comparing Center1 images before and after the upgrade. Error bars show the standard deviation of the relative mean difference. The average relative mean differences of the within Center1 measurements were also added for the comparison purposes.

surface depends in contrast and contrast to noise) it is important that measures are included that assess the "down stream" effects of image quality on image analysis as well as simple acquisition-related measures. The results indicated that the performance of FreeSurfer for reconstructing the surfaces was higher for MPRAGE sequences than the FLASH sequences. This is consistent with the results of Tardif et al. [42] and Deichmann et al. [43] that showed that because of their higher CNR images, MPRAGE sequences improve the accuracy of tissue classification. Therefore MPRAGE sequences are better options for segmentation tools such as FreeSurfer and VBM. Consequently, the FLASH sequence (protocol A) was rejected from further analysis, and from the remaining MPRAGE sequences we selected the two with the highest total summary data quality ranks (protocols C and F).

The top performing T1-weighted volumes were optimized in order to generate artefact-free protocols while retaining high image quality as assessed by FreeSurfer. We did this by applying a combination of changes in the parameter settings of the protocols including changing

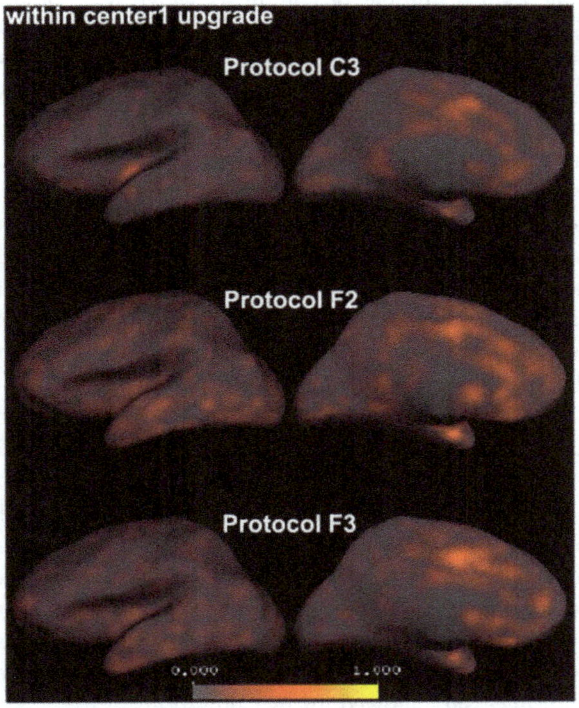

Figure 7 Average absolute cortical thickness differences between before and after scanner upgrade images in Center1 calculated for each vertex on the left cortical surface (right hemisphere is similar). All the protocols show low average absolute cortical thickness differences and therefore high reproducibility.

the phase encoding direction and/or adding flow compensation and/or saturation band. The extracted data quality measures indicated that image quality remained high enough (compared to *"Bert"* dataset and to the initial T1-weighted protocols) for all the 7 protocols in this dataset and we therefore visually inspected the images in order to select the best three artefact-free protocols to take forward for further testing. This dataset demonstrated that relatively minor changes to the protocol could have measurable effects on overall data quality, and emphasised the necessity for optimisation of protocols for the particular analysis to be performed.

Within-center comparisons of the quantitative measures from the short-term two-center and long-term two-center datasets with a scan interval of 1.5 year (Figure 2 and 3) indicated that for Center 2 cortical thickness comparisons, protocols F2 (with right-left phase encoding direction) and F3 (with right-left phase encoding direction and saturation band) showed low reproducibility in frontal, cingulate and parietal regions whereas all the regions were highly reproducible when using protocol C3 (with right-left phase encoding direction and flow compensation). In Center 1, on the other hand, all the protocols showed a high reproducibility for within-center cortical thickness comparisons. Within-center comparisons of a selection of subcortical structure volumes also indicated differences in the performance of the protocols, with protocol C3 showing higher reproducibility in most regions for measurements from both centers. VBM total volume results also showed lower reproducibility for GM measurements acquired using F2 and F3 than C3 and WM measurements acquired using C3 than F2 and F3. Whole brain volume measurements found to be more reproducible using C3 than the other protocols for both centers. These findings not only suggest that, for this study, protocol C3 gave the highest reproducible with respect to quantitative measures after a 1.5 year scan interval, but also highlights the importance of evaluating reproducibility at all sites in multi-center studies. While the Center 2 and Center 1 scanners are nominally identical, performance varied between these sites. Takao et al. [31] have reported similar findings, showing that even with scanners of exactly the same model (3 T General Electric scanners in their case) scanner drift and inter-scanner variability could cancel out the effects of genuine longitudinal brain volume changes. Since the PIQT data of the QA protocol did not show any significant difference between the two centers, the fact that all the protocols performed better at Center1 than at Center2 might reflect a subtle bias due to the fact that the optimization steps were performed for Center1 and the protocols then simply transferred to the other site. In this study, because of considerations of cost and time we chose to perform the initial comparison of T1-weighted volumes at one center and to use the best performing protocols from this center at both centers. However the ideal procedure for a multi-center study would be to: 1) perform and compare the QA information from the different centers, 2) acquire the first two steps at all sites and chose the best performing artefact-free protocols at all centers and then 3) perform the reproducibility tests. Furthermore, within-center variations were found comparing test and retest measurements at each of the centers which were highest for some of the protocols. One of the goals of the present study was thus to highlight the importance of reproducibility studies such as these, since this kind of within-center variation is not predictable a-priori. Han et al. [24] and Jovicich et al. [25] reported similar small variations in cortical and subcortical measurements, in their case comparing the scans from two different sessions with a 2-week scan interval (short-term scan interval). In the current study we compared the measurements after a long-term scan interval and showed that although some of the measurements showed lower reproducibility, it was possible to find a protocol and set of scan parameters that gave reproducible measures even over this longer interval.

Between-center comparison of cortical thickness from the short-term two-center comparison indicated that, with protocols F2 and F3 the reproducibility was lower for frontal, cingulate and parietal regions. However, with these two protocols, the differences in these regions were less in the long-term two-center retest comparisons. The reproducibility of all the regions in both the between-center test and in the between-center retest was higher using protocol C3. In the subcortical comparisons, the reproducibility of several volumes were low for protocols F2 and F3 in the initial between-center test scans while protocol C3 showed highly reproducible results. For the between-center retest scans also low reproducibility was found in several volumes using protocols F2 and F3 and protocol C3 found to be the most reproducible one. With respect to VBM total volume measurements, GM and WM measurements of the retest scans acquired using all the protocols were highly reproducible and for the GM and WM of the test scans and also WBV of both test and retest scans, protocol C3 found to be the most reproducible protocol. Again, these findings are important since they indicate that although both centers were equipped with the scanners of the same field strength and from the same manufacturer, the reproducibility was not always high and can be improved by carefully selecting the acquisition protocol.

The reproducibility of the quantitative measures was also examined after a scanner upgrade at Center 1. The reproducibility of all the protocols was relatively high for all the quantitative measures, even in problematic regions and structures, for both the within-center and between-center comparisons. These results are in line with reports from Han et al. [24], Stonnington et al. [44] and Jovicich et al. [25] in which the morphometric brain measurements did not significantly vary after even major scanner upgrades. Our results of between-center comparisons also indicate that the cortical thickness and VBM measurements difference across the centers were reduced after scanner upgrade at Center1. We speculate that this may be because of general servicing and tuning of the scanner during the upgrade but were not able to specifically assess this.

Ideally in large-scale multi-center and longitudinal studies which involve scanning very large number of subjects in several different centers, such as the Alzheimer's Disease Neuroimaging Initiative (ADNI) study [13] and Schizophrenia Twin and Relatives (STAR) study [45], using several human subjects for calibration procedure is preferred to get more precise results. In relatively small studies like ours (http://www.neuroimaging-did.com), however, which only involves scanning 50 subjects in each of the two centers, scanning a large number of calibration subjects is not feasible in terms of cost or time. Therefore, we decided to perform the calibration study using a small number of volunteers which is a potential limitation of this study. An additional potential confound is the impact of subject motion on the Euler number and other assessment measures; in the current study we control this by visual assessment of scans, but with a larger number of calibration subjects and scans, more quantitative methods could be applied to assess the effects.

Another important issue to consider is that of longitudinal studies. As was shown in the current study, within-center long-term reproducibility precision may vary to some extent depending on the MR protocol and these variations could be confounding factors. Systematic differences between scans acquired at different times could be mis-interpreted as real brain volumetric changes. Therefore, longitudinal studies need to consider performing reproducibility tests with a larger sample size and on a regular basis, and need to be appropriately powered. They also need more robust techniques than cross sectional measurements, which is particularly important when more than one center is involved in a longitudinal study. The results of such studies may also allow inter-site differences in accuracy to be assessed and if necessary allowed for by calibrations [45].

To summarize, our results showed that while several of the protocols showed promise, with high FreeSurfer performance/image quality and being artefact-free, one of the protocols (C3) gave the highest reproducibility. Determining this a-priori would have been impossible without acquiring and assessing these datasets. Since we scanned only three participants in the current study, we chose not to statistically compare the quantitative measures, but were nevertheless able to draw useful conclusions from the results.

The approach described here could be applied to protocol optimization across centers for other multi-center studies. These findings suggest researchers planning to perform multicenter studies should consider performing assessments such as these to ensure that by pooling data from different centers they are not unnecessarily reducing the power of their study due to variance from unexpected inter- or intra-site differences.

Conclusions

In conclusion, in this study assessing the summary data quality measures helped us to find the protocols with the best reconstructed surface and the highest contrast-to-noise ratio (important for brain morphometric analysis, especially when using FreeSurfer). Evaluating the quantitative measures assisted us to specify the protocol with the highest reproducibility both for within- and between-center comparisons, which is crucial not only in multi-center but also in longitudinal studies. We strongly recommend assessing both quantitative and summary quality measures within and across the centers for multi-center studies, in order to ensure optimal behaviour of FreeSurfer, VBM and other similar methodologies, and to therefore enhance the trustworthiness of the final results.

Abbreviations

MRI: Magnetic Resonance Imaging; sMRI: structural MRI; VBM: Voxel Based Morphometry; MPRAGE: Magnetization Prepared Rapid Gradient Echo; FLASH: Fast low Angle Shot; GM: Gray Matter; WM: White Matter; CSF: Cerebrospinal Fluid; WBV: Whole Brian Volume; CNR: Contrast to Noise Ratio; T: Thalamus; C: Caudate; PU: Putamen; PA: Pallidum; H: hippocampus; A: amygdala.

Competing interests

The authors declare that they have no competing interests.

Authors' contributions

All the co-authors have made substantial contributions to one or more of the following: the conception and design of the study; acquisition of data; analysis and interpretation of data. All have also been involved in drafting and revising the article, and have approved the final version to be published.

Acknowledgements

A.A.T. Simone Reinders is supported by the Netherlands Organization for Scientific Research (www.nwo.nl), NWO-VENI grant no. 451-07-009. Andrew Simons was supported by funding from the NIHR Biomedical Research Centre for Mental Health at South London and Maudsley NHS Foundation Trust and Institute of Psychiatry, King's College London. The authors would like to thank Eline Vissia and Mechteld Giesen for their participation as volunteers in the scanning procedures, and Mrs. A.J. Sibeijn-Kuiper for her help in data acquisition and Dr. R. Renken and Dr. M. Caan for their help in phantom data assessment.

Author details

[1]Department of Neuroscience, University Medical Center Groningen, and BCN Neuroimaging Center, University of Groningen, Groningen, The Netherlands. [2]King's College London, Institute of Psychiatry, Department of Psychosis Studies, London, UK. [3]King's College London, Institute of Psychiatry, Department of Neuroimaging, London, UK. [4]Biomedical Research Centre for Mental Health at South London and Maudsley NHS Foundation Trust and Institute of Psychiatry, King's College London, London, UK. [5]Centre for Neurodegeneration Research, King's College London, London, UK. [6]Department of Radiology, University Medical Center Groningen, University of Groningen, Groningen, The Netherlands.

References

1. Hogg RC, Raggenbass M, Bertrand D: **Nicotinic acetylcholine receptors: From structure to brain function.** *Rev Physiol Biochem Pharmacol* 2003, **147**:1–46.
2. Hermann BP, Seidenberg M, Bell B: **The neurodevelopmental impact of childhood onset temporal lobe epilepsy on brain structure and function and the risk of progressive cognitive effects.** *Prog Brain Res* 2002, **135**:429–438.
3. Bremner JD, Vythilingam M, Vermetten E, Southwick SM, McGlashan T, Nazeer A, Khan S, Vaccarino LV, Soufer R, Garg PK, Ng CK, Staib LH, Duncan JS, Charney DS: **MRI and PET study of deficits in hippocampal structure and function in women with childhood sexual abuse and posttraumatic stress disorder.** *Am J Psychiatry* 2003, **160**(5):924–932.
4. Als H, Duffy FH, McAnulty GB, Rivkin MJ, Vajapeyam S, Mulkern RV, Warfield SK, Huppi PS, Butler SC, Conneman N, Fischer C, Eichenwald EC: **Early experience alters brain function and structure.** *Pediatrics* 2004, **113**(4):846–857.
5. Sowell ER, Peterson BS, Thompson PM, Welcome SE, Henkenius AL, Toga AW: **Mapping cortical change across the human life span.** *Nat Neurosci* 2003, **6**(3):309–315.
6. Lerch JP, Pruessner JC, Zijdenbos A, Hampel H, Teipel SJ, Evans AC: **Focal decline of cortical thickness in alzheimer's disease identified by computational neuroanatomy.** *Cereb Cortex* 2005, **15**(7):995–1001.
7. Thompson PM, Hayashi KM, de Zubicaray G, Janke AL, Rose SE, Semple J, Herman D, Hong MS, Dittmer SS, Doddrell DM, Toga AW: **Dynamics of gray matter loss in alzheimer's disease.** *J Neurosci* 2003, **23**(3):994–1005.
8. Sailer M, Fischl B, Salat D, Tempelmann C, Schonfeld MA, Busa E, Bodammer N, Heinze HJ, Dale A: **Focal thinning of the cerebral cortex in multiple sclerosis.** *Brain* 2003, **126**(Pt 8):1734–1744.
9. Charil A, Dagher A, Lerch JP, Zijdenbos AP, Worsley KJ, Evans AC: **Focal cortical atrophy in multiple sclerosis: Relation to lesion load and disability.** *Neuroimage* 2007, **34**(2):509–517.
10. Rimol LM, Hartberg CB, Nesvag R, Fennema-Notestine C, Hagler DJ Jr: **Pung CJ, Jennings RG, Haukvik UK, Lange E, Nakstad PH, Melle I, Andreassen OA, Dale AM, Agartz I: Cortical thickness and subcortical volumes in schizophrenia and bipolar disorder.** *Biol Psychiatry* 2010, **68**(1):41–50.
11. Narr KL, Bilder RM, Toga AW, Woods RP, Rex DE, Szeszko PR, Robinson D, Sevy S, Gunduz-Bruce H, Wang YP, DeLuca H, Thompson PM: **Mapping cortical thickness and gray matter concentration in first episode schizophrenia.** *Cereb Cortex* 2005, **15**(6):708–719.
12. Mueller SG, Stables L, Du AT, Schuff N, Truran D, Cashdollar N, Weiner MW: **Measurement of hippocampal subfields and age-related changes with high resolution MRI at 4 T.** *Neurobiol Aging* 2007, **28**(5):719–726.
13. Jack CR Jr, Shiung MM, Weigand SD, O'Brien PC, Gunter JL, Boeve BF, Knopman DS, Smith GE, Ivnik RJ, Tangalos EG, Petersen RC: **Brain atrophy rates predict subsequent clinical conversion in normal elderly and amnestic MCI.** *Neurology* 2005, **65**(8):1227–1231.
14. Kantarci K, Jack CR Jr: **Quantitative magnetic resonance techniques as surrogate markers of alzheimer's disease.** *NeuroRx* 2004, **1**(2):196–205.
15. Douaud G, Gaura V, Ribeiro MJ, Lethimonnier F, Maroy R, Verny C, Krystkowiak P, Damier P, Bachoud-Levi AC, Hantraye P, Remy P: **Distribution of grey matter atrophy in huntington's disease patients: A combined ROI-based and voxel-based morphometric study.** *Neuroimage* 2006, **32**(4):1562–1575.
16. Peinemann A, Schuller S, Pohl C, Jahn T, Weindl A, Kassubek J: **Executive dysfunction in early stages of huntington's disease is associated with striatal and insular atrophy: A neuropsychological and voxel-based morphometric study.** *J Neurol Sci* 2005, **239**(1):11–19.
17. Makris N, Goldstein JM, Kennedy D, Hodge SM, Caviness VS, Faraone SV, Tsuang MT, Seidman LJ: **Decreased volume of left and total anterior insular lobule in schizophrenia.** *Schizophr Res* 2006, **83**(2–3):155–171.
18. Ecker C, Suckling J, Deoni SC, Lombardo MV, Bullmore ET, Baron-Cohen S, Catani M, Jezzard P, Barnes A, Bailey AJ, Williams SC, Murphy DG, MRC AIMS Consortium: **Brain anatomy and its relationship to behavior in adults with autism spectrum disorder: a multicenter magnetic resonance imaging study.** *Arch Gen Psychiatry* 2012, **69**(2):195–209.
19. van Haren NE, Cahn W, Hulshoff Pol HE, Schnack HG, Caspers E, Lemstra A, Sitskoorn MM, Wiersma D, van den Bosch RJ, Dingemans PM, Schene AH, Kahn RS: **Brain volumes as predictor of outcome in recent-onset schizophrenia: A multi-center MRI study.** *Schizophr Res* 2003, **64**(1):41–52.
20. Schnack HG, van Haren NE, Brouwer RM, van Baal GC, Picchioni M, Weisbrod M, Sauer H, Cannon TD, Huttunen M, Lepage C, Collins DL, Evans A, Murray RM, Kahn RS, Hulshoff Pol HE: **Mapping reliability in multicenter MRI: Voxel-based morphometry and cortical thickness.** *Hum Brain Mapp* 2010, **31**(12):1967–1982.
21. Teipel SJ, Ewers M, Wolf S, Jessen F, Kolsch H, Arlt S, Luckhaus C, Schonknecht P, Schmidtke K, Heuser I, Frolich L, Ende G, Pantel J, Wiltfang J, Rakebrandt F, Peters O, Born C, Kornhuber J, Hampel H: **Multicentre variability of MRI-based medial temporal lobe volumetry in alzheimer's disease.** *Psychiatry Res* 2010, **182**(3):244–250.
22. Hsu YY, Schuff N, Du AT, Mark K, Zhu X, Hardin D, Weiner MW: **Comparison of automated and manual MRI volumetry of hippocampus in normal aging and dementia.** *J Magn Reson Imaging* 2002, **16**(3):305–310.
23. Song T, Angelini E, Mensh B, Laine A: **Comparison study of clinical 3D MRI brain segmentation evaluation.** *Conference Proceedings of IEEE Eng Med Biol Soc* 2004, **3**:1671–1674.
24. Han X, Jovicich J, Salat D, van der Kouwe A, Quinn B, Czanner S, Busa E, Pacheco J, Albert M, Killiany R, Maguire P, Rosas D, Makris N, Dale A, Dickerson B, Fischl B: **Reliability of MRI-derived measurements of human cerebral cortical thickness: The effects of field strength, scanner upgrade and manufacturer.** *Neuroimage* 2006, **32**(1):180–194.

25. Jovicich J, Czanner S, Han X, Salat D, van der Kouwe A, Quinn B, Pacheco J, Albert M, Killiany R, Blacker D, Maguire P, Rosas D, Makris N, Gollub R, Dale A, Dickerson BC, Fischl B: **MRI-derived measurements of human subcortical, ventricular and intracranial brain volumes: Reliability effects of scan sessions, acquisition sequences, data analyses, scanner upgrade, scanner vendors and field strengths.** *Neuroimage* 2009, **46**(1):177–192.
26. Kruggel F, Turner J, Muftuler LT: **Alzheimer's Disease Neuroimaging Initiative. Impact of scanner hardware and imaging protocol on image quality and compartment volume precision in the ADNI cohort.** *Neuroimage* 2010, **49**(3):2123–2133.
27. Ewers M, Teipel SJ, Dietrich O, Schonberg SO, Jessen F, Heun R, Scheltens P, van de Pol L, Freymann NR, Moeller HJ, Hampel H: **Multicenter assessment of reliability of cranial MRI.** *Neurobiol Aging* 2006, **27**(8):1051–1059.
28. Filippi M, van Waesberghe JH, Horsfield MA, Bressi S, Gasperini C, Yousry TA, Gawne-Cain ML, Morrissey SP, Rocca MA, Barkhof F, Nijeholt GJ La, Bastianello S, Miller DH: **Interscanner variation in brain MRI lesion load measurements in MS: Implications for clinical trials.** *Neurology* 1997, **49**(2):371–377.
29. Wonderlick JS, Ziegler DA, Hosseini-Varnamkhasti P, Locascio JJ, Bakkour A, van der Kouwe A, Triantafyllou C, Corkin S, Dickerson BC: **Reliability of MRI-derived cortical and subcortical morphometric measures: Effects of pulse sequence, voxel geometry, and parallel imaging.** *Neuroimage* 2009, **44**(4):1324–1333.
30. Kempton MJ, Underwood TS, Brunton S, Stylios F, Schmechtig A, Ettinger U, Smith MS, Lovestone S, Crum WR, Frangou S, Williams SC, Simmons A: **A comprehensive testing protocol for MRI neuroanatomical segmentation techniques: Evaluation of a novel lateral ventricle segmentation method.** *Neuroimage* 2011, **58**(4):1051–1059. Epub 2011 Jul 30.
31. Takao H, Hayashi N, Ohtomo K: **Effect of scanner in longitudinal studies of brain volume changes.** *J Magn Reson Imaging* 2011, **34**(2):438–444.
32. Dewey J, Hana G, Russell T, Price J, McCaffrey D, Harezlak J, Sem E, Anyanwu JC, Guttmann CR, Navia B, Cohen R, Tate DF: **HIV Neuroimaging Consortium: Reliability and validity of MRI-based automated volumetry software relative to auto-assisted manual measurement of subcortical structures in HIV-infected patients from a multisite study.** *Neuroimage* 2010, **51**(4):1334–1344.
33. Morey RA, Selgrade ES, Wagner HR 2nd, Huettel SA, Wang L, McCarthy G: **Scan-rescan reliability of subcortical brain volumes derived from automated segmentation.** *Hum Brain Mapp* 2010, **31**(11):1751–1762.
34. Ashburner J, Friston KJ: **Voxel-based morphometry–the methods.** *Neuroimage* 2000, **11**(6 Pt 1):805–821.
35. Good CD, Johnsrude IS, Ashburner J, Henson RN, Friston KJ, Frackowiak RS: **A voxel-based morphometric study of ageing in 465 normal adult human brains.** *Neuroimage* 2001, **14**(1 Pt 1):21–36.
36. Ashburner J, Friston KJ: **Unified segmentation.** *Neuroimage* 2005, **26**(3):839–851.
37. Fischl B, Salat DH, Busa E, Albert M, Dieterich M, Haselgrove C, van der Kouwe A, Killiany R, Kennedy D, Klaveness S, Montillo A, Makris N, Rosen B, Dale AM: **Whole brain segmentation: Automated labeling of neuroanatomical structures in the human brain.** *Neuron* 2002, **33**(3):341–355.
38. Dale AM, Fischl B, Sereno MI: **Cortical surface-based analysis.** *I. segmentation and surface reconstruction. Neuroimage* 1999, **9**(2):179–194.
39. Fischl B, Salat DH, van der Kouwe AJ, Makris N, Segonne F, Quinn BT, Dale AM: **Sequence-independent segmentation of magnetic resonance images.** *Neuroimage* 2004, **23**(Suppl 1):S69–S84.
40. Fischl B, Dale AM: **Measuring the thickness of the human cerebral cortex from magnetic resonance images.** *Proceedings of Natl Acad Sci USA* 2000, **97**(20):11050–11055.
41. Lee JK, Lee JM, Kim JS, Kim IY, Evans AC, Kim SI: **A novel quantitative cross-validation of different cortical surface reconstruction algorithms using MRI phantom.** *Neuroimage* 2006, **31**(2):572–584.
42. Tardif CL, Collins DL, Pike GB: **Sensitivity of voxel-based morphometry analysis to choice of imaging protocol at 3 T.** *Neuroimage* 2009, **44**(3):827–838.
43. Deichmann R, Good CD, Josephs O, Ashburner J, Turner R: **Optimization of 3-D MP-RAGE sequences for structural brain imaging.** *Neuroimage* 2000, **12**(1):112–127.
44. Stonnington CM, Tan G, Kloppel S, Chu C, Draganski B, Jack CR Jr, Chen K, Ashburner J, Frackowiak RS: **Interpreting scan data acquired from multiple scanners: A study with alzheimer's disease.** *Neuroimage* 2008, **39**(3):1180–1185.
45. Schnack HG, van Haren NE, Hulshoff Pol HE, Picchioni M, Weisbrod M, Sauer H, Cannon T, Huttunen M, Murray R, Kahn RS: **Reliability of brain volumes from multicenter MRI acquisition: A calibration study.** *Hum Brain Mapp* 2004, **22**(4):312–320.

5

Utility of cardiac magnetic resonance in assessing right-sided heart failure in sarcoidosis

Jacob Lønborg[1,2], Michael Ward[1,3], Anthony Gill[5], Stuart M Grieve[1,4] and Gemma A Figtree[1,3*]

Abstract

Background: Cardiac involvement in sarcoidosis is associated with a poor prognosis. In patients with right sided heart failure, differentiating between cor-pulmonale, or cardiac sarcoidosis has important implications to management.

Case presentation: We present the case of a patient with severe but stable pulmonary sarcoidosis and new onset right sided heart failure despite only mild elevations of pulmonary artery pressure. CMR demonstration of extensive right ventricular fibrosis with associated dilatation and hypokinesis was a key finding for prognosis and management of the patient.

Conclusion: Cardiac magnetic resonance (CMR) is the preferred investigation in the diagnosis of cardiac sarcoidosis, allowing assessment of myocardial inflammation and fibrosis, as well as function, in a manner not matched by other technologies.

Keywords: Myocardial sarcoidosis, Cardiac magnetic resonance, Heart failure, Cardiomyopathy

Background

Sarcoidosis is a multi-organ disease characterised by the formation of granulomas. The lungs are most commonly affected. Although cardiac involvement is clinically detected in only 2% of patients, underdiagnosis is a major issue of considerable clinical importance. Recent autopsy data suggest that the heart is, in fact, involved in 20-25% of patients [1], and is directly responsible for up to 25-80% of deaths attributed to sarcoidosis [2].

In patients with identified cardiac sarcoidosis the left ventricle (LV) is involved in 98% and the right ventricle (RV) in up to 40%, usually in the context of biventricular involvement [3]. Cardiac sarcoidosis affecting predominantly the RV is rare. In a patient with severe, but stable pulmonary sarcoidosis, we illustrate the important role of CMR in the diagnosis and management of new onset RV failure. CMR is able to identify granulomatous infiltration of the RV, providing evidence for sarcoidosis as the cause of primary RV failure rather than cor pulmonale as the cause of the patients presentation.

Case presentation

A 42-yr old man initially presented with exertional dyspnoea and cough. He had no previous medical history of significance and was a non-smoker. The clinical examination and biochemistry were unremarkable, except for elevated serum angiotensin converting enzyme (ACE). Chest x-ray showed bulky hilar lymphadenopathy with extensive reticulonodular and mass like opacities in both lungs with a middle zone predominance (Figure 1). A non-contrast computed tomography (CT) scan of the thorax demonstrated numerous nodules in a perilymphatic distribution (subpleural and peribronchovascular) together with perihilar conglomerate masses (Figure 2). Several enlarged partly calcified hilar, paratracheal and subcarinal mediastinal lymph nodes were evident. Histopathology of a transbronchial lung biopsy showed numerous well-formed, non-necrotising epithelioid granulomas (Figure 3), but tests for bacilli, fungi and tuberculosis were negative. Based on clinical, radiological and pathological findings the diagnosis of pulmonary sarcoidosis was made.

Five years after initial presentation the patient represented with dyspnoea and peripheral edema. ACE was

* Correspondence: gfigtree@med.usyd.edu.au
[1]North Shore Heart Research Group, Kolling Institute of Medical Research, University of Sydney, Sydney, Australia
[3]Department of Cardiology, Royal North Shore Hospital, St Leonards, NSW 2065, Australia
Full list of author information is available at the end of the article

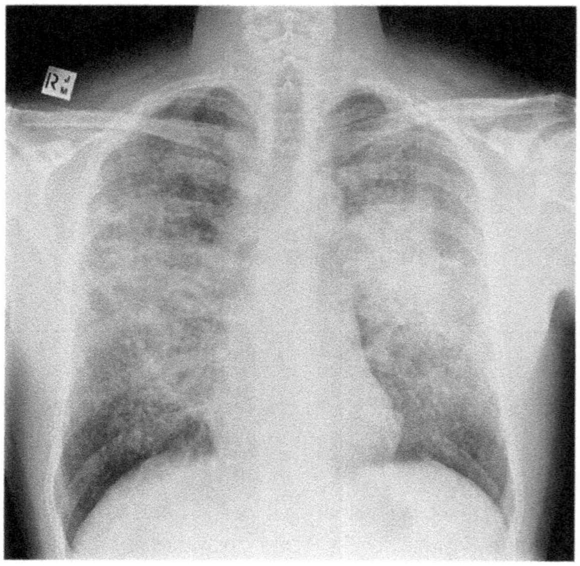

Figure 1 A frontal chest x-ray showing changes consistent sarcoidosis. There is bilateral bulky hilar and paratracheal lymphadenopathy together with extensive, confluent reticulonodular opacities with a characteristic distribution in the mid and upper zones.

within normal limits and electrocardiogram (EKG) was normal. Findings on chest x-ray and CT scan showed minimal change compared to previous imaging. Transthoracic echocardiography showed normal LV function, and a severely dilated RV with moderately impaired contractile function. Pulmonary pressures were only mildly elevated as measured by both echocardiography and right-heart catheterisation. A cardiac magnetic resonance (CMR) scan confirmed a dilated RV with impaired systolic function (Figure 4), RV ejection fraction (EF) was 34% (normal 44–63%). Extensive, patchy delayed gadolinium enhancement was observed in the RV free wall, as well as subtle mid-wall delayed enhancement in the interventricular and the interatrial septum (Figure 5). The CMR findings led to a diagnosis of right heart failure secondary to sarcoidosis infiltration of the RV wall. The evidence of RV infiltration by sarcoidosis led to immediate immunosuppressive therapy in accordance with general recommendations for cardiac sarcoidosis, and insertion of an implantable cardioverter-defibrillator (AICD). Follow-up interrogation of the AICD revealed an episode of non-sustained fast ventricular tachycardia.

Discussion

The diagnosis of cardiac sarcoidosis is often problematic due to non-specific manifestations, as seen in the present case. These findings include non-specific EKG changes, clinical heart failure, abnormal non-specific echocardiography findings, elevated serum ACE and sudden death [1]. A multimodality approach has traditionally been used to determine cardiac involvement [4]. Dyspnoea from LV heart failure may be attributed to primary pulmonary sarcoidosis. Signs of right heart failure may be put down to pulmonary hypertension secondary to pulmonary sarcoidosis and cor pulmonale. The diagnosis of cardiac sarcoidosis predominantly involving the RV may be even more problematic and may need to be distinguished from arrhythmogenic RV cardiomyopathy. Abnormalities on diagnostic tests such as EKG and echocardiography do not differentiate cardiac sarcoidosis from other cardiac diseases. However, in a patient with sarcoidosis any abnormal findings on EKG or echocardiography should lead to further investigations.

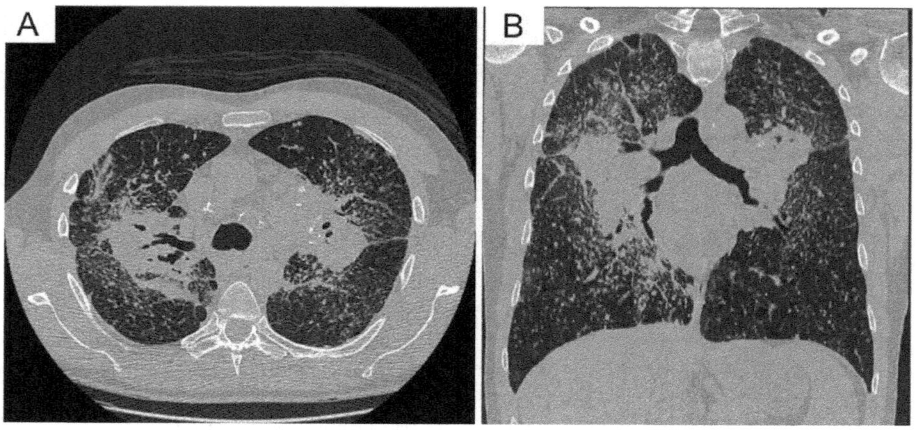

Figure 2 Selected axial (A) and high resolution coronal (B) reformats from a non-contrast helical CT shows striking bilateral bulky hilar and mediastinal adenopathy. Mass-like fibrosis is encasing the hila and central bronchi causing traction bronchiectasis. There are several partially calcified hilar lymph nodes. There are also extensive perivascular and perilymphatic nodules throughout both lobes with relative sparing of the lower zones and right upper lobe bullae.

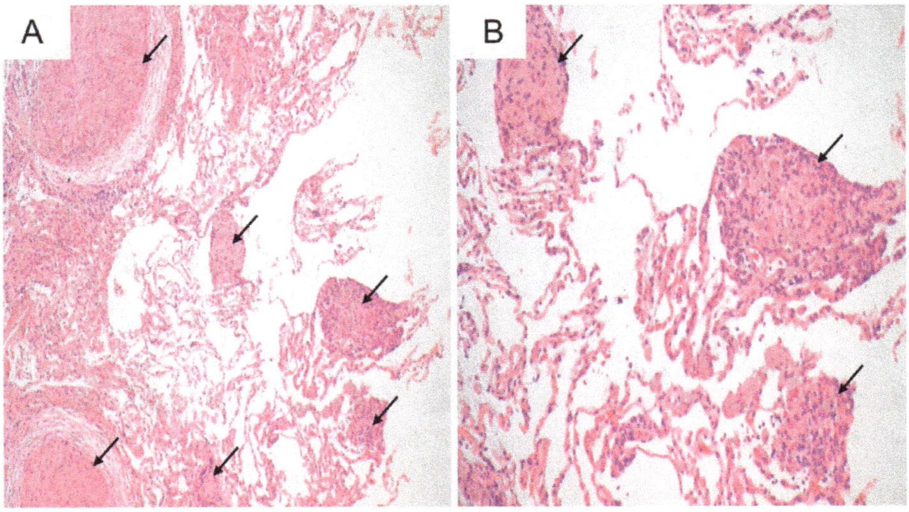

Figure 3 Histology H&E images, original magnifications 200x (A) and 400x (B), of specimen from the transbronchial lung biopsy. It identified numerous well-formed, non-necrotising epithelioid granulomas (arrows) at both low (**A**) and intermediate (**B**) power.

Recently, advanced imaging techniques have been used to identify and characterise cardiac sarcoidosis, with both positron emission tomography (PET) and CMR shown to be superior to the previously recommended scintigraphy [5,6]. CMR has a sensitivity of 100% and a specificity of 78% for the diagnosis of cardiac sarcoidosis [6]. CMR allows for accurate assessment of cardiac function and comprehensive tissue characterisation. Functional CMR images assess ventricular volumes, function and focal wall motion abnormalities; T2 weighted black blood images can be used to identify oedema and the presence of active inflammation; and delayed gadolinium enhancement images detect scarring with great accuracy [7]. New emerging pre- and postcontrast T1 mapping CMR techniques may provide information regarding interstitial fibrosis and extracellular matrix volume [8]. However, these new techniques are not yet performed routinely in clinical practice. The pattern of oedema or myocardial late enhancement is used to differentiate between non-ischemic and ischemic scarring. Typical cardiac sarcoidosis lesions seen with CMR are focal mid-myocardial or sub-epicardial scarring, whereas sub-endocardial lesions, typical for coronary artery related infarction, is rare with sarcoidosis [6]. CMR is the optimal method of imaging the RV, both in regards to its contractile function, as well as the presence of sarcoid infiltration with late enhancement,

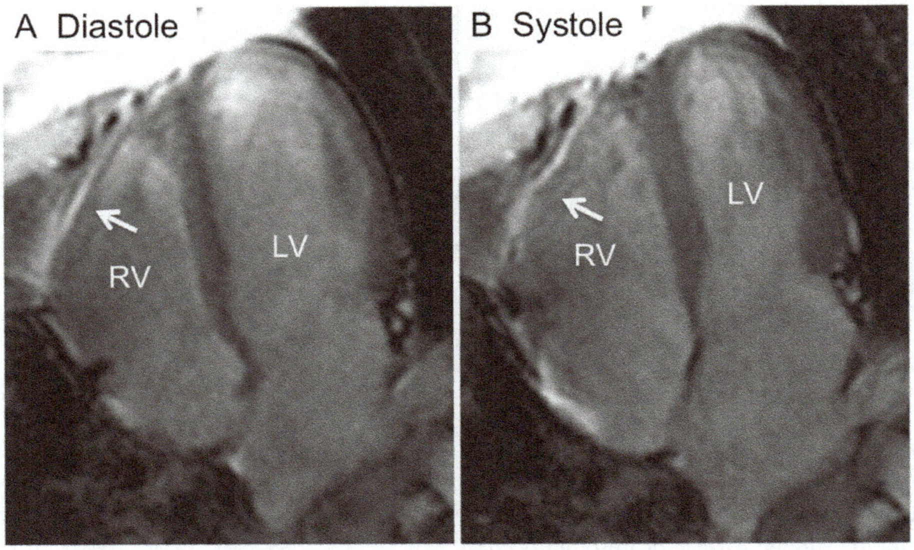

Figure 4 Functional (cine) cardiac magnetic resonance images in the four-chamber image plane in diastole (A) and systole (B). The images show poor contraction of the right ventricle (RV) free wall (arrows in **A** and **B**), but normal contraction of the left ventricle (LV).

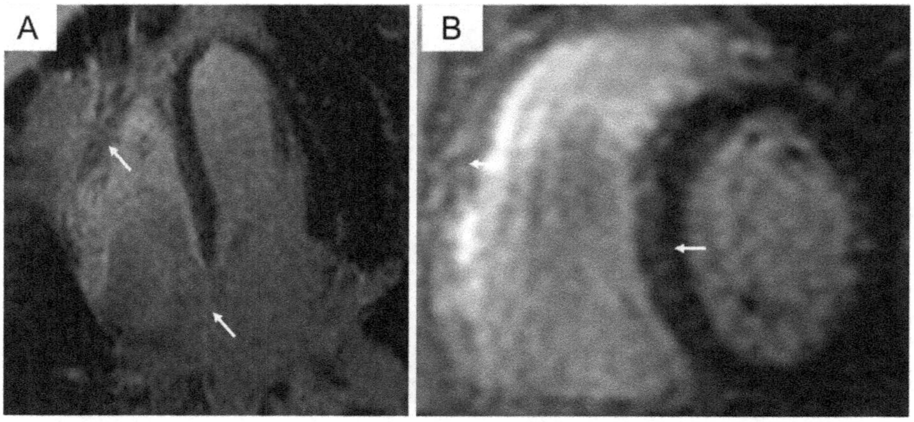

Figure 5 Delayed enhancement cardiac magnetic resonance images in the four-chamber (A) and short axis (B) image plane. The images show a patchy pattern of delayed enhancement (arrows) in the subepicardial and mid-wall of the right ventricle free wall, interventricular and interatrial septum. The myocardium of the left ventricle free wall is normal.

as demonstrated by this case. Serial CMR is also useful in the evaluation of anti-inflammatory treatment [6]. The high sensitivity of 18F-FDG PET for active inflammatory lesions is partially countered by the reduced specificity of 18F-FDG in the heart due to the high metabolic rate of the myocardium. However, it is very likely that a complementary role for PET and CMR in the Clinic will be defined in the near future.

Limitations of CMR include significant claustrophobia in up to 5% of patients and contraindication to gadolinium administration in patients with impaired renal function, and inability to image patients with non-MRI compatible pacemakers or AICDs. Furthermore, although CMR is superior to echocardiography in imaging RV structure and function, the thin walled nature of the RV makes delayed enhancement difficult to discriminate from artefact. This is even more problematic when using T2 based imaging sequences to identify oedema in the RV.

Although patients with cardiac sarcoidosis are at risk of adverse cardiac events including ventricular tachycardia (VT) and CMR is predictive of this [9], the role of prophylactic AICD is not well defined. It is clear that all patients with established VT should receive an AICD and anti-arrhythmic therapy. The patient presented received an AICD due to the extensive nature of RV involvement, with associated dilatation and impaired systolic function. The recorded episode of rapid ventricular tachycardia suggests that this was an appropriate management decision.

Conclusion

CMR is critical in differentiating the cause of new onset right heart failure in a patient with stable pulmonary sarcoidosis, but no significant pulmonary hypertension. Major cardiac events, including sudden cardiac death often occur in patients despite normal EKG and echocardiography. The excellent sensitivity of CMR, its ability to predict cardiac events, and its lack of ionizing radiation has led to the proposal by many experts that CMR should be part of the routine work-up in any patient with sarcoidosis.

Consent

Written informed consent was obtained from the patient for publication of this case and any accompanying images. A copy of the written consent is avaliable for review by the Series Editor of this journal.

Abbreviations

ACE: Angiotensin converting enzyme; CMR: Cardiac magnetic resonance; CT: Computed tomography; EF: Ejection fraction; EKG: Elektrocardiogram; LV: Left ventricle; PET: Positron emission tomography; RV: Right ventricle.

Competing interests

There were no competing interests.

Authors' contributions

JL participated in the concept and design; contributed to the imaging analysis; and drafted the manuscript. MSG, MW and GAF participated in the design and concept; contributed to the imaging analysis; and revised the manuscript critically. All authors have read and approved the final manuscript.

Acknowledgements

This work was supported by North Shore Heart Research Foundation; Sydney Medical Foundation. JL was supported by Danish Heart Foundation; Danish Cardiovascular Research Academy; Rigshospitalet Research Foundation. GF was supported by a Chapman Fellowship from the Sydney Medical School Foundation.

Author details

[1]North Shore Heart Research Group, Kolling Institute of Medical Research, University of Sydney, Sydney, Australia. [2]Department of Cardiology, Rigshospitalet, Copenhagen, Denmark. [3]Department of Cardiology, Royal North Shore Hospital, St Leonards, NSW 2065, Australia. [4]Department of Radiology, Royal Prince Alfred Hospital, Sydney, Australia. [5]Department of Pathology, Royal North Shore Hospital, Sydney, Australia.

References

1. Dubrey SW, Falk RH: **Diagnosis and management of cardiac sarcoidosis.** *Prog Cardiovasc Dis* 2010, **52:**336–346.
2. Kim JS, Judson MA, Donnino R, Gold M, Cooper LT Jr, Prystowsky EN, Prystowsky S: **Cardiac sarcoidosis.** *Am Heart J* 2009, **157:**9–21.
3. Roberts WC, McAllister HA Jr, Ferrans VJ: **Sarcoidosis of the heart. A clinicopathologic study of 35 necropsy patients (group 1) and review of 78 previously described necropsy patients (group 11).** *Am J Med* 1977, **63:**86–108.
4. Soejima K, Yada H: **The work-up and management of patients with apparent or subclinical cardiac sarcoidosis: with emphasis on the associated heart rhythm abnormalities.** *J Cardiovasc Electrophysiol* 2009, **20:**578–583.
5. Patel MR, Cawley PJ, Heitner JF, Klem I, Parker MA, Jaroudi WA, Meine TJ, White JB, Elliott MD, Kim HW, Judd RM, Kim RJ: **Detection of myocardial damage in patients with sarcoidosis.** *Circulation* 2009, **120:**1969–1977.
6. Smedema JP, Snoep G, van Kroonenburgh MP, van Geuns RJ, Dassen WR, Gorgels AP, Crijns HJ: **Evaluation of the accuracy of gadolinium-enhanced cardiovascular magnetic resonance in the diagnosis of cardiac sarcoidosis.** *J Am Coll Cardiol* 2005, **45:**1683–1690.
7. Figtree GA, Lonborg J, Grieve SM, Ward MR, Bhindi R: **Cardiac magnetic resonance imaging for the interventional cardiologist.** *JACC Cardiovasc Interv* 2011, **4:**137–148.
8. White SK, Sado DM, Flett AS, Moon JC: **Characterising the myocardial interstitial space: the clinical relevance of non-invasive imaging.** *Heart* 2012, **98:**773–779.
9. Azuma A, Kim HW, Parker M, Kim RJ: **Prognostic value of delayed enhancement cardiovascular magnetic resonance in patients with sarcoidosis.** *J Cardiovasc Magn Reson* 2012, **14**(Suppl 1):O13.

6

Lesion detection and assessment of extrahepatic findings in abdominal MRI using hepatocyte specific contrast agents – comparison of Gd-EOB -DTPA and Gd-BOPTA

Kristina I Ringe[1,2*], Daniel T Boll[2], Daniela B Husarik[2], Mustafa R Bashir[2], Rajan T Gupta[2] and Elmar M Merkle[2,3]

Abstract

Background: To evaluate the contrast agent performance of Gd-EOB-DTPA and Gd-BOPTA for detection and assessment of extrahepatic findings, semi-quantitatively and qualitatively.

Methods: 13 patients with 19 extrahepatic lesions underwent liver MRI with Gd-EOB-DTPA and Gd-BOPTA. Quantitative and relative SNR measurements were performed in each dataset in the arterial and portalvenous phase within the extrahepatic lesion, aorta, inferior vena cava, portal vein, spleen, pancreas and renal cortex. Further, relative CNR measurements were performed. Three readers assessed contrast quality using a five-point scale and choosing the preferred image dataset. Statistical analysis consisted of a Student's t-test with $p < 0.05$ deemed significant, a weighted kappa statistic for assessment of interobserver variability and an ROC analysis.

Results: Mean SNR after injection of Gd-BOPTA was significantly higher compared with Gd-EOB-DTPA for all measurements ($p < 0.05$). Mean relative SNR was also higher for Gd-BOPTA, but without being statistically significant. There was no significant difference in relative CNR. Interobserver agreement for selection of image preference was moderate (mean weighted kappa 0.485). The area under the curve for the ROC-analysis regarding contrast agent performance was 0.464.

Conclusion: Even though mean SNR is significantly higher after injection of Gd-BOPTA compared with Gd-EOB -DTPA, there is no significant difference in relative CNR with extrahepatic lesions being assessed equally well. Visual impression may differ after injection of Gd-EOB-DTPA, but does not influence image interpretation. Extrahepatic findings can be assessed similarly to MRI after injection of Gd-BOPTA.

Keywords: Gd-EOB-DTPA, Gadoxetate disodium, Gd-BOPTA, Extrahepatic

Background

Gadoxetate disodium (Gd-EOB-DTPA, gadoxetic acid, Eovist® or Primovist®, Bayer HealthCare, Wayne, NJ) is a liver-specific contrast agent, which has recently become available for detection and characterization of focal hepatic lesions. Pharmacokinetic and pharmacodynamic properties of Gd-EOB-DTPA differ not only from other non-specific contrast agents used in MR imaging, but also from more established liver-specific contrast agents such as Gd-BOPTA (gadobenate dimeglumine, Multihance®, Bracco, Princeton, NJ) [1,2].

In contrast to pure extracellular contrast agents, both substances show a partial specific uptake by hepatocytes and subsequently biliary excretion, allowing for data acquisition in the hepatocyte phase in addition to the usual dynamic phases. Whereas hepatic uptake and biliary elimination for gadobenate dimeglumine is only 3-5%, excretion through the hepatobiliary pathway is approximately 50% for gadoxetate disodium [1,3]. In addition, the characteristic pharmacodynamic properties of Gd-EOB-DTPA allow a lower dosage compared with other

* Correspondence: ringe.kristina@mh-hannover.de
[1]Department of Diagnostic and Interventional Radiology, Hannover Medical School, Carl-Neuberg Str. 1, 30625 Hannover, Germany
[2]Department of Radiology, Duke University Medical Center, Box 3808, Durham, North Carolina 27710, USA
Full list of author information is available at the end of the article

gadolinium chelates [4]. A dosage of 0.025 mmol/kg body weight is approved by the FDA. This dosage is equivalent to one quarter of the gadolinium dose recommended for all other MRI contrast agents approved by the FDA for liver imaging. However, the approved dosage of 0.025 mmol/kg body weight for Gd-EOB-DTPA is currently under debate with some radiologists preferring twice that dosage.

Recapitulating, it is known that the distinct pharmacokinetic and pharmacodynamic properties of Gd-EOB -DTPA may result in a different image appearance especially of primary and secondary liver lesions [5,6], as well as other parenchymal organs and vessels [7,8], compared with other established MRI contrast agents such as Gd-BOPTA [9]. As comprehensive MR imaging of the liver usually includes imaging of the upper abdomen, this leads to the question, whether image interpretation of incidental extrahepatic findings may be influenced unknowingly. It has been suggested that further clinical studies in patients with various tumors are needed to clarify this circumstance and to establish more routine [8]. Thus, the purpose of our study was to evaluate the contrast agent performance of Gd-EOB-DTPA and Gd-BOPTA for detection and assessment of extrahepatic findings both, semi-quantitatively and qualitatively.

Methods

This retrospective study was approved from the local institutional review board of Duke University Medical Center with a waiver of consent granted.

Patients

A total of 13 patients (8 male, 5 female; mean age 57.4 -years, range 37–73 years) were included in this study, who met the inclusion criteria. The patients were chosen from a database consisting of a total of 552 patients in whom MRI was performed including the administration of Gd-EOB-DTPA at our institution between October 2008 and January 2010. All patients were referred for liver MR imaging, including administration of a hepatocyte specific contrast agent. Due to a change in clinical routine patients received different contrast agents over time and for clinical follow-up. Inclusion criteria were as follows: age of at least 18 years, availability of a comparison study within one year and administration of either Gd-EOB-DTPA or Gd-BOPTA, and presence of an extrahepatic finding seen on both imaging studies.

The extrahepatic lesions were as follows: 4 adrenal lesions (adenoma n = 3, metastasis n = 1), 5 kidney lesions (angiomyolipoma n = 1, metastasis n = 4), 5 splenic lesions (hemangioma n = 5), 2 pulmonary lesions (hamartoma n = 2), 1 pancreatic lesion (microcystic cystadenoma n = 1), 2 spinal lesions (metastasis n = 2). Parenchymal lesions showed no change in size (mean lesion size: 2.15 cm; range: 1–4.32 cm) and appearance between comparative studies. Patient characteristics are summarized in Table 1.

MR imaging technique

MR examinations were all performed on 1.5 T systems. Including the administration of Gd-EOB-DTPA examinations were performed on following scanners: Magnetom Avanto (Siemens, Erlangen, Germany), n = 5; Signa HDx (GE Healthcare, Milwaukee, USA), n = 8. Comparison studies including the administration of Gd-BOPTA were performed on the same scanners (Magnetom Avanto; Siemens (n = 5) or Signa HDx; GE Healthcare (n = 8)).

In all patients, dedicated multidetector surface coils that covered the abdomen were used. All patients underwent a clinical routine image protocol of the liver including the administration of either 0.025 mmol/ kg Gd-EOB-DTPA or 0.1 mL/ kg Gd-BOPTA at a rate of 2 mL/ sec followed by a saline flush using a dual power injector. The MR pulse sequence protocol for all examinations included a T2w HASTE (half-Fourier single shot turbo spin-echo) and a T1w gradient dual echo sequence before contrast injection, as well as a dynamic contrast series including the acquisition of a triple arterial phase (3D T1w gradient echo sequence) with a fixed scan delay (15 seconds in patients <60 years and 20 seconds in patients >60 years, respectively) and a portal venous phase (3D T1w gradient echo sequence) after contrast injection, which was acquired approximately 15–20 seconds after completion after the arterial phase data acquisition. These imaging sequences and parameters were the same between imaging platforms and comparative studies.

Image evaluation

a. Quantitative analysis: In each patient signal-to-noise ratio (SNR; signal intensity / standard deviation

Table 1 Patient characteristics and assessed extrahepatic findings

Gender (male / female)	8 / 5
Age (years)	37-73 (mean 57.4)
Extrahepatic lesion	
Adrenal adenoma	3
Adrenal metastasis	1
Angiomyolipoma kidney	1
Kidney metastasis	4
Splenic hemangioma	5
Pulmonary hamartoma	2
Pancreatic cystadenoma	1
Spinal metastasis	2

noise) measurements were obtained in each dataset (Gd-EOB-DTPA and Gd-BOPTA) in the arterial and portal venous phase in corresponding positions. Noise estimates were derived in each dataset from a region outside the body in the vicinity of the liver. Measurements were all conducted by two radiologists in consensus (KIR, fifth year radiology resident and EMM, fellowship-trained radiologist with a focus on abdominal imaging and 13 years of experience after board certification) who where blinded to the type of dataset. By placing an oval region of interest (ROI) measurements were performed in the aorta, inferior vena cava, portal vein, pancreas, spleen, renal cortex and the extrahepatic lesion. The size of the ROI was adjusted to the size of the lesion and the same for comparative studies. In addition, relative SNR ((SNR $_{\text{post contrast}}$ - SNR $_{\text{pre contrast}}$) / SNR $_{\text{pre contrast}}$) and relative contrast to noise (CNR; relative SNR $_{\text{lesion}}$ - relative SNR $_{\text{organ}}$) measurements were obtained in the same position of each dataset and examination.

b. Qualitative analysis: Of each dataset (Gd-EOB-DTPA and Gd-BOPTA) representative T1w non contrast, arterial and portal venous phase images were prepared for blinded reading and opposed for comparison (dataset A and dataset B). Three independent readers performed the qualitative image analysis in terms of assessing lesion detectability and contrast quality using a five-point scale: 1, non diagnostic; 2, poor; 3, acceptable; 4, good; 5, very good. The group of readers comprised a junior abdominal imaging attending one year post fellowship training (RTG), an abdominal imaging fellow (MRB) and a fifth year radiology resident (DBH). In addition, each reader was asked to choose the preferred imaging dataset.

c. Statistical analysis: Statistical analysis was performed with SPSS software (version 17; SPSS, Chicago, Illinois). Results of the quantitative analyses were compared with a two-sided unpaired student's T-test, with $p < 0.05$ deemed significant. Interobserver variability was assessed by means of a weighted kappa statistic and an ROC analysis. Interobserver agreement was classified as follows: a κ value of less than 0.20 indicated poor agreement; a κ value of 0.21-0.40, fair agreement; a κ value of 0.41-0.60, moderate agreement; a κ value of 0.61-0.80, good agreement; a κ value of 0.81-1.00, excellent agreement [10].

Results

All patients underwent MR imaging of the upper abdomen using Gd-BOPTA and Gd-EOB-DTPA. Mean time interval between both examinations was 165 days (range 23–265 days).

a. Quantitative analysis: Mean SNR after injection of Gd-BOPTA was significantly higher compared with Gd-EOB-DTPA for all lesions, vessels and organs, in the arterial as well as in the portal venous phase ($p < 0.05$) (Figures 1, 2). Mean SNR for assessed lesions in the arterial phase was 266.7 (range 50–528) for Gd-EOB -DTPA and 567.5 (range 52–1956) for Gd-BOPTA, respectively. Mean SNR for evaluated lesions in the portal venous phase was 221.4 (range 72–428) for Gd-EOB-DTPA and 617.6 (range 88–2502) for Gd-BOPTA, respectively. Mean relative SNR was also higher for Gd-BOPTA, but without being statistically significant (e.g. mean relative SNR for assessed lesions in the arterial phase was 0.9 (range 0.1-3.3) for Gd-EOB-DTPA and 1.0 (range 0.1-3,8) for Gd-BOPTA; mean relative SNR for evaluated lesions in the portal venous phase was 0.6 (range 0.1-2.4) for Gd-EOB -DTPA and 1.1 (range 0.1-4,5) for Gd-BOPTA, respectively). For all measurements there was no significant difference in relative CNR, neither in the arterial nor in the portal venous phase ($p > 0.05$).

b. Qualitative analysis: For all readers there were no significant differences in image quality comparing imaging with Gd-BOPTA and Gd-EOB-DTPA (Figure 3). Interobserver variability regarding the assessment of image quality was fair for Gd-EOB -DTPA and Gd-BOPTA with a mean weighted kappa of 0.245 and 0.316, respectively. Interobserver agreement for selection of image preference was moderate (mean weighted kappa 0.485). The area under the curve for the ROC-analysis was 0.464, implying that there was no significant difference comparing imaging with Gd-EOB-DTPA and Gd-BOPTA.

Discussion

Extracellular contrast agents, such as gadopentetate dimeglumine (Gd-DTPA, Magnevist, Bayer HealthCare), have been in clinical use for more than two decades and are well established. More recently, liver-specific contrast agents have become available for the detection and characterization of focal hepatic lesions. Whereas Gd-BOPTA has been approved for liver imaging by the European authorities several years ago and certain experience and routine is available, Gd-EOB-DTPA is fairly new and has gained FDA approval only in 2008.

Brismar et al. compared liver vessel and liver parenchymal enhancement after the injection of Gd-EOB -DTPA and Gd-BOPTA using a bolus technique in ten healthy volunteers. Results showed a higher maximum of enhancement of the hepatic artery, portal vein and middle hepatic vein during the arterial, portal venous phase and delayed phase for Gd-BOPTA, while there was no significant difference in liver parenchymal

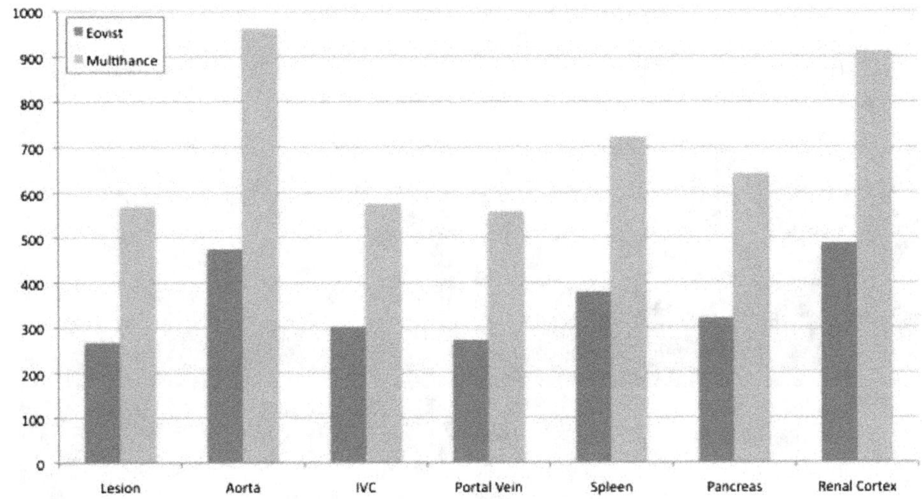

Figure 1 Comparison of SNR measurements using Gd-EOB-DTPA (Eovist™, Bayer HealthCare, Wayne, NJ) and Gd-BOPTA (Multihance™, Bracco, Princeton, NJ) in the arterial phase. Shown is the mean SNR for the extrahepatic lesion, as well as for different vessels and organs.

contrast enhancement [7]. So far only few studies have compared the performance of Gd-EOB-DTPA with other more established contrast agents regarding the assessment of extrahepatic tissues and vessels. Kühn et al. compared the enhancement patterns of solid organs and the abdominal aorta after the injection of gadobutrol and gadoxetate disodium in 50 patients. Mean enhancement indexes were higher for gadobutrol except for the abdominal aorta, and it has been suggested that early dynamic MRI of the upper abdomen benefits from the higher gadolinium concentration of gadobutrol than in the organ-specific contrast agent gadoxetic acid [11]. However, patients in the two compared contrast agents groups were not the same. These results were similar to those gained by Zizka et al. earlier [12]. A more recent intraindividual comparison of liver, abdominal and pulmonary vessel enhancement in staging for rectal carcinoma showed comparable contrast enhancement after gadoxetic acid to gadobutrol [13]. Tamada et al. compared enhancement patterns of solid abdominal organs and vessels in 13 healthy volunteers after the injection of Gd-DTPA (Magnevist) and Gd-EOB-DTPA. It has been proposed that lower arterial vascular and parenchymal enhancement with Gd-EOB-DTPA as compared with

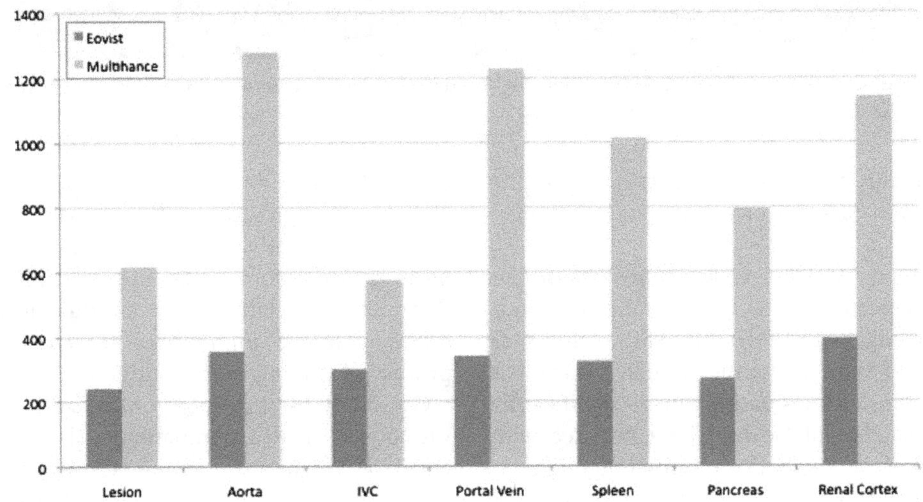

Figure 2 Comparison of SNR measurements using Gd-EOB-DTPA (Eovist™, Bayer HealthCare, Wayne, NJ) and Gd-BOPTA (Multihance™, Bracco, Princeton, NJ) in the portal venous phase. Shown is the mean SNR for the extrahepatic lesion, as well as for different vessels and organs.

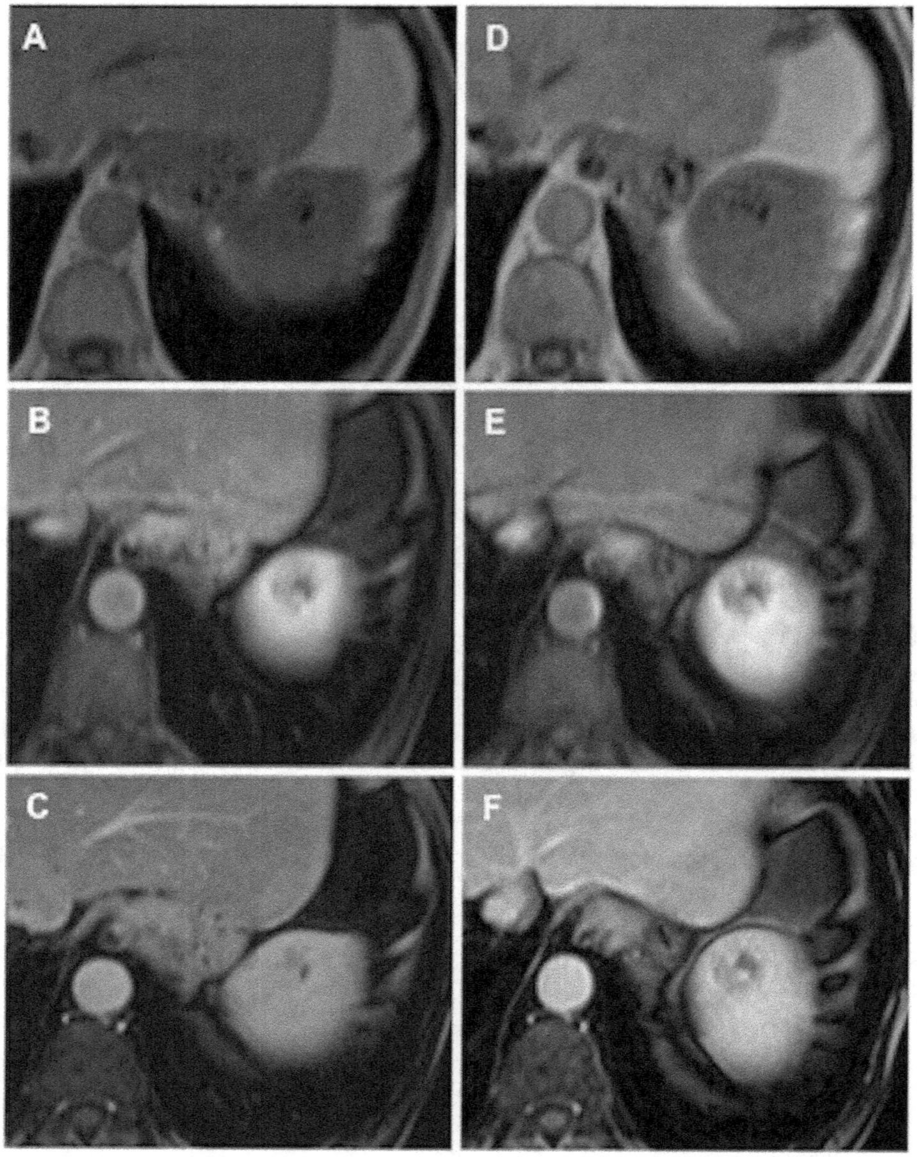

Figure 3 Comparison of Gd-BOPTA (A-C) and Gd-EOB-DTPA (D-E) for detection and characterization of a splenic hemangioma. Pre contrast T1w images (**A**,**D**; top row), arterial phase images (**B**,**E**; middle row) and portal venous phase images (**C**,**F**; bottom row).

GD-DTPA may require reassessment of its dose, despite the higher late venous phase liver parenchymal enhancement [8].

To the best of our knowledge, no study has so far compared the enhancement effect of extrahepatic findings in MR imaging with Gd-EOB-DTPA and Gd-BOPTA. Our results show that even though mean SNR in extrahepatic lesions, vessels and organs is significantly higher after the injection of Gd-BOPTA compared with Gd-EOB-DTPA, there is no significant difference in relative CNR with extrahepatic lesions being assessed adequately. Thus, visual impression may differ after injection of Gd-EOB-DTPA, but does not influence image interpretation, and extrahepatic findings can be assessed similarly to MRI after injection of Gd-BOPTA. The circumstance that interobserver variability for Gd-BOPTA is slightly better than for Gd-EOB-DTPA may be justified to some extent by the fact, that gadoxetate disodium is a relatively new contrast agent resulting in a different image impression and that we are in the process of gaining more routine [5-8].

Our study has a number of limitations. The time interval between MRI examination with Gd-EOB-DTPA and Gd-BOPTA was fairly long in some patients (mean 165 - days). On the other hand, evaluated parenchymal lesions showed no change in size and appearance between comparative studies, so that evaluation especially of metastatic lesions could not be influenced by these factors.

Also, comparative studies were performed on the same scanners using identical imaging parameters. Another limitation is the small sample size and heterogeneity of incidentally detected lesions (malignant as well as benign). As the same lesion was evaluated on two different studies, we think that this intralesional comparison is valid.

Conclusions

In conclusion, hepatocyte-specific contrast agents are increasingly used for comprehensive MR imaging of the liver. Incidental extrahepatic parenchymal findings are common and need to be appraised when imaged. It is known that the distinct pharmacokinetic and pharmacodynamic properties of Gd-EOB-DTPA may result in a different image appearance especially of primary and secondary liver lesions. Therefore assessment of extrahepatic findings may unknowingly be influenced as well, and a comparison of contrast agent performance is clinically important. The results of our study show, that visual impression of incidental extrahepatic findings may differ after injection of Gd-EOB-DTPA compared with Gd-BOPTA, but does not influence image interpretation. Reliable assessment of extrahepatic findings is feasible using the hepatocyte-specific contrast agent Gd-EOB -DTPA, although results need to be validated in future studies with larger patient cohorts.

Competing interests

The authors declare that they have no competing interests.

Authors' contributions

KIR and EMM conceived and designed the experiments. KIR, DTB, DBH, MRB, RTG and EMM performed the experiments and acquisition of data. KIR, DTB and EMM analyzed the data. All authors participated in writing and revising the manuscript.

Author details

[1]Department of Diagnostic and Interventional Radiology, Hannover Medical School, Carl-Neuberg Str. 1, 30625 Hannover, Germany. [2]Department of Radiology, Duke University Medical Center, Box 3808, Durham, North Carolina 27710, USA. [3]University Hospital Basel, Radiology and Nuclear Medicine, Petersgraben 4, CH-4031 Basel, Switzerland.

References

1. Schuhmann-Giampieri G, Schmitt-Willich H, Press WR, Negishi C, Weinmann HJ, Speck U: **Preclinical evaluation of Gd-EOB-DTPA as a contrast agent in MR imaging of the hepatobiliary system.** *Radiology* 1992, **183**:59–64.
2. Hamm B, Staks T, Mühler A, Bollow M, Taupitz M, Frenzel T, Wolf KJ, Weinmann HJ, Lange L: **Phase I clinical evaluation of Gd-EOB-DTPA as a hepatobiliary contrast agent: safety, pharmacokinetics, and MR imaging.** *Radiology* 1995, **195**:785–792.
3. Kirchin MA, Pirovano GP, Spinazzi A: **Gadobenate dimeglumine (Gd-BOPTA) - An overview.** *Invest Radiol* 1998, **33**:798–809.
4. Reimer P, Rummeny EJ, Shamsi K, Balzer T, Baldrup HE, Tombach B, Hesse T, Berns T, Peters PE: **Phase II clinical evaluation of Gd-EOB-DTPA: dose, safety aspects, and pulse sequence.** *Radiology* 1996, **199**:177–183.
5. Ringe KI, Husarik DB, Sirlin CB, Merkle EM: **Gadoxetate-disodium enhanced MRI of the liver: Part 1, Protocol optimization and lesion appearance in the non-cirrhotic liver.** *AJR Am J Roentgenol* 2010, **195**:13–28.
6. Cruite I, Schröder M, Merkle EM, Sirlin CB: **Gadoxetate-disodium enhanced MRI of the liver: Part 2, Protocol optimization and lesion appearance in the cirrhotic liver.** *AJR Am J Roentgenol* 2010, **195**:29–41.
7. Brismar TB, Dahlstrom N, Edsborg N, Persson A, Smedby O, Albiin N: **Liver vessel enhancement by Gd-BOPTA and Gd-EOB-DTPA: a comparison in healthy volunteers.** *Acta Radiol* 2009, **50**:709–715.
8. Tamada T, Ito K, Sone T, Yoshida K, Kakuba K, Tanimoto D, Higashi H, Yamashita T: **Dynamic contrast-enhanced magnetic resonance imaging of abdominal solid organ and major vessel: comparison of enhancement effect between Gd-EOB-DTPA and Gd-DTPA.** *J Magn Reson Imaging* 2009, **29**:636–640.
9. Goodwin MD, Dobson JE, Sirlin CB, Lim BG, Stella DL: **Diagnostic pitfalls and challenges in MR imaging with hepatocyte-specific contrast agents.** *Radiographics* 2011, **31**:1547–1568.
10. Lim JS, Kim MJ, Myoung S, Park MS, Choi JY, Choi JS, Kim SI: **MR cholangiography for evaluation of hilar branching anatomy in transplantation on the right hepatic lobe from a living donor.** *AJR Am J Roentgenol* 2008, **191**:537–545.
11. Kuhn JP, Hegenscheid K, Siegmund W, Froehlich CP, Hosten N, Puls R: **Normal dynamic MRI enhancement patterns of the upper abdominal organs: gadoxetic acid compared with gadobutrol.** *AJR Am J Roentgenol* 2009, **193**:1318–1323.
12. Zizka J, Kizo L, Ferda J, Mrklovsky M, Bukac J: **Dynamic and delayed contrast enhancement in upper abdominal MRI studies: comparison of gadoxetic acid and gadobutrol.** *Eur J Radiol* 2007, **62**:186–191.
13. Huppertz A, Franiel T, Wagner M, Püttcher O, Wagner J, Rief M, Schwenke C, Hamm B, Strassburg J: **Whole-body MRI with assessment of hepatic and extraabdominal enhancement after administration of gadoxetic acid for staging of rectal carcinoma.** *Acta Radiol* 2010, **52**:842–850.

7

Incidental discovery of circle contact lens by MRI: you can't scan my poker face, circle contact lens as a potential MRI hazard

Hiroyuki Tokue*, Ayako Taketomi-Takahashi, Azusa Tokue and Yoshito Tsushima

Abstract

Background: Circle contact lenses, also known as color contact lenses and big eye contact lenses, are a type of cosmetic contact lens. It is not generally known that a circle contact lens usually contains iron oxide and other metals, which means their use during magnetic resonance imaging (MRI) is a potential hazard.

Case presentation: We present a rare case of incidental discovery of circle contact lenses by MRI and MRI images of circle lenses in vitro.

Conclusions: Circle contact lenses usually contain iron oxide, which is a known source of susceptibility artifact on MRI. Not only radiologists and radiographers but also referring physicians should be familiar with the imaging findings and potential risk of scanning circle contact lenses by MRI.

Keywords: Circle contact lenses, Color contact lenses, Magnetic resonance imaging (MRI), Susceptibility artifact

Background

Circle contact lenses, also known as color contact lenses and big eye contact lenses, are a type of cosmetic contact lens. Circle contact lenses make one's eyes appear larger and come in a variety of colors and effects. They have received rather limited attention outside the Asian population until recently, but trends such as music videos of doll eyed pop stars have, reportedly, led to their increased use [1]. It is not generally known that a circle contact lens usually contains iron oxide and other metals [2], which means their use during MRI is a potential hazard.

We present a rare case of incidental discovery of circle contact lenses on MRI. Additionally, we recreated the image of circle contact lenses in vitro.

Case presentation

A 28 year-old woman who had a cervical desmoid underwent a follow-up MRI. MRI showed an artifact in the globes (Figure 1). She had experienced no discomfort or local heat or pain in her eyes during the examination. We asked her about her eyes, and it was proved that she wore circle contact lenses while being imaged in the 3.0 Tesla (3.0 T) MRI scanner (Magnetom Trio, Siemens Medical Systems, Erlangen, Germany). One year after this examination, she has not had any eye symptoms.

In vitro study

We placed circle contact lenses [2-hydroxyethyl methacrylate (HEMA) with iron oxide] in a gelatin phantom and obtained T1 weighted images (WI), T2WIs and T2*WIs in our institution's clinical 3.0 T MRI scanner. The diameter of the circle contact lenses was 14.2 mm, and the thickness was 0.08 mm. We measured a temperature change of circle contact lenses after MRI scan.

Methods

MR imaging protocol

T1-weighted fast spin-echo images were acquired using the following parameters: repetition time (TR), 600 msec; echo time (TE), 10 msec; flip angle, 90°. T2-weighted fast spin-echo images were acquired using the following parameters: TR, 4000 msec; echo TE, 80 msec; flip angle, 90°. T2*-weighted gradient-echo images were acquired using the following parameters: TR, 680 msec; TE, 20 msec; flip angle, 90°. For all sequences, matrix was 256 × 256;

* Correspondence: tokue@s2.dion.ne.jp
Department of Diagnostic and Interventional Radiology, Gunma University Hospital, 3-39-22 Showa-machi, Maebashi, Gunma 371-8511, Japan

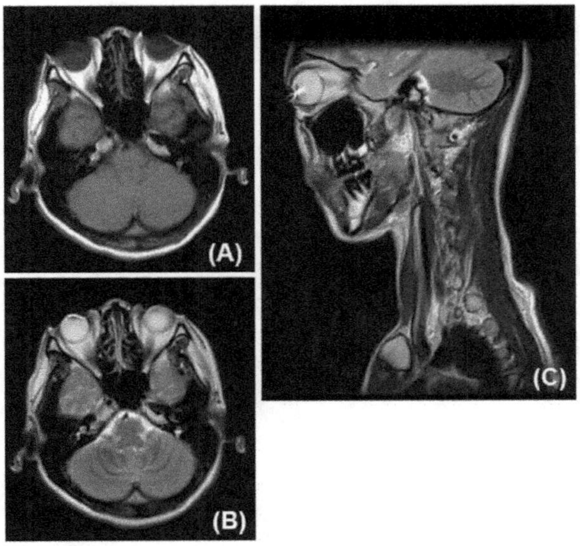

Figure 1 A 28-year-old woman who wore circle contact lenses. MRI showed a susceptibility artifacts in her eyes. **A**. T1-weighted fast spin-echo axial image: TR/TE, 545/15 (msec). **B**. T2-weighted fast spin-echo axial image: TR/TE, 4130/83 (msec). **C**. T2-weighted PROPELLER sagittal image: TR/TE, 3000/83 (msec). TR: repetition time, TE: echo time, PROPELLER: Periodically Rotated Overlapping Parallel Lines with Enhanced Reconstruction.

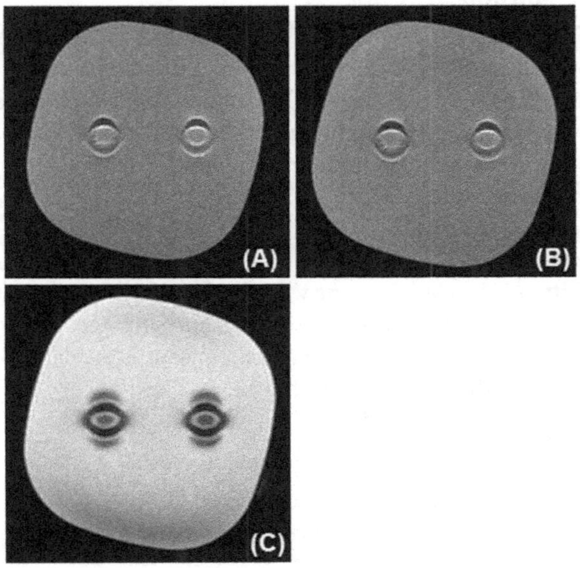

Figure 2 MRI of gelatin phantom containing circle contact lenses showed susceptibility artifacts consistent with extra-wide outer rim of the lens. A. T1-weighted fast spin-echo image: TR/TE, 600/10 (msec). **B**. T2-weighted fast spin-echo image: TR/TE, 4000/80 (msec). **C**. T2*-weighted gradient-echo image: TR/TE, 680/20 (msec).

Field of view (FOV) 220 × 220 mm; number of excitations (NEX), one; section thickness, 3 mm.

Results

MRI of the gelatin phantom containing circle contact lenses showed susceptibility artifact consistent with extra-wide outer rim of the lenses (Figure 2). The circle contact lenses was not deformed nor moved after the MRI scan. The total MRI scanning time was 8 minutes. After the MRI scan, the temperature of circle contact lenses rose 1.0 degree Celsius (°C).

Discussion

Circle contact lenses have gained popularity in the younger population for their tendency to enlarge and draw attention to the iris. The diameter of regular contact lenses is similar to the diameter of the cosmetic circle contact lenses. The difference between the two types of lenses is that circle contact lenses are tinted not only in the area that covers the iris of the eye, but also has a rim slightly outside this area, usually in a darker color. The result is the appearance of a bigger, wider iris, which creates an illusion of large, doll-like eyes [1]. However, the extra-wide outer rim of the lens usually contains iron oxide, a known source of susceptibility artifact in MRI scans [3]. Indeed, the circle contact lenses showed susceptibility artifact consistent with extra-wide outer rim of the lenses in our in vitro case. However, the resolution of the clinical scanner used to image the circle contact lenses in vitro (0.86 mm in plane, 3 mm slice) was larger than the thickness of the circle contact lenses (0.08 mm), so that the images in Figure 2 might show the extent of the susceptibility artifacts rather than the circle contact lenses themselves.

There have been no reports in the English literature about the imaging findings of circle contact lenses in vitro and in vivo on MRI. There was only one Japanese report about the interactions of MR equipment with circle contact lenses [4]. They reported that a circle contact lens was not likely to be affected by the power of absorption by 3.0 T MRI. However, they did not verify the extent of temperature change during MRI scan.

Clinical MRI services should be aware of circle contact lenses as a source of decreased image quality as well as the theoretical risk of burns to the globe [5]. The cosmetic effects of circle contact lenses are much more subtle than the intended audience of computer graphics-enhanced music videos might be led to believe, and it is in fact sometimes difficult to tell they are being worn. Information on the content ratio of iron or other metals in circle lenses has not been made public. Several types of colored contact lenses are available and some of manufactures have revealed the contents, to some extent. Some colored contact lenses do not contain iron oxide. Currently, products of unknown origins may be also distributed. Removal of all contact lenses prior to an MRI examination should continue to be enforced, as it seems the only realistic way to prevent patients from being scanned while still wearing circle lenses.

Conclusions

We presented a rare case of incidental discovery of circle contact lenses on MRI and the MRI imaging finding of circle lenses in a phantom. Not only physicians but also radiographers and referring physicians should be familiar with the imaging findings and potential risk of scanning circle contact lenses by MRI.

Consent

Written informed consent was obtained from the patient for publication of this Case report and any accompanying images. A copy of the written consent is available for review by the Editor of this journal.

Competing interests

The authors declare that they have no competing interests.

Authors' contributions

HT participated in the design of the study and carried out the clinical examination. All authors read and approved the final manuscript.

References

1. *What Big eyes You have, dear, but Are those contacts risky?* The New York Times; 2010. http://www.nytimes.com/2010/07/04/fashion/04lenses.html (accessed 1st July 2010).
2. *Color additives in medical devices.* U.S. Food and Drug Administration; 2012. http://www.fda.gov/MedicalDevices/DeviceRegulationandGuidance/HowtoMarketYourDevice/PremarketSubmissions/PremarketApprovalPMA/ucm142716.htm (accessed 1st July 2010).
3. Sacco DC, Steiger DA, Bellon EM, Coleman PE, Haacke EM: **Artifacts caused by cosmetics in MR imaging of the head.** *Am J Roentgenol* 1987, **148:**1001–1004.
4. Amauchi H: **Educational-industrial complex research on interactions of MR equipments with contact lenses.** *Nihon Hoshasen Gijutsu Gakkai Zasshi* 2007, **63:**390–393 (in Japanese).
5. Wagle WA, Smith M: **Tattoo-induced skin burn during MR imaging.** *Am J Roentgenol* 2000, **175:**1795.

Lipomatous metaplasia identified in rabbits with reperfused myocardial infarction by 3.0 T magnetic resonance imaging and histopathology

Yuanbo Feng[1,2], Feng Chen[1,2], Yi Xie[3], Huaijun Wang[1,2], Marlein Miranda Cona[1,2], Jie Yu[1,2], Junjie Li[1,2], Jan Bogaert[1], Stefan Janssens[4], Raymond Oyen[1] and Yicheng Ni[1*]

Abstract

Background: Cardiac lipomatous metaplasia (LM) occurs in patients with chronic ischemic heart disease and heart failure with unclear mechanisms. We studied coronary occlusion/reperfusion-induced myocardial infarction (MI) in rabbits during a 9-months follow-up using 3.0 T magnetic resonance scanner, and confirmed the presence of MI in acute phase and LM in chronic phase using histopathology.

Methods: MI was surgically induced in 10 rabbits by 90-min coronary artery occlusion and reperfusion. Forty-eight hours later, multiparametric cardiac magnetic resonance imaging (cMRI) was performed at a 3.0 T clinical scanner for MI diagnosis and cardiac function analysis. Afterwards, seven rabbits were scarified for histochemical staining with triphenyltetrazolium chloride (TTC), and hematoxylin-eosin (HE), and 3 were scanned with cMRI at 2 days, 2 weeks, 2 months and 9 months for longitudinal observations of morphological and functional changes, and the fate of the animals. Post-mortem TTC, HE and Masson's trichrome (MTC) were studied for chronic stage of MI.

Results: The size of acute MI correlated well between cMRI and TTC staining (r^2=0.83). Global cardiac morphology-function analysis showed significant correlation between increasing acute MI size and decreasing ejection fraction ($p<0.001$). During 9 months, cMRI documented evolving morphological and functional changes from acute MI to chronic scar transformation and fat deposition with a definite diagnosis of LM established by histopathology.

Conclusions: Acute MI and chronic LM were induced in rabbits and monitored with 3.0 T MRI. Studies on this platform may help investigate the mechanisms and therapeutic interventions for LM.

Keywords: Acute myocardial infarction, Animal model, Chronic ischemia, Cardiovascular magnetic resonance imaging, Lipomatous metaplasia

Background

The moderate size rabbit model of occlusion/reperfusion-induced myocardial infarction (MI) has been used in cardiac imaging research [1-3]. In particular, its versatile advantages have been demonstrated in cardiac magnetic resonance imaging (cMRI) studies at a 1.5 T clinic magnet [2]. 3.0 T MRI scanner with 8-channels or more cardiac array coils can obtain cardiac images with higher signal-to-noise-ratio, temporal and spatial resolutions, and shorter acquisition time compared to the conventional 1.5 MRI scanner [4,5]. However, there are few reports on the evaluation of rabbit model of occlusion/reperfusion-induced MI by 3.0 T scanner. In this experiment, we applied a 3.0 T magnet to re-evaluate the rabbit model on both the acute and chronic phases of MI.

Myocardial fat develops with aging and is commonly seen at right ventricular (RV) free wall and RV outflow tract in humans. Substitution of myocardial tissue by fat is less common in the left ventricle, except for some pathologic conditions such as healed MI, dysplasia, cardiac lipoma, tuberous sclerosis complex, dilated and dystrophic cardiomyopathy, etc. [6]. Myofibroblasts are supposed to play an important role in myocardial healing after MI. These cells produce collagen to constitute scar tissue,

* Correspondence: yicheng.ni@med.kuleuven.be
[1]Radiology Section, Department of Imaging and Pathology, University Hospitals, KU Leuven, Belgium
Full list of author information is available at the end of the article

prevent infarct expansion, and stabilize ventricular wall of the heart [7]. Cardiac lipomatous metaplasia (LM) refers to the adipose tissue present in the cardiac wall to replace scar tissue within an infarcted territory. Recently, one clinical report showed that the LM occurred more often in hyperlipoproteinaemia patients and in 11% patients with chronic ischemic heart disease (CIHD) [8]. Another paper indicates that 68% of scars associated with CIHD showed the LM on autopsy [9]. How the collagen fiber degenerates into adipose tissue is still unclear. Findings of LM have been seldom described in veterinary subjects [10], yet never established by both *in vivo* and *ex vivo* animal research.

The purposes of this study were as follows: a) longitudinal evaluation of MI by a 3.0 T MRI scanner, and b) comparison of MI between MRI and histopathology findings on both acute and chronic phase. This way, we incidentally identified the presence of LM in rabbits. In this report, we describe such findings and further discuss their implications for translational cardiologic research by cross-referencing pertinent literature.

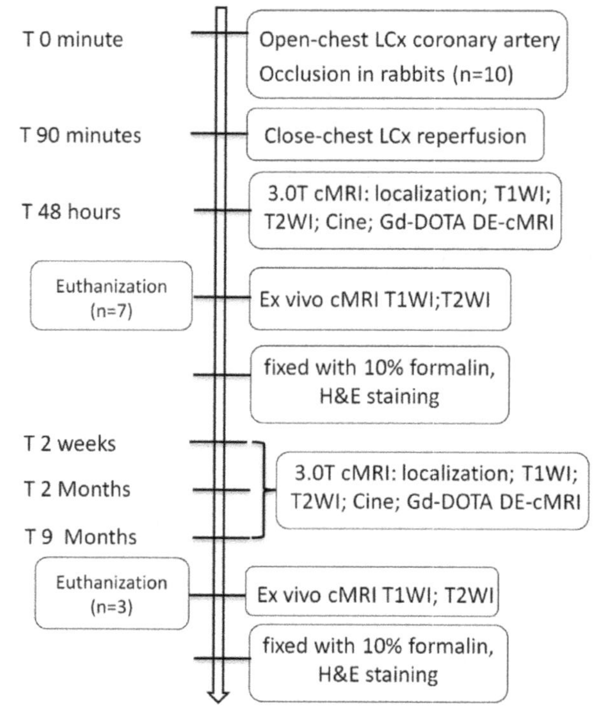

Figure 1 Flowchart of experimental procedure. LCx: left circumflex; cMR: cardiac magnetic resonance; T1WI: T1 weighted imaging; T2WI: T2 weighted imaging; DE: delayed enhancement; HE: hematoxylin and eosin.

Methods

Animal models

This study was approved by the institutional ethical committee for animal care and use. Ten male New Zealand white rabbits (Animal House, K.U. Leuven, Belgium) weighing 3.0 kg were sedated, endotracheally intubated and mechanically ventilated. The rabbit received intravenous (i.v.) injection of pentobarbital (Nembutal; Sanofi Sante Animale, Brussels, Belgium) at 40 mg/kg/h to maintain anesthesia during the open-chest operation. A left-side thoracotomy was performed at the fourth intercostal space and a suture was placed underneath the left coronary artery. Reperfused MI was induced by tying the suture with a single detachable knot. Ninety minutes after coronary occlusion and sixty minutes after closure of thoracic cavity, the knot was detached outside the thorax by pulling the exteriorized end of suture in the closed-chest condition [2]. As shown in the flowchart of the experimental procedure (Figure 1), all the animals were imaged for acute phase evaluation with cMRI, 3 rabbits were randomly served as chronic MI models and underwent cMRI 48 hours, 2 weeks, 2 months and 9 months after acute MI for longitudinal observations on morphological and functional changes as well as the fate of the animals.

cMRI

The rabbit was gas-anesthetized with 2% isoflurane in the mixture of 20% oxygen and 80% room air, through a mask connected via a tube to a ventilation instrument (Holliston, MA, USA) and placed supinely in a holder. Using a commercial 8-channal phased array knee coil, cMRI was performed at a 3.0 T clinical MRI scanner (Trio, Siemens, Erlangen, Germany) with a maximum gradient capability of 45 mT/m. The acquisition of cMRI was triggered by ECG and gated by the respiration using a small animal monitoring and gating system (SA Instruments, Inc. Stony Brook, New York). The two surface ECG electrodes were attached to the shaved thorax skin of apparent apical pulse and the left leg. The respiration control sensor was attached on the middle of the abdomen. As shown in Table 1, cardiac morphology and edema were inspected with T1 weighted imaging (T1WI) and T2 weighted imaging (T2WI), respectively. The cine-MR images were acquired in the short-axis, vertical long-axis and horizontal long-axis planes for displaying cardiac contraction. Each cine-MRI consisted of 25 frames, spaced equally across the cardiac cycle, with the acquisition time of 2.5 min. To evaluate MI, 3D delayed-enhancement (DE-cMRI) was acquired 20 min after bolus iv injection of Gd-DOTA (Dotarem, Guerbet, France) at 0.1 mmol/kg. The ex vivo cMRI on rabbit heart was described previously [2].

Postmortem histochemical staining

After the cMRI scans at day 2 and month 9, the rabbits were euthanized with overdosed pentobarbital. The excised heart was imbedded in and filled with 3% agar solution of 40°C in a Plexiglas heart matrix for ex vivo cMRI after cooling at −20°C for 15 min. After MRI, the

Table 1 Parameters of cMRI sequences with a 3.0 T clinic scanner without respiration holding

	T1WI In vivo	T2WI In vivo	Cine-MRI In vivo	DE-MRI In vivo	T1WI Ex vivo	T2WI Ex vivo
Sequence type	TSE	TSE	True-FISP	IR-turbo-FLASH	SE	SE
Repetition time (ms)	621	750	357	396	2300	3200
echo time (ms)	15	74	1.6	1.54	4.12	490
Field of view (mm^2)	240×195	240×195	240×195	240×180	512×464	512×464
Filp angle (°)	180	180	60	15	9	0
Bandwidth (Hz/Px)	305	235	751	300	350	434
In-plane resolution (mm^2)	0.9×0.9	0.9×0.9	1.2×0.9	1.1×0.8	0.5×0.5	0.6×0.6
Slice thickness (mm)	3.0	3.0	3.0	3.0	0.5	0.6
Slices	8	8	1	10 (3D)	64 (3D)	52 (3D)
Number of averages	6	6	3	1	1	4
Inversion time (ms)	(–)	(–)	(–)	360	900	(–)
Fat suppress	No	No	Yes	Yes	Yes(Figure 6) No(Figure 7)	Yes
Total acquisition time	15 min 5 s	7 min 32 s	2 min 50s	1 min	5 min 21 s	10 min 10 s
Phase			25 frames/cycle			
Contrast agent (mmol/kg)				0.1		

TSE Tubo Spin echo, *True-FISP*: true fast imaging with steady-state precession; *IR-turbo-FLASH*: A segmented k-space inversion recovery turbo fast low angle shot.

imbedded heart was cut into 3 mm short axis slices similar to that with *in vivo* cMRI. The slices were incubated at 37°C in 2% triphenyltetrazolium chloride (TTC) solution for 15 min and fixed with 10% formalin for 24 hours. The heart sections in the fresh condition, shortly after TTC staining, and 24 hours after formalin fixation were photographed with a digital camera. One day later, heart sections were imbedded into paraffin-blocks, which were then cut into 5 micron thick slices and stained with Masson's trichrome (MTC) and hematoxylin -eosin (HE) for microscopic assessment. MTC staining is used for the detection of collagen fibers in the heart, where the collagen fibers are stained blue and the nuclei are stained black and the background myocardium is stained red. HE and MTC macro- and microscopic photographs were further co-localized and interpreted cross-referencing cMRI findings.

Data analysis

The global LV parameters including end-diastolic volume (EDV), end-systolic volume (ESV), stroke volume (SV), ejection fraction (EF), cardiac output (CO), and LV-mass were determined by tracing the endocardial and epicardial contours on end-distolic and end-systolic cine images with a commercially available software Syngo Argus (Siemens, Germany). The papillary muscles were included in LV mass measurement. Mass in grams was calculated assuming a specific gravity of 1.05 g/cm3.

The planimetry of the percent of MI size on DE-cMRI and postmortem digital photographs were estimated on built in software of the system (SyngoMR A30) and the software Image J 1.38x (Research Services Branch, NIH, Bethesda, MD, USA). All the images were in different order, the estimation of MI size on cMRI and on pathology was performed by two authors separately.

The MI size per slice by MRI was assessed semiautomatically by computer counting of all enhanced pixels within the short-axis image. Enhanced pixels were defined as pixels with signal intensities more than two standard deviations above the mean of image intensities in the remote normal myocardial region on the same images [11]. The sum of enhanced pixels from each of the 6 to 8 short-axis images divided by the total number of pixels within the LV myocardium multiplied by 100%. The global MI size was determined as a percent of left ventricle mass volume (%LV).

The signal intensity (SI) ratio refers to myocardial lesion comparable to normal myocardium on T1WI and T2WI, which was performed on the Siemens workstation using the built-in software by two authors with consensus. For the quantification of SI ratios, a round of region of interesting about 1 cm2 was drawn on the lesion and normal myocardium.

Statistical analyses

Data were reported as mean ± standard deviation (SD). Statistical analysis was performed with Graphpad Prism 5 software. The correlation relationship between EF and MIS was compared by the linear correlation analysis. The agreement between DE-cMRI and TTC measurements of infarct size was assessed by linear correlation analysis. A difference was considered statistically significant if the P value was less than 0.05.

Results

General conditions

All rabbits tolerated well the procedures including systemic anesthesia, open-chest surgery, and cMRI. Seven rabbits were used for acute phase and 3 for chronic phase of MI studies. The presence of MI was evident by typical ECG alterations initially, on cMRI during follow-up and with histomorphology at the end. The 3 rabbits gained body weight from 3.0 to 4.2 kg during the 9 months after the MI insult. They manifested normal behaviors and diet without symptoms of heart failure such as dyspnea, tachycardia, tachypnea, cyanosis, stupor, arrhythmia, and hypothermia. There was no apparent difference that allowed distinguishing one from the other rabbits.

cMRI and histopathology findings 48 hours after acute MI

Cardiac global morphology-function analysis on cine-MRI and DE-cMRI showed that the increasing MI size significantly correlates with the decreasing EF (r^2=0.95; p<0.001), confirming a successful model of AMI (Figure 2).

The average sizes of MI (% LV) on DE-cMRI and TTC were 35.41% ± 12.2% and 31.62%± 13.74%, respectively with no significant difference between them (p=0.8). The representative MI on DE-MRI and histopathology of acute MI were shown in Figure 3. A hyperenhanced transmural zone with sporadic hypointense spots at the anterior lateral wall on DE-MRI (Figure 3A). The pale region with dark red spots on TTC histochemically stained section (Figure 3B) corresponded to hyperenhanced region with hypointense spots on DE-MRI (Figure 3A). Microscopic view of HE stained slide proved the presence of acute reperfused hemorrhagic MI (Figure 3C). The linear regression correlation test showed the high correspondence (r^2=0.83) on MRI and TTC (Figure 4).

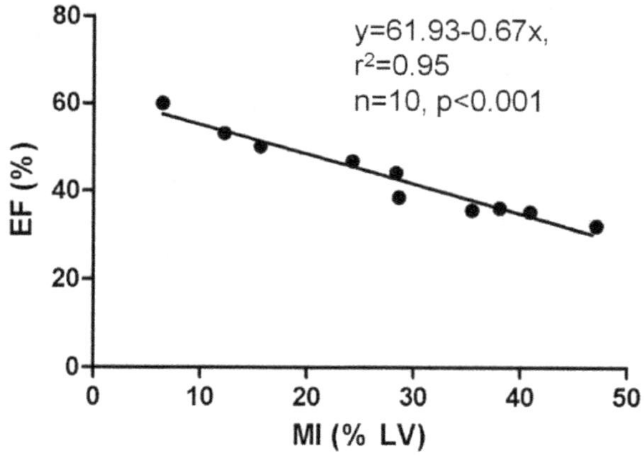

Figure 2 Cardiac global morphology-function analysis. In vivo cMRI enabled to establish the relationship between MI (hyperenhanced region on DE-cMRI) and EF (global LV function measured on cine-MRI) in rabbits with reperfused MI at 48 hours. The increasing MI size correlates significantly with the decreasing EF (p<0.001), confirming a successful model of acute reperfused MI.

Longitudinal cMRI findings during 9 months

The global functional parameters of EDV, ESV, SV, CO, EF and LV-mass were derived from cine cMRI for 48 hours and 9 months after MI and listed in Table 2. Although the small sample size did not allow comprehensive statistical analyses, a considerable increase of the EF was noticed in these 3 rabbits after 9 months of MI.

The longitudinal changes of SI ratio on T1WI and T2WI averaged from three LM animals were showed in Figure 5. On T1WI, the SI ratio was closed to 1 from 48 hours and 2 weeks after MI, the ratio dropped below 1 in 2 months, but rebounded to about 1.5 after 9 months. On T2WI, the SI ratios were about 2.5 and 2 on 48 hours and 2 weeks due to the serious edema during the first two weeks, decreased to about 1 on 2 months as a result of fibrosis; and increased to 1.5 after 9 months with the LM formation. The ratio changes on both T1WI and T2WI display a step-by-step evolution from myocardial necrosis through fibrosis to adipose substitution.

The gradual identification of LM formation was shown in Figure 6.

Acute MI stage (Figure 6 A1-A5): 48 hours after reperfused MI, the infarcted region appeared almost isointense on T1WI, but hyperintense to a larger extent at the lateral and inferior wall involving a papillary muscle (LCx supplied area) on T2WI. DE-cMRI revealed a hyperenhanced area at the lateral and inferior wall, which was smaller than that shown on T2WI (Figure 6 A2). Cine-cMR showed homogenous signal but hypokinetic on the lateral wall (Figure 6 A4, A5). These were similar to what have been described for rabbits with acute MI [10].

Early chronic MI (Figure 6 B1-B5): 2 weeks after MI, the infarct remained isointense on T1WI and hyperintense on T2WI, but the hyperintense area on T2WI became smaller than that at 48 hours (Figure 6 B2 vs. A2), suggesting resolved edema. DE-cMRI showed hyperenhancement both at the lateral wall and papillary muscle (Figure 6 B3), which was thinner than that seen at 48 hours (Figure 6 A3). Cine-cMRI confirmed dyskinesia of the lateral wall (Figure 6 B4, B5).

Chronic MI (Figure 6 C1-C5): 2 months after MI, the lesion became slightly hypointense on T1WI (Figure 6 C1) and almost isointense on T2WI with irregular, blurred boundary (Figure 6 C2). DE-cMRI showed moderately enhanced signal on the scar tissue (Figure 6 C3). With impaired motion and thickening at the lateral and inferior wall, the lesion signal was partially lost on the fat suppressed cine-images, suggesting the initiation of LM.

LM after MI (Figure 6 D1-D5, E1, E2): 9 months after MI, T1WI exhibited hyperintense signal with clear

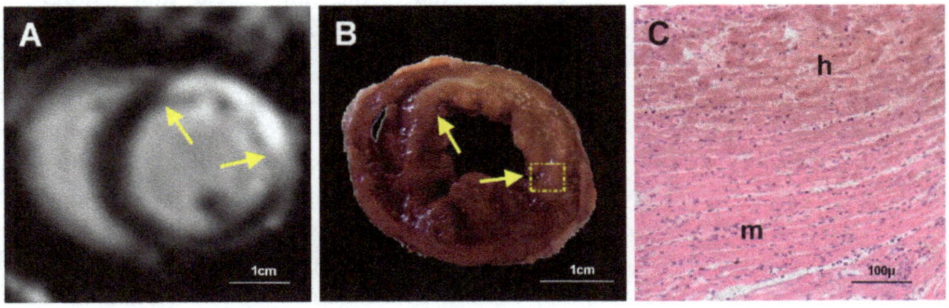

Figure 3 A short axis midventricular section shown on cMRI and histopathology in a rabbit with 48-hours reperfused MI. A: DE-MRI shows a hyperenhanced transmural zone at the anterior lateral wall with sporadic hypointense spots corresponding to intramural hemorrhage. **B**: The pale region with dark red spots on TTC histochemically stained section corresponds to hyperenhanced region with hypointense spots on DE-MRI. Dashed square indicates where microscopy was focused. **C**: microscopic view (magnification×100) of HE stained slide proves the presence of reperfused hemorrhagic acute MI. h: hemorrhagic infarction; m: adjacent myocardium with inflammatory infiltration.

boundary at the lateral wall (Figure 6 D1), along with a dramatic signal drop on *ex vivo* fat suppressed T1WI (Figure 6 E1). T2WI showed moderately hyperintense signal (Figure 6 D2) correspondent to the signal-void area on *ex vivo* fat suppressed T2WI (Figure 6 E2). DE-cMRI did not reveal apparent contrast enhancement of this healed MI (Figure 6 D3). On fat suppressed cine-images, the signal was lost at the lesion, of which the area was enlarged relative to that 5 months ago (Figure 6 D4 and D5 vs. C4 and C5), suggesting the formation of LM.

Pathological findings after 9 months MI

Macroscopically (Figure 6 F1-F3), cardiac sections including the fresh section (Figure 6 F1) and the same section 15 min (Figure 6 F2) and 24 hours (Figure 6 F3) after TTC staining corresponded well with cMRI. The thickness of the lateral and inferior wall appeared almost the same as that of the normal ventricular wall. The MI territory looked whitish and was not stained by TTC, suggesting that the scar has been extensively substituted by fat tissue. Part of posterior papillary muscle was also replaced by adipose tissue.

Low-power H&E (Figure 6 G1) and MTC (Figure 6 G3) slides confirmed the above gross inspection, and demonstrated the clear, definable interface between normal myocardium and LM of the ventricular wall. High-power H&E (Figure 6 G2) and MTC (Figure 6 G4) photomicrographs revealed that high densities of the adipose cells were surrounded by few fibers, and macrophages infiltrated the interstitial space.

In this case, the final LM sizes were approximately 25.13%, 24.87%, and 24.14% of the ventricular volume as quantified by in vivo T1WI, ex vivo T1WI and TTC.

The other 2 rabbits manifested smaller LM 9 months after MI as exemplified on Figure 7. Interestingly, although LM was hardly detectable by cMRI in this case (Figure 7 A-E), photomicrographs do demonstrate sporadic or patchy presence of adipose deposition in the lateral ventricular wall and posterior papillary muscle (Figure 7 E1-E3), suggesting LM change to a lesser extent.

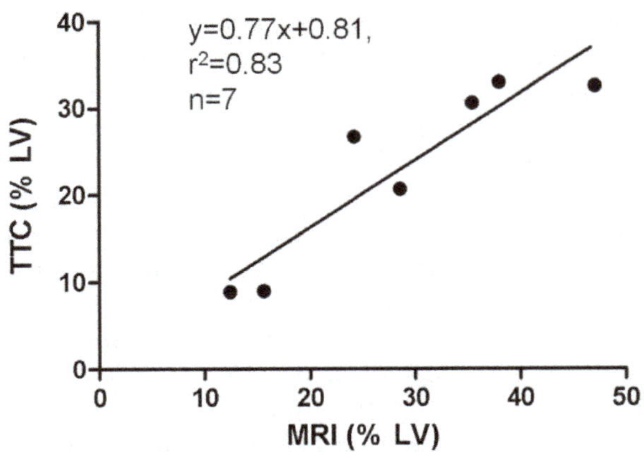

Figure 4 Comparing the global MI size between in vivo cMRI and TTC histochemical staining in rabbits with reperfused MI at 48 hours. The linear regression correlation test shows the high correspondence on MI (% LV) between MRI and TTC.

Table 2 Quantitative parameters of global LV function on 48 hours and 9 months

	48 Hours	9 Months
Parameters	Mean ± SD	Mean ± SD
HR (bpm)	134±16	123±15
EDV (ml)	4.36±0.94	4.71±1.04
ESV (ml)	2.97±0.77	2.75±0.57
SV (ml)	1.35±0.11	1.95±0.38
CO (l/min)	0.18±0.04	0.24±0.08
EF (%)	29.63±2.73	41.69±1.93
Myoc.m(g)	3.31±0.38	2.71±0.72

HR heart rate, *EDV* end diastolic volume, *ESV* end systolic volume, *SV* stroke volume, *CO* cardiac output, *EF* ejection fraction, *Myoc.m* myocardial mass. HR acquired under anesthesia.

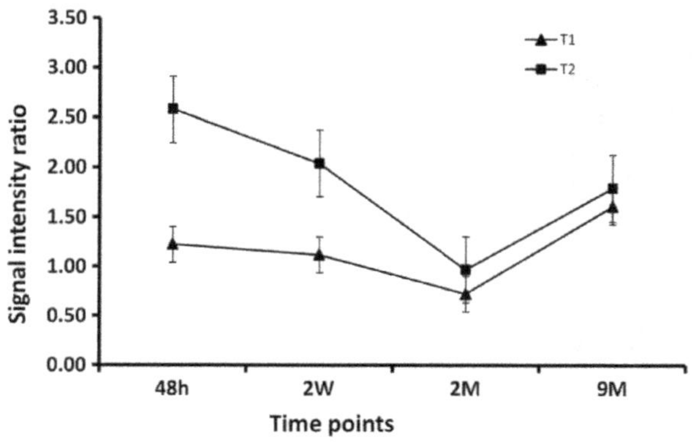

Figure 5 The changes of signal intensity (SI) ratio with time on T1WI and T2WI of three LM cases. On T1WI, the SI ratio remained almost the same on 48 hours and 2 weeks after MI, decreased 2 months later indicating the formation of fibrotic scar; but elevated drastically after 9 months suggesting the substitution of fibrosis with the LM. On T2WI, the high SI ratio declined gradually from 48 hours to 2 weeks reflecting the serious to resolved edema, followed by a normalized ratio on 2 months due to fibrosis. The ratio after 9 months increased again due to the LM. The ratio changes on both T1WI and T2WI display a step-by-step evolution from myocardial necrosis through fibrosis to adipose substitution.

After 9 months of MI, all cases failed to show typical delayed enhancement on DE-MRI (Figures 6 and 7), suggesting ceased tissue reactions in the healed MI.

Discussion

With an increasing importance in cardiovascular medicine, cMRI has been widely recognized as an accurate and reliable means for assessing cardiac anatomy and function, and for identifying different infarct components such as edema, necrotic tissue, fibrotic scar, fat or calcium after MI [8,12-15]. The black-blood spin echo sequences with T1WI and T2WI, the bright-blood steady-state sequences on cine MRI, and the contrast-enhanced cMRI are most useful for determining the presence, extent, and underlying pathophysiological changes in acute, subacute and chronic MI.

In this study, by using a clinic 3.0 T MRI scanner, we imaged rabbit MI models on both acute and chronic phases. The excellent correspondence of cMRI and histopathology confirmed the useful model of reperfused MI in rabbits and its application in cMRI studies at a clinic 3.0 T magnet. We were able to follow up the MI by cMRI for 9 months. The T2WI showed well demarcated hyperintensity in the acute MI as a result of cytotoxic and vasogenic edema 24 hours after the insult. This hyperintense region was larger than the contrast-enhanced region on DE-cMRI. The latter is regarded as the irreversible core of necrosis. Edema is generally maximal at 48 to 72 hours beyond myocardial ischemia and resolved over 2 weeks, as revealed on T2WI [11,16]. The infarct did not appear much differently on T1WI between 24 hours and 2 weeks, but became hypointense on T1WI at 2 months and was moderately enhanced on DE-cMRI, suggesting the formation of fibrotic scar. The signal intensity of MI remained enhanceable from acute through subacute until chronic stage at 2 months, but became unenhanced on DE-cMRI at 9 months. The functional studies of cine-MRI confirmed the systolic dysfunction of the left ventricle, showing a marked thinning and hypokinetic movement of the lateral and inferior wall. At month 9, the bright signal intensity characteristic of LM was demonstrated on both T1WI and T2WI, suggesting locally enriched fatty tissue of high proton density. This hyperintensity was drastically reduced by using a fat suppression technique as seen on *ex vivo* cMRI, indicating the presence of adipose LM. The diagnosis of LM was finally established by using the gold-standard histological staining methods that revealed the underlying adipose component in infarcted territories.

Since fibrotic scar was almost completely substituted by adipose tissue, the infarct could no longer be enhanced on DE-cMRI, which is in line with what was found in a patient [17,18]. Using MR fat-water separation imaging to evaluate chronic MI, the fat deposition was predominately found at mid myocardia or mid pericardia [19]. Other CT studies suggest that fat deposition often affects the subendocardium [20-22]. Interestingly, it was shown in our animal study that little fibrotic tissue was left and the fat infiltrated entirely from endocardium to epicedium within the infarct over several months. Therefore, the location and extension of adipose deposition in LM vary depending likely on the exact situations of individual MI patients, without a common pattern. Clinically, transformation of a compact scar into compressible and "sliding' adipose tissue may worsen ventricular wall function, thus facilitating and/or aggravating aneurysm formation [9]. However, this concern was not evident in our rabbit experiment, probably due to the difference of induced MI in a healthy heart from rabbits versus spontaneous MI in atherosclerotic human patients.

Although the lineage of adipocytes still remains unclear, preadipocytes are undifferentiated fibroblasts that could be stimulated to form adipocytes [23,24], or pluripotent myofibroblasts may differentiate into adipocytes. Not only the etiology and pathophysiology but also clinical aspects of the LM deserve research attentions. It is unclear whether the LM affects long-term prognosis. Substitution of scar tissue by LM is often associated with severe heart failure and is more frequently and extensively seen in CIHD [9]. It has been suggested that therapeutic approaches (e.g. ACE inhibitors and statins) in the management of IHD may promote the development of adiposity within scar tissue [24]. If confirmed, this also raises the intriguing possibility to therapeutically modify the

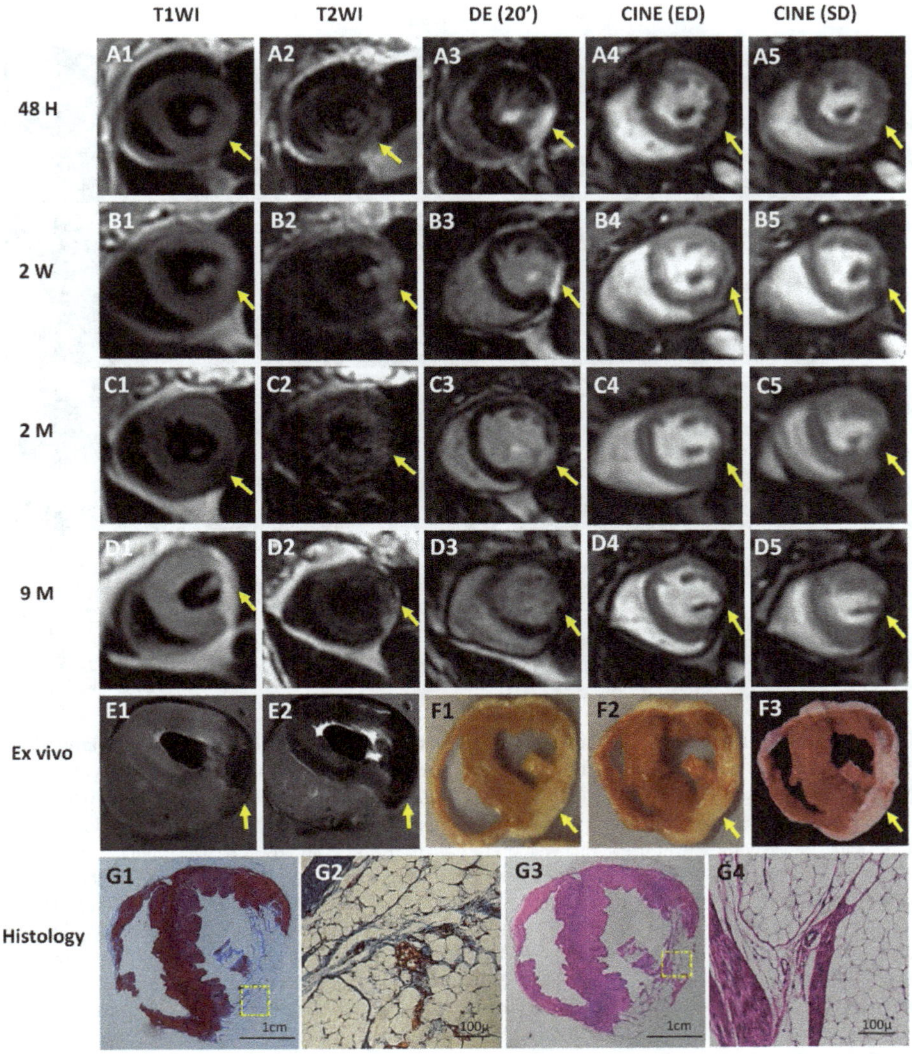

Figure 6 Longitudinal evaluation of progressive changes from infarcted myocardium to large LM (arrows) by in vivo, ex vivo cMRI and histological study. Serial images of the midcardiac slice by T1WI (A1-D1), T2WI (A2-D2), DE-MRI (A3-D3) and Cine-MRI (A4-D4 and A5-D5) were taken at 48 hours (A1-A5), 2 weeks (B1-B5), 2 months (C1-C5) and 9 months (D1-D5), respectively. Acute (48 hours) MI (A1-A5): The infarct appeared isointense on T1WI (A1); hyperintense including papillary muscle on T2WI (A2); hyperenhanced on DE-cMRI (A3); and isointense but hypokinetic on Cine-MRI (A4, A5). Early (2 weeks) chronic MI (B1-B5): The infarct remained isointense on T1WI (B1); hyperintense but smaller on T2WI (B2); hyperenhanced transmural on DE-MRI, thinner than before (B3); and dyskinesia of the lateral wall on Cine-MRI (B4, B5). Chronic (2 months) MI (C1-C5): slightly hypointense on T1WI (C1); almost isointense with irregular, boundary on T2WI (C2); moderately enhanced on DE-MRI (C3); partially signal lost on the fat suppression Cine-MRI, suggesting the initiation of LM (C4, C5). Healed (9 months) MI (D1-D5): hyperintense with clear boundary on T1WI (D1); moderately hyperintense on T2WI (D2); lack of contrast enhancement on DE-MRI (D3); and signal void on cine-MRI with fat suppression (D4, D5). Postmortem T1WI and T2WI MRI with fat suppression (E1, E2): drastic signal losses corresponded to the high signal on in vivo T1WI and T2WI (D1, D2), suggesting large LM. Macroscopies (F1: fresh section; F2: 15 min after TTC staining; F3: 24 hours after TTC staining) corresponded well with MR images. Fat extensively occupied TTC-negative region. Histology (G1-G4): MTC stained photograph (G1) and photomicrograph (G2) (magnification, ×100) and H&E stained photograph (G3) and photomicrograph (G4) (magnification, ×100) demonstrated clearly LM, with high densities of the adipose cells surrounded by few fibers and macrophages. Dashed square indicates where microscopy was focused.

underlying processes to promote myocyte, rather than adipocyte, generation. Our rabbit model may also be used in research for this purpose.

By combining *in vivo* longitudinal cMRI with postmortem histological verification, we were able to experimentally describe, for the first time to our knowledge, the LM phenomena. We noticed 1) the infarcted ventricular wall did not become thinning at 9 months after MI as expected; 2) the LM region was stained whitish by TTC in contrast to brick-red normal myocardium, which was confused with acute MI and left a question about its histological nature; 3) H&E photomicrographs indicate that damaged myocardium is replaced by large quantity of adipocytes infiltrated with macrophages, i.e. the MI

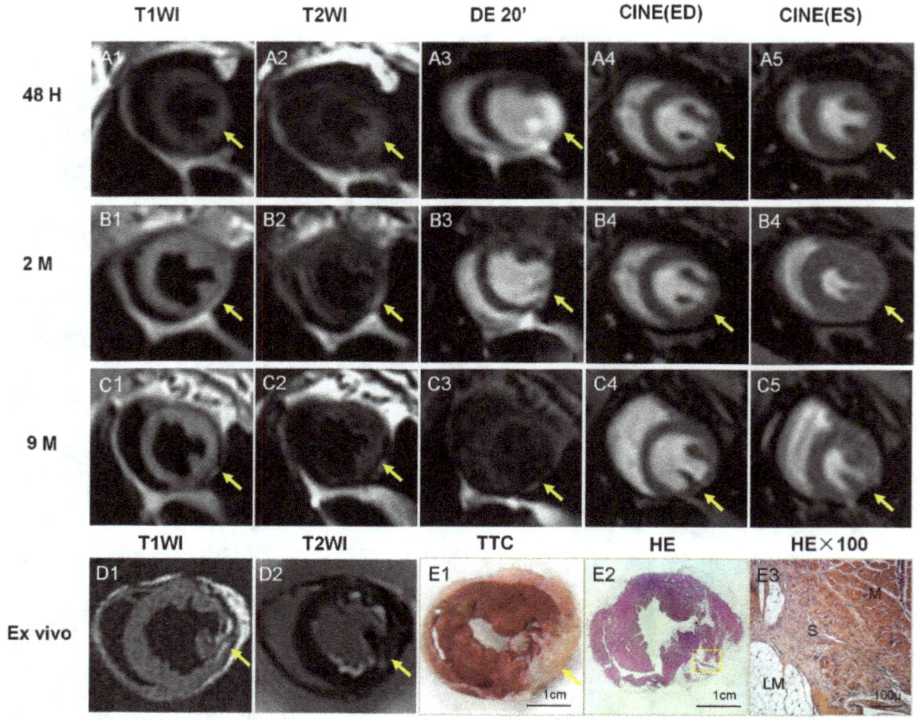

Figure 7 Longitudinal evaluation of the changes of damaged myocardium (arrows), which progressively changed into scar tissue with moderate LM by in vivo and ex vivo cMRI in combination with postmortem histomorphology. Serial images of the midcardiac slice by T1WI (A1-C1), T2WI (A2-C2), DE-MRI (A3-C3) and Cine-MRI (A4-C4; A5-C5), respectively, taken at 48 hours (A1-A5), 2 months (B1-B5) and 9 months (C1-C5). Acute (48 hours) MI (A1-A5): The infarct appeared as isointense region on T1WI (A1); more extensive hyperintense region on T2WI (A2); hyperenhanced area including papillary muscle at the lateral wall on DE-MRI (A3); and isointense but hypokinetic region at the lateral wall on Cine-MRI (A4, A5). Chronic (2 months) MI (B1-B5): The lesion became almost isointense on both T1WI (B1) and T2WI (B2); moderately enhanced with blurred edge on DE-MRI (B3); and almost normal contraction and signals on the fat suppression Cine-MRI (B4, B5). Healed (9 months) MI (C1-C5): The lesion appeared slightly hyperintense on T1WI (C1) and T2WI (C2); no contrast enhancement on DE-MRI (C3); and partially lost signals on the fat suppression Cine-images, suggesting occurrence of little LM (C4, C5). Ex vivo T1WI without fat suppression (D1): there exist patching high signals on the later wall. Ex vivo T2WI with fat suppress (D2): the signal void area corresponded to the region with high signal on T1 WI, indicating the region of little LM. Photograph of macroscopic TTC section (E1): the clear distinction between normal myocardium and TTC negative region is observed. Photograph of macroscopic HE stained slide (E2): the region corresponding to TTC negative area appeared inhomogeneous, suggesting mixed scar tissues. Dashed square indicates where microscopy was focused. Photomicrograph of HE staining (E3) proves the presence of the adipose cells mixed with fibrotic scar (magnification, ×100). N: normal myocytes; S: scar tissue; LM: lipomatous metaplasia.

was entirely substituted by LM; and 4) MTC stained photomicrographs reveal few collagen fibers left.

Post-infarct LM is increasingly reported in clinical patients with very limited histological evidence. It usually occurs several years or over one decade after MI [8,17,22,25,26], much longer than the cases in this animal study. This should not be surprising, because 9 months in rabbits approximate 8 years in humans to form LM, considering their lifespans in proportion. Therefore, the faster evolution of MI in rabbits may provide a good opportunity to study the mechanisms of LM and to develop new therapeutic interventions.

The rabbit appears an ideal animal for cardiac research [1,3,10,27]. Comparing to large animals such as pigs, sheep, and dogs, the mid-size rabbit can be easily handled in addition to its inexpensiveness. Small animals such as rats and mice need dedicated higher field MRI facilities, which are not universally available. We believe multiparametric capabilities of cMRI at a standard clinical magnet in combination with a rabbit model make it an ideal modality to noninvasively identify cardiac pathologies including LM *in vivo*.

Study limitations

The major weakness of this work is the small sample size and only 3 rabbits with chronic MI were studied longitudinally with cMRI, partially due to the constrains of animal protection and limited housing space. Secondly, this study was not by intention to address the LM, and therefore only some cMRI sequences were applied for detection of fat. The LM was only recognized incidentally at 9 months after MI induction. Nevertheless, the collected evidences especially from the evolving features on cMRI and the characteristic changes on pathological specimens do justify this reliable finding of the LM in rabbits.

Conclusion

We validated 3.0 T cMRI for evaluation of acute and chronic MI in rabbits and presented a new finding of the LM in rabbits with chronic MI after a longitudinal (from 48 hours to 9 months) follow-up using cMRI in correlation with histopathology. The *in vivo* cMRI corresponded well to *ex vivo* MRI and histomorphology, suggesting a promising animal model and research platform for further study on the mechanisms and possible therapeutic interventions of LM.

Competing interests

All authors claim no conflict of interest what so ever in the context.

Authors' contributions

All the authors 1) have made substantial contributions to conception and design, or acquisition of data, or analysis and interpretation of data; 2) have been involved in drafting the manuscript or revising it critically for important intellectual content; and 3) have given final approval of the version to be published.

Acknowledgements

This study was partially supported by the grants awarded by the KU Leuven Molecular Small Animal Imaging Center MoSAIC (KUL EF/05/08); the center of excellence In vivo Molecular Imaging Research (IMIR) of KU Leuven; and the EU project Asia-Link CfP 2006-EuropeAid/123738/C/ACT/Multi-Proposal No. 128-498/111. The corresponding author Yicheng Ni is currently a Bayer Lecture Chair holder. All authors declare no conflict of interest regarding the content of the paper.

Author details

[1]Radiology Section, Department of Imaging and Pathology, University Hospitals, KU Leuven, Belgium. [2]Molecular Small Animal Imaging Center (MoSAIC), Biomedical Sciences Group, University Hospitals, KU Leuven, Belgium. [3]Departments of Electronics and Information System (ELIS), Ghent University, Ghent, Belgium. [4]Department of Cardiovascular Diseases, University Hospitals, KU, Leuven, Belgium.

References

1. Fonge H, Vunckx K, Wang H, Feng Y, Mortelmans L, Nuyts J, *et al*: **Non-invasive detection and quantification of acute myocardial infarction in rabbits using mono-[123I]iodohypericin microSPECT.** *Eur Heart J* 2008, **29**(2):260–269.
2. Feng Y, Xie Y, Wang H, Chen F, Ye Y, Jin L, *et al*: **A modified rabbit model of reperfused myocardial infarction for cardiac MR imaging research.** *Int J Cardiovasc Imaging* 2009, **25**(3):289–298.
3. Feng Y, Xie Y, Wang H, Chen F, Marchal G, Ni Y: **Animal models of ischemic heart disease for cardiac MR imaging research.** *International Journal of Modelling, Identification and Control* 2010, **9**:288–310.
4. Greenman RL, Shirosky JE, Mulkern RV, Rofsky NM: **Double inversion black-blood fast spin-echo imaging of the human heart: a comparison between 1.5T and 3.0T.** *J Magn Reson Imaging* 2003, **17**(6):648–655.
5. Hinton DP, Wald LL, Pitts J, Schmitt F: **Comparison of cardiac MRI on 1.5 and 3.0 Tesla clinical whole body systems.** *Invest Radiol* 2003, **38**(7):436–442.
6. Kimura F, Matsuo Y, Nakajima T, Nishikawa T, Kawamura S, Sannohe S, *et al*: **Myocardial fat at cardiac imaging: how can we differentiate pathologic from physiologic fatty infiltration?** *Radiographics* 2010, **30**(1):1587–1602.
7. van den Borne SWM, Diez J, Blankesteijn WM, Verjans J, Hofstra L, Narula J: **Myocardial remodeling after infarction: the role of myofibroblasts.** *Nat Rev Cardiol* 2010, **7**(1):30–37.
8. Lucke C, Schindler K, Lehmkuhl L, Grothoff M, Eitel I, Schuler G, *et al*: **Prevalence and functional impact of lipomatous metaplasia in scar tissue following myocardial infarction evaluated by MRI.** *Eur Radiol* 2010, **20**(9):2074–2083.
9. Baroldi G, Silver MD, De Maria R, Parodi O, Pellegrini A: **Lipomatous metaplasia in left ventricular scar.** *Can J Cardiol* 1997, **13**(1):65–71.
10. Agudelo CF, Fictum P, Skoric M, Kazbundova K, Svoboda M, Scheer P: **Unusual massive fatty infiltration of the heart in a British cat: a case report.** *Vet Med* 2011, **56**(3):145–147.
11. Choi SH, Kang JW, Kim ST, Lee BH, Chun EJ, Schuleri KH, *et al*: **Investigation of T2-weighted signal intensity of infarcted myocardium and its correlation with delayed enhancement magnetic resonance imaging in a porcine model with reperfused acute myocardial infarction.** *Int J Cardiovasc Imaging* 2009, **25**(Suppl 1):111–119.
12. Saeed M, Lee RJ, Weber O, Do L, Martin A, Ursell P, *et al*: **Scarred myocardium imposes additional burden on remote viable myocardium despite a reduction in the extent of area with late contrast MR enhancement.** *Eur Radiol* 2006, **16**(4):827–836.
13. Aquaro GD, Nucifora G, Pederzoli L, Strata E, De Marchi D, Todiere G, *et al*: **Fat in left ventricular myocardium assessed by steady-state free precession pulse sequences.** *Int J Cardiovasc Imaging* 2012, **28**(4):813–821.
14. Okayama S, Uemura S, Sugimoto H, Enomoto S, Onoue K, Omori S, *et al*: **Dual gradient-echo in-phase and opposed-phase magnetic resonance imaging to evaluate lipomatous metaplasia in patients with old myocardial infarction.** *Magn Reson Med Sci* 2010, **9**(2):85–89.
15. Okayama S, Uemura S, Watanabe M, Morikawa Y, Onoue K, Soeda T, *et al*: **Novel application of black-blood echo-planar imaging to the assessment of myocardial infarction.** *Heart Vessels* 2010, **25**(2):104–112.
16. Arai AE: **Magnetic resonance imaging for area at risk, myocardial infarction, and myocardial salvage.** *J Cardiovasc Pharmacol Ther* 2011, **16**(3–4):313–320.
17. Valle-Munoz A, Estornell-Erill J, Corbi-Pascual M, Ridocci-Soriano F: **Lipomatous metaplasia. Two chronic infarcts in the same patient detected by cardiac magnetic resonance.** *Rev Esp Cardiol* 2009, **62**(7):830–831.
18. Arnold JR, Karamitsos TD, Pegg TJ, Francis JM, Neubauer S: **Left ventricular lipomatous metaplasia following myocardial infarction.** *Int J Cardiol* 2009, **137**(1):e11–e12.
19. Goldfarb JW, Roth M, Han J: **Myocardial fat deposition after left ventricular myocardial infarction: assessment by using MR water-fat separation imaging.** *Radiology* 2009, **253**(1):65–73.
20. Wheeler LD, Wood AM: **Re: CT imaging features and frequency of left ventricular myocardial fat in patients with CT findings of chronic left ventricular myocardial infarction.** *Clin Radiol* 2008, **63**(10):1184–1185. author reply 1185.
21. Zafar HM, Litt HI, Torigian DA: **CT imaging features and frequency of left ventricular myocardial fat in patients with CT findings of chronic left ventricular myocardial infarction.** *Clin Radiol* 2008, **63**(3):256–262.
22. Ichikawa Y, Kitagawa K, Chino S, Ishida M, Matsuoka K, Tanigawa T, *et al*: **Adipose tissue detected by multislice computed tomography in patients after myocardial infarction.** *JACC Cardiovasc Imaging* 2009, **2**(5):548–555.
23. Lehmann GM, Woeller CF, Pollock SJ, O'Loughlin CW, Gupta S, Feldon SE, *et al*: **Novel anti-adipogenic activity produced by human fibroblasts.** *Am J Physiol Cell Physiol* 2010, **299**(1):c672–c681.
24. Su L, Siegel JE, Fishbein MC: **Adipose tissue in myocardial infarction.** *Cardiovasc Pathol* 2004, **13**(2):98–102.
25. Schmitt M, Samani N, McCann G: **Images in cardiovascular medicine. Lipomatous metaplasia in ischemic cardiomyopathy: a common but unappreciated entity.** *Circulation* 2007, **116**(1):e5–e6.
26. McKeag NA, Harbinson MT, McKeown PP, Roberts MJ: **Lipomatous metaplasia within an old anterior myocardial infarction.** *Qjm-an International Journal of Medicine* 2011, **104**(12):1101–1102.
27. van der Laarse A, van der Wall EE: **Rabbit models: ideal for imaging purposes?** *Int J Cardiovasc Imaging* 2009, **25**(3):299–301.

9

Comparison of T_2 and T_2^*-weighted MR molecular imaging of a mouse model of glioma

Barbara Blasiak[1,2], Samuel Barnes[4], Tadeusz Foniok[1], David Rushforth[1], John Matyas[5], Dragana Ponjevic[5], Wladyslaw P Weglarz[2], Randy Tyson[8], Umar Iqbal[7], Abedelnasser Abulrob[6,7], Garnette R Sutherland[1], Andre Obenaus[4] and Boguslaw Tomanek[1,2,3*]

Abstract

Background: Standard MRI has been used for high-grade gliomas detection, albeit with limited success as it does not provide sufficient specificity and sensitivity to detect complex tumor structure. Therefore targeted contrast agents based on iron oxide, that shorten mostly T2 relaxation time, have been recently applied. However pulse sequences for molecular imaging in animal models of gliomas have not been yet fully studied. The aim of this study was therefore to compare contrast-to-noise ratio (CNR) and explain its origin using spin-echo (SE), gradient echo (GE), GE with flow compensation (GEFC) as well as susceptibility weighted imaging (SWI) in T2 and T2* contrast-enhanced molecular MRI of glioma.

Methods: A mouse model was used. U87MGdEGFRvIII cells (U87MG), derived from a human tumor, were injected intracerebrally. A 9.4 T MRI system was used and MR imaging was performed on the 10 day after the inoculation of the tumor. The CNR was measured prior, 20 min, 2 hrs and 24 hrs post intravenous tail administration of glioma targeted paramagnetic nanoparticles (NPs) using SE, SWI, GE and GEFC pulse sequences.

Results: The results showed significant differences in CNR among all pulse sequences prior injection. GEFC provided higher CNR post contrast agent injection when compared to GE and SE. Post injection CNR was the highest with SWI and significantly different from any other pulse sequence.

Conclusions: Molecular MR imaging using targeted contrast agents can enhance the detection of glioma cells at 9.4 T if the optimal pulse sequence is used. Hence, the use of flow compensated pulse sequences, beside SWI, should to be considered in the molecular imaging studies.

Keywords: Contrast-to-noise ratio, MRI, Molecular MRI, Contrast agents, Glioma

Background

MRI has been widely recognized as a diagnostic tool for early cancer detection, treatment monitoring and image guided surgery. Of particular interest is imaging of high-grade gliomas due to their rapid growth [1] and very poor prognosis with a median survival rate of only 9 months [2].

Standard contrast enhanced MRI, including application of Gd-based T_1 contrast agents [3,4] do not provide sufficiently high specificity for tumor diagnosis and thus require targeted contrast agents which can be applied to provide information on tumor status (e.g. [5-7]). One approach to apply a molecular contrast agent which is usually composed of a superparamagnetic core and a shell of varying composition and size [8,9]. The superparamagnetic core reduces T_2, T_2*, and to a lesser degree, T_1 relaxation times while the shell of the contrast agent is typically utilized to decrease toxicity and to allow nanoparticle (NP) functionalization [10]. Furthermore, increased core size increases T_2 shortening and decreases T_2/T_1 ratio [11]. The small size of iron based NPs (usually 5–20 nm) and their strong impact on T_2 and T_2*, even in very small concentrations, make them ideal compounds for application to molecular imaging. Their T_2 relaxivity can be up to 20 times that of Gd-DTPA [12].

While the impact of the size and composition of targeted contrast agents on MR properties have been

* Correspondence: tomanekb22@gmail.com
[1]Department of Clinical Neurosciences and Radiology, University of Calgary, 3330 Hospital Dr NW, Calgary, Alberta T2N 4N1, Canada
[2]Polish Academy of Sciences, Institute of Nuclear Physics, Krakow,152 Radzikowskiego, Krakow, Malopolska 31-342, Poland
Full list of author information is available at the end of the article

studied using standard pulse sequences, optimization of pulse sequences for molecular imaging in animal models of gliomas have not been yet fully characterized. The competing requirements of molecular contrast imaging are to minimize cytotoxicity and maximize signal detection *in vivo*, and thus, require application of low concentrations of the contrast combined with an imaging technique that provides optimum contrast-to-noise ratio (CNR) enabling clinical application. While optimum pulse parameters for *ex vivo* experiments, when T_2 and T_2* are known, are relatively easy to establish, *in vivo* experiments are more complex as they include physiological parameters such as respiration, heart rate or blood flow that are very difficult to predict theoretically and to include into pulse sequence parameters. While there are methods for reducing motion artifacts, such as gating (e.g. [13]), data post processing [14] or ordered phase encoding [15] these methods do not address spin dephasing between excitation pulses and data acquisition due to fluid flows. To overcome these MR sequence shortfalls, we applied a pulse sequence that uses flow compensating gradients, known as gradient moment nulling (GMN) [16-18]. The goal of our studies was to optimize CNR using spin echo (SE), gradient echo (GE) and gradient echo with flow compensation (GEFC) in contrast-enhanced molecular MRI at 9.4 T. As susceptibility weighted imaging (SWI) [19,20] is frequently used for molecular MRI we also converted GE images into SWI as reference images. An *in vivo* model was used for evaluating CNR of antibody-targeted iron nanoparticles in transplanted glioma using a range of pulse sequences to assess the vascular density of the tumor.

Materials and methods

Tumor cell preparation

Details of the tumor and cell preparation have been previously published (e.g. [1]). Briefly, the U87MGdEGFRvIII cell line (U87MG) was derived from a human tumor known to express high levels of vascular endothelial growth factor and epidermal growth factor receptor [21]. This cell line was provided by the Ludwig Institute for Cancer Research (La Jolla, California, USA). The U87MG implants grow as solid, nonencapsulated spheroidal tumors. The tumor displays a dense vascular network, with many of the characteristics of glioblastoma vessels [3,7] including tortuous vessels with abnormal vascular basement membranes and increased permeability.

U87MG cells were cultured in DMEM solution supplemented with 10% fetal calf serum and maintained in a humidified 5% CO_2 atmosphere at 37°C. Cells were harvested by trypsinization in ethylenediaminetetraacetic acid (EDTA)/trypsin, washed in phosphate-buffered saline (PBS), and centrifuged three times at 200 G. Viability was assessed using a 0.4% trypan blue exclusion test. After cell density was determined, cells were brought into suspension at a final concentration of 5×10^4/2.5 μL and mixed with 2.5 μL of matrigel for a total volume of 5 μL. Cells were kept on ice until inoculation.

Tumor model

Six CD-1 nude mice (male, 6 weeks old, Charles River, Canada) were anesthetized by intraperitoneal injection of a mixture of ketamine (8 mg/kg) and xylazine (6 mg/kg) and placed in a stereotactic head frame (Kopf Instruments, Tujunga, CA). Tumor cells were inoculated using procedures described previously [1,3,7]. Briefly, the scalp was shaved and swabbed with iodine and alcohol. The skin was incised and a 0.18 mm diameter hole was drilled in the skull. Approximately 5×10^4 U87MGdEGFRvIII glioma cells, suspended in a total volume of 5 μL, were injected intracerebrally into the frontal lobe of each mouse with a chromatography syringe at a depth of 2.5-3 mm (1 mm anterior and 1.8 mm lateral to the bregma). Subsequently, the bony calvarium was sealed by a droplet of bone wax to prevent reflux and the skin was sutured. After the surgery, animals were allowed to recover from the anesthesia and were placed in their cages. All animal procedures were approved by the local Animal Care Committee.

Contrast agent synthesis and injection

Commercially available iron oxide NPs were used (Nanotech-Ocean, USA). The NP consists of the mean core Fe_3O_4 diameter of 20 nm embedded in dextran matrix, with a hydrodynamic diameter of about 63 nm [21-23]. The NPs were functionalized with IGFBP7-sdAb [24,25], an antibody that binds with high specificity to glioma vasculature. Intravenous tail injection was used to deliver the contrast agent after the first series of MR images was obtained.

Histology

To confirm accumulation of the contrast within the tumor, histology was performed at the end of the experiment. Mice were sacrificed by intracardiac perfusion with heparinzed saline and their brains were excised and fixed in formalin (Figure 1). Coronal sections (50 μm) were obtained using a Vibratome (Ted Pella, Redding, California). Brain tissue sections were examined for the presence of iron nanoparticles by an Iron Stain Kit (Sigma) as per manufacturer's instructions. Briefly, the sections were incubated for 30 min at room temperature with iron staining solution (a 1:1 mixture of 4% potassium ferrocyanide and 4% hydrochloric acid). Sections were then washed in deionized water and incubated for 3 min with 1% pararosaniline solution diluted 1/50 in water, followed by additional washing with deionized water. Tissue sections were then mounted on Superfrost

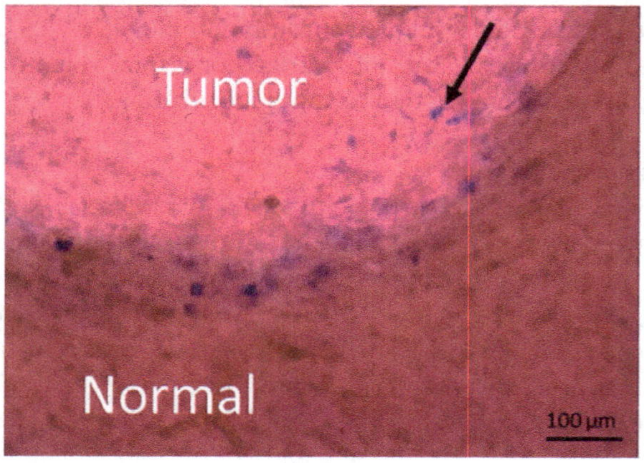

Figure 1 Microscopic images of mouse glioma sections obtained using Prussian Blue staining collected after the last MRI session (24 hours after intravenous injection of the targeted contrast agent). The image shows accumulation of the iron within the tumor (as indicated by the black arrow). Blue spots indicate iron, red - nuclei and pink - cytoplasm.

Plus microscope slides (Fisher Scientific, Nepean, ON, Canada), cover slipped using mounting media and examined under a light microscope.

MRI protocol

The MRI sessions started 10 days after cell inoculation when the tumor was about 2 mm in diameter. A 9.4 T/ 21 cm horizontal bore magnet (Magnex, UK) with a Biospec console (Bruker, Germany) was used. A volume (3 cm diameter, 2.5 cm long) radio-frequency coil was placed over the animal's head covering the region of interest namely frontal cortices. For *in vivo* MRI experiments, a 2 mg Fe/ml concentration of the functionalized contrast agent was used [26] and 200 μl of the contrast agent was slowly (2–3 min) administered via tail vein using a 0.5-ml insulin syringe with a 27-gauge fixed needle (vehicle, 0.9% saline).

Three pulse sequences were tested: spin echo (SE), gradient echo (GE) and GE with flow compensation (GEFC). The MRI session started with SE 20 min after contrast injection (SE lasted 10 minutes) and it was followed by GE and GEFC CNR was calculated for each pulse sequence and eight echo times (TE) for each pulse sequence were tested to find the TE that provided maximum CNR. T_2- and T_2*-weighted axial images were acquired at the level of the tumor. FOV = 2 × 2 cm and slice thickness of 1 mm were used for each pulse sequence. For 2D GE we used the following parameters: TR = 50 ms, 10 continuous slices, 10 averages, 78 kHz bandwidth (BW), 1 ms Hermit selective pulse with a 15 degree flip angle, echo time (TE) 3, 7, 11, 15 and 19 ms. For 2D GEFC: TR = 50 ms, TE = 7 ms, 1 ms sin10h selective pulse with a flip angle 15°, BW = 50 kHz, 2 continuous slices, 10 averages were applied. A multiecho 2D SE sequence was used with TR = 5000 ms, 1 average, 10 continuous slices, 16 echoes, 10 ms apart each, first echo at 10 ms. Matrix size was 256 × 256 for SE and 128 × 128 for GE and GEFC. Total data acquisition time was 10 min for SE, 1 min for GE and 1 min for GEFC.

The SW images, for both GE and GEFC data, were processed as described by Haacke et al. [19]. The raw time-domain data were zero filled to 512 × 512 prior to 2D Fourier transformation and a phase image generated in the frequency domain. A high-pass filter was used to remove the low-spatial-frequency phase as follows: the central 48 × 48 points were used to create a phase image which was then used to subtract out the low-frequency phase components of the original 512 × 512 phase image. A mask was then calculated to multiply the 512 × 512 magnitude image using the following rule designed to enhance pixels of positive phase:

$$f(x,y) = \frac{\pi - \phi(x,y)}{\pi} \quad for \quad \pi > \phi(x,y) > 0 \qquad (1)$$
$$f(x,y) = 1 \quad otherwise$$

This mask was multiplied with original magnitude image four times to produce the final SW image.

The applied GEFC pulse sequence uses first order flow compensation gradients in three directions. The flow compensation gradients reduce the signal loss due to flow. In our study TE = 7 ms was found to provide the maximum CNR thus that value was used for all scans. SNR and CNR were calculated as follows:

$$SNR(t) = \frac{SI(t)}{Noise} \qquad (2)$$

$$CNR = \frac{SI(t) - SI(b)}{Noise} \qquad (3)$$

where *SI(t) and SI(b)* are the averaged signal intensities within the tumor and a normal brain region respectively; *Noise* is the averaged noise outside the rodent head (in the air) ROIs for tumor and brain were selected using pre-contrast SE pulse sequence, as areas within the tumor and the corresponding contralateral brain region (see Figure 2). Due to the different bandwidths (50 kHz vs 78 kHz) used for the GE and GEFC sequences which would result in a SNR advantage for GEFC all SNR and CNR values for GEFC were scaled by a factor of 0.8 ($\sqrt{50/78}$) to correct for this advantage.

Results

Several pilot experiments with different TEs for each pulse sequence were performed to optimize CNR. The optimum CNR was found to be TE = 7 ms for GE and GEFC pulse sequences and TE = 60 ms for SE. Examples of pre- and post-contrast MRIs using SE, GE and GEFC

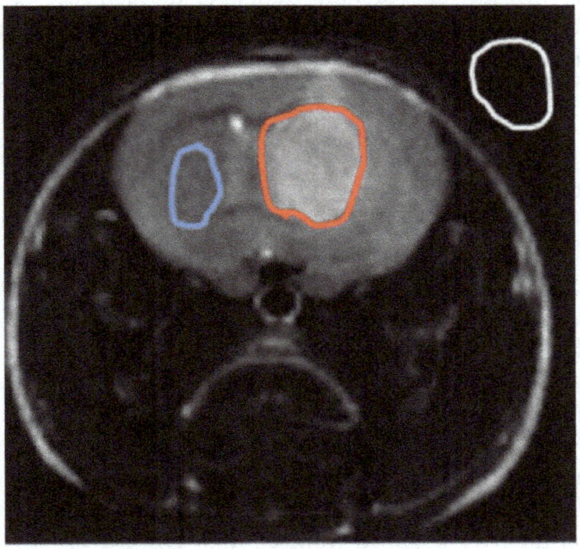

Figure 2 **A method of calculating CNR using ROIs.** ***SI(t) and SI(b)*** **are the averaged signal intensities within the tumor (red line) and a normal brain (blue line) region respectively;** ***Noise*** **was measured outside the mouse head (white line).** ROIs were selected using pre-contrast SE pulse sequence.

pulse sequences as well as SWI are presented in Figure 3. The pulse parameters remained unchanged for each MRI session. Pre-injection GE, GEFC and SW MR images showed very low contrast while pre-injection SE MRI showed good contrast between tumor and healthy brain tissues. The pre-injection CNR for each pulse sequence were significantly ($p < 0.05$) different from each other. Following contrast agent administration, CNR increased significantly for SWI, GE and GEFC pulse sequences, but decreased for SE. The absolute values of CNR for GE and SE were not significantly different at 20 min after injection, however the contrast was reversed: tumor was darker than normal tissue in GE and brighter in SE MRI.

CNR was higher for GEFC 310 and 131 min after injection when compared to GE at 30 and 130 min, and SE at 20 and 120 min, but it was not significantly higher 24 hrs after injection when compared to SE. The changes in the absolute CNR values for each pulse sequence averaged over 6 animals are shown in Figure 4, while the corresponding CNR values are presented in Table 1. The contrast remained positive (tumor brighter)

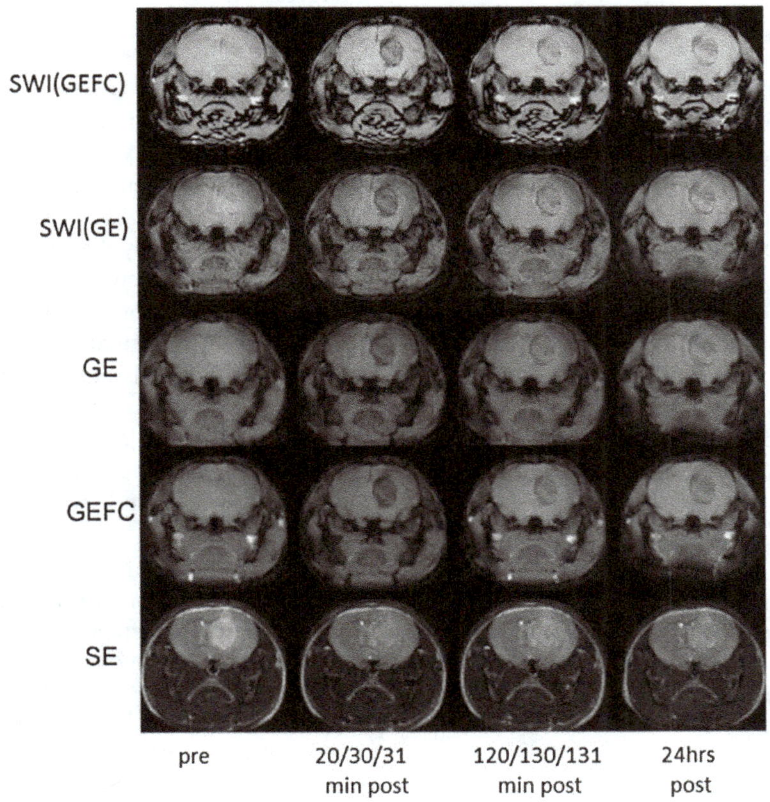

Figure 3 **MR images of the tumor bearing mouse using GE, GEFC, SE as well as SWI(GE) and SWI(GEFC) at the following time points after intravenous tail injection of targeted contrast agents: prior, 20, 120 min and 24 hrs post for SE; prior, 30, 130 min and 24 hrs for GE and prior, 31, 131 min and 2 hrs for GEFC.** TR/TE = 50/7 ms for GE and GEFC. TR/TE = 5000/60 ms for SE. FOV = 2 × 2 cm for each MRI. Note the increased negative contrast for GE and GEFC after contrast agent injection.

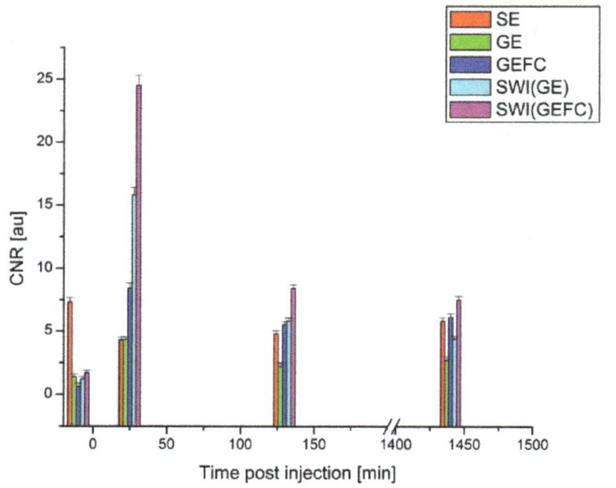

Figure 4 Absolute CNR values for SE, GE, GEFC obtained prior, 20/30/31, 120/130/131 and 1440/1450/1451 min (~24 hrs) post intravenous tail contrast injection respectively. SWI obtained from GE and GEFC data are also shown for comparison. Note the two-fold increase in CNR with the GEFC pulse sequence and even larger increase for SWI after injection of the targeted NP. (The sequence durations are not to scale for clarity.)

for SE and negative (tumor darker) for both GE and GEFC at each time point.

In addition, based on multi-echo GE and single exponent echo train fitting, we measured T_2^* of tumor and brain areas. T_2^* within the tumor area decreased almost two fold (from about 15 ms to about 7 ms) following injection. Brain T_2^* decreased by about 15% (from about 16 ms to 14 ms) in the same time. While the T_2* of the blood could not be directly measured it was estimated based on the expected contrast agent concentration. We injected 0.4 mg Fe into the mouse with an approximate total blood volume of 1.9 ml resulting in an estimated iron concentration of 3.7 mM. The R_2 relaxivity of the contrast agent is about 100 mM^{-1} s^{-1} at 9.4 T based on other agents with a similar core and hydrodynamic size [26]. Therefore, if the blood initially had a T_2^* value of ~10 ms, just after administration of the contrast agent the T_2^* would be about 2 ms and would gradually increase towards its initial value at the later time points.

There is a lack of signal from arteries in GEFC MRI 31 min after injection caused by the high concentration of iron oxide in the blood due to the extremely short T_2^*. Such a short relaxation time overwhelms the usual time-of-flight inflow enhancement seen in the arteries in the other flow compensated images. The brain and tumor signal-to-noise (SNR) before and at different time points after injection was about 10% higher for GEFC than for GE (Table 2) after correcting for the bandwidth difference.The SNR of the brain for SE decreased 20 min after injection by about 20%: from 34.3 to 27.8 for brain. The CNR (Table 1 and Figure 4) was almost twofold higher for GEFC 31 and 131 min after injection than for GE at 30 and 131 min, and 3.7 and 5.7 times higher after injection for SWI obtained from GE and GEFC respectively when compared to either the SE or GE sequences. The CNR decreased about 3 times for both SWI(GE) and SWI(GEFC) 130 min post injection and 4 times after 24 hrs yet remained about 2–3 times higher than GE or GEFC. This demonstrates that SWI based on GEFC indeed provides superior CNR for glioma detection when a targeted NP is utilized.

Table 1 Comparison of CNR between the tumor and brain regions using GEFC, GE and SE pulse sequences as well as SWI at the respective time points: 20, 120 min and 24 hrs for SE; 30, 130 min and 24 hrs for GE; 31, 131 min and 24 hrs for GEFC post *iv* tail injection of the targeted contrast agent

	Pre	20/30/31 min	120/130/131 min	24 hrs
GEFC	−0.6	−8.4	−5.5	−6.1
GE	1.4	−4.3	−2.2	−2.7
SE	7.3	4.3	4.8	5.8
SWI (GE)	−1.2	−15.8	−5.8	−4.4
SWI (GEFC)	−1.7	−24.5	−8.4	−6.9

The negative CNR value indicates that tumor is darker than normal brain.

Discussion

Early detection of glioma, when the tumor is about a millimeter in size, may be associated with long-term survival [27,28]. However, conventional anatomical imaging techniques based on SE providing T_1 and T_2-weighted MRI typically can only detect neoplasias of several millimeters or larger, which contain approximately 1 million cells. Such large tumor size greatly decreases the odds of survival [28-31]. Furthermore, current clinical tumor segmentation methods require a trained operator's input and is based on manual marking of tumor edges on T_2-weighted MRI [29,30]. Therefore, early detection of the tumor and precise, accurate and fast determination of the tumor position and its boundaries are of particular clinical importance.

Table 2 Comparison of SNR from the normal brain for SE, GE and GEFC pulse sequences pre, and at the respective time points: 20, 120 min and 24 hrs for SE; 30, 130 min and 24 hrs for GE; 31, 131 min and 24 hrs for GEFC post *iv* tail injection of the targeted contrast agent

	Pre	20/30/31 min	120/130/131 min	24 hrs
SE	25.3	19.7	25.9	26.2
GE	29.0	18.7	24.5	25.4
GEFC	31.2	21.1	25.9	29.8

The standard deviation was smaller than ±1.3 for each measurement. The SNR for GE is corrected for the bandwidth difference (0.8).

Application of SE pulse sequence allows tumor to be brighter before contrast application due to longer T_2 tumor values. The elevated T_2 values of high-grade gliomas involve many processes within tumor cells and their associated tumor blood vessels [29-32]. High-grade glioma angiogenesis results in hypervascularization, tortuous vessels exhibiting increased permeability, vasogenic edema, retention of plasma fluids and proteins within the extracellular space [1,3,7,33-37]. Furthermore, overexpression of CXCR4, a chemokine receptor known to mediate glioma cells invasiveness, has been correlated with increased T_2 [30]. All these factors contribute to a longer T_2 value within the tumor compared to healthy brain tissues thus leading to tumor hyperintensity and high positive contrast in SE T_2-weighted images. This is in contrast to GE based techniques which have very little innate contrast. GE, GEFC and SW MR images prior to injection of the NP in our study showed very low contrast between tumor and healthy brain tissues.

Application of a superparamagnetic contrast agent reduces T_2 and T_2^* of both brain and tumor decreasing their SNR. It has been previously reported that the high intravascular blood volume and vessel leakage in glioma causes more contrast to be delivered and accumulate in the tumor than in the brain [3,38,39] decreasing the T_2 and T_2^* of the tumor more than that of the brain [40,41]. This decreases the CNR in SE sequences (which start with positive contrast) and generates high negative contrast in GE sequences. This observation was verified with post-injection images demonstrating significantly increased absolute CNR for the GE, GEFC and SW(GE) and SW(GEFC) images (by 2.9, 7.8, 14.8 and 22.2 respectively), but decreased CNR for SE (by 3.0). It should also be noted, that acquisition time of SE is much longer than GE-based technique which makes SE less suitable for molecular imaging.

The best CNR was achieved with the SW images processed from the GEFC sequence at 30 min post injection, but similar contrast was obtained at the 131 min and 24 hour time point. This is expected as SWI is known to be very sensitive to superparamagnetic iron based contrast agents [19,20]. The GEFC images also showed better contrast compared to the GE images. This result is likely caused by at least two phenomena, that each contributes to the overall significant differences between GE and GEFC. We partially attribute the results to an increased SNR in the GEFC images due to the action of the flow compensation gradients and to an increased cancelation between signals from the blood and brain tissues. The increase of SNR in GEFC depends mostly on the efficacy of the applied compensating gradients, namely their proper balancing. The signal cancelation from the brain and blood should be considered in the terms of contrast agents containing superparamagnetic NPs that cause a local susceptibility effect leading to a phase shift within the blood vessels [42,43]. This phase shift can cause the signal from the blood to cancel with the signal from the tissue at appropriate echo times [42-47]. The increased signal intensity of the blood vessels due to the flow compensation may enhance this signal cancelation leading to lower signal intensities in voxels that contain both tissue and blood vessels. However, the estimated very short T_2^* value (~2 ms) of blood at the 30 min time point would virtually eliminate any signal from the blood and therefore prevent any significant cancelation at this time point. While some cancelation could occur at later time points, the GEFC shows higher CNR at all time-points, which makes signal cancelation unlikely to be the main cause for the improved CNR. Likewise, measured SNR values only showed a difference of about 10% between GE and GEFC after correction due to the different receiver bandwidths. The CNR changes observed were significantly larger than 10% and cannot be wholly attributed to a simple increase in the SNR of the GEFC scan.

It should be also noted, that magnetic susceptibility difference between blood vessels and surrounding tissue impacts signal of both GE and GEFC. For vessels that are not parallel to the main magnetic field (B_0), the susceptibility difference creates extravascular field inhomogeneities, thus strong T_2^* decrease independent of the blood flow. Considering isotropic distribution of tumor vessels' orientation and preferred direction introduced by B_0, a substantial fraction of the vessels is oriented at angles larger than 50° with respect to the main magnetic field [48]. The field inhomogeneities at larger angles reach far beyond the actual vessel [47,49] thus the flow compensation is more efficient enhancing contrast due to the signal cancelation in the direction parallel rather than perpendicular to the main magnetic field diminishing overall contrast improvement that would be expected solely from the cancellation between blood and surrounding tissue. As seen above there are various potential mechanisms that may be responsible for the improved CNR for GEFC when compared to GE. However neither of these putative mechanisms can sufficiently explain the observed changes. While the above discussion provides some explanation further studies into the origin of these changes are warranted.

We presume that the decrease in CNR for both GE and GEFC (with a post-injection time of 2 and 24 hrs) but sustaining CNR above pre-injection levels, could be due to preferential retention of superparamagnetic NPs within the tumor compared to the normal brain tissue due to selective immunoaffinity of the targeted contrast agent. These observations are important not only for glioma detection within an experimental setting, but are also applicable for clinical diagnosis. The results of these studies with targeted superparamagnetic contrast agents suggest that the best CNR is provided by SWI(GEFC) compared to SE and GE pulse sequences. It should be however noted that GE based pulse sequences and hence SWI are prone to artifacts, in areas such as auditory canal or frontal lobes, due to their sensitivity to susceptibility effects. Our results also demonstrate that molecular MR imaging using targeted contrast agents can enhance the detection of a relatively small number of glioma cells if an improved and optimal pulse sequence is used. Of particular interest is also the fact that CNR is higher just after injection and remains higher at 24 hrs point for GEFC and thus SWI(GEFC). This is important for imaging comparing non-targeted and targeted iron based contrast agents. The first time point (~20-30 min) is important as then non selective accumulation occurs. At the last time point (~24 hrs) targeted contrast agent accumulation can be observed as more NPs are expected to selectively bind to the tumor unlike non-target NPs that are washed out by that time. Thus the results could also be used for improved differentiation between targeted and non-targeted contrast agents at diagnostically important time points.

Conclusion

The appropriate use of SWI and flow compensated pulse sequences needs to be considered in the ongoing development of molecular imaging, particularly in vasculature rich tissues.

Competing interest

The authors declare that they have no competing interests.

Authors' contributions

BB designed the study, performed MRI experiments, statistical data analysis and prepared manuscript; SB, AO analyzed SWI data, provided explanation of the results; TF optimized pulse sequences, obtained preliminary data; DR performed cell inoculation; WPW, GS provided input on the experimental design and data interpretation; JM, DP performed cell culture and tumor model; RT performed SWI; UI, AA provided histology and synthetized contrast agents; BT conceived the idea and participated in data analysis, supervised the study; all authors revised the article critically, read and approved the final manuscript.

Acknowledgements

The work was supported by the Canadian Institutes of Health Research Team Grant RMF-79031 and FP7-PEOPLE-IRSES-2008.

Author details

[1]Department of Clinical Neurosciences and Radiology, University of Calgary, 3330 Hospital Dr NW, Calgary, Alberta T2N 4N1, Canada. [2]Polish Academy of Sciences, Institute of Nuclear Physics, Krakow,152 Radzikowskiego, Krakow, Malopolska 31-342, Poland. [3]Thunder Bay Regional Research Institute, 980 Oliver Road, Thunder Bay, Ontario P7B 6V4, Canada. [4]Departments of Radiation Medicine, Radiology, Pediatrics, Loma Linda University Chan Shun Pavilion, Room A101011175 Campus Street, Loma Linda, California 92354, USA. [5]Faculty of Veterinary Medicine, University of Calgary, 3330 Hospital Dr NW, Calgary, Alberta T2N 4N1, Canada. [6]Department of Cellular and Molecular Medicine, Faculty of Medicine, University of Ottawa, 451 Smyth Road, Ottawa, Ontario K1H 8M5, Canada. [7]Human Health Therapeutics Portfolio, National Research Council of Canada, Ottawa K1A 0R6, Ontario, Canada. [8]Alberta Innovates – Technology Futures, 3608 33 Street NW, Calgary T2L 2A6, Alberta, Canada.

References

1. Blasiak B, Tomanek B, Abulrob A, Iqbal U, Stanimirovic D, Albaghdadi H, Foniok T, Lun X, Forsyth P, Sutherland RG: **Detection of T_2 changes in an early mouse brain tumor.** *Magn Res Imag* 2010, **28:**784–789.
2. Ohagaki H, Kleihues P: **Population-based studies on incidence, survival rates, and genetic alterations in astrocytic and oligodendroglial gliomas.** *J Neuropathol Exp Neurol* 2005, **64:**479–489.
3. Ellegala DB, Leong-Poi H, Carpenter JE, Klibanov AL, Kaul S, Shaffrey ME, Sklenar J, Lindner JR: **Imaging tumor angiogenesis with contrast ultrasound and microbubbles targeted to $\alpha_v\beta_3$.** *Circulation* 2003, **108:**336–341.
4. Aghi M, Gaviani P, Henson JW, Batchelor TT, David N, Louis DN, Barker FG II: **Magnetic resonance imaging characteristics predicts epidermal growth factor receptor amplification status in glioblastomas.** *Clin Cancer Res* 2005, **11:**8600–8605.
5. Veish O, Gunn JW, Zhang M: **Design and fabrication of magnetic nanoparticles for targeted drug delivery and therapy.** *Adv Drug Deliv Rev* 2010, **62:**284–304.
6. Figuerola A, Di Corato R, Manna L, Pelligrino T: **From iron oxide nanoparticle towards advanced iron-based inorganic materials designed for biomedical applications.** *Pharmacol Res* 2010, **26:**126–143.
7. Tomanek B, Iqbal U, Blasiak B, Abulrob A, Albaghdadi H, Matyas JR, Ponjevic D, Sutherland GR: **Evaluation of brain tumor vessels specific contrast agents for glioblastoma imaging.** *Neuro Oncol* 2012, **14**(1):53–63.
8. Das GK, Johnson NJJ, Cramen J, Blasiak B, Latta P, Tomanek B, van Veggel FCJM: **NaDyF4 nanoparticle as T2 contrast agent for ultra-high field magnetic resonance imaging.** *J Phys Chem Lett* 2012, **3:**524–529.
9. Dong C, Korinek A, Blasiak B, Tomanek B, van Veggel F: **Cation exchange: a facile method to make NaYF4:Yb, Tm-NaGdF4 core-shell nanoparticles with a thin, tunable, and uniform shell.** *Chem Mater* 2012, **24**(7):1297–1305.
10. LaConte LE, Nitin N, Zurkiya O, Caruntu D, O'Connor CJ, Hu X, Bao G: **Coating thickness of magnetic iron oxide nanoparticles affects R2 relaxivity.** *J Magn Reson Imag* 2007, **26:**1634–1641.
11. Wang YX, Hussain SM, Krestin GP: **Superparamagnetic iron oxide contrast agents: physicochemical characteristics and applications in MR imaging.** *Eur Radiol* 2001, **11:**2319–2331.
12. Gambarota G, van Laarhoven HW, Phillipens M, Lok J, van der Kogel A, Punt CJA, Heerschap A: **Assessment of absolute blood volume in carcinoma by USPIO contrast-enhanced MRI.** *Magn Reson Imag* 2006, **24:**279–286.
13. Runge VM, Clanton JA, Partian CL, James AE Jr: **Respiratory gating in magnetic resonance imaging at 0.5 Tesla.** *Radiology* 1984, **151:**521–523.
14. Haacke EM, Patrick JL: **Reducing motion artifacts in two-dimensional Fourier transform imaging.** *Mag Reson Imaging* 1986, **4:**359–376.
15. Bailes DR, Gilderdale DJ, Bydder GM, Collins AG, Firmin DN: **Respiratory ordered phase encoding (ROPE): a method for reducing motion artefacts in MR imaging.** *J Comput Assist Tomogr* 1985, **9:**835–838.
16. Ehman RL, Felmlee FP: **Flow artifact reduction in MRI: a review of the roles of gradients moment nulling and spatial presaturation.** *Magn Reson Med* 1990, **14:**293–307.
17. Haacke EM, Lenz GW: **Improving MR image quality in the presence of motion by using rephrasing gradients.** *AJR Am J Roentgenol* 1987, **148:**1251–1258.
18. Pattaney PM, Philips JJ, Chiu LC, Lipcamon JD, Duerk JL, McNally JM, Mohapatra SN: **Motion artifacts suppression technique (MAST) for MR imaging.** *J Comput Assist Tomogr* 1987, **11:**369–377.
19. Haacke EM, Mittal S, Wue Z, Neelavalli J, Cheng Y-CN: **Susceptibility-weighted imaging: technical aspects and clinical applications, part 1.** *AJNR* 2009, **30:**19–30.
20. Reichenbach JR, Venkatesan R, Schillinger DJ, Kido DK, Haacke EM: **Small vessels in the human brain: MR venography with deoxyhemoglobin as an intrinsic contrast agent.** *Radiology* 1997, **204:**272–277.
21. Nishikawa MM, Sant'Anna OD, Lazera MS, Wanke B: **Use of D-proline assimilation and CGB medium for screening Brazilian Cryptococcus neoformans.** *J Med Vet Mycol* 1996, **34:**365–366.

22. Corot C, Robert P, Idee J-M, Port M: **Recent advances in iron oxide nanocrystal technology for medical imaging.** *Adv Drug Deliv Rev* 2006, **58**:1471–1504.
23. Gupta AK, Gupta M: **Synthesis and surface engineering of iron oxide nanoparticles for biomedical applications.** *Biomaterials* 2005, **26**(18):3995–4021.
24. Amstad E, Zurcher S, Mashaghi A, Wong JY, Textor M, Reimhult E: **Surface functionalization of single superparamagnetic iron oxide nanoparticles for targeted magnetic resonance imaging.** *Small* 2009, **5**:1334–1342.
25. Abulrob N, Veres T, Iqbal U, Stanimirovic D, Tomanek B: *Single-domain antibody targeted formulations with superparamagnetic nanoparticles for cancer imaging.* US: Provisional Patent; 2009. 61/118,205.
26. Moller-Hartmann W, Herninghaus S, Krings T, Marquardt G, Lanfermann H, Pilatus U, Zanella FE: **Clinical application of proton magnetic resonance spectroscopy in the diagnosis of intracranial mass lesions.** *Neuroradiology* 2002, **44**:371–381.
27. Lee N, Kim H, Choi SH, Park M, Kim D, Kim HC, Choi Y, Lin S, Kim BH, Jung HS, Kim H, Park KS, Moon WK, Hyeona T: **Magnetosome-like ferrimagnetic iron oxide nanocubes for highly sensitive MRI of single cells and transplanted pancreatic islets.** *Proc Natl Acad Sci USA* 2011, **108**(7):2662–2667.
28. Provias J, Claffey K, DelAguila L, Nelson L, Matthias F, Abhijit G: **Meningiomas: role of vascular endothelial growth factor/vascular permeability factor in angiogenesis and peritumoral edema.** *Neurosurgery* 1997, **40**:1016–1026.
29. Etzioni R, Urban N, Ramsey S, McIntosh M, Schwartz S, Reid B, Radich J, Anderson G, Hartwell L: **The case for early detection.** *Nat Rev Cancer* 2003, **3**:243–252.
30. Stevenson CB, Ehtesham M, McMillan MK, Valadez JG, Edgeworth ML, Price RR, Abel TW, Mapara KY, Thompson RC: **CXCR4 expression is elevated in glioblastoma multiforme and correlates with an increase in intensity and extent of peritumoral T2-weighted magnetic resonance imaging signal abnormalities.** *Neurosurgery* 2008, **63**:560–569.
31. Ehtesham M, Winston JA, Kabos P, Thompson RC: **CXCR4 expression mediates glioma cell invasiveness.** *Oncogene* 2006, **25**:2801–2806.
32. Skong J, Wurdinger T, van Rijn S, Meijer DH, Gainche L, Curry WT, Carter BS Jr, Krichevsky AM, Breakefield XO: **Glioblastoma microvesicles transport RNA and proteins that promote tumor growth and provide diagnostic biomarkers.** *Nat Cell Biol* 2008, **10**:1470–1476.
33. Hammoud MA, Sawaya R, Shi W, *et al*: **Prognostic significance of preoperative MRI scan in gliobliastoma multiforme.** *J Neurooncol* 1996, **27**:65–73.
34. Claes A, Idema AJ, Wesseling P: **Diffuse glioma growth: a guerilla war.** *Acta Neuropathol* 2007, **114**:443–458.
35. Tozer GM, Ameer-Beg SM, Baker J, Barber PR, Hill SA, Hodgkiss RJ, Locke R, Prise VE, Wilson I, Vojnovic B: **Intravital imaging of tumor vascular networks using multi-photon fluorescence microscopy.** *Adv Drug Deliver Rev* 2005, **57**:135–152.
36. Kuroiwa T, Cahn R, Juhler M, Goping G, Campbell G, Klatzo I: **Role of extracellular proteins in the dynamics of vasogenic brain edema.** *Acta Neuropathol* 1985, **66**:3–11.
37. Reulen HJ, Graham R, Spatz M, Klatzo I: **Role of pressure gradients and bulk flow in dynamics of vasogenic brain edema.** *J Neurosurgery* 1977, **46**:24–35.
38. Strugar J, Rothbart D, Harrington W, Criscuolo GR: **Vascular permeability factor in brain metastases correlation with vasogenic brain edema and tumor angiogenesis.** *J Neurosurgery* 1994, **81**:560–566.
39. Martin-Villalba A, Okuducu AF, von Deimling A: **The evolution of our understanding on glioma.** *Brain Pathol* 2008, **18**:455–463.
40. Gambarota G, Leenders W, Maass C, Wesseling P, van der Kogel B, van Tellingen O, Heerschap A: **Characterisation of tumor vasculature in mouse brain by USPIO contrast-enhanced MRI.** *Br J Cancer* 2008, **98**:1784–1789.
41. Dennie J, Mandeville JB, Boxerman JL, Packard SD, Rosen BR, Weisskoff RM: **NMR imaging of changes in vascular morphology due to tumor angiogenesis.** *Magn Reson Med* 1998, **40**:793–799.
42. Kennan RP, Zhong J, Gore JC: **Intravascular susceptibility contrast mechanisms in tissues.** *Magn Reson Med* 1994, **31**:9–21.
43. Oostendorp M, Post MJ, Backes WH: **Vessel growth and function: depiction with contrast-enhanced MR imaging.** *Radiology* 2009, **251**:317–335.
44. Lin W, Mukherjee P, An H, Yu Y, Wang Y, Vo K, Lee B, Kido D, Haacke EM: **Improving high-resolution MR bold venographic imaging using a T1 reducing contrast agent.** *J Magn Reson Imag* 1999, **10**:118–123.
45. Urchuk SN, Plewes DB: **Mechanisms of flow-induced signal loss in MR angiography.** *J Magn Reson Imag* 1992, **2**:453–462.
46. Weisskoff RM, Kihne S: **MRI susceptometry: image-based measurement of absolute susceptibility of MR contrast agents and human blood.** *Magn Reson Med* 1992, **24**:375–383.
47. Sedlacik J, Rauscher A, Reichenbach JR: **Obtaining blood oxygenation levels from MR Signal behavior in the presence of single venous vessels.** *Magn Reson Med* 2007, **58**:1035–1044.
48. Denk C, Torres EH, MacKay A, Rauscher A: **The influence of white matter fibre orientation on MR signal phase and decay.** *NMR Biomed* 2011, **24**:246–252.
49. Deistung A, Rauscher A, Sedlacik J, Stadler J, Witoszynskyj S, Reichenbach JR: **Susceptibility weighted imaging at ultra high magnetic field strengths: theoretical considerations and experimental results.** *Magn Reson Med* 2008, **60**:1155–1168.

10

Added value of Gd-EOB-DTPA-enhanced Hepatobiliary phase MR imaging in evaluation of focal solid hepatic lesions

Michael Haimerl[1*], Max Wächtler[1], Ivan Platzek[2], Rene Müller-Wille[1], Christoph Niessen[1], Patrick Hoffstetter[1], Andreas Georg Schreyer[1], Christian Stroszczynski[1] and Philipp Wiggermann[1]

Abstract

Background: Correct characterization of focal solid hepatic lesions has always been a challenge and is of great diagnostic and therapeutic relevance. The purpose of this study was to determine the added value of hepatobiliary phase images in Gd-EOB-DTPA-enhanced magnetic resonance imaging (MRI) for differentiating focal solid hepatic lesions.

Methods: In this retrospective trial 84 consecutive patients underwent Gd-EOB-DTPA-enhanced MR examinations. MRI was conducted for 64 patients with malignant focal hepatic lesions (34 hepatocellular carcinoma (HCC), 30 metastases) and for 20 patients with benign hepatic lesions (14 focal nodular hyperplasia (FNH), 3 adenoma, 3 hemangioma). Five radiologists independently reviewed three sets of MR images by means of a 5-point confidence scale from score 1 (definitely benign) to score 5 (definitely malignant): set 1: unenhanced images; set 2: unenhanced and Gd-EOB-DTPA-enhanced dynamic images; set 3: hepatobiliary phase images in addition to set 2. Accuracy was assessed by the alternative free-response receiver operating characteristic curve (A_z) and the index of diagnostic performance was calculated.

Results: Diagnostic accuracy was significantly improved by the addition of Gd-EOB-DTPA-enhanced dynamic images: A_z in set 1 was 0.708 and 0.833 in set 2 ($P = 0.0002$). The addition of hepatobiliary phase images increased the A_z value to 0.941 in set 3 (set 3 vs set 2, $P < 0.0001$; set 3 vs set 1, $P < 0.0001$). The index of diagnostic performance was lowest in set 1 (45%), improved in set 2 (71%), and highest in set 3 (94%).

Conclusions: Hepatobiliary phase images obtained after Gd-EOB-DTPA-enhanced dynamic MRI improve the differentiation of focal solid hepatic lesions.

Keywords: Magnetic resonance imaging, Focal hepatic lesions, Gd-EOB-DTPA-enhanced MR imaging, Hepatobiliary, Diagnostic performance, Characterization

Background

Focal solid hepatic lesions include primary liver malignancies, metastases, and benign tumor-like lesions. The detection and accurate characterization of such lesions is of high clinical importance for surgical interventions and minimally invasive tumor therapies. MR imaging (MRI) of the liver with an extracellular contrast medium, such as gadopentetate dimeglumine (Gd-DTPA) and particularly liver-specific contrast agents, has been shown to increase the detection rate and the diagnostic accuracy of focal solid hepatic lesions in comparison to other noninvasive modalities including ultrasonography (US) and computed tomography (CT) [1-4]. Over the past 10 years, several liver-specific MRI contrast media have been developed, for example, superparamagnetic iron oxide particles targeting Kupffer cells and gadobenate dimeglumine (Gd-BOPTA) or mangafodipir trisodium (Mn-DPDP), which are taken up by hepatocytes. These contrast agents have been investigated in clinical trials with the objective of increasing the performance of

* Correspondence: michael.haimerl@ukr.de
[1]Department of Radiology, University Medical Center Regensburg, Regensburg 93042, Germany
Full list of author information is available at the end of the article

MR liver imaging [5-7]. Recently, the liver-specific hepatobiliary contrast agent Gadolinium ethoxybenzyl diethylenetriaminepentaacetic acid (Gd-EOB-DTPA, gadoxetic acid disodium, Primovist, Schering, Berlin, Germany) has been introduced for hepatic MRI examinations. Gd-EOB-DTPA is a hydrophilic, paramagnetic, highly water-soluble, and therefore bolus-injectable Gd-DTPA derivate for T1-weighted MRI that allows the evaluation of delayed hepatocyte uptake and biliary excretion [8,9]. Approximately 50% of the injected dose is taken up by functioning hepatocytes and excreted in bile compared to a hepatocellular uptake rate of 3% to 5% for gadobenate dimeglumine [10].

In principle, injected Gd-EOB-DTPA accumulates in hepatocytes during the hepatobiliary phase. Consecutive normal areas of the liver — in contrast to malignant focal hepatic lesions, such as metastases — exhibit T1-shortening. Gd-EOB-DTPA produces both dynamic perfusion and liver-specific hepatobiliary MR images, thus combining the properties of an extracellular fluid contrast agent and a hepatobiliary agent [11,12].

Recent studies showed that Gd-EOB-DTPA-enhanced hepatobiliary phase MR images can help differentiating hepatocellular carcinoma (HCC) from arterial enhancing pseudolesions and that combined reading with pre-contrast and Gd-EOB-DTPA-enhanced MR images may improve the diagnostic performance for the diagnosis of HCCs [13-15].

The purpose of this trial was to determine the value of hepatobiliary phase post-contrast images in gadoxetic acid-enhanced MRI in addition to unenhanced and contrast-enhanced dynamic MRI for obtaining the highest possible accuracy in characterizing such lesions in the clinical routine of a university hospital.

Methods

Patients

The Ethics Committee deemed approval of this retrospective trial unnecessary. Between January 2009 and September 2010, 194 consecutive patients with focal hepatic lesions diagnosed using US or CT examination underwent hepatic gadoxetic acid disodium-enhanced MRI to confirm or rule out malignancy. Exclusion criteria were portal vein thrombosis, as well as obvious malignancies, such as disseminated liver metastases, peritoneal carcinomatosis, or local lymph node metastases. Other exclusion criteria were history of chemotherapy including transcatheter arterial chemoembolization (TACE), history of thermal ablation, presence of hemosiderosis or hemochromatosis. Eighty-four patients, i.e. 54 men (mean age: 66.7; age range: 43 to 86 years) and 30 women (mean age: 53.2; age range: 21 to 83 years), met the inclusion criteria of this trial. Figure 1 summarizes the patient flowchart.

Standard of reference

Diagnosis of HCC was either confirmed by histology, based on surgical findings (n = 5) or on results of percutaneous biopsies (n = 24), or obtained from pathologically elevated α-fetoprotein (AFP) values (>196 ng/ml) (n = 5). The diameter of the 34 HCCs ranged from 0.8 cm to 14 cm. Diagnosis of hepatic metastases was based on resection (n = 8), percutaneous biopsy (n = 8), or typical image analysis if the primary tumor was known (n = 14). Twenty lesions were considered benign (focal nodular hyperplasia (FNH) n = 14, hemangioma n = 3, adenoma n = 3) because of the absence of interval changes in the follow-up CT or MR images for more than 6 months without treatment. Figure 1 summarizes how diagnosis of hepatic lesions was confirmed.

MR Imaging

Gadoxetic acid-enhanced MRI was conducted for all patients by means of a 1.5-T system (Magnetom Symphony, Siemens, Erlangen, Germany) with the manufacturer's body and spine array coils. The entire liver was imaged in the transverse plane.

First, we obtained respiratory-triggered single-shot T2-weighted turbo spin-echo images (repetition time (TR)/echo time (TE): 1000/85; flip angle: 150°; slice thickness: 6 mm; matrix: 180 × 320) followed by two different breath-hold fast-spoiled gradient-echo images, i. e. T1-weighted in-phase (repetition time (TR)/echo time (TE): 87/4.8; flip angle: 60°; slice thickness: 6 mm; matrix: 154 × 320) and T1-weighted out-of-phase images (repetition time (TR)/echo time (TE): 100/2.7; flip angle: 70°; slice thickness: 6 mm; matrix: 154 × 320).

Then, we conducted a three-dimensional T1-weighted gradient-echo sequence (repetition time (TR)/echo time (TE): 4.0/1.5; flip angle: 10°; slice thickness: 6 mm; matrix: 174 × 320) using the fat suppression technique. After the administration of 10 ml Gd-EOB-DTPA (Primovist; Bayer Schering, Berlin, Germany), the same sequence was repeated with dynamic contrast-enhanced MRI. The contrast material was injected with a power injector as a bolus at a rate of 2 mL/s via a 22-gauge intravenous cubital line flushed with 15 mL of saline. Dynamic contrast-enhanced MRI was initiated after the start of the bolus injection to obtain multi-phasic images (arterial, portal, and equilibrium phases). Additionally, hepatobiliary phase images were obtained after 20 min using the same dynamic contrast-enhanced MR sequence. Also, respiratory-triggered T2-weighted turbo spin-echo images with fat suppression (repetition time (TR)/echo time (TE): 2220/79; flip angle: 140°; slice thickness: 6 mm; matrix: 320 × 320) and respiratory-triggered diffusion-weighted images (repetition time (TR)/echo time (TE): 1900/72; slice thickness: 6 mm; matrix: 144 × 192) were obtained between the late phase

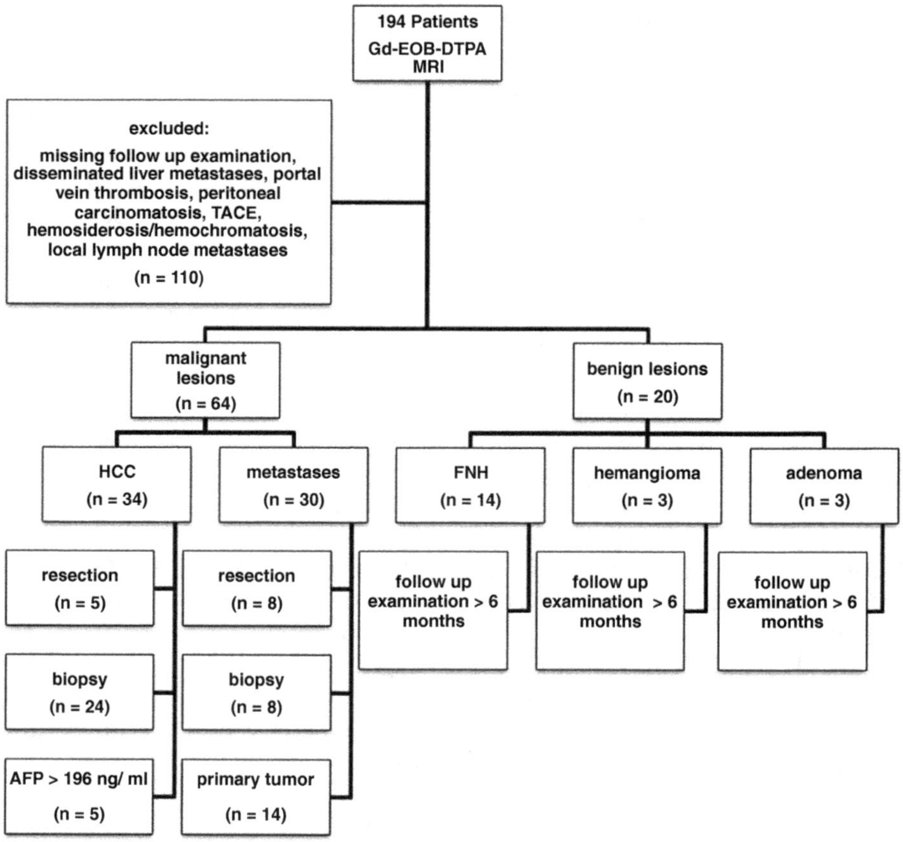

Figure 1 Flowchart of patients and lesions included in this trial. 194 patients underwent Gd-EOB-DTPA-enhanced MRI of the liver. 110 patients were excluded, mainly because of missing follow-up examinations, and 84 consecutive patients were included. Malignant lesions (n = 64) were proven by histology (n = 45), or diagnosis was either based on AFP > 196 ng/ml (n = 5) or knowledge of the primary tumor in case of metastases (n = 14). Benign lesions (n = 20) showed no change on follow-up examinations for more than 6 months.

and the hepatobiliary phase as part of the routine liver MRI protocol (Table 1).

Imaging analysis

Five radiologists (with 1, 5, 6, 10, and 16 years of experience in abdominal imaging respectively) independently reviewed 3 sets of MR images in random order: set 1, unenhanced (precontrast T1- and T2-weighted) images; set 2, unenhanced and gadoxetic acid-enhanced dynamic images (arterial, portal, and equilibrium phases); set 3, unenhanced, gadoxetic acid-enhanced dynamic images (arterial, portal, and equilibrium phases) and hepatobiliary phase images 20 min after Gd-EOB-DTPA bolus injection. The 5 observers were blinded to laboratory

Table 1 MR imaging parameter

Parameter	T2-weighted imaging unenhanced	T1-weighted imaging unenhanced	Contrast-enhanced imaging
Sequence	Fast spin-echo	Gradient-echo, FLASH	Gradient-echo, FLASH
Respiratory-triggered	Yes	No	No
Matrix	180 × 320	174 × 320	174 × 320
Section thickness (mm)	6	6	6
Flip angle (degrees)	150	10	10
Field of view	285 × 380	344 × 380	344 × 380
Repetition time (ms)	1000	4.0	4.0
Echo time (ms)	85	1.5	1.5
Acquisition time	>79 s	17 s	17 s

results, patient histories, findings of other imaging modalities, and final diagnoses. The interval between the reviews of the 3 sets of images was at least 3 weeks.

Each observer used a 5-point confidence rating scale for the respective set to evaluate each lesion as follows: score 1: definitely benign, score 2: preferentially benign, score 3: unclear; score 4: preferentially malignant; score 5: definitely malignant.

Statistical analysis

Statistical analyses were done with a commercially available software program (MedCalc, version 12.1.4, MedCalc Software, Mariakerke, Belgium). The means of age between men and women were compared with the Mann–Whitney U-test. A receiver operating characteristic analysis with the maximum likelihood estimation program (ROCKIT DBMMRMC 2.2 B3, C.E. Metz, University of Chicago, Chicago, Ill) was conducted to show the diagnostic performance with dynamic gadoxetic acid-enhanced MRI. For each observer, diagnostic accuracy (area under the alternative free-response receiver operating characteristic curve (Az)) was calculated and compared.

The index of diagnostic performance was determined as the sum of lesions correctly rated as definitely benign (1) or preferentially benign (2) among benign lesions and as preferentially malignant (4) or definitely malignant (5) among malignant lesions.

Results

Az values for each observer are shown in Table 2. For all 5 observers, Az values for combined unenhanced and gadoxetic acid-enhanced dynamic and hepatobiliary phase images (set 3; observer 1: 0.890; observer 2: 0.923; observer 3: 0.934; observer 4: 0.975; observer 5: 0.984 were significantly higher than those for unenhanced images (set 1; observer 1: 0.677 (P = 0.002); observer 2: 0.695 (P = 0.002); observer 3: 0.634 (P < 0.0001); observer 4: 0.725 (P = 0.0001); observer 5: 0.810 (P = 0.002)). Four out of the 5 observers achieved higher Az values for combined unenhanced and gadoxetic acid-enhanced dynamic images (set 2; observer 1: 0.659; observer 2: 0.837, observer 3: 0.789; observer 4: 0.892; observer 5: 0.989) than for unenhanced images (set 1); for one observer, values were not statistically significant. Furthermore, 4 out of 5 observers got higher Az values for additional hepatobiliary phase images, and 3 out of these 4 observers achieved a significant increase (observer 1: P = 0.001; observer 3: P = 0.009; observer 4: P = 0.004;). The mean Az value of all observers in set 2 (mean Az = 0.833; 95% confidence interval (CI) = 0.788-0.863) was significantly higher than in set 1 (mean Az = 0.708; 95% CI = 0.655-0.745; P = 0.0002). The mean Az value of all observers in set 3 (mean Az = 0.941; 95% CI = 0.908-0.958) was significantly higher than in set 2 (P < 0.0001) (Figure 2 and Table 3).

Table 2 A_z values for characterization of focal solid hepatic lesions for each observer (Sets are defined in the Methods section)

Observer	Set 1	Set 2	Set 3	p value Set 1 vs. Set 2	p value Set 2 vs. Set 3
Observer 1	0.677	0.659	0.890	0.835	0.001
Observer 2	0.695	0.837	0.923	0.112	0.081
Observer 3	0.634	0.789	0.934	0.047	0.009
Observer 4	0.725	0.892	0.975	0.014	0.004
Observer 5	0.810	0.989	0.984	0.0004	0.748

The index of diagnostic performance regarding the differentiation between benign and malignant lesions was 45% in unenhanced T1- and T2-weighted images (Set 1). Accuracy improved in unenhanced and gadoxetic acid-enhanced dynamic images (Set 2; 71%) and was highest in set 3 with additional hepatobiliary phase images (94%).

With unenhanced T1- and T2-weighted images (set 1), 37.9% of the lesions were rated as unclear (score 3). With dynamic phase images (set 2), this rate could be lowered to 18.1%. The combination of unenhanced images, dynamic images, and additional hepatobiliary phase images (set 3) further decreased this rate to 6.7%.

A representative image of each benign and malignant focal solid hepatic lesion is shown in Figure 3. Imaging findings of respective benign and malignant lesions are shown in Table 4.

Discussion

The early detection and characterization of hepatic lesions has become increasingly important because surgical and

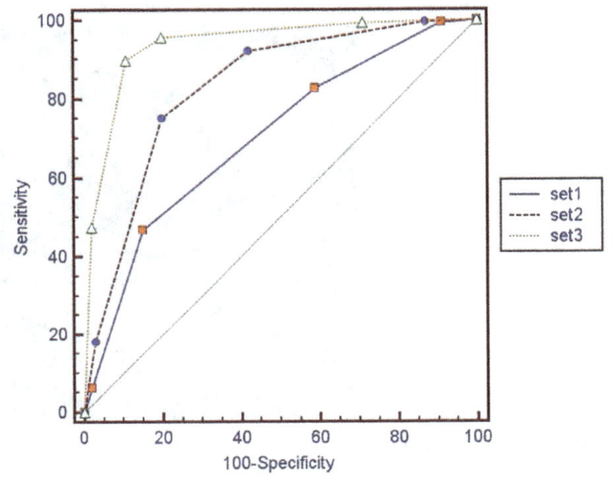

Figure 2 ROC analysis of each set for all observers. Areas under the curve were 0.708 for set 1, 0.833 for set 2, and 0.941 for set 3.

Table 3 Diagnostic performance of all observers (mean A_z) for imaging sets

	Set 1	Set 2	Set 3	p value set 1 vs. set 2	p value set 2 vs. set 3
Mean A_Z	0.708	0.833	0.941	0.0002	<0.0001
95% CI	0.655-0.745	0.788-0.863	0.908-0.958		

minimally invasive interventional techniques may cure or at least improve diagnosis [16].

Several trials have proven that contrast-enhanced MRI is more sensitive in the detection of hepatic metastases and HCC than dynamic contrast-enhanced CT, probably because of the superior delineation of the contrast between lesion and liver and a more subtle depiction of the different tissue properties [3,11,17,18].

Therefore, numerous magnetic resonance contrast agents are available to facilitate the detection and characterization of hepatic lesions in MRI. Among these agents, Gd-EOB-DTPA has become increasingly more important because this contrast medium is able to create both dynamic phase images as well as liver specific (hepatocyte phase) MR images within the same examination [19].

In non-cirrhotic patients, the liver-specific hepatocyte phase can be scanned as early as 10 min after the injection of the contrast medium; however, many patients undergoing liver MRI suffer from liver cirrhosis that results in delayed Gd-EOB-DTPA hepatocyte uptake. Thus, a 20 min delay appears to be more appropriate [20]. Several trials have shown the best liver-to-lesion contrast 20 min after the injection of Gd-EOB-DTPA without any significant improvement in hepatobiliary phase images later than 20 min post-injectionem [12,21].

In early dynamic images, hypervascular benign hepatic lesions (e.g. hemangioma, FNH, adenoma) have to be distinguished from hypervascular metastases and HCCs that show arterial enhancement. Thus, if extracellular contrast agents are used, HCCs frequently appear isointense on equilibrium phase images, which might impede correct differentiation [22,23]. In the majority of cases in our trial, however, the use of gadoxetic acid-enhanced MR images led to rapid and strong enhancement of the liver parenchyma that showed arterial enhancement and clear wash-out during the late dynamic images, which increased diagnostic accuracy. However, enhancement patterns of HCCs on dynamic phase images and hepatobiliary phase images are dependent from type and progression of hepatocarcinogenesis. HCCs with atypical enhancement patterns in terms of missing arterial hypervascularity and consecutive missing wash-out pattern in delayed phase are shown in majority of cases to have a lower histologic grade, lower tumor aggressiveness, and a consecutive better clinical outcome [24]. However, atypical HCCs carry the risk to be overlooked in dynamic phase images and Gd-EOB-DTPA-enhanced hepatobiliary phase images have been shown to improve both detection and characterization of those lesions [15]. Only recently the malignant potential of hypointense lesions detected in the hepatobiliary phase of Gd-EOB-DTPA-enhanced MRI has been shown emphasizing its clinical benefit [25].

MRI is widely used for the differential diagnosis of benign hepatic lesions, such as FNH and hepatocellular adenoma (HCA). Both types of lesions are managed rather differently: whereas FNH do usually not require resection and are treated conservatively, HCA are commonly surgically removed to avoid serious clinical

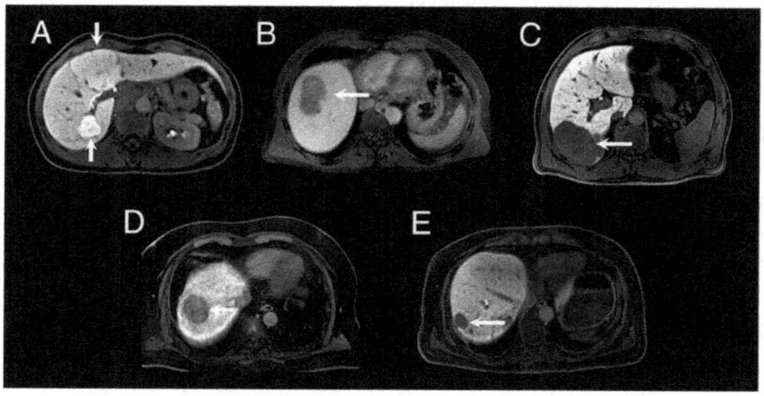

Figure 3 Hepatobiliary phase images of benign and malignant focal solid hepatic lesions. A-E, Transverse 3D fat-suppressed T1-weighted gradient-echo sequence (TR/TE: 4.0/1.5; flip angle: 10°; slice thickness: 6 mm) obtained 20 min after Gd-EOB-DTPA administration in hepatobiliary phase: white arrows depict **(A)** hyperintense FNHs with central scar, **(B)** hypointense adenoma, **(C)** hypointense hemangioma, **(D)** hypointense HCC and **(E)** hypointense metastasis.

Table 4 Imaging findings at Gadoxetic acid-enhanced MRI

	HCC (n = 34)	Metastasis (n = 30)	FNH (n = 14)	Hemangioma (n = 3)	Adenoma (n = 3)
Arterial phase imaging					
Hyperintense	23	2	14	0	3
Isointense	8	12	0	0	0
Hypointense	3	16	0	3	0
Portal venous phase imaging					
Hyperintense	7	0	7	0	2
Isointense	12	9	7	0	1
Hypointense	15	21	0	3	0
Equilibrium phase imaging					
Hyperintense	5	0	7	0	2
Isointense	10	8	7	0	1
Hypointense	19	22	0	3	0
Hepatobiliary phase imaging					
Hyperintense	1	0	7	0	0
Isointense	7	3	6	1	0
Hypointense	26	27	1	2	3

consequences [26]. The two benign tumors appear as hypervascular lesions on enhanced dynamic images, which leads to diagnostic problems in differential diagnosis. However, it could be shown recently that Gd-EOB-DTPA-enhanced hepatobiliary phase MRI facilitates the accurate differentiation between FNH and HCA: whereas FNH lesions appeared hyperintens in comparison to the adjacent liver parenchyma, adenoma were markedly hypointens in hepatobiliary phase images [27].

Furthermore, other trials have shown that Gd-EOB-DTPA-enhanced hepatobiliary phase MRI is superior to CT or standard gadolinium chelates, particularly in the differential diagnosis of hypervascular lesions and in the detection of small metastases, because detection rates and correct characterization have increased [8,19,28].

The results of our trial show the significant advantage of Gd-EOB-DTPA-enhanced MRI in evaluating hepatic tumor specimens:

The diagnostic performance of 4 out of 5 observers was better with early dynamic phase images than with plain T1- and T2-weighted images, whereas the diagnostic performance of 1 observer did not improve after the addition of dynamic images (Az set 1: 0.677; Az set 2: 0.659).

However, the additional information on tissue structure gained from Gd-EOB-DTPA-enhanced MRI during the hepatobiliary phase is of high importance for the interpretation of focal solid hepatic lesions, thus this tool still aids diagnostic accuracy. In our trial, the Az value could be increased with additional hepatobiliary phase images for 4 out of 5 observers. However, the observer whose performance did not improve with hepatobiliary phase images (observer 5) had already shown the highest diagnostic performance with Gd-EOB-DTPA-enhanced dynamic images (Az Set 2: 0.989). Regarding the fact that observer 5 had 16 years of experience in abdominal imaging and observer 1 was the most inexperienced of the 5 observers, the added value of Gd-EOB-DTPA-enhanced hepatobiliary phase images seems to be most apparent for radiologists who are not only specialized in abdominal MRI. Therefore, Gd-EOB-DTPA-enhanced dynamic imaging might be a crucial tool for quotidian use in a university hospital, where most radiologists are expected to run several imaging-units simultaneously.

The index of diagnostic performance showing a mean overall accuracy of the respective set for all 5 observers was significantly higher with dynamic images (71%) compared to T1- and T2- weighted images (45%) and highest with the addition of hepatobiliary phase images in set 3 (94%). This increase was very likely caused by the constant decrease of score 3, meaning "unclear" in subsequent sets ranging from 38% in set 1 to 7% in set 3.

Our trial has several limitations. First, we did not conduct a needle biopsy of every hepatic nodule. The majority of malignant lesions was either proven by histology or based on surgical findings or on results of percutaneous biopsy. There was only a low number of benign lesions and benign lesions were not histologically confirmed but regarded as benign if they remained unchanged at the follow-up examinations for more than 6 months without treatment in combination with typical imaging findings in previous examinations. Second, Gd-EOB-DTPA-enhanced MRI was conducted regardless of the liver function; delayed hepatocyte uptake concurs with diminished liver function, which might have influenced the diagnostic performance, particularly in case of HCC on cirrhosis. Consequently, it may be difficult to clearly define the value of contrast-enhanced dynamic and hepatobiliary phase images.

Conclusion

The results of our trial support the conclusion that Gd-EOB-DTPA contrast-enhanced hepatobiliary phase MRI has an additional diagnostic value for the differential diagnosis of focal solid hepatic lesions in clinical routine and therefore the potential to improve diagnostic performance; notably, the added diagnostic value of Gd-EOB-DTPA-enhanced hepatobiliary phase MRI became more apparent particularly for radiologists with less experience in liver MRI.

In summary, Gd-EOB-DTPA-enhanced MRI is a useful tool for assessing the possible malignancy of focal solid hepatic lesions in clinical routine and therefore for the staging of malignant disease prior to surgery or percutaneous interventional therapies.

Abbreviations

AFP: α-fetoprotein; A_z: Area under the alternative free-response receiver operating characteristic curve; CT: Computed tomography; FNH: Focal nodular hyperplasia; HCA: Hepatocellular adenoma; HCC: Hepatocellular carcinoma; MRI: Magnetic resonance imaging; US: Ultrasonography.

Competing interests

The authors declare that they have no competing interest.

Authors' contribution

MH performed the statistical analysis, did the literature search, interpretated data and drafted the manuscript. MW and IP participated in its design, collected the data and edited the manuscript. RM and CN helped in data acquisition, literature search and interpretation of data. PH and AS revised the manuscript critically for important intellectual content and made substantial contributions to data analysis. CS and PW participated in its design, coordination and statistical analysis and helped to draft the manuscript. All authors read and approved the final manuscript.

Author details

[1]Department of Radiology, University Medical Center Regensburg, Regensburg 93042, Germany. [2]Department of Radiology, University Hospital Carl Gustav Carus Dresden, Dresden, Germany.

References

1. Hagspiel KD, Neidl KF, Eichenberger AC, Weder W, Marincek B: **Detection of liver metastases: comparison of superparamagnetic iron oxide-enhanced and unenhanced MR imaging at 1.5 T with dynamic CT, intraoperative US, and percutaneous US.** *Radiology* 1995, **196**:471–478.
2. Kim YK, Park G, Kim CS, Yu HC, Han YM: **Diagnostic efficacy of gadoxetic acid-enhanced MRI for the detection and characterisation of liver metastases: comparison with multidetector-row CT.** *Br J Radiol* 2012, **85**:539–547.
3. Semelka RC, Martin DR, Balci C, Lance T: **Focal liver lesions: comparison of dual-phase CT and multisequence multiplanar MR imaging including dynamic gadolinium enhancement.** *J Magn Reson Imaging* 2001, **13**:397–401.
4. Hwang J, Kim SH, Lee MW, Lee JY: **Small (</= 2 cm) hepatocellular carcinoma in patients with chronic liver disease: comparison of gadoxetic acid-enhanced 3.0 T MRI and multiphasic 64-multirow detector CT.** *Br J Radiol* 2012, **85**:e314–e322.
5. Koh DM, Brown G, Riddell AM, Scurr E, Collins DJ, Allen SD, Chau I, Cunningham D, deSouza NM, Leach MO, Husband JE: **Detection of colorectal hepatic metastases using MnDPDP MR imaging and diffusion-weighted imaging (DWI) alone and in combination.** *Eur Radiol* 2008, **18**:903–910.
6. Petersein J, Spinazzi A, Giovagnoni A, Soyer P, Terrier F, Lencioni R, Bartolozzi C, Grazioli L, Chiesa A, Manfredi R, Marano P, Van Persijn Van Meerten EL, Bloem JL, Petre C, Marchal G, Greco A, McNamara MT, Heuck A, Reiser M, Laniado M, Claussen C, Daldrup HE, Rummeny E, Kirchin MA, Pirovano G, Hamm B: **Focal liver lesions: evaluation of the efficacy of gadobenate dimeglumine in MR imaging–a multicenter phase III clinical study.** *Radiology* 2000, **215**:727–736.
7. Ros PR, Freeny PC, Harms SE, Seltzer SE, Davis PL, Chan TW, Stillman AE, Muroff LR, Runge VM, Nissenbaum MA, *et al*: **Hepatic MR imaging with ferumoxides: a multicenter clinical trial of the safety and efficacy in the detection of focal hepatic lesions.** *Radiology* 1995, **196**:481–488.
8. Bluemke DA, Sahani D, Amendola M, Balzer T, Breuer J, Brown JJ, Casalino DD, Davis PL, Francis IR, Krinsky G, Lee FT Jr, Lu D, Paulson EK, Schwartz LH, Siegelman ES, Small WC, Weber TM, Welber A, Shamsi K: **Efficacy and safety of MR imaging with liver-specific contrast agent: U.S. multicenter phase III study.** *Radiology* 2005, **237**:89–98.
9. Hamm B, Staks T, Muhler A, Bollow M, Taupitz M, Frenzel T, Wolf KJ, Weinmann HJ, Lange L: **Phase I clinical evaluation of Gd-EOB-DTPA as a hepatobiliary MR contrast agent: safety, pharmacokinetics, and MR imaging.** *Radiology* 1995, **195**:785–792.
10. Bartolozzi C, Crocetti L, Lencioni R, Cioni D, Della Pina C, Campani D: **Biliary and reticuloendothelial impairment in hepatocarcinogenesis: the diagnostic role of tissue-specific MR contrast media.** *Eur Radiol* 2007, **17**:2519–2530.
11. Hammerstingl R, Huppertz A, Breuer J, Balzer T, Blakeborough A, Carter R, Fuste LC, Heinz-Peer G, Judmaier W, Laniado M, Manfredi RM, Mathieu DG, Muller D, Mortele K, Reimer P, Reiser MF, Robinson PJ, Shamsi K, Strotzer M, Taupitz M, Tombach B, Valeri G, van Beers BE, Vogl TJ: **Diagnostic efficacy of gadoxetic acid (Primovist)-enhanced MRI and spiral CT for a therapeutic strategy: comparison with intraoperative and histopathologic findings in focal liver lesions.** *Eur Radiol* 2008, **18**:457–467.
12. Reimer P, Schneider G, Schima W: **Hepatobiliary contrast agents for contrast-enhanced MRI of the liver: properties, clinical development and applications.** *Eur Radiol* 2004, **14**:559–578.
13. Sun HY, Lee JM, Shin CI, Lee DH, Moon SK, Kim KW, Han JK, Choi BI: **Gadoxetic acid-enhanced magnetic resonance imaging for differentiating small hepatocellular carcinomas (< or =2 cm in diameter) from arterial enhancing pseudolesions: special emphasis on hepatobiliary phase imaging.** *Invest Radiol* 2010, **45**:96–103.
14. Ahn SS, Kim MJ, Lim JS, Hong HS, Chung YE, Choi JY: **Added value of gadoxetic acid-enhanced hepatobiliary phase MR imaging in the diagnosis of hepatocellular carcinoma.** *Radiology* 2010, **255**:459–466.
15. Sano K, Ichikawa T, Motosugi U, Sou H, Muhi AM, Matsuda M, Nakano M, Sakamoto M, Nakazawa T, Asakawa M, Fujii H, Kitamura T, Enomoto N, Araki T: **Imaging study of early hepatocellular carcinoma: usefulness of gadoxetic acid-enhanced MR imaging.** *Radiology* 2011, **261**:834–844.
16. Kim SH, Lee J, Kim MJ, Jeon YH, Park Y, Choi D, Lee WJ, Lim HK: **Gadoxetic acid-enhanced MRI versus triple-phase MDCT for the preoperative detection of hepatocellular carcinoma.** *AJR Am J Roentgenol* 2009, **192**:1675–1681.
17. de Ledinghen V, Laharie D, Lecesne R, Le Bail B, Winnock M, Bernard PH, Saric J, Couzigou P, Balabaud C, Bioulac-Sage P, Drouillard J: **Detection of nodules in liver cirrhosis: spiral computed tomography or magnetic resonance imaging? A prospective study of 88 nodules in 34 patients.** *Eur J Gastroenterol Hepatol* 2002, **14**:159–165.
18. Ichikawa T, Saito K, Yoshioka N, Tanimoto A, Gokan T, Takehara Y, Kamura T, Gabata T, Murakami T, Ito K, Hirohashi S, Nishie A, Saito Y, Onaya H, Kuwatsuru R, Morimoto A, Ueda K, Kurauchi M, Breuer J: **Detection and characterization of focal liver lesions: a Japanese phase III, multicenter comparison between gadoxetic acid disodium-enhanced magnetic resonance imaging and contrast-enhanced computed tomography predominantly in patients with hepatocellular carcinoma and chronic liver disease.** *Invest Radiol* 2010, **45**:133–141.
19. Zech CJ, Herrmann KA, Reiser MF, Schoenberg SO: **MR imaging in patients with suspected liver metastases: value of liver-specific contrast agent Gd-EOB-DTPA.** *Magn Reson Med Sci* 2007, **6**:43–52.
20. Tanimoto A, Lee JM, Murakami T, Huppertz A, Kudo M, Grazioli L: **Consensus report of the 2nd International Forum for Liver MRI.** *Eur Radiol* 2009, **19**(Suppl 5):S975–S989.
21. Tschirch FT, Struwe A, Petrowsky H, Kakales I, Marincek B, Weishaupt D: **Contrast-enhanced MR cholangiography with Gd-EOB-DTPA in patients with liver cirrhosis: visualization of the biliary ducts in comparison with patients with normal liver parenchyma.** *Eur Radiol* 2008, **18**:1577–1586.
22. Hayashida M, Ito K, Fujita T, Shimizu A, Sasaki K, Tanabe M, Matsunaga N: **Small hepatocellular carcinomas in cirrhosis: differences in contrast enhancement effects between helical CT and MR imaging during multiphasic dynamic imaging.** *Magn Reson Imaging* 2008, **26**:65–71.
23. van den Bos IC, Hussain SM, Dwarkasing RS, Hop WC, Zondervan PE, de Man RA, JN IJ, Walker CW, Krestin GP: **MR imaging of hepatocellular carcinoma: relationship between lesion size and imaging findings, including signal intensity and dynamic enhancement patterns.** *J Magn Reson Imaging* 2007, **26**:1548–1555.
24. Choi JW, Lee JM, Kim SJ, Yoon JH, Baek JH, Han JK, Choi BI: **Hepatocellular carcinoma: imaging patterns on gadoxetic acid-enhanced MR Images and their value as an imaging biomarker.** *Radiology* 2013, **267**:776–786.
25. Akai H, Matsuda I, Kiryu S, Tajima T, Takao H, Watanabe Y, Imamura H, Kokudo N, Akahane M, Ohtomo K: **Fate of hypointense lesions on Gd-EOB-DTPA-enhanced magnetic resonance imaging.** *Eur J Radiol* 2012, **81**:2973–2977.
26. Cherqui D, Rahmouni A, Charlotte F, Boulahdour H, Metreau JM, Meignan M, Fagniez PL, Zafrani ES, Mathieu D, Dhumeaux D: **Management of focal nodular hyperplasia and hepatocellular adenoma in young women: a**

series of 41 patients with clinical, radiological, and pathological correlations. *Hepatology* 1995, **22**:1674–1681.

27. Grazioli L, Bondioni MP, Haradome H, Motosugi U, Tinti R, Frittoli B, Gambarini S, Donato F, Colagrande S: **Hepatocellular adenoma and focal nodular hyperplasia: value of gadoxetic acid-enhanced MR imaging in differential diagnosis.** *Radiology* 2012, **262**:520–529.
28. Huppertz A, Balzer T, Blakeborough A, Breuer J, Giovagnoni A, Heinz-Peer G, Laniado M, Manfredi RM, Mathieu DG, Mueller D, Reimer P, Robinson PJ, Strotzer M, Taupitz M, Vogl TJ: **Improved detection of focal liver lesions at MR imaging: multicenter comparison of gadoxetic acid-enhanced MR images with intraoperative findings.** *Radiology* 2004, **230**:266–275.

11

Reproducibility of small animal cine and scar cardiac magnetic resonance imaging using a clinical 3.0 tesla system

Robert Manka[1,2,3*†], Cosima Jahnke[4†], Thomas Hucko[5], Thore Dietrich[5], Rolf Gebker[5], Bernhard Schnackenburg[6], Kristof Graf[5] and Ingo Paetsch[4]

Abstract

Background: To evaluate the inter-study, inter-reader and intra-reader reproducibility of cardiac cine and scar imaging in rats using a clinical 3.0 Tesla magnetic resonance (MR) system.

Methods: Thirty-three adult rats (Sprague–Dawley) were imaged 24 hours after surgical occlusion of the left anterior descending coronary artery using a 3.0 Tesla clinical MR scanner (Philips Healthcare, Best, The Netherlands) equipped with a dedicated 70 mm solenoid receive-only coil. Left-ventricular (LV) volumes, mass, ejection fraction and amount of myocardial scar tissue were measured. Intra-and inter-observer reproducibility was assessed in all animals. In addition, repeat MR exams were performed in 6 randomly chosen rats within 24 hours to assess inter-study reproducibility.

Results: The MR imaging protocol was successfully completed in 32 (97%) animals. Bland-Altman analysis demonstrated high intra-reader reproducibility (mean bias%: LV end-diastolic volume (LVEDV), -1.7%; LV end-systolic volume (LVESV), -2.2%; LV ejection fraction (LVEF), 1.0%; LV mass, -2.7%; and scar mass, -1.2%) and high inter-reader reproducibility (mean bias%: LVEDV, 3.3%; LVESV, 6.2%; LVEF, -4.8%; LV mass, -1.9%; and scar mass, -1.8%). In addition, a high inter-study reproducibility was found (mean bias%: LVEDV, 0.1%; LVESV, -1.8%; LVEF, 1.0%; LV mass, -4.6%; and scar mass, -6.2%).

Conclusions: Cardiac MR imaging of rats yielded highly reproducible measurements of cardiac volumes/function and myocardial infarct size on a clinical 3.0 Tesla MR scanner system. Consequently, more widely available high field clinical MR scanners can be employed for small animal imaging of the heart e.g. when aiming at serial assessments during therapeutic intervention studies.

Background

The accurate and reproducible assessment of cardiac function by measurement of leftventricular (LV) volumes, ejection fraction, and the amount of myocardial scar tissue is fundamental for evaluating heart diseases in cardiovascular research. A great advantage of cardiac magnetic resonance (CMR) imaging is the inherently high soft tissue contrast, and the possibility to image cardiac and vascular anatomy in a three-dimensional manner. The accuracy of CMR imaging for the evaluation of LV volumes, mass and scar amount has been validated in several human and small animal studies [1-6]. However, most animal studies have been conducted on dedicated ultra-high field small animal MR systems which are not widely available [6-8]. Thus, cardiac imaging in rodents using conventional clinical MR scanners would be highly desirable but remains technically demanding since imaging at high heart rates (> 300/min) will inadvertently limit the required high spatial and temporal resolution [9]. Recently, clinical MR scanners have been successfully employed to overcome these difficulties [10-12]. Cardiovascular research generally relies on reliable and accurate imaging protocols and such imaging

* Correspondence: robert.manka@usz.ch
†Equal contributors
[1]Department of Cardiology, University Hospital Zurich, Rämistrasse 100, 8091, Zurich, Switzerland
[2]Institute for Biomedical Engineering, University and ETH Zurich, Zurich, Switzerland
Full list of author information is available at the end of the article

protocols are mandatory for small animal examinations either; in particular the exact determination of LV volumes/mass and myocardial infarct size plays a pivotal role in therapeutic intervention studies [13]. In order to facilitate accurate and reproducible cardiac small animal imaging on commonly available clinical MR scanners, the present study determined inter-study, inter-reader and intra-reader reproducibility for the evaluation of LV volumes, mass and myocardial scar size in rats using a clinical 3.0 Tesla MR system.

Methods

Animal preparation

The study was approved by the Charité Institutional Review Board. Thirty-three adult Sprague–Dawley rats (7–16 weeks old) with a mean weight of 355.5 ± 91.8 g (range 269–589 g) were included in our study protocol. For surgical intervention, the animals were anesthetized with 0.3 ml Domitor® (1 mg/1 mL) + 0.8 ml Dormicum® (5 mg/1 mL)/kg BW. After thoracotomy, the left anterior descending coronary artery (LAD) was occluded on the level of the first diagonal branch by placing a snare ligature around the artery and a small portion of the surrounding myocardium. All animals underwent CMR imaging within 24 hours after surgery.

CMR imaging

CMR imaging was performed using a clinical 3.0 Tesla MR system (Philips Healthcare, Best, The Netherlands) equipped with a Quasar Dual gradient system (40 mT/m, slew rate 200 T/m/sec) using a dedicated 70 mm solenoid receive-only coil placed perpendicular to B0 providing a high signal-to-noise ratio (Philips Research Laboratory, Hamburg, Germany). Anaesthesia was induced and maintained during the CMR examination with 3% isoflurane administered by a nasal cone. The animals were placed in a specially-designed cradle with four neonatal ECG electrodes (3 M™ Red Dot™ 2269 T) being attached to the paws in order to record an electrocardiogram for triggering of image data acquisition (see Figure 1). A dedicated software patch (GyroTools Ltd., Zurich Switzerland) installed on the scanner console enabled triggered image data acquisition up to heart rates of 400 beats per minute which constituted the only modification applied to the commercially available standard software of the scanner system. A multi-stack, multi-slice, segmented, spoiled gradient echo (GRE) pulse sequence was performed for localization of the heart in the three standard planes (transverse, sagittal, and coronal). For the assessment of LV volumes/mass whole heart coverage with contiguous short-axis cine imaging (8–10 slices) was carried out followed by acquisition of standard 4-and 2-chamber views.

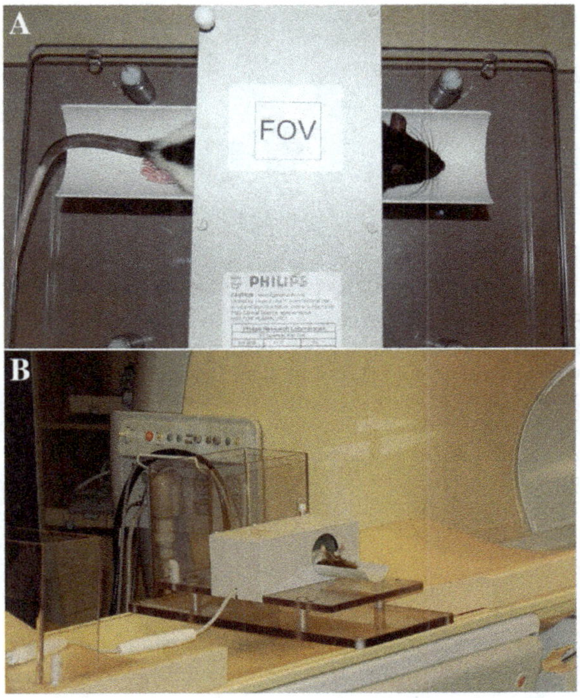

Figure 1 Experimental Setup for CMR imaging of small animals (rat). A specifically designed solenoid coil **(A)**, Philips Research Laboratory, Hamburg, Germany) with a diameter of 70 mm was placed perpendicular to the B_0 field of the MR scanner **(B)** and favourably provided a high signal-to-noise ratio.

For cine imaging a segmented gradient echo sequence was applied (turbo field echo; repetition time/echo time, 9.0 ms/4.2 ms; flip angle, 15°; temporal resolution 9.9 ms; in-plane spatial resolution, 0.4 x 0.4 mm^2; slice thickness, 1.5 mm; field-of-view, 64 mm^2; matrix, 159; total scan time approximately 20 minutes). Following cine imaging, a bolus of gadolinium-DTPA (dosage, 0.5 mmol/100 g BW) was administered via a catheter placed in a tail vein. After a 15 minute waiting period, full left-ventricular coverage, three-dimensional late enhancement (LE) imaging was performed in identical short axis geometry using an inversion prepared segmented gradient-echo-sequence (data acquisition window, 32 ms; time between 180° pulses = 2 heart beats; echo time, 3.3 ms; flip angle, 15°; in-plane spatial resolution, 0.3 x 0.3 mm^2; slice thickness, 1.6 mm; field-of-view, 55 mm^2; matrix, 188; total scan time approximately 14 minutes). The delay of the inversion prepulse was determined from an inversion prepared cine scan (Look-Locker sequence) and individually adjusted to optimally suppress signal from normal myocardium. All acquisitions were performed during free breathing with respiratory motion being partially compensated for by employing signal averaging (Number of Signal Averages, NSA = 5 for cine imaging and NSA = 2 for LE imaging).

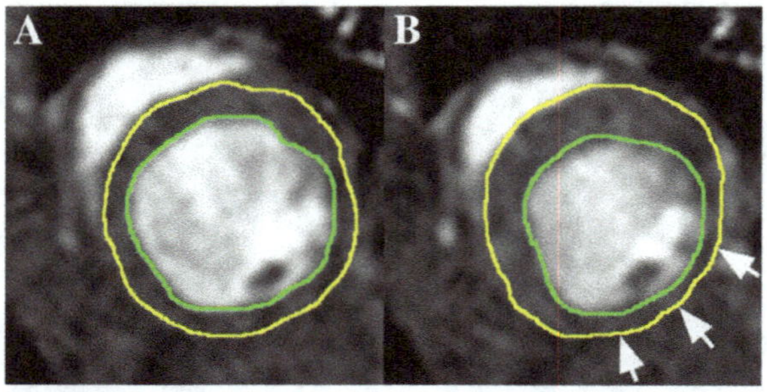

Figure 2 Representative imaging example of endo-and epicardial contour delineation. LV endocardial contours of the heart were traced manually at end-diastole **(A)** and end-systole **(B)** to calculate LV volumes according to Simpson's rule. In addition, LV epicardial contours were traced manually to calculate LV mass; papillary muscles were excluded. White arrows indicate akinetic myocardial segments due to myocardial infarction.

Image analysis

All data sets were evaluated using a standard analysis software (ViewForum Release 5.1, Philips Healthcare, Best, The Netherlands).

Assessment of LV volumes

Endocardial borders were traced manually at end-diastole and end-systole (Figure 2) with endocardial trabeculae being excluded; basal short axis slices demonstrating > 50% of visible circumferential LV myocardium were included in the analysis. LV end-diastolic volume (LVEDV) and LV end-systolic volume (LVESV) were calculated by applying Simpson's rule with LV ejection fraction (LVEF) derived accordingly. In addition, end-diastolic epicardial borders were traced manually for measurement of end-diastolic LV mass (specific myocardial density, 1.05 g/cm3). LV end-diastolic diameter (LVEDD) was measured in a basal short-axis view according to standard definitions.

Assessment of LV scar amount

Endo-and epicardial borders were manually traced on LE images. The amount of scar was quantified by manual segmentation with the signal intensity threshold set to >2 standard deviations above the mean signal intensity of a remote myocardial region (Figure 3). The volume of enhanced myocardium was determined according to the disc summation method and provided in microliter (μl); in addition percentage of scar of total LV mass was calculated.

Reproducibility

The intra-reader and inter-reader reproducibility of LV volumes and mass were evaluated in all animals. To assess intra-reader reproducibility, left-ventricular contours were redrawn by the original observer (T.H., >4 years experience in reading >500 CMR studies per year) one month after the initial analysis. In order to assess inter-reader reproducibility an additional observer (R.M., >7 years experience in reading >600 CMR studies per year) carried out a separate analysis. For the assessment of inter-study reproducibility, 6 randomly chosen animals were scanned twice within 24 hours and evaluated by the first observer being blinded to the animal data.

Statistical analysis

Statistical analyses were performed using SPSS, version 17.0, software (SPSS, Chicago). Values are reported as means ± standard deviations. The mean bias between the reads and their limits of agreement were determined according to the method described by Bland and Altman [14] and by calculating Lin's concordance coefficient [15] using MedCalc® Version 9.2.1.0 (MedCalc Software, Belgium). In addition, the coefficient of variability (CV) was derived [16]. All tests were two sided, and $P < 0.05$ was considered to indicate statistical significance.

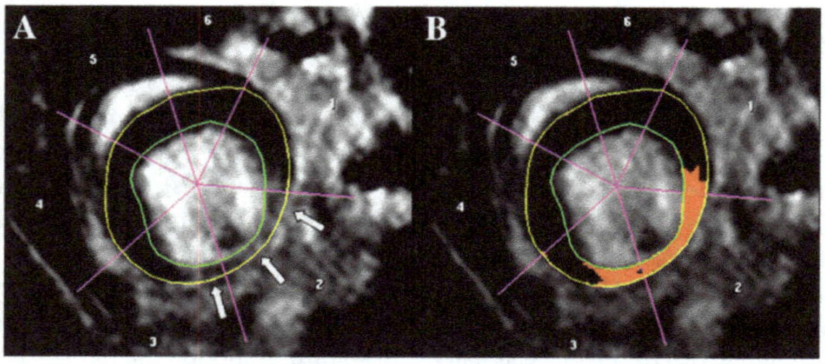

Figure 3 Representative imaging example of endo-and epicardial contour delineation for the assessment of myocardial scar amount. White arrows indicate infarcted region **(A)**. Red-coloured overlay represents segmented myocardial scar tissue **(B)**.

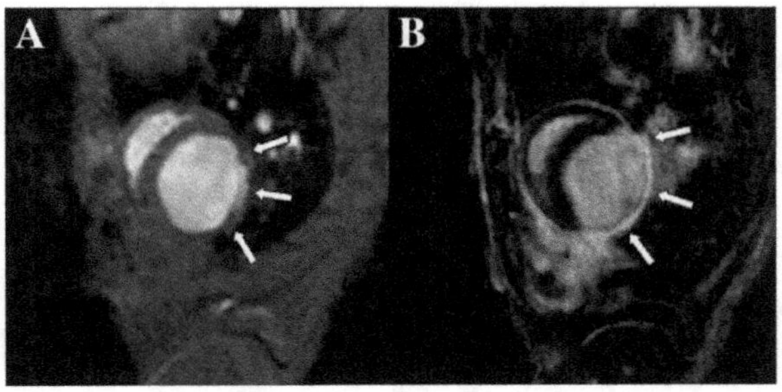

Figure 4 Comparison of cine and late enhancement imaging (identical slice geometry). Representative example showing an end-diastolic cine short-axis frame **(A)** and the corresponding late enhancement image **(B)**. White arrows indicate the akinetic **(A)** and infarcted region **(B)**; see also movie 1 (see additional file 1).

Results

Study population

Image data acquisition was successfully completed in 32 out of 33 animals (97%) and in all 6 animals (100%) undergoing repeat CMR examinations. Heart rate ranged from 270 to 310 beats per minute (bpm), one CMR examination suffered from ECG-related triggering problems and could not be finalized. All 32 completed CMR examinations were of diagnostic image quality and constituted the final study population for analysis (for a representative imaging example see Figure 4 and Additional file 1).

Left ventricular measurements

LVEF, LVEDV and LVEDD ranged from 23.0 to 68.8%, 257.0 to 609.2 µl and 5.3 to 8.7 mm, respectively; LV mass demonstrated values between 199.4 and 450.4 mg and myocardial scar volume ranged from 0 to 99.9 µl. The absolute values of all parameters are summarized in Table 1.

Intra- and inter-reader reproducibility

Bland-Altman plots of intra-and inter-reader agreement are shown in Figure 5A and B, respectively. Calculation of Lin's concordance correlation coefficient confirmed a substantial intra-reader agreement with regard to LV volume assessment and myocardial scar amount (range, 0.92 to 0.97); inter-reader agreement for the assessment of LV volumes and scar amount was moderate (range, 0.82 to 0.95, see Table 1).

Inter-study reproducibility

The bias of repeat CMR examinations was found to be minimal for all left-ventricular parameters (Table 2). In addition, calculation of Lin's concordance correlation coefficient resulted in a substantial inter-study agreement for the assessment of LV volumes and scar amount (range, 0.84 to 0.96, see Table 2).

Discussion

The present study validated the use of a clinical 3.0 Tesla MR system for cardiac cine and scar imaging in small animals. Primarily, small rodent imaging is performed on dedicated animal MR systems with field strengths ≥ 4.7 Tesla with gradient and coil systems especially developed for small animal imaging. However, these MR scanner systems are not widely available and

Table 1 Intra- and inter-reader reproducibility in 32 rats

Intra-reader reproducibility of left ventricular measurements in 32 rats							
	Read 1 [mean ± SD]	**Read 2 [mean ± SD]**	**% Bias**	**[95% - CI]**	**Lins's, *Pc***	**[95% - CI]**	**CV**
LVEDV [µl]	453.0 ± 96.6	464.0 ± 113.8	-1.7	[-17.3; 14.0]	0.92	[0.84; 0.96]	0.09
LVESV [µl]	244.4 ± 105.8	250.5 ± 109.3	-2.2	[-25.7; 21.3]	0.97	[0.94; 0.99]	0.1
LVEF [%]	47.9 ± 14.9	47.6 ± 15.2	1.0	[-17.6; 19.5]	0.96	[0.91; 0.98]	0.09
LVEDD [mm]	7.6 ± 0.9	7.8 ± 1.0	-3.3	[-20.2; 13.6]	0.72	[0.52; 0.85]	0.09
LV mass [mg]	306.4 ± 54.8	315.0 ± 57.2	-2.7	[-23.7; 18.2]	0.82	[0.67; 0.91]	0.1
LV scar [µl LV mass]	41.8 ± 27.6	43.2 ± 28.2	-1.2	[-36.9; 34.6]	0.97	[0.94; 0.99]	0.15
LV scar [% LV mass]	14.4 ± 9.4	14.3 ± 9.5	2.1	[29.1; 33.4]	0.97	[0.94; 0.99]	0.15
Inter-reader reproducibility of left ventricular measurements in 32 rats							
	Reader 1 [mean ± SD]	**Reader 2 [mean ± SD]**	**% Bias**	**[95% - CI]**	**Lins's, *Pc***	**[95% - CI]**	**CV**
LVEDV [µl]	453.0 ± 96.6	440.4 ± 105.1	3.3	[-23.5; 30.1]	0.82	[0.66; 0.91]	0.13
LVESV [µl]	244.4 ± 105.8	234.1 ± 108.6	6.2	[-24.0; 36.4]	0.93	[0.89; 0.97]	0.14
LVEF [%]	47.9 ± 14.9	49.5 ± 13.6	-4.8	[-31.6; 21.9]	0.93	[0.87; 0.96]	011.
LVEDD [mm]	7.6 ± 0.9	7.8 ± 1.0	-3.5	[-17.5; 10.5]	0.81	[0.65; 0.90]	0.07
LV mass [mg]	306.4 ± 54.8	313.9 ± 64.0	-1.9	[-50.1; 45.7]	0.83	[0.68; 0.91]	0.11
LV scar [µl LV mass]	41.8 ± 27.6	43.3 ± 28.7	-1.8	[-35.7; 32.1]	0.94	[0.89; 0.97]	0.22
LV scar [% LV mass]	14.4 ± 9.4	14.1 ± 9.5	3.8	[-31.7; 39.2]	0.93	[0.86; 0.97]	0.25

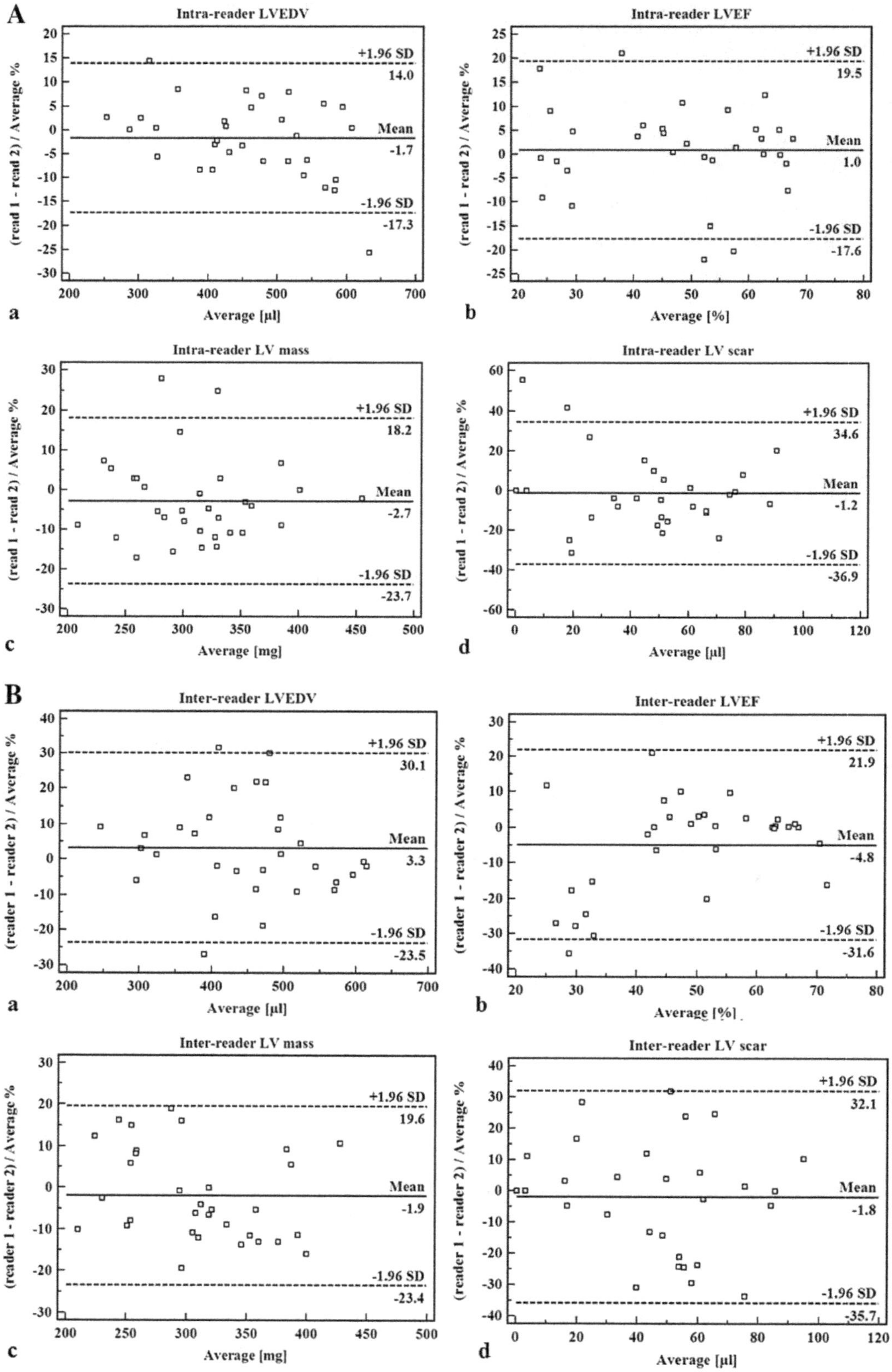

Figure 5 Bland-Altman plots. Intra-reader **(A)** and inter-reader **(B)** agreement for the assessment of **(a)** left ventricular end-diastolic volume, **(b)** left ventricular ejection fraction, **(c)** left ventricular mass, and **(d)** left ventricular scar volume, respectively.

Table 2 Inter-study reproducibility assessed in 6 randomly chosen rats

Inter-study reproducibility of left ventricular measurements in 6 rats							
	Study 1 [mean ± SD]	Study 2 [mean ± SD]	% Bias	[95% - CI]	Lin's *Pc*	[95% - CI]	CV
LVEDV [μl]	524.9 ± 29.4	525.1 ± 39.7	0.1	[-7.6; 7.8]	0.84	[0.39; 0.97]	0.04
LVESV[μl]	296.5 ± 74.3	302.7 ± 79.0	-1.8	[-14.0; 10.4]	0.96	[0.79; 0.99]	0.06
LVEF [%]	43.6 ± 13.8	42.8 ± 12.6	1.0	[-20.8; 22.9]	0.95	[0.71; 0.99]	0.1
LVEDD [mm]	8.4 ± 0.5	8.5 ± 0.5	-1.0	[-7.2; 5.2]	0.85	[0.29; 0.98]	0.03
LV mass [mg]	361.7 ± 127.5	379.8 ± 128.6	-4.6	[-38.2; 29.0]	0.89	[0.42; 0.98]	0.16
LV scar [μl LV mass]	66.6 ± 44.1	69.6 ± 39.6	-6.2	[-43.3; 31.0]	0.94	[0.64; 0.99]	0.22
LV scar [% LV mass]	19.2 ± 8.1	19.5 ± 8.7	-1.6	[-24.2; 21.0]	0.95	[0.72; 0.99]	0.13

beyond that, require expensive investments. To overcome these restrictions, clinical MR systems may have the potential to represent a valuable alternative for accurate assessment of cardiovascular anatomy and function in small rodents. However, several key items need to be considered when performing CMR examinations in small animals: First, robust ECG monitoring is essential to ensure reliably triggered image data acquisition. Second, anaesthesia and animal temperature have to be monitored and maintained throughout the complete CMR examination in particular when aiming at serial examinations. Finally, in order to achieve an optimal signal-to-noise ratio resulting in high quality CMR images, high magnetic field strengths need to be combined with dedicated small animal radiofrequency receiver coils. In the present study, a clinically employed 3.0 Tesla system was introduced for the purpose of small animal imaging. In order to increase image SNR and minimize breathing artefacts, signal averaging was mandatory thereby accepting an increased total scan duration. In addition, for cine imaging a segmented gradient echo sequence was chosen over the commonly used steady-state free precession (SSFP) sequence type since the latter resulted in poor image quality mainly due to flow-/bloodpool-related artifacts with impairment of endocardial visibility (e.g. in the region of mitral inflow/aortic root). However, small animal CMR imaging at 3.0 Tesla proved to be feasible with a success rate of >97%. Recently, Saleh et al. [10] proved that long-term left ventricular remodelling in rat hearts after myocardial infarction can be rapidly and accurately assessed using a clinical 3.0 Tesla System with a dedicated small animal coil and a gradient echo sequence. In addition, quantitative assessment of cardiac volumes, mass and infarct size provided robust results with high inter-study, inter-reader and intra-reader reproducibility. The high reproducibility for the quantification of left-ventricular volumes and mass was in accordance to previously published data by Montet-Abou et al. [17] who investigated nine normal rats with four standard MR fast gradient- echo sequences using a 1.5 Tesla MR system. However, inter-, and intra-reader reproducibility was limited to four rats. Jones et al. [18] investigated 11 rats in an ischemia-reperfusion model and showed similar inter-study (3.3% vs. 4.8%) and intra-study (1.6% vs. 1.0%) reproducibility for the assessment of LVEF.

Accurate depiction of myocardial infarct size in animal models of cardiac diseases is crucial; hence, late enhancement imaging was incorporated in the current study protocol. Recently, Voelkl et al. [12] showed that widely available clinical 1.5 Tesla scanners enable high quality and accurate assessment of infarct size and functional parameters in mice. In our study quantitative analysis of myocardial infarct size demonstrated high inter-study, inter-reader and intra-reader reproducibility. The overall high reproducibility of quantitative CMR measurements may allow for the reliable and accurate assessment of even small treatment effects during serial examinations with the additional benefit of reducing sample size. In general, CMR imaging has been proposed the imaging method of choice to assess treatment effects in clinical and animal studies due to its high accuracy and low inter-study variability [6,16]. Based on the results of the present study conducted with the use of a conventional clinical 3.0 Tesla MR system a more widespread use of CMR imaging in small animal studies can be encouraged. In particular, the combined protocol of functional and morphological imaging of the rat heart is advantageous and can be integrated in pharmacological or interventional treatment studies in small animals.

Limitations

Even though clinical MR scanners are more abundant than dedicated animal MR scanners, they may not always be available for animal studies and/or local rules may prevent their use. Image quality of small animal imaging on clinical scanners is generally restricted by limited shim capabilities which may be addressed by introducing high-order shimming. In addition, for small objects like rats and mice, the noise not only arises from physiological and thermal object noise but is rather dominated by noise from the electronic pathways; hence, a fully digital broadband system with analog to digital signal conversion in the radiofrequency coil may prove beneficial. Taking advantage of such technical improvements may allow for example to use steady-state free precession imaging sequences.

Conclusions

The present study showed that a conventional clinical 3.0 Tesla MR scanner environment can be adapted to achieve high quality functional and morphological cardiac MR imaging of rats in vivo. Measurements of LV functional parameters and scar amount were highly reproducible. Consequently, the performance of therapeutic interventions aiming at the improvement of contractile function and the reduction of myocardial scar amount (e.g. stem cell therapy) may be studied in small animal models using widely available clinical CMR scanners.

Competing interests
The authors declare that they have no competing interests.

Authors' contributions
RM, CJ, IP, BS and KG conceived of the study, participated in its design and coordination and performed the statistical analysis. RM, CJ, RG and IP carried out the imaging studies and drafted the manuscript. RM and TH carried out image analysis. TH and TD carried out animal preparation and experimental setup. All authors read and approved the final manuscript.

Author details
[1]Department of Cardiology, University Hospital Zurich, Rämistrasse 100, 8091, Zurich, Switzerland. [2]Institute for Biomedical Engineering, University and ETH Zurich, Zurich, Switzerland. [3]Institute of Diagnostic and Interventional Radiology, University Hospital Zurich, Zurich, Switzerland. [4]Department of Cardiology, University Hospital RWTH Aachen, Aachen, Germany. [5]Department of Cardiology, German Heart Institute Berlin, Berlin, Germany. [6]Philips Healthcare, Hamburg, Germany.

References

1. Daire JL, Jacob JP, Hyacinthe JN, Croisille P, Montet-Abou K, Richter S, Botsikas D, Lepetit-Coiffe M, Morel D, Vallee JP: **Cine and tagged cardiovascular magnetic resonance imaging in normal rat at 1.5 T: a rest and stress study.** *J Cardiovasc Magn Reson* 2008, **10:**48.
2. Fieno DS, Jaffe WC, Simonetti OP, Judd RM, Finn JP: **TrueFISP: assessment of accuracy for measurement of left ventricular mass in an animal model.** *J Magn Reson Imaging* 2002, **15:**526–531.
3. Goetti R, Kozerke S, Donati OF, Surder D, Stolzmann P, Kaufmann PA, Luscher TF, Corti R, Manka R: **Acute, subacute, and chronic myocardial infarction: quantitative comparison of 2D and 3D late gadolinium enhancement MR imaging.** *Radiology* 2011, **259:**704–711.
4. Kim RJ, Chen EL, Lima JA, Judd RM: **Myocardial Gd-DTPA kinetics determine MRI contrast enhancement and reflect the extent and severity of myocardial injury after acute reperfused infarction.** *Circulation* 1996, **94:**3318–3326.
5. Rehr RB, Malloy CR, Filipchuk NG, Peshock RM: **Left ventricular volumes measured by MR imaging.** *Radiology* 1985, **156:**717–719.
6. Yang Z, Berr SS, Gilson WD, Toufektsian MC, French BA: **Simultaneous evaluation of infarct size and cardiac function in intact mice by contrast-enhanced cardiac magnetic resonance imaging reveals contractile dysfunction in noninfarcted regions early after myocardial infarction.** *Circulation* 2004, **109:**1161–1167.
7. Krombach GA, Saeed M, Higgins CB, Novikov V, Wendland MF: **Contrast-enhanced MR delineation of stunned myocardium with administration of MnCl(2) in rats.** *Radiology* 2004, **230:**183–190.
8. Dietrich T, Hucko T, Bourayou R, Jahnke C, Paetsch I, Atrott K, Stawowy P, Grafe M, Klein C, Schnackenburg B, *et al*: **High resolution magnetic resonance imaging in atherosclerotic mice treated with ezetimibe.** *Int J Cardiovasc Imaging* 2009, **25:**827–836.
9. Vallee JP, Ivancevic MK, Nguyen D, Morel DR, Jaconi M: **Current status of cardiac MRI in small animals.** *MAGMA* 2004, **17:**149–156.
10. Saleh MG, Sharp SK, Alhamud A, Spottiswoode BS, van der Kouwe AJ, Davies NH, Franz T, Meintjes EM: **Long-term left ventricular remodelling in rat model of nonreperfused myocardial infarction: sequential MR imaging using a 3 T clinical scanner.** *J Biomed Biotechnol* 2012, **2012:**504037.
11. Campan M, Lionetti V, Aquaro GD, Forini F, Matteucci M, Vannucci L, Chiuppesi F, Di Cristofano C, Faggioni M, Maioli M, *et al*: **Ferritin as a reporter gene for in vivo tracking of stem cells by 1.5-T cardiac MRI in a rat model of myocardial infarction.** *Am J Physiol Heart Circ Physiol* 2011, **300:**H2238–2250.
12. Voelkl JG, Haubner BJ, Kremser C, Mayr A, Klug G, Loizides A, Muller S, Pachinger O, Schocke M, Metzler B: **Cardiac imaging using clinical 1.5 t MRI scanners in a murine ischemia/reperfusion model.** *J Biomed Biotechnol* 2011, **2011:**185683.
13. Gilson WD, Kraitchman DL: **Cardiac magnetic resonance imaging in small rodents using clinical 1.5 T and 3.0 T scanners.** *Methods* 2007, **43:**35–45.
14. Bland JM, Altman DG: **Statistical methods for assessing agreement between two methods of clinical measurement.** *Lancet* 1986, **1:**307–310.
15. Lin LI: **A concordance correlation coefficient to evaluate reproducibility.** *Biometrics* 1989, **45:**255–268.
16. Grothues F, Smith GC, Moon JC, Bellenger NG, Collins P, Klein HU, Pennell DJ: **Comparison of interstudy reproducibility of cardiovascular magnetic resonance with two-dimensional echocardiography in normal subjects and in patients with heart failure or left ventricular hypertrophy.** *Am J Cardiol* 2002, **90:**29–34.
17. Montet-Abou K, Daire JL, Ivancevic MK, Hyacinthe JN, Nguyen D, Jorge-Costa M, Morel DR, Vallee JP: **Optimization of cardiac cine in the rat on a clinical 1.5-T MR system.** *MAGMA* 2006, **19:**144–151.
18. Jones JR, Mata JF, Yang Z, French BA, Oshinski JN: **Left ventricular remodeling subsequent to reperfused myocardial infarction: evaluation of a rat model using cardiac magnetic resonance imaging.** *J Cardiovasc Magn Reson* 2002, **4:**317–326.

Diffusion-weighted MRI characteristics of the cerebral metastasis to brain boundary predicts patient outcomes

Rasheed Zakaria[1,2,6*], Kumar Das[3], Mark Radon[3], Maneesh Bhojak[3], Philip R Rudland[2], Vanessa Sluming[4] and Michael D Jenkinson[1,5]

Abstract

Background: Diffusion-weighted MRI (DWI) has been used in neurosurgical practice mainly to distinguish cerebral metastases from abscess and glioma. There is evidence from other solid organ cancers and metastases that DWI may be used as a biomarker of prognosis and treatment response. We therefore investigated DWI characteristics of cerebral metastases and their peritumoral region recorded pre-operatively and related these to patient outcomes.

Methods: Retrospective analysis of 76 cases operated upon at a single institution with DWI performed pre-operatively at 1.5T. Maps of apparent diffusion coefficient (ADC) were generated using standard protocols. Readings were taken from the tumor, peritumoral region and across the brain-tumor interface. Patient outcomes were overall survival and time to local recurrence.

Results: A minimum ADC greater than 919.4×10^{-6} mm^2/s within a metastasis predicted longer overall survival regardless of adjuvant therapies. This was not simply due to differences between the types of primary cancer because the effect was observed even in a subgroup of 36 patients with the same primary, non-small cell lung cancer. The change in diffusion across the tumor border and into peritumoral brain was measured by the "ADC transition coefficient" or ATC and this was more strongly predictive than ADC readings alone. Metastases with a sharp change in diffusion across their border (ATC >0.279) showed shorter overall survival compared to those with a more diffuse edge. The ATC was the only imaging measurement which independently predicted overall survival in multivariate analysis (hazard ratio 0.54, 95% CI 0.3 – 0.97, p = 0.04).

Conclusions: DWI demonstrates changes in the tumor, across the tumor edge and in the peritumoral region which may not be visible on conventional MRI and this may be useful in predicting patient outcomes for operated cerebral metastases.

Keywords: Cerebral metastasis, Brain neoplasms, Secondary, Neoplasm invasiveness, Diffusion-weighted imaging, Apparent diffusion coefficient, MRI

Background

Cerebral metastases are an increasingly common problem with an incidence ten times that of primary brain tumors and the diagnosis is often made by general radiologists [1,2]. Traditionally MRI has been used for assessing the site and number of metastases, planning for surgery or radiosurgery and assessing the response to therapy [3,4]. Newer MRI techniques have been applied to help distinguish solitary cerebral metastases from mimics such as high grade glioma or abscess. One common example is by measuring the ADC of the lesion but these readings have more recently been suggested to have some *prognostic* value as well as diagnostic [5,6]. When comparing cerebral metastases to glioma considerable attention has focused on the peritumoral region around the lesion [7-14]. A number of metrics from DWI including ADC values have been directly measured

* Correspondence: rzakaria@nhs.net
[1]Department of Neurosurgery, The Walton Centre NHS Foundation Trust, Liverpool, UK
[2]Institute of Integrative Biology, University of Liverpool, Liverpool, UK
Full list of author information is available at the end of the article

in this region and the "normal" range of values for a metastasis determined [15]. The interaction of cerebral metastases and the surrounding brain tissue would be expected to be crucial to the development of therapies aimed at preventing further spread and invasion. Work on different methods of invasion - either co-opting existing blood vessels or inducing new blood vessel formation - has already led to anti-angiogenesis drugs for certain cerebral metastases [16,17]. Furthermore, the degree of invasion of metastases may affect the margin used in existing treatments such as surgery and radiosurgery. Despite this potential clinical importance little has been done to investigate the invasiveness of cerebral metastases using MRI and nobody has compared the tumor and peritumoral ADC readings *within* a group of metastases. We therefore examined the MRI characteristics of the tumor, tumor boundary and peritumoral region for a series of patients with cerebral metastases who had undergone pre-operative MRI with DWI followed by surgery. We investigate whether patient outcomes such as survival and recurrence may be predicted by different DWI metrics.

Methods

Patients

Patients with a diagnosis of cerebral metastasis were identified from a histopathology archive spanning the period 2007 – 2012 at a single institution. Records were searched and cases with a diffusion-weighted MRI scan of the brain prior to first neurosurgical intervention were selected. Recursive Partitioning Analysis (RPA) [18] class and Graded Prognostic Assessment (GPA) [19] score were determined; these are validated predictive measures in cerebral metastasis patients and are based on information such as control of the primary cancer, extra-cranial metastases, number of metastases and general health or "performance status" of the patient. Post-operative clinical course and oncology care including administration of whole brain radiotherapy (WBRT) or the use of adjuvant systemic chemotherapy were recorded from tumor board and patient notes as these were potential confounding factors. This study was conducted in accordance with the principles of the declaration of Helsinki and ethical approval was granted as an internal project within the institution's research tissue bank (National Research Ethics Service # 11/WNo03/2).

Histological analysis

All cases had been reviewed by a consultant neuropathologist in the course of routine clinical care. A histological diagnosis of metastasis was made and primary tumor type suggested by review of H & E sections, tumor specific immuno-histo-cytochemistry and clinical correlation. Where original material was available an additional automated assessment of cellularity was then made "blind" to the clinical and imaging data. Five separate 200× magnification fields were photographed avoiding gross haemorrhage or necrotic material on the H & E slide. Using Image J software (U. S. National Institutes of Health, Bethesda, Maryland, USA 2007-2012) with no additional plugins the percentage nuclear area in each field was determined using the measure function and a mean taken. A second independent observer, a cellular pathology researcher of 30 years' experience then repeated this analysis manually using a grid and microscopy.

MRI acquisition and analysis

All patients had undergone preoperative MRI brain scans on different whole body systems at 1.5T with a single channel head coil at local institutions before transfer to the Regional Neuroscience Centre (of the 76 cases: 11 on GE Signa HD, 6 on a GE Discovery, 43 on Philips Achieva and 16 on a Siemens Avanto). All patients had received at least 24-48 hours of dexamethasone treatment (of at least 4mg twice daily orally) prior to MR imaging. The imaging included DWI using one acquisition over 90 seconds through single-shot echo planar imaging with two b values of 0 and 1000 second/mm^2 in all cases. MR parameters were similar between scanners and in the following range: slice thickness 6mm for all, TR 2515 - 3513 msec, TE 71-94 msec. Trace-weighted imaging and ADC trace maps were calculated and subsequent readings taken using the post processing software package GE FuncTool version 4.5.5 (General Electric Co., Maryland, USA). All patients had also undergone a fast spoiled gradient echo (FSPGR) or equivalent sequence with gadolinium contrast, again variable between institutions but most commonly TR 25 msec, TE 6.1 msec, flip angle 20 degrees.

Conventional MRI measures were taken on this post-contrast T1-weighted sequence including the number of lesions, maximum diameter on axial slices and volume (using three orthogonal measurements of diameter). The largest, operated metastasis only was assessed for those with multiple lesions (note that in general the cases with more than one metastasis included a dominant lesion with only small additional lesions). A number of different assessments of diffusion were made for each metastasis from the DWI scan and resulting ADC map. Figure 1 demonstrates the position of regions of interest (ROI) for recording these different ADC metrics. We have previously reported excellent intra and inter-observer reliability taking the readings below on this software for 12 of the 76 patients described, with one observer a clinical research fellow in neurosurgery and the second a clinician of 10 years specialised training in neuroradiology [20].

- **ADCmin**: The axial slice with the largest area of tumor was identified and a freehand ROI created using the tumor border on postcontrast T1-weighted

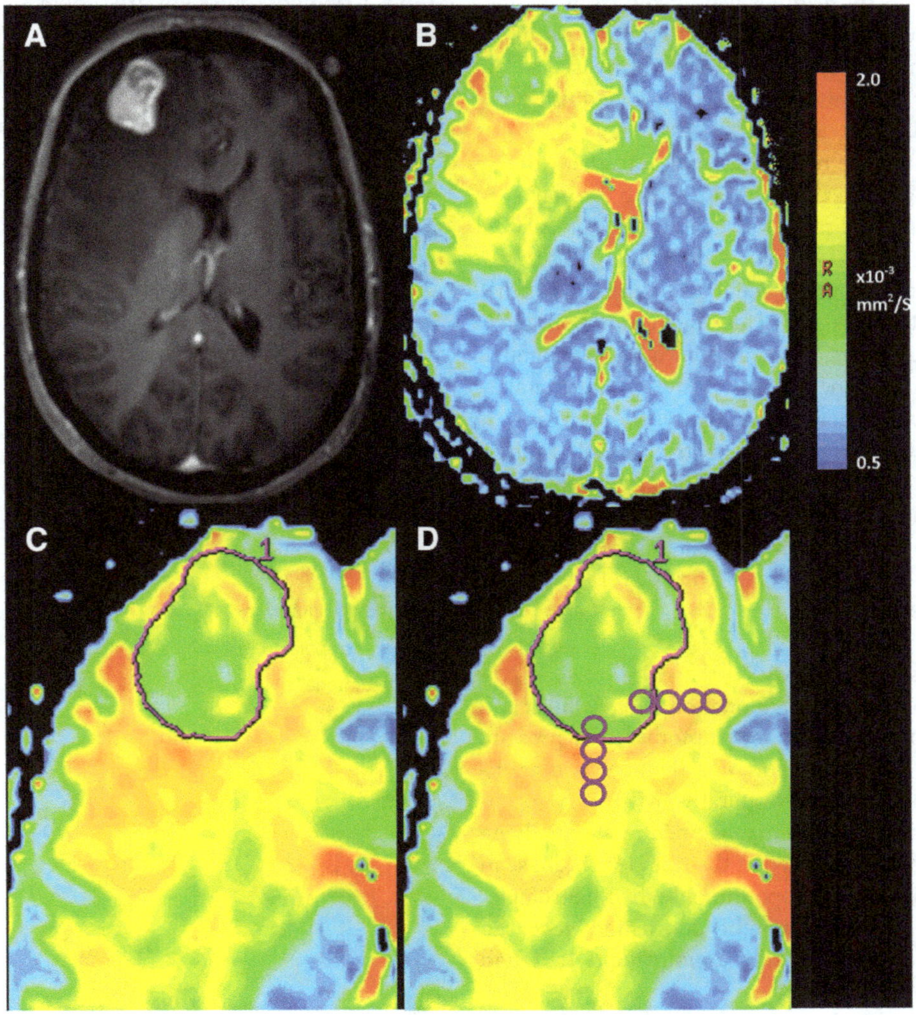

Figure 1 Measurement of ADC metrics from brain metastases on diffusion-weighted MRI scans. A patient with a history of lung adenocarcinoma presents with headache and focal neurological deficit. **A.** Postcontrast T1-weighted sequence demonstrates a right frontal lesion, which was confirmed as a metastasis after excision. **B.** An ADC map is generated from B = 0.1000 images using post processing software. On this color map, blue areas represent low ADC and red higher ADC. **C.** A freehand region of interest is traced around the tumor border using the postcontrast T1-weighted sequence as reference on the axial slice with the largest tumor area and those immediately above and below. The ADCmin is the lowest bin of a histogram of ADC values for all pixels contained within this ROI, averaged over these three slices. Three ROI are placed within the tumor on the axial slice with the largest area, avoiding necrosis, haemorrhage, cyst and the mean taken to give ADCmean. **D.** To assess change of ADC across the tumor border, four ROI are placed starting just inside the tumor border and extending out into the peritumoral region. The slope of the four ADC values is taken as the "ADC transition coefficient" or ATC. This is repeated in 3 orthogonal directions, avoiding structures such as ventricle or falx and then repeated on two slices above and below, with the ATC being the mean of the 9 readings.

sequence. This was repeated on the slices immediately above and below using the same method. The software then gives the maximum and minimum reading for the given ROI and the mean of the three minimum values across the three slices was used.

- **ADCmean**: Three to five circular ROIs of 50 mm^2 were placed within the borders of the tumor on each axial slice, avoiding areas of cyst, necrosis or haemorrhage. A number of metastases show haemorrhage and the T1-, T2- weighted and b0 sequence were all assessed for evidence of intratumoral bleeding. Cases were also excluded at this stage if >50% of the tumor was affected by haemorrhage.
- **Peritumoral region**: The "peritumoral region" was taken to be the extent of signal abnormality on the T2-weighted sequence and "near" as <1 cm from the tumor edge (as assessed by the co-registered post-contrast T1-weighted sequence) versus "far" as ≥1 cm from the edge. Readings of the near (ADCnear) and far (ADCfar) peritumoral region were taken using three circular 50 mm^2 ROIs on up to three on contiguous slices.

- Up to four control readings were taken from the unaffected contralateral white matter and a mean obtained. The above readings were normalised to this in order to minimise differences in acquisition parameters used at different institutions.
- **ATC**: To assess the metastasis-brain interface, the gradient of change of the ADC which we have called the "ADC Transition Coefficient" or ATC was calculated. As previously described [21] this involves placing four adjacent ROI (area: 22 mm^2) in a line with the first inside the tumor boundary and the rest in brain. This was done along orthogonal trajectories across the anterior, posterior and lateral tumor tumor borders (avoiding cysts, necrosis and anatomical boundaries: ventricle, skull vault, cortex, falx cerebri). The gradient of a linear regression line (which provided the best fit) through the four ADC values of the four ROI was derived and all the trajectories averaged to generate the ATC.

Table 1 Demographics and treatment summary for the series (76 patients)

Age at diagnosis/years (mean & range)	**60.6 (35.9 – 81.4)**	
Gender	**36 male : 40 female**	
Size of operated lesion	27 (9 – 70)	Diameter/mm
(Median & range)	8.9 (0.3 – 130)	Volume/cc
Disease information	Number	%
Primary cancer type		
Non-small cell lung	36	47.4
Small cell lung	6	7.9
Breast	10	13.7
Melanoma	5	6.6
Gastrointestinal	5	6.6
Urogenital	4	5.3
Ovarian	4	5.3
Squamous cell tonsil	1	1.3
Unknown primary	5	6.6
Location of operated lesion		
Supratentorial	64	84.2
Infratentorial	12	15.8
Number of brain mets		
Solitary	56	73.7
2 lesions	11	14.5
>2 lesions	9	11.8
RPA class		
I	19	25
II	51	67.1
III	6	7.9
GPA score		
<1.0	6	7.9
1.5-2	20	26.3
2.5-3.0	39	51.3
>3.0	11	14.5
Neurosurgery		
Gross total resection	67	88.2
Partial resection/Biopsy	9	11.8
Adjuvant chemotherapy for systemic cancer	45	59.2
Whole brain radiotherapy after neurosurgery (30 Gy/5# as standard)	56	73.7

Follow up & statistical methods

Patients were followed up in regional oncology clinics and repeat MRI brain taken only if symptoms were present. Local recurrence or progression was defined as demonstrable brain disease on a post-operative MRI with appropriate clinical correlation and management; patients dying before that point were censored at the last clear brain scan (CT or MRI) or last clinical appointment when neurologically well. Patients who could not be confirmed deceased were censored at the last clinic appointment that had been recorded.

Data were analysed and graphs generated using Statistica version 6 (StatSoft, Inc. 2003) and SPSS version 20.0 (IBM co., 2011). For analysis of survival, the Kaplan-Meier product limit method was used and life tables with survival curves plotted. Log rank tests were applied to detect differences between paired groups and Wilcoxon modification (the Breslow chi square test) used in cases where hazard did not appear to be proportional. For multivariate analysis Cox regression was used. Standard tests were used for comparisons of means and analysis of variance and descriptive statistics, distributions were plotted for all variables to check assumptions. The level of significance was set at 95% to reject the null hypothesis and all p-values and confidence intervals are stated in the Results section.

Results

Clinical outcomes

The demographic details of the cohort of 76 patients are summarised in Table 1. The median survival from first diagnosis of cerebral metastasis to death was 9.3 months (range 0.9 – 34.3 months). 11 cases were censored, mainly due to death by other causes or loss of follow up suggesting the length of the follow up period was adequate. It was not appropriate to analyse local recurrence where the tumor was not fully resected; in the 66 cases where gross total resection was performed, local recurrence occurred in 16 patients (24%) at a median of 17.7 months from presentation (95% CI 10.9 – 24.6). The factors associated with overall and progression free survival, including standard MRI measures such as tumor size, volume and number, are summarised in Table 2.

ADC readings from the metastases & tumor cellularity

The median ADCmean for cerebral metastases in this series was 1148.1 × 10^{-6} mm^2/s and the median ADCmin was 919.4 × 10^{-6} mm^2/s. There were significant differences in ADC between cerebral metastases from different primary cancers by one-way ANOVA ($F = 2.797$, $p = 0.025$). On post hoc comparison, this was seen to be because metastases from the so-called "poorly differentiated" cancers such as melanoma (n = 5) and small cell lung carcinoma (n = 6) had a lower ADC compared to the metastases from carcinomas such as breast (n = 10), ovarian (n = 4) and colorectal (n = 4), as shown in Figure 2.

Tissue was only available for 16 of 76 cases. Cellularity assessment by ImageJ software as compared to pathologist assessment appeared to be valid with consistency between the two observers (intraclass correlation coefficient = 0.61, $p < 0.05$). The mean cellularity was negatively correlated with both the ADCmin and the ADCmean and could be fitted to either of these with a simple linear regression model which was highly significant (for ADCmin, $F = 7.99$, $p = 0.013$ and for ADCmean $F = 5.56$, $p = 0.033$). ATC was strongly correlated with cellularity as shown in Figure 3 and was predicted by it using a simple linear regression model ($F = 9.84$, $p = 0.007$).

Relation of tumor ADC to patient outcomes

For survival analysis, the patients were grouped based on each of the DWI characteristics of their cerebral metastases and the two groups compared. The cases having a higher than median ADCmin (>919.4 × 10^{-6} mm^2/s) showed a longer overall survival, median 9.7 months (95% CI: 8.5 – 11.0) versus those with a lower ADCmin (median survival 6.2 months, 95% CI: 3.7 – 8.8, Breslow Chi square 3.87, $p = 0.049$). There was no difference in the proportion of patients receiving WBRT in the high versus the low ADCmin groups that would confound the effect on survival (Chi square = 3.49, $p = 0.062$). The effect was also seen if the median ADCmean was used as the cutoff to define the two groups but was not statistically significant: OS 9.7 months, 95% CI 7.9 – 11.5 for patients with metastases having a higher ADCmean (>1148.1 × 10^{-6} mm^2/s) versus 6.7 months for lower ADCmean, 95% CI 4.9 – 8.5, Breslow Chi square = 2.83, $p = 0.093$.

Regarding local control, the median progression free survival was 11.3 months (95% 5.8 – 16.8) in those cases with a low ADCmean reading versus 18.4 months (95% CI 11.6 – 25.1) in those with a high ADCmean (Log rank test, Chi Square 4.263, $p = 0.039$). This is illustrated in Figure 4. This effect was also seen when the median ADCmin was used as the cutoff to define the two groups but did not reach statistical significance (high ADCmin, progression free survival 18.4 months, 95% CI 13.2 – 23.6 versus low ADCmin, progression free survival 11.3 months, 95% CI 8.4 – 14.3, Log rank = 2.93, $p = 0.087$).

Non-small cell lung cancer metastases represented the largest group of cases from a single primary cancer (although further detail was not known, even within this group there would be expected to be subdivisions such as adenocarcinoma and squamous cell carcinoma; it is at least more uniform than any previous analysis which includes multiple different primary sites) and this subgroup of 36 cases was therefore analysed separately in order to confirm that the ADC has value in and of itself as a prognostic marker not simply as a surrogate of the primary tumor type. Overall survival was significantly longer for non-small cell lung cancer cases with a high tumor ADCmin at 9.7 months (CI 6.7 – 12.6) versus 5.3 months (CI 2.2 – 8.5) for those with low ADCmin, Log rank Chi square = 4.008, $p = 0.045$. The same effect was observed and was significant using median ADCmean as the cutoff because higher ADC group had median OS 10.5months (CI 7.7 – 13.2) versus 5.8 months, (CI 3.2 – 8.4) for low ADC group, Log rank = 4.135, $p = 0.042$.

ADC changes at the brain-metastasis interface

The change in diffusion across the brain-metastasis interface might be expected to relate to changes at the cellular level and hence even reflect tumor-stroma interactions. We have previously devised and applied a measure of the changing ADC at the metastasis-brain boundary, called the "ADC transition coefficient" or ATC. This could be calculated for 70 cases (as described in the Methods there needs to be a boundary to surrounding tissue to measure and calculate a reading) and found the ATC to have a median value of 0.279 (range 0.063 - 0.453). The ATC showed no relationship to the primary cancer type on one-way ANOVA (df 11, $F = 0.348$, $p = 0.9$) and weak negative correlation with ADCmean and ADCmin (Pearson correlation coefficient -0.39 and -0.33 respectively, $p > 0.05$) suggesting it was measuring a different feature rather than just acting as a surrogate of the other ADC characteristics or the primary cancer.

The group was divided into two based on the ATC, and those patients with a metastasis showing high ATC (> median) and therefore a *sharp* boundary on the ADC map had a shorter overall survival 6.8 months (95% CI 5.3 – 8.4) as compared to those with a low ATC and hence diffuse boundary on ADC map (11.2 months, 95% CI 8.3 – 14.0, Log rank Chi-Square = 4.19, $p = 0.041$). This is illustrated more clearly in the conventional MRI scans and accompanying ADC maps in Figure 5. There was also a tendency to earlier local recurrence in high ATC cases versus low ATC but this was not statistically significant (shown in Table 2).

Table 2 Clinical and radiological factors associated with survival and progression

Factor	Overall survival median/months	95% CI	Significance on univariate analysis	Progression free survival median/months	95% CI	Significance on univariate analysis
GPA score						
< 1.0	5.3	0.4 – 10.2	0.306	Not reached		0.936
1.5-2	6.8	0 – 14.0		18.4	-	
2.5-3.0	9.3	8.0 – 10.6		17.8	6.1 – 29.4	
> 3.0	9.8	7.8 – 11.7		13.1	9.0 – 17.2	
RPA class						
I	14.0	6.1 – 22.0	0.030*	17.7	14.6 – 20.9	0.636
II	8.4	5.1 – 11.8		13.1	9.7 – 16.6	
III	2.0	0 – 6.2		Not reached		
Primary cancer						(too many censored cases in each category for analysis)
Lung non-small cell	9.2	2.0 – 19.8	0.061	Not reached		
Lung small cell	4.5	1.0 – 28.9		10.5	-	
Breast	10.4	0.9 – 21.2		9.2	5.6 – 12.9	
Colorectal	6.8	5.3 – 12.3		Not reached		
Melanoma	11.5	2.4 – 14.7		7.3	4.9 – 9.7	
Urological	4.0	1.1 – 9.6		Not reached		
Ovarian	11.2	4.7 – 30		17.8	-	
Unknown	5.6	1.5 – 22.8		18.4	-	
Location						
Supratentorial	9.6	8.2 – 11.1	0.070	17.7	10.8 – 24.6	0.872
Infratentorial	4.4	0 – 10.1		Not reached		
Surgery						
Biopsy	5.9	0 – 16.4	0.091			
Resection	9.6	8.1 – 11.0				
Adjuvant whole brain radiotherapy						
Yes	10.5	8.9 - 12	0.000*	17.7	10.9 – 24.6	0.000*
No	2.4	1.5 – 3.3		Not reached		
Adjuvant chemotherapy						
Yes	10.5	8.2 – 12.7	0.001*	15.7	10.7 – 20.6	0.240
No	5.3	3.0 – 7.6		Not reached		
Diffusion MR metrics						
ADCmin > 919 × 10^{-6} mm^2/s	9.7	8.5 – 11.0	0.049*	18.4	13.2 – 23.6	0.087
ADCmin < 919 × 10^{-6} mm^2/s	6.2	3.7 – 8.8		11.3	8.4 – 14.3	
ADCmean > 1148 × 10^{-6} mm^2/s	9.7	7.9 – 11.5	0.093	18.4	11.6 – 25.1	0.039*
ADCmean < 1148 × 10^{-6} mm^2/s	6.7	4.9 – 8.5		11.3	5.8 – 16.8	
ATC > 0.279	6.8	5.3 – 8.4	0.041*	11.3	8.2 – 14.4	0.072
ATC < 0.279	11.2	8.3 – 14.0		Not reached		
Standard MRI measures						
Diameter > 30 mm	6.7	2.4 – 11.0	0.246	13.1	9.7 – 16.6	0.551
Diameter < 30 mm	9.6	8.8 – 10.4		17.8	14.7 – 20.1	
Volume > 8.9 cc	6.7	1.9 – 11.5	0.077	13.1	9.2 – 17.1	0.158
Volume < 8.9 cc	9.6	8.8 – 10.3		17.8	13.7 – 21.8	

Table 2 Clinical and radiological factors associated with survival and progression *(Continued)*

Solitary	8.42	5.3 – 11.5	0.101	15.7	10.3 – 21.0	0.673
2 lesions	14.1	10.7- 17.6		11.3	0.85 – 21.8	
> 2 lesions	6.1	5.1 – 12.2		Not reached		

Log rank tests were applied to detect differences between categories with Wilcoxon modification (the Breslow chi square test) in cases where hazard did not appear to be proportional. In all comparisons *indicates $p < 0.05$.

ADC readings in the peritumoral region

Initially we did not find a large variability in the ADC around a given metastasis and for the 76 cases together, the mean "near" peritumoral ADC was 2028.4 × 10^{-6} mm^2/s which did not differ significantly from the mean "far" peritumoral ADC of 1994.9 × 10^{-6} mm^2/s. There was no significant variation of either variable by primary cancer type on one-way ANOVA. There was also no significant differences in patient outcomes (overall survival, local recurrence) when the cohort was divided into two "high" and "low" groups by either near peritumoral ADC, far peritumoral ADC or near:far ADC ratio and actuarial survival analysis performed.

When visually inspecting the ADC maps for the 76 cases, however, it appeared that for a minority of metastases, in particular those from melanoma primaries, diffusion *did* vary greatly between the near and far peritumoral regions. The values of ADC at each point going out from the tumor towards normal white matter were plotted for illustrative purposes to show the "ADC signature" for that type of metastasis and an example of this is given in Figure 6. It was relevant to directly compare such patterns of ADC change in two types of cancer known to show differing mechanisms of brain invasion, as outlined in Discussion. The ratio of the near and far ADC values were therefore calculated for metastases of melanoma and non-small cell

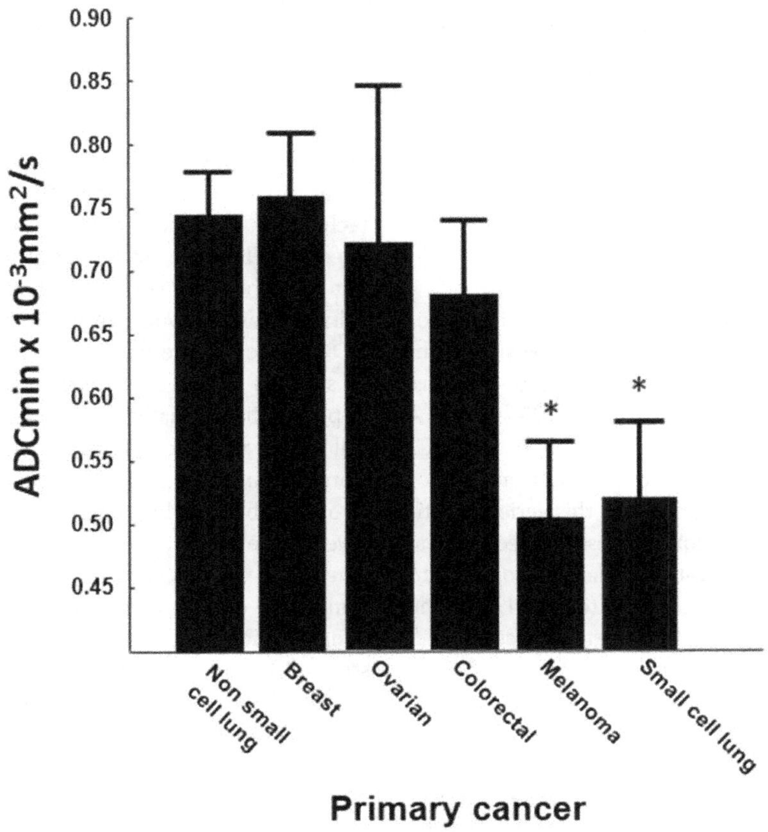

Figure 2 ADC values of 76 brain metastases by primary cancer of origin. The mean ADCmin value for each primary cancer type is shown +/- standard error and *indicates significant difference from the group at $p < 0.05$ by independent student t-test. All histological diagnoses were confirmed by neuropathology assessment after biopsy or resection and correlation with clinical data.

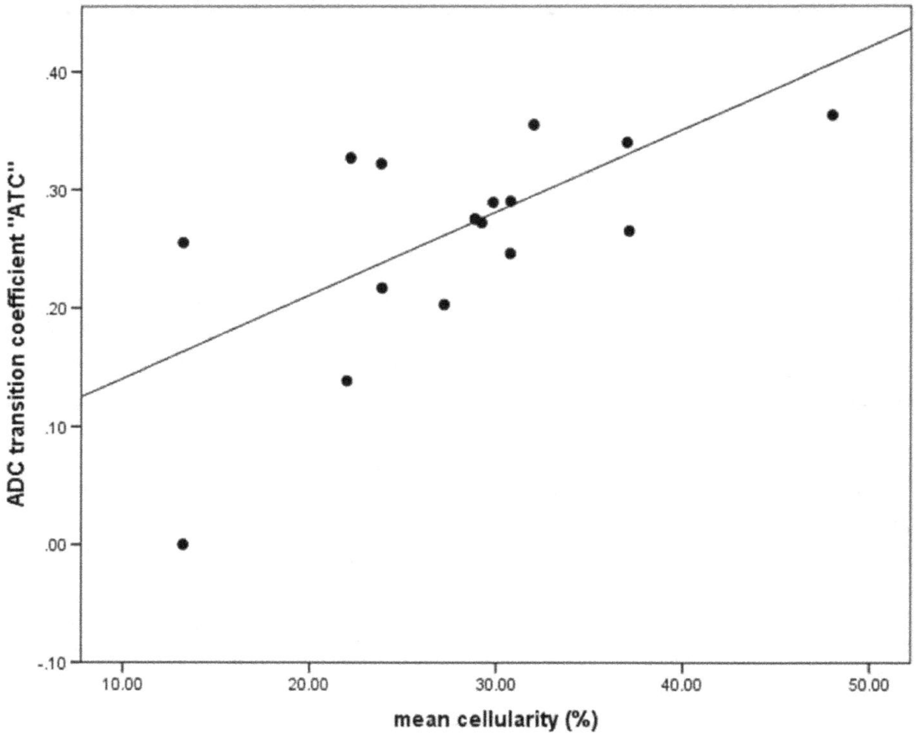

Figure 3 The gradient in change of ADC across the tumor border on preoperative DWI for brain metastases, called the ATC (see Methods) was strongly predictive of the cellularity, as shown in the scatterplot above. Cellularity was assessed in a semi-automated fashion using ImageJ software from five different high power fields and ATC measured as shown in Figure 1. The line shows a simple linear regression model which was highly significant (ATC = 0.007* mean cellularity + 0.07, ANOVA $F = 9.84$, $p < 0.001$).

lung cancer and it was seen that for melanoma metastases this ratio was significantly higher (independent 2-tailed t test = 2.259, df 36, $p = 0.03$).

Multivariate analysis

A Cox regression model was generated using the radiological and non-radiological factors found to be significant discriminators of overall survival in univariate analysis. Only post-operative WBRT (hazard ratio 3.1, 95% CI 1.5 – 6.8, p =0.004) and low ATC (hazard ratio 0.54, 95% CI 0.3 – 0.97, $p = 0.04$) were found to be significantly associated with prolonged overall survival in this series. Multivariate analysis was attempted for progression free survival however modelling was inaccurate with large errors due to the high proportion of censored data (only 24% of the group or 16 cases developed local recurrence, as stated).

Discussion

The value of tumor ADC in cerebral metastases

This is the largest examination of diffusion-weighted MRI and cerebral metastases to date. The numerical values for tumor ADC are in line with previous investigations of cerebral metastases which would be expected given the standard methods and protocols used for imaging and analysis [6,7,10,13,14,22,23]. We used a variety of methods of taking measurements from the ADC maps so as not to miss an effect due to our measurement technique. We have confirmed that ADC varies between cerebral metastases from different primary cancers but like others not sufficiently to distinguish the individual primary cancer type [24,25]. This may be because the ADC reflects more general characteristics like cellularity. In support of this, ADC values were lower for the group of poorly differentiated metastases of melanoma and small cell lung cancer compared to the group of metastases from carcinomas (including breast and colorectal). We also corroborate the suggestion that tumor cellularity is inversely related to tumor ADC for a sample of our cases where tissue was available, whether measured by the minimum or the mean ADC. This is logical as more densely packed cells would broadly be expected to restrict diffusion, with the caveat that this coarse method of calculating ADC maps does not reflect the more subtle distinctions between intra and extracellular diffusion that others have derived using more advanced models in animals [26,27]. However it has also been shown in cerebral metastases *post mortem* that a dense extracellular matrix correlates with low ADC, similarly suggesting a role for the tumor-stroma interaction we discuss later in human cases [6].

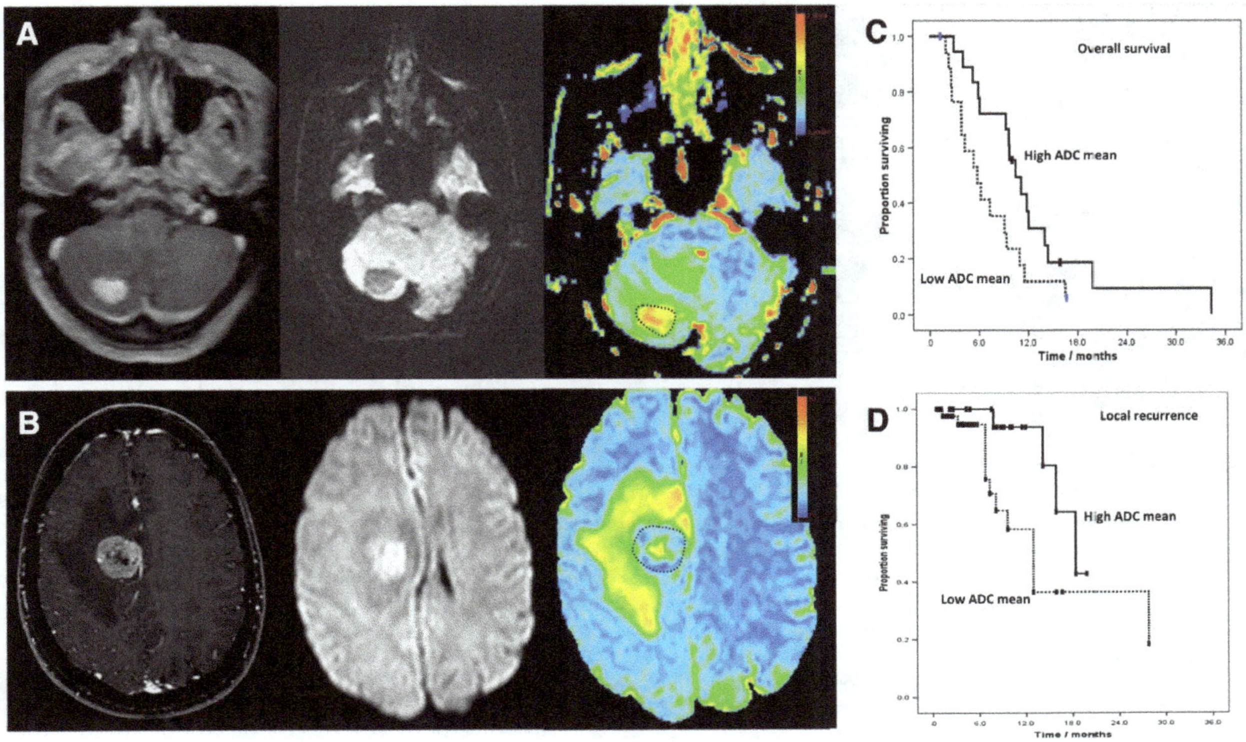

Figure 4 ADC of the metastasis predicts subsequent patient outcomes. Cases such as that in **A**. an enhancing lesion with hypo-intense DWI signal and higher than median ADC were compared to those such as **B**. an enhancing lesion but with hyper-intense DWI signal and corresponding low readings on ADC map. **C**. The largest group of metastases (n = 36) from a single primary - lung non-small cell carcinoma – were stratified into two groups by these readings of tumor ADC. Overall survival was significantly longer for cases with a high tumor ADCmean (10.5 months, CI 7.7 – 13.2) versus a low tumor ADCmean (5.8 months, CI 3.2 – 8.4, Log rank = 4.135, p = 0.042). **D**. For the 66 cases where gross total resection was performed, local recurrence in the brain occurred in 16. Metastases with a higher ADC showed significantly longer progression free survival, 18.4 months (95% CI 11.6 – 25.1) versus 11.3 months (95% 5.8 – 16.8) in those with a low ADCmean (Log rank test, Chi Square 4.263, p = 0.039).

Our survival analyses generally support the finding of this smaller study [6] that the pre-operative mean ADC of a cerebral metastasis is correlated with subsequent overall patient survival and we have now demonstrated this for a single tissue type; non-small cell lung carcinoma. We did not find that this effect persists in multivariate analysis. This may be due to including oligometastatic disease in this series but it seemed reasonable to include such cases as they all had a single larger, dominant lesion and we included the number of lesions as a confounding factor as it forms part of the GPA score. These findings that ADC predicts prognosis are in keeping with a number of reports from other brain tumors where DWI has been applied to predict stage and prognosis [28-30] as well as other organ systems such as renal, rectal, head and neck or cervical tumors [31-35]. In our series, in addition to whole brain radiotherapy - which is a treatment – it was only the *change* in diffusion across the tumor boundary which we call the ADC transition coefficient (ATC) that independently predicted the overall survival in multivariate analysis despite all other clinical factors. Why should this be?

The brain-metastasis interface

We have shown that changes in ADC across the brain-metastasis interface can be used to define the "sharpness" of this boundary, yielding additional information compared to assessing the boundary on postcontrast T1-weighted sequences alone. Rather than a low ATC and diffuse boundary on ADC map being associated with poor survival - as one might expect if this simply represented a more infiltrative pattern of growth - the reverse was true. A high ATC may in fact reflect high cellularity at the leading edge of the metastasis and hence greater tendency to recur locally. In support of this, the ATC was strongly linearly related to tumor cellularity in a sample of cases where tissue was available. One might predict that these cases may benefit from more aggressive local adjuvant treatments, such as wider surgical margins or radiosurgery "boost" to the cavity. Previous work on the interface between cerebral metastases and the surrounding brain has been conducted using histological methods on surgically resected or *post mortem* specimens [36-38] and this has certainly suggested that there are different patterns and depths of invasion, even if this has not been related to clinical outcomes. Furthermore,

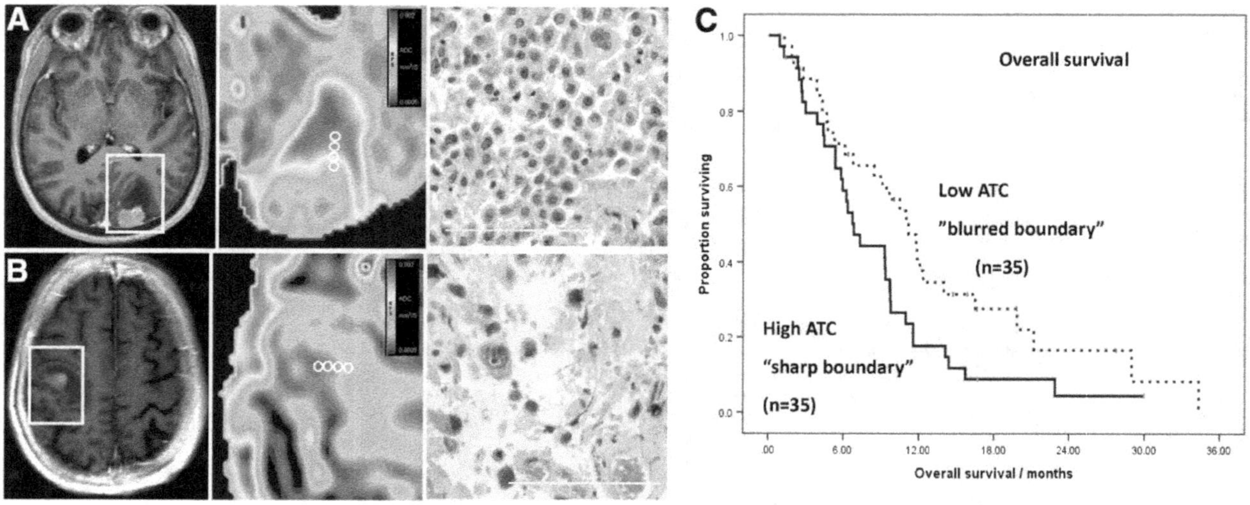

Figure 5 Analysing the brain-metastasis interface. Metastases could be stratified by the sharpness of the tumor border on ADC maps. Panel **A**. demonstrates a lesion with a high ATC or "ADC transition coefficient" implying a sharp border. This type of metastasis tended to have a high cellularity (H & E section x200). Panel **B**. demonstrates a case which looks superficially similar on postcontrast T1-weighted sequence but actually has a much more diffuse border on the ADC map and hence a low ATC, with lower cellularity. **C**. These metastases differ in their outcomes and the cases with a high ATC (> median) and therefore a sharp boundary had a shorter overall survival 6.8 months (95% CI 5.3 – 8.4) as compared to those with a low ATC and hence diffuse boundary (11.2 months, 95% CI 8.3 – 14.0, Log rank Chi-Square = 4.19, p = 0.041). This effect was significant even in multivariate analysis incorporating traditional clinical predictors.

it has been shown that wider resection margins may improve clinical survival [39] and that ADC changes across the border of another brain tumor - oligodendroglioma - may predict growth pattern and aggressiveness [21]. Novel therapies acting at the brain-metastasis interface are being developed [40], therefore more accurate non-invasive, radiological methods may be needed to assess the degree of invasion of cerebral metastases and characterise the tumor boundary changes seen at diffusion-weighted MRI.

The peritumoral region

The MRI characteristics of the peritumoral region of cerebral metastases have previously been examined only in order to distinguish these tumors from glioma and abscess [15,41,42]. In this context the contrast enhancing margin has been taken as the reference and the near peritumoral region has been taken as being within 1 cm of this edge. We have shown that for some metastases the ADC varies considerably from the core of the tumor, toward the leading edge and out into both the near and far peritumoral regions. It is known that the extent of T2-weighted oedema (over 1 cm in width from the tumor edge +/- midline shift) may be a prognostic factor [43] and the different peritumoral ADC values in different metastases may be due to differences in the intensity of peritumoral oedema and/or underlying vascular permeability due to different patterns of infiltration. Melanoma metastases, for example, showed a significantly higher near:far peritumoral ADC ratio than non-small cell lung cancer metastases in this study. These tumors are known to show different patterns of growth [16]; melanoma metastases co-opt existing vessels whereas lung adenocarcinoma (the most common non-small cell lung cancer) stimulates neoangiogenesis and the pattern of peritumoral ADC changes might reflect this. In animal models peritumoral ADC changes are seen *before* postcontrast T1-weighted enhancement as micro-metastasis formation and multiplication occurs [44]. Tissue samples with paired radiological data would be needed to confirm what the correlate of these ADC changes are in humans, however it is unlikely that one would be practically able to gather tissue from deep within the region of peritumoral oedema around a metastasis as has been done for glioma [45]. The brain-metastasis boundary is therefore a more fruitful area to investigate in the first instance. One could ask what the biological differences in pattern of infiltration, vascularity, protein expression and inflammatory response are around metastases with a sharp versus a diffuse ADC border and therefore could the ATC or similar measures of diffusion change be used as a surrogate of such biological activity.

Limitations and future directions

A prospective study with image guided sampling in the course of routine resection would provide matched MRI and tissue data within and around cerebral metastases (as has been done with glioma and in animal models [44]) and should confirm the underlying biological changes which account for the ADC patterns seen. This was a

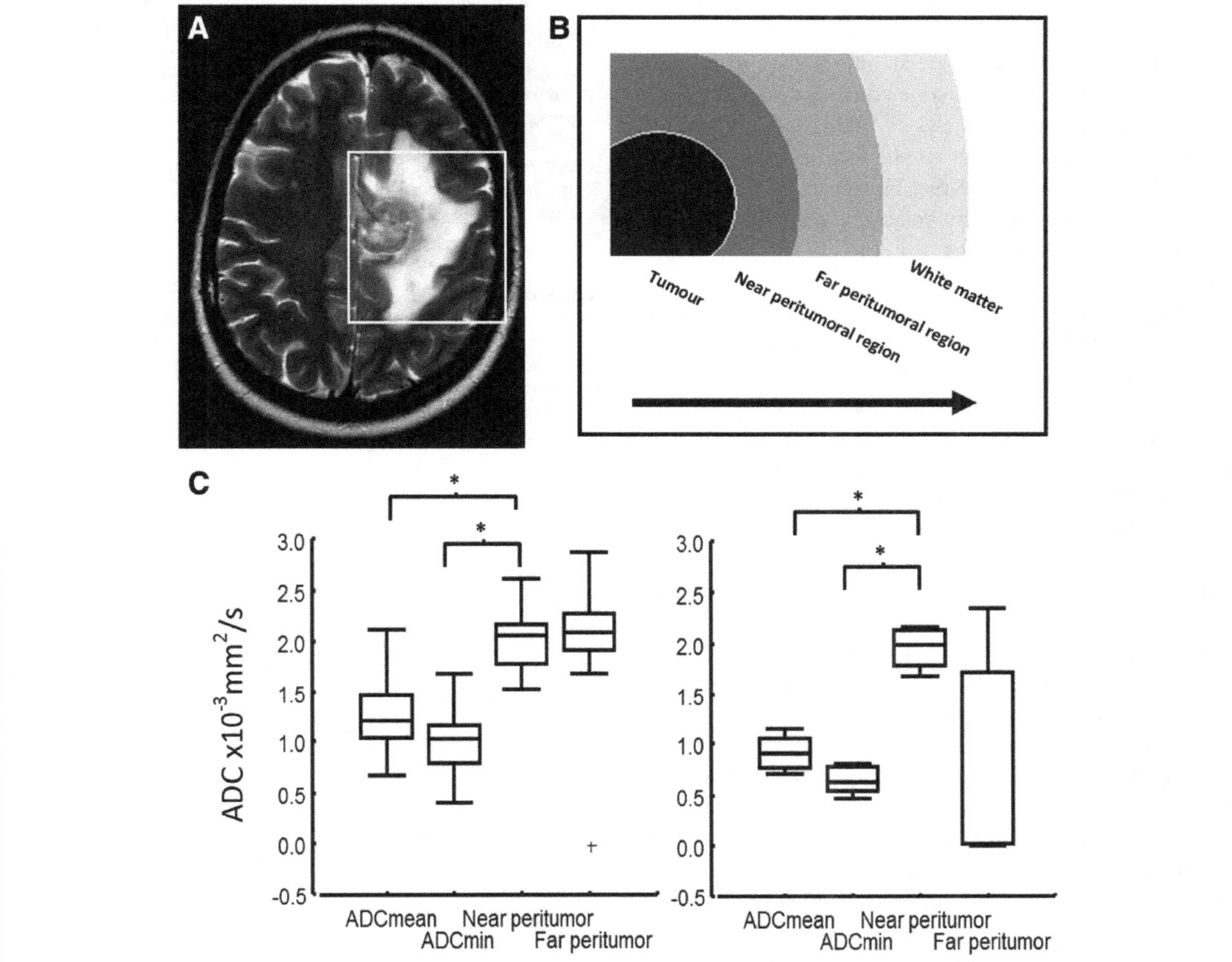

Figure 6 Changes in diffusion around a brain metastasis. A solitary metastasis in a patient with known renal cell carcinoma is shown in **(A)** with a clear boundary, necrotic centre and surrounding oedema, visible on the T2-weighted sequence. What is happening in the region around the metasasis? There is substantial evidence that this region consists of vasogenic oedema, higher diffusion and lower perfusion when compared to high grade glioma for example, but what about comparing *within* a group of metastases. **(B)**. One can place serial regions of interest and measure and plot the ADC changes from the necrotic centre of the tumor through the leading edge and into the peritumoral regions. **(C)** Box and whisker plots showing the median, interquartile range and outliers for ADC readings in and around melanoma (n = 5) and non-small cell lung cancer (n = 36) metastases demonstrates differences in this ADC signature between the two groups and within them but the biological correlate of these differences needs to be investigated.

retrospective study and therefore tissue was not universally available and was in paraffin embedded blocks from non-specific areas of the tumor, hence such an analysis was not possible. This study only examined ADC maps as more gradient directions were not available (again due to the MRI data having already been acquired and the analysis being retrospective) but ideally, more MRI sequences would be analysed pre-operatively including assessment of anisotropic diffusion, via fractional anisotropy. Disruption of white matter tracts is traditionally only seen in infiltrating tumors such as glioblastoma [46] and it would be important to observe if more infiltrative brain metastases as described pathologically [47] show different fractional anisotropy values in the peritumoral region. These findings are also cautioned by the need for validated, reproducible methods when measuring DWI metrics. In particular, we found differences in "tumor ADC" between measuring whole tumor values, minimum values and taking the mean of multiple ROIs. We have previously described good inter and intra-observer agreement measuring ADC metrics with various ROI methods in brain metastases on different post processing platforms [20]. A logical step would be to validate these metrics – in particular the ATC - on a separate, larger dataset and perhaps integrate MRI measures with conventional predictive models such as RPA and GPA.

Different MRI protocols from different vendors have had to be combined in this series due to a need for sufficient power for survival analysis. Again, data gathered in a prospective fashion on a single scanner with uniform protocols would be preferable. However ADC maps are theoretically and practically relatively resistant to variations in MR parameters (for example diffusion is insensitive to B_1 errors). More sophisticated DWI parameters, including assessment of anisotropic diffusion (fractional anisotropy) which we would intend to study next, present more variation between centres. The use of phantoms and comparison of normal white matter readings may be needed to reduce and quantify between centre variation respectively [48]. The precise dosing and timing of corticosteroid therapy could also be established in a prospective series and effects on DWI parameters assessed.

The prevalence of intratumoral haemorrhage in many brain metastasis types is a problem and reduces the number of cases which are suitable for analysis (cases with overwhelming haemorrhage were excluded as stated in the Methods) as well as potentially making these findings less relevant to cases which tend to bleed such as melanoma and renal. Nonetheless a reasonable spread of common histological types was used here. Newer systemic therapies for treating cerebral metastases may lead to significant differences in survival between different tumor types and comprehensive clinical data with large numbers would be needed to stratify cases in future, for example by HER2 responsiveness in breast carcinoma metastases. This makes large scale biomarker studies practically difficult and the need for collaboration between centres paramount.

Conclusions

Diffusion-weighted MRI demonstrates changes in the tumor, across the tumor edge and in the peritumoral region which may not be visible on standard MRI and this may be useful in predicting patient outcomes for cerebral metastases.

Abbreviations

ADC: Apparent diffusion coefficient; ATC: Apparent diffusion coefficient transition coefficient; DWI: Diffusion-weighted imaging; H & E: Haematoxylin and eosin; GPA: Graded prognostic assessment; ROI: Region of interest; RPA: Recursive partitioning analysis; WBRT: Whole brain radiotherapy.

Competing interests

The authors declare that they have no competing interests.

Authors' contributions

RZ, MR, MB and PR gathered data. KD, MR, MB, VS assisted and advised on image analysis. PR, VS and MDJ were involved in devising and supervising the work. RZ analysed data and wrote the final manuscript and all authors made substantial changes. All authors read and approved the final manuscript.

Acknowledgements

Rasheed Zakaria is supported by a Clinical Research Fellowship grant (MR/L017342/1) from the Medical Research Council, UK and research capacity funding from the Walton Centre NHS Foundation Trust, Liverpool, UK. With thanks to Carol Walker PhD, Neurosciences Research Centre, Liverpool for advice and assistance.

This data has been presented at different stages at the Society for Neuro-Oncology meeting (SNO), San Francisco, November 2013 and the British Society of Neurosurgeons meeting, London, February 2014 and published in abstract form as proceedings of these meetings.

Author details

[1]Department of Neurosurgery, The Walton Centre NHS Foundation Trust, Liverpool, UK. [2]Institute of Integrative Biology, University of Liverpool, Liverpool, UK. [3]Department of Neuroradiology, The Walton Centre NHS Foundation Trust, Liverpool, UK. [4]Magnetic resonance and image analysis research centre (MARIARC), University of Liverpool, Liverpool, UK. [5]Institute of Translational Medicine, University of Liverpool, Liverpool, UK. [6]Neurosciences Research Centre, The Walton Centre NHS Foundation Trust, Liverpool L9 7LJ, UK.

References

1. Jenkinson MD, Haylock B, Shenoy A, Husband D, Javadpour M: **Management of cerebral metastasis: evidence-based approach for surgery, stereotactic radiosurgery and radiotherapy.** *Eur J Cancer* 2011, **47**(5):649–655.
2. Nussbaum ES, Djalilian HR, Cho KH, Hall WA: **Brain metastases. Histology, multiplicity, surgery, and survival.** *Cancer* 1996, **78**(8):1781–1788.
3. Young RJ, Sills AK, Brem S, Knopp EA: **Neuroimaging of metastatic brain disease.** *Neurosurgery* 2005, **57**(5 Suppl):S4-10–S14-23.
4. Fink KR, Fink JR: **Imaging of brain metastases.** *Surg Neurol Int* 2013, **4**(Suppl 4):S209–S219.
5. Kim YJ, Chang KH, Song IC, Kim HD, Seong SO, Kim YH, Han MH: **Brain abscess and necrotic or cystic brain tumor: discrimination with signal intensity on diffusion-weighted MR imaging.** *AJR Am J Roentgenol* 1998, **171**(6):1487–1490.
6. Berghoff AS, Spanberger T, Ilhan-Mutlu A, Magerle M, Hutterer M, Woehrer A, Hackl M, Widhalm G, Dieckmann K, Marosi C, Birner P, Prayer D, Preusser M: **Preoperative diffusion-weighted imaging of single brain metastases correlates with patient survival times.** *PLoS One* 2013, **8**(2):e55464.
7. Wang S, Kim S, Chawla S, Wolf RL, Zhang WG, O'Rourke DM, Judy KD, Melhem ER, Poptani H: **Differentiation between glioblastomas and solitary brain metastases using diffusion tensor imaging.** *Neuroimage* 2009, **44**(3):653–660.
8. Tsuchiya K, Fujikawa A, Nakajima M, Honya K: **Differentiation between solitary brain metastasis and high-grade glioma by diffusion tensor imaging.** *Br J Radiol* 2005, **78**(930):533–537.
9. Toh CH, Wei KC, Ng SH, Wan YL, Lin CP, Castillo M: **Differentiation of brain abscesses from necrotic glioblastomas and cystic metastatic brain tumors with diffusion tensor imaging.** *AJNR Am J Neuroradiol* 2011, **32**(9):1646–1651.
10. Stadnik TW, Chaskis C, Michotte A, Shabana WM, van Rompaey K, Luypaert R, Budinsky L, Jellus V, Osteaux M: **Diffusion-weighted MR imaging of intracerebral masses: comparison with conventional MR imaging and histologic findings.** *AJNR Am J Neuroradiol* 2001, **22**(5):969–976.
11. Lu S, Ahn D, Johnson G, Law M, Zagzag D, Grossman RI: **Diffusion-tensor MR imaging of intracranial neoplasia and associated peritumoral edema: introduction of the tumor infiltration index.** *Radiology* 2004, **232**:221–228.
12. Lee EJ, terbrugge K, Mikulis D, Choi DS, Bae JM, Lee SK, Moon SY: **Diagnostic value of peritumoral minimum apparent diffusion coefficient for differentiation of glioblastoma multiforme from solitary metastatic lesions.** *AJR Am J Roentgenol* 2011, **196**(1):71–76.
13. Chen XZ, Yin XM, Ai L, Chen Q, Li SW, Dai JP: **Differentiation between brain glioblastoma multiforme and solitary metastasis: qualitative and quantitative analysis based on routine MR imaging.** *AJNR Am J Neuroradiol* 2012, **33**(10):1907–1912.
14. Byrnes TJ, Barrick TR, Bell BA, Clark CA: **Diffusion tensor imaging discriminates between glioblastoma and cerebral metastases in vivo.** *NMR Biomed* 2011, **24**(1):54–60.

15. Sternberg EJ, Lipton ML, Burns J: **Utility of Diffusion Tensor Imaging in Evaluation of the Peritumoral Region in Patients with Primary and Metastatic Brain Tumors.** *AJNR Am J Neuroradiol* 2014, **35**(3):439–444.
16. Kienast Y, von Baumgarten L, Fuhrmann M, Klinkert WE, Goldbrunner R, Herms J, Winkler F: **Real-time imaging reveals the single steps of brain metastasis formation.** *Nat Med* 2010, **16**(1):116–122.
17. Leenders WP, Kusters B, Verrijp K, Maass C, Wesseling P, Heerschap A, Ruiter D, Ryan A, de Waal R: **Antiangiogenic therapy of cerebral melanoma metastases results in sustained tumor progression via vessel co-option.** *Clin Canc Res* 2004, **10**(18 Pt 1):6222–6230.
18. Gaspar L, Scott C, Rotman M, Asbell S, Phillips T, Wasserman T, McKenna WG, Byhardt R: **Recursive partitioning analysis (RPA) of prognostic factors in three Radiation Therapy Oncology Group (RTOG) brain metastases trials.** *Int J Radiat Oncol Biol Phys* 1997, **37**:745–751.
19. Sperduto PW, Berkey B, Gaspar LE, Mehta M, Curran W: **A new prognostic index and comparison to three other indices for patients with brain metastases: an analysis of 1,960 patients in the RTOG database.** *Int J Radiat Oncol Biol Phys* 2008, **70**(2):510–514.
20. Zakaria R, Das K, Bhojak M, Radon M, Sluming V, Walker C, Jenkinson MD: **The reliability of routine clinical post-processing software in assessing potential diffusion-weighted MRI "biomarkers" in brain metastases.** *Magn Reson Imaging* 2014, **32**(3):291–296.
21. Jenkinson MD, Smith TS, Brodbelt AR, Joyce KA, Warnke PC, Walker C: **Apparent diffusion coefficients in oligodendroglial tumors characterized by genotype.** *J Magn Reson Imaging* 2007, **26**(6):1405–1412.
22. Calli C, Kitis O, Yunten N, Yurtseven T, Islekel S, Akalin T: **Perfusion and diffusion MR imaging in enhancing malignant cerebral tumors.** *Eur J Radiol* 2006, **58**(3):394–403.
23. Chiang IC, Kuo YT, Lu CY, Yeung KW, Lin WC, Sheu FO, Liu GC: **Distinction between high-grade gliomas and solitary metastases using peritumoral 3-T magnetic resonance spectroscopy, diffusion, and perfusion imagings.** *Neuroradiology* 2004, **46**(8):619–627.
24. Duygulu G, Ovali GY, Calli C, Kitis O, Yunten N, Akalin T, Islekel S: **Intracerebral metastasis showing restricted diffusion: correlation with histopathologic findings.** *Eur J Radiol* 2010, **74**(1):117–120.
25. Hayashida Y, Hirai T, Morishita S, Kitajima M, Murakami R, Korogi Y, Makino K, Nakamura H, Ikushima I, Yamura M, Kochi M, Kuratsu JI, Yamashita Y: **Diffusion-weighted imaging of metastatic brain tumors: comparison with histologic type and tumor cellularity.** *AJNR Am J Neuroradiol* 2006, **27**(7):1419–1425.
26. Iima M, Reynaud O, Tsurugizawa T, Ciobanu L, Li JR, Geffroy F, Djemai B, Umehana M, Le Bihan D: **Characterization of Glioma Microcirculation and Tissue Features Using Intravoxel Incoherent Motion Magnetic Resonance Imaging in a Rat Brain Model.** *Invest Radiol* 2014, **49**(7):485–490.
27. Panagiotaki E, Walker-Samuel S, Siow B, Johnson SP, Rajkumar V, Pedley RB, Lythgoe MF, Alexander DC: **Noninvasive quantification of solid tumor microstructure using VERDICT MRI.** *Cancer Res* 2014, **74**(7):1902–1912.
28. Porto L, Jurcoane A, Schwabe D, Kieslich M, Hattingen E: **Differentiation between high and low grade tumours in paediatric patients by using apparent diffusion coefficients.** *Eur J Paediatr Neurol* 2013, **17**(3):302–307.
29. Mahmoud OM, Tominaga A, Amatya VJ, Ohtaki M, Sugiyama K, Sakoguchi T, Kinoshita Y, Takeshima Y, Abe N, Akiyama Y, El-Ghoriany AI, Abd Alla AK, El-Sharkawy MA, Arita K, Kurisu K, Yamasaki F: **Role of PROPELLER diffusion-weighted imaging and apparent diffusion coefficient in the evaluation of pituitary adenomas.** *Eur J Radiol* 2011, **80**(2):412–417.
30. Barajas RF Jr, Rubenstein JL, Chang JS, Hwang J, Cha S: **Diffusion-weighted MR imaging derived apparent diffusion coefficient is predictive of clinical outcome in primary central nervous system lymphoma.** *AJNR Am J Neuroradiol* 2010, **31**(1):60–66.
31. Somoye G, Harry V, Semple S, Plataniotis G, Scott N, Gilbert FJ, Parkin D: **Early diffusion weighted magnetic resonance imaging can predict survival in women with locally advanced cancer of the cervix treated with combined chemo-radiation.** *Eur Radiol* 2012, **22**(11):2319–2327.
32. Frankel TL, Gian RK, Jarnagin WR: **Preoperative imaging for hepatic resection of colorectal cancer metastasis.** *J Gastrointest Oncol* 2012, **3**(1):11–18.
33. Squillaci E, Manenti G, Di Stefano F, Miano R, Strigari L, Simonetti G: **Diffusion-weighted MR imaging in the evaluation of renal tumours.** *J Exp Clin Canc Res* 2004, **23**:39–45.
34. Lambregts DM, Beets GL, Maas M, Curvo-Semedo L, Kessels AG, Thywissen T, Beets-Tan RG: **Tumour ADC measurements in rectal cancer: effect of ROI methods on ADC values and interobserver variability.** *Eur Radiol* 2011, **21**(12):2567–2574.
35. Matoba M, Tuji H, Shimode Y, Toyoda I, Kuginuki Y, Miwa K, Tonami H: **Fractional Change in Apparent Diffusion Coefficient as an Imaging Biomarker for Predicting Treatment Response in Head and Neck Cancer Treated with Chemoradiotherapy.** *AJNR Am J Neuroradiol* 2014, **35**(2):379–385.
36. Raore B, Schniederjan M, Prabhu R, Brat DJ, Shu HK, Olson JJ: **Metastasis infiltration: an investigation of the postoperative brain-tumor interface.** *Int J Radiat Oncol Biol Phys* 2011, **81**(4):1075–1080.
37. Baumert BG, Rutten I, Dehing-Oberije C, Twijnstra A, Dirx MJ, Debougnoux-Huppertz RM, Lambin P, Kubat B: **A pathology-based substrate for target definition in radiosurgery of brain metastases.** *Int J Radiat Oncol Biol Phys* 2006, **66**(1):187–194.
38. Neves S, Mazal PR, Wanschitz J, Rudnay AC, Drlicek M, Czech T, Wustinger C, Budka H: **Pseudogliomatous growth pattern of anaplastic small cell carcinomas metastatic to the brain.** *Clin Neuropathol* 2001, **20**(1):38–42.
39. Patel AJ, Suki D, Hatiboglu MA, Abouassi H, Shi W, Wildrick DM, Lang FF, Sawaya R: **Factors influencing the risk of local recurrence after resection of a single brain metastasis.** *J Neurosurg* 2010, **113**(2):181–189.
40. Goodman SL, Picard M: **Integrins as therapeutic targets.** *Trends Pharmacol Sci* 2012, **33**(7):405–412.
41. Mills SJ, Thompson G, Jackson A: **Advanced magnetic resonance imaging biomarkers of cerebral metastases.** *Cancer Imaging* 2012, **12**:245–252.
42. Price SJ, Gillard JH: **Imaging biomarkers of brain tumour margin and tumour invasion.** *Br J Radiol* 2011, **84**(2):S159–S167.
43. Spanberger T, Berghoff AS, Dinhof C, Ilhan-Mutlu A, Magerle M, Hutterer M, Pichler J, Wohrer A, Hackl M, Widhalm G, Hainfellner JA, Dieckmann K, Marosi C, Birner P, Prayer D, Preusser M: **Extent of peritumoral brain edema correlates with prognosis, tumoral growth pattern, HIF1a expression and angiogenic activity in patients with single brain metastases.** *Clin Exp Metastasis* 2013, **30**(4):357–368.
44. Serres S, Martin CJ, Sarmiento Soto M, Bristow C, O'Brien ER, Connell JJ, Khrapitchev AA, Sibson NR: **Structural and functional effects of metastases in rat brain determined by multimodal MRI.** *Int J Cancer* 2014, **134**(4):885–896.
45. Kelly PJ, Daumas-Duport C, Scheithauer BW, Kall BA, Kispert DB: **Stereotactic histologic correlations of computed tomography- and magnetic resonance imaging-defined abnormalities in patients with glial neoplasms.** *Mayo Clin Proc* 1987, **62**(6):450–459.
46. Price SJ, Pena A, Burnet NG, Jena R, Green HA, Carpenter TA, Pickard JD, Gillard JH: **Tissue signature characterisation of diffusion tensor abnormalities in cerebral gliomas.** *Eur Radiol* 2004, **14**(10):1909–1917.
47. Berghoff AS, Rajky O, Winkler F, Bartsch R, Furtner J, Hainfellner JA, Goodman SL, Weller M, Schittenhelm J, Preusser M: **Invasion patterns in brain metastases of solid cancers.** *Neuro Oncol* 2013, **15**(12):1664–1672.
48. Tofts PS, Collins DJ: **Multicentre imaging measurements for oncology and in the brain.** *Br J Radiol* 2011, **84**(2):S213–S226.

13

Valid and efficient manual estimates of intracranial volume from magnetic resonance images

Niklas Klasson[1*], Erik Olsson[1], Mats Rudemo[2], Carl Eckerström[1], Helge Malmgren[1,3] and Anders Wallin[1]

Abstract

Background: Manual segmentations of the whole intracranial vault in high-resolution magnetic resonance images are often regarded as very time-consuming. Therefore it is common to only segment a few linearly spaced intracranial areas to estimate the whole volume. The purpose of the present study was to evaluate how the validity of intracranial volume estimates is affected by the chosen interpolation method, orientation of the intracranial areas and the linear spacing between them.

Methods: Intracranial volumes were manually segmented on 62 participants from the Gothenburg MCI study using 1.5 T, T_1-weighted magnetic resonance images. Estimates of the intracranial volumes were then derived using subsamples of linearly spaced coronal, sagittal or transversal intracranial areas from the same volumes. The subsamples of intracranial areas were interpolated into volume estimates by three different interpolation methods. The linear spacing between the intracranial areas ranged from 2 to 50 mm and the validity of the estimates was determined by comparison with the entire intracranial volumes.

Results: A progressive decrease in intra-class correlation and an increase in percentage error could be seen with increased linear spacing between intracranial areas. With small linear spacing (≤15 mm), orientation of the intracranial areas and interpolation method had negligible effects on the validity. With larger linear spacing, the best validity was achieved using cubic spline interpolation with either coronal or sagittal intracranial areas. Even at a linear spacing of 50 mm, cubic spline interpolation on either coronal or sagittal intracranial areas had a mean absolute agreement intra-class correlation with the entire intracranial volumes above 0.97.

Conclusion: Cubic spline interpolation in combination with linearly spaced sagittal or coronal intracranial areas overall resulted in the most valid and robust estimates of intracranial volume. Using this method, valid ICV estimates could be obtained in less than five minutes per patient.

Keywords: Intracranial volume, Manual estimation, Magnetic resonance imaging, Validity

Background

Intracranial volume (ICV) estimated by magnetic resonance images (MRI) is often used as a proxy variable for premorbid brain volume in brain volumetric studies. ICV normalization has been used to reduce interindividual variance in both whole brain volume [1] and regional brain volumes, e.g. hippocampus [2,3]. To save time, estimates of ICVs are commonly calculated by the sum of linearly spaced intracranial areas (ICA) multiplied by the distance between those areas. Eritaia et al. evaluated how the validity of such estimates decreases as the linear spacing increases using sagittal ICAs [4]. They found that the validity not only decreased with increased linear spacing, but also grew more uncertain due to an oscillation in the functions reported. To avoid this uncertainty it has been common to use small linear spacings of no more than 10 mm between sagittal ICAs e.g. [5,6]. In these cases the validity of the estimates should be high, with an intra-class correlation of about 0.999 [4]. However, the adoption of the method is often hard to appraise as it tends to be sparsely reported, e.g. leaving out choice of linear spacing [7-10].

Information about the shape and volume of an intracranial vault is lost when only a few ICAs are segmented.

* Correspondence: niklas.klasson@neuro.gu.se
[1]Institute of Psychiatry and Neurochemistry, Department of Neuroscience and physiology, The Sahlgrenska Academy, University of Gothenburg, Box 430, SE-405 30 Göteborg, Sweden
Full list of author information is available at the end of the article

From the known ICAs this lost information can be approximated by different means. When multiplying the sum of ICAs by the linear spacing between them, a piecewise constant interpolation is made (Figure 1,a-b). This is the simplest form of interpolation method, and the oscillation seen in the study by Eritaia et al. reflects its irregular performance [4]. If we also, besides the linear spacing, note the order of the known ICAs, better approximations of the lost ICAs may be achieved. In this case we can assume that ICAs between two known ICAs follow a linear function or other polynomial functions. These assumptions can be implemented using so called piecewise polynomial interpolations (Figure 1c). The possibility of achieving more valid ICV estimates by using piecewise polynomial interpolation seems not to have been investigated before. Further, the validity of ICV estimates using linearly spaced ICAs in coronal or transversal orientation is still unknown.

While the method evaluated by Eritaia et al. [4] has been used both to evaluate other ICV estimation methods [11,12] and to correct for differences in premorbid brain volume [5,6], the original study itself has not been validated. The aim of the present study was therefore to 1) replicate the study by Eritaia et al., in a different sample, in order to validate their findings, 2) evaluate the validity of ICV estimates from coronal and transversal ICAs, and 3) evaluate different interpolation methods that could improve the validity of the ICV estimates.

Methods

Participants

The present study is part of the Gothenburg MCI (mild cognitive impairment) study from which a subsample of 38 patients and 32 controls with 1.5 T MRI scans was included. The patients, who were referred to the memory clinic in Mölndal with subjective or objective cognitive impairment, were first included in the Gothenburg MCI study if they did not fulfill any of the exclusion criteria. Exclusion criteria were severe somatic or psychiatric disorder, alcohol or substance abuse, confusion caused by drugs, and pseudodementia. Patients were classified into one of four stages using the global deterioration scale (GDS) for assessment of primary degenerative dementia [13], where stage 1 means no cognitive decline, stage 2 is subjective cognitive impairment, stage 3 is mild cognitive impairment and stage 4 indicates dementia. Controls were mainly recruited from organizations for senior citizens and were excluded if they had any sign of cognitive impairment. To participate in the Gothenburg MCI study both patients and controls had to give their written informed consent. The Gothenburg MCI study has previously been described [14] and has been approved by the ethics committee of Gothenburg University (diary number: L091-99, 1999; T479-11, 2011).

Eight of the 70 participants in the present substudy were excluded because parts of the intracranial vault had not been covered in the MRI scans. Of the excluded subjects two (25 percent) were women. Two had GDS 4, three had GDS 2–3 and three were controls. Of the remaining 62 participants, 39 (63 percent) were women. Twenty-five had GDS 4, eight had GDS 2–3 and 29 were controls. The excluded and the remaining subjects did not differ significantly with respect to age, education or MMSE, but differed significantly regarding gender. The complete demographics of the remaining participants can be viewed in Table 1.

MRI acquisition

Coronal, T_1-weighted, 3D IR/GR (inversion recovery/gradient echo) MRI scans, obtained from a 1.5 T

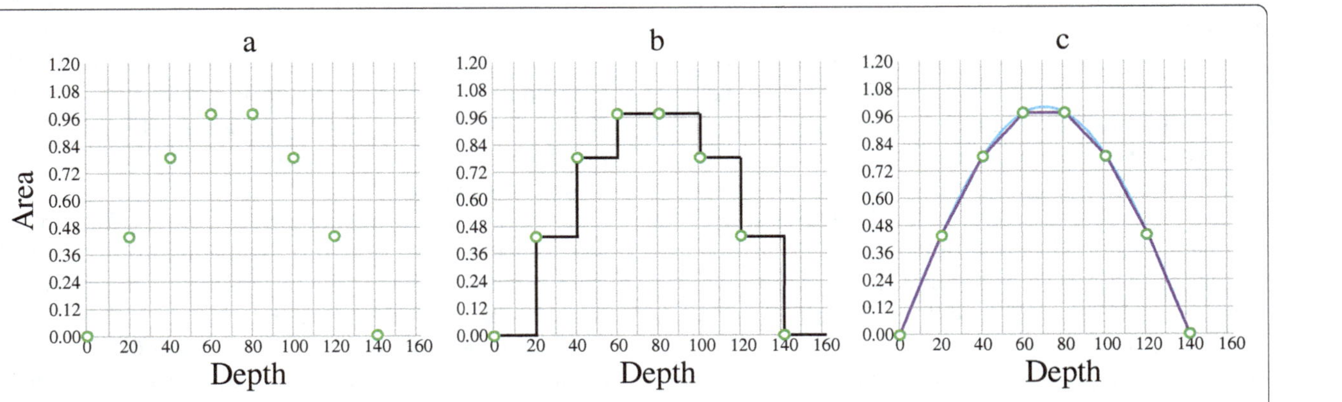

Figure 1 Estimating a volume by linearly spaced areas. a) The green dots illustrate known, linearly spaced, areas from an unknown volume. The Y-axis gives the size of these areas and the X-axis at which depth, in the unknown volume, they were measured. **b)** By multiplying each known area by the linear spacing, the lost areas are approximated (black border), a piecewise constant interpolation is made. The area under the curve is the estimate of the unknown volume. **c)** The lost areas approximated by two piecewise polynomial interpolations, a piecewise linear interpolation (purple graph) and a cubic spline interpolation (blue graph).

Table 1 Study demographics for the remaining participants

Group belonging	N	Gender (m/f)	Age	Education	MMSE
Controls	29	8/21	66.4 ± 7.5	11.5 (7.0, 15.0)	30 (27, 30)
Patients, GDS 2-3	8	4/4	66.7 ± 8.2	12.0 (6.5, 20)	28.5 (26.0, 29.0)
Patients, GDS 4	25	11/14	65.5 ± 8.8	10.0 (6.0, 23.0)	25 (16, 30)

Study demographics for the remaining controls, patients with a global deterioration scale (GDS) score of 2–3 and patients with GDS score of 4. N gives the number of participants and the gender ratio is given as males (m) per females (f). Age is described with means and standard deviations while education and mini-mental state examination (MMSE) are described with medians with minimum and maximum values enclosed in parentheses.

Siemens Symphony scanner, were used for the ICV segmentations. The coronal plane was aligned perpendicular to the longitudinal axis of hippocampus during the MRI examinations. All MRI examinations were performed at Sahlgrenska University Hospital, Mölndal radiology department. The acquisition parameters were: echo time = 2.38 ms, field of view = 250 x 203 mm, flip angle = 15°, inversion time = 820 ms, matrix size = 512 × 416, pixel spacing = 0.49 × 0.49 mm, repetition time = 1610 ms, slice thickness = 1 mm, bit depth = 12.

Image analysis

The ICV segmentations were performed manually using a MacBook Pro 13" with an Intel Core i7 processor, an Intel HD Graphics 3000 graphic card, and an external Wacom DTU-2231 interactive pen display with about 102 pixels per inch resolution and a system gamma of 1.8. The segmentations were acquired using a custom built software (MIST) developed by N. Klasson for manual segmentation of MRI volumes.

The MRI scans were reformatted into 1 mm cubic voxels using linear interpolation, but no realignment of the images was done to correct for head tilt. A simple method was used to adjust the MRI scans to the same intensity level. Essentially, the mean intensity of each MRI scan was adjusted in brightness so that it matched the pre-adjustment mean intensity of all MRI scans. However, if the amount of background in a scan is large (e.g. due to a small head), its mean intensity tends to be lower compared to a scan with less background (e.g. due to a large head). The mean intensity would in this case reflect the amount of background rather than the brightness of the MRI scan. To avoid this bias the mean intensity of each image was calculated from the middle 80 % of the tonal range. To improve the visibility of the dura, the total tonal range was then expanded by compressing 10 % of the brightest and darkest voxels to their respective extremes. Further, the images were made brighter by a gamma correction with gamma set to 0.8. The gamma correction was performed using the function $y = b * (x/b)^{\gamma}$ where y = output data, b = bit depth, x = input data, and γ = gamma value. Finally, the image size on the screen was scaled to 0.25 (0.5 × 0.5) times the true size of data, which meant that a 1 mm horizontal or vertical line on the screen corresponded to 2 mm in the image data.

The segmentations were performed in sagittal orientation by tracing the dural margins using the landmarks described by Eritaia et al. [4]. If the dura was not visible its location was estimated by visual extrapolation guided by the cerebral contour and surrounding dura mater. The segmentation crosses the foramen magnum at the arches of the atlas (C1), continuing along the clivus and excluding the pituitary gland by traversing the sella turcica from the dorsum sellae to the jugum sphenoidale. Further on, the inferior surface of the frontal lobe is followed. Using these landmarks the superior sagittal sinus, the confluence of sinuses, the transverse sinuses, the sigmoid sinuses and the occipital sinus were included. All measurements started at the slice near the longitudinal fissure where the cerebral aqueduct was most prominent and continued laterally in both directions until the last traces of the meninges disappeared. The software enables markers to be placed in coronal orientation, which then appear in sagittal orientation. In the present study such markers were used to guide the segmentation at the lateral ends of the dura. The mean number of sagittal slices was 136 per MRI scan with a standard deviation of 5 slices, and the segmentations took on average a little over two and a half hours per scan. N. Klasson performed the segmentations.

Using the MATLAB (version R2012b) function inpolygon, each voxel within the sagittal ICAs was traced resulting in a 3D matrix of voxels describing the intracranial vault. This 3D matrix was then used to calculate ICAs in coronal and transversal orientation. That is, ICV segmentations were reconstructed as if they had been segmented in coronal and transversal orientation. This was done to evaluate how the linear spacing affects not only ICV estimates based on sagittal ICA segmentations, but also those based on coronal and transversal ICAs. An illustration of the initial sagittal segmentation and its coronal and transversal reconstructions can be viewed in Figure 2.

New sagittal segmentations were performed six months after the first ICV segmentations to enable intra-rater reliability analysis. This was done in two sessions by first re-segmenting every 10th mm on 31 randomly selected MRI scans and then every 40th mm on the remaining 31 scans. The image settings were the same as during the first segmentation process and the segmentations began at the sagittal slice where the cerebral aqueduct was most prominent. The segmentations took on average 13 ½ minutes when segmenting every 10th mm, and 4 ½ minutes when segmenting every 40th mm. Using

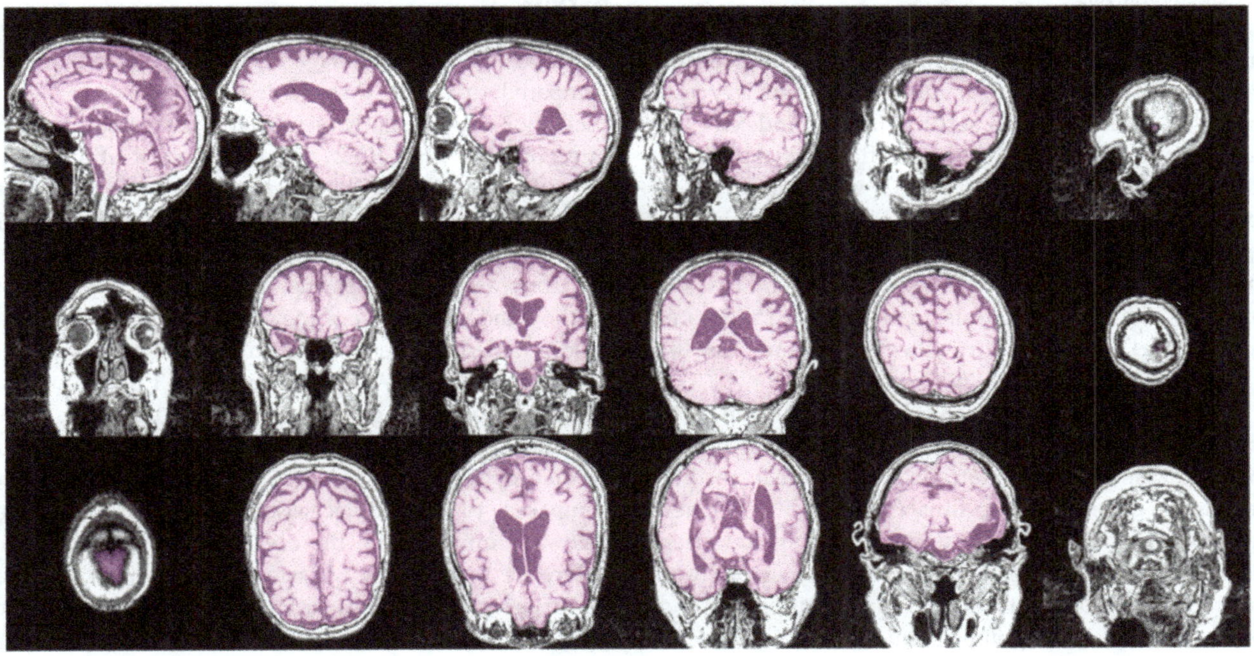

Figure 2 Illustration of a segmentation. The first row shows a sagittal segmentation from the intracranial area where the cerebral aqueduct was most prominent to one of the lateral ends of the cranial vault. The second row shows the coronal reconstruction of the same segmentation, and the third row the transversal reconstruction; both reconstructions are visualized from the first to the last slice where at least one voxel has been classified as intracranial volume.

the same procedure and group selection as in the intra-rater analysis, one additional rater (S. Skau) performed segmentations for inter-rater reliability. On average these segmentations took 22 ½ minutes when segmenting every 10th mm and 5 minutes when segmenting every 40th mm. Both raters were blinded to participant age, gender, and cognitive status as well as to previous segmentations during all ICV segmentations.

Estimate calculation

ICV estimates were derived from the ICV segmentations, following and extending the procedure of Eritaia et al. [4]. Briefly, subsamples of linearly spaced ICAs were interpolated into ICV estimates with the position of the first ICA restricted to be within one linear spacing from the outermost ICA. Thus, using a linear spacing of n results in n possible subsamples of ICAs and therefore n possible estimates for each of the 62 ICV segmentations. To calculate the validity of the estimates, combinations containing one estimate for each ICV segmentation were used. Such a combination can be derived in n^{62} ($n_{ICV1} * n_{ICV2} * n_{ICV3}... * n_{ICV62}$) different ways (the multiplication principle). The validity of each of the combinations depends on which estimates were chosen, and then not only on the linear spacing, but also on which positions were used for the first ICAs. Therefore, to describe the validity of estimates only due to linear spacing, independently of the position of the first ICA, the validity of all possible combinations must be described. As it is practically impossible to evaluate all of these n^{62} combinations of estimates, 2000 combinations were chosen randomly for each linear spacing. The randomization was done by randomly choosing one estimate out of the n possible for each ICV segmentation to construct one combination, and then this procedure was repeated 2000 times.

The whole process was carried out for the sagittal, coronal and transversal ICAs separately and was done using linear spacings ranging from 2 mm up to 50 mm. The first coronal ICAs were chosen anteriorly and the first transversal ICAs superiorly.

Three different interpolation methods were evaluated using the same randomly chosen combinations of ICA subsamples for each orientation. The methods were 1) a piecewise constant interpolation, 2) a piecewise linear interpolation and 3) a cubic spline interpolation. The last two are different kinds of piecewise polynomial interpolation methods and were implemented using the MATLAB functions interp1 and spline respectively. To assure interpolation up to the sagittal borders of the intracranial vaults, zeros (indicating an ICA of zero mm^2) were added at the positions were the intracranial vaults ended. This addition of zero ICAs is not useful for the piecewise constant interpolation.

Statistical analysis

A total of 441 (3 interpolation methods * 3 ICA orientations * 49 linear spacings) unique estimation settings were evaluated using 2000 combinations of ICV estimates for each. For each setting, Jaccard index values, Pearson's linear correlation coefficients, and intra-class correlation coefficients (ICC) were calculated for each of the 2000 combinations in relation to the ICV segmentations. Percentage errors for all estimates in these combinations were also calculated. The ICC calculations were performed using a two-way random effects model for single measurements and absolute agreement [15].

To evaluate if the percentage errors of the cubic spline interpolation differed significantly from those of the piecewise constant interpolation, the mean absolute percentage error of the n estimates of each ICV segmentation was calculated for each linear spacing and orientation. These mean absolute percentage errors were then compared between the two interpolation methods for each linear spacing and orientation using Student's t-tests for paired data.

Intra- and inter-rater ICCs were calculated by comparing the re-segmentations with the corresponding subsamples of sagittal ICAs obtained from the first ICV segmentations, excluding all other ICAs. These ICC values were calculated using a two-way mixed effects model for single measurements and absolute agreement.

As a way of evaluating the ICV segmentations, associations of ICV to age, gender and group belonging (controls, GDS 2, 3 or 4) were analyzed. The possible correlation between ICV and age was evaluated using Pearson's linear correlation coefficient, gender difference was evaluated using an independent-samples t-test, and difference due to group belonging by a Kruskal-Wallis test. As the male to female ratio differed between controls and patients, the Kruskal-Wallis test was also performed for males and females separately.

All statistics were performed in MATLAB (version R2012b) and p values less than or equal to 0.05 were regarded as statistically significant. Pearson's correlations were calculated using the MATLAB function corr, t-test was performed using the function ttest, and the Kruskal-Wallis tests using the function kruskalwallis. ICC values were calculated using the external MATLAB function ICC written by Arash Salarian that is available online at the MATLAB file exchange homepage [16], and Jaccard index values by the function $\left(\sum_{n=1}^{62}\min(x_n, y_n)\right)/\left(\sum_{n=1}^{62}\max(x_n, y_n)\right)$ [17], where x is a vector containing the 62 actual ICVs and y a vector containing the given combination of corresponding ICV estimates.

Results

Figure 3 shows the ICCs, Pearson's correlations, Jaccard index values, and percentage errors of the ICV estimates compared to the ICV segmentations. Except for some oscillations, particularly visible for piecewise constant interpolation, the ICCs, Pearson's correlations, and Jaccard index values generally decreased and the percentage errors increased with increased linear spacing. Similarly, the variance of these validity measures increased with increased linear spacing regardless of interpolation method and orientation of the ICAs. Still, the decrease in validity differed depending on interpolation method and orientation of the ICAs, as seen in Figure 3.

With linear spacings above or equal to 12 mm, the t-test analyses revealed that cubic spline interpolation with coronal or sagittal ICAs decreased the percentage error compared to using piecewise constant interpolation. Below 12 mm, or with the use of transversal ICAs, the difference was not always significant. Using transversal ICAs, cubic spline interpolation could even result in larger percentage errors compared to when using piecewise constant interpolation. Means and confidence intervals of the percentage error differences between the two interpolation methods are presented in Figure 4.

The ICC value for intra-rater reliability in the present study was 0.996, both when segmenting every 10th and when segmenting every 40th mm. The inter-rater reliability was 0.991 in the case of every 10th mm and 0.987 in the case of every 40th mm.

No correlation between ICV and age could be seen (p = 0.376). Further, the distributions of the ICVs did not differ due to group belonging (p_{all} = 0.977, $p_{females}$ = 0.458, p_{males} = 0.672), while a difference in mean ICV could be seen by gender ($p < 0.001$) where the females had a mean ICV of 1416955 mm^3 (standard deviation: 91678 mm^3) and the males a mean ICV of 1658268 mm^3 (standard deviation: 115535 mm^3). In Figure 5 the ICVs are displayed in relation to age, group belonging and gender.

Discussion

The present study shows that a high validity of ICV estimates, calculated by linearly spaced ICAs, could be maintained also at larger linear spacings if using cubic spline interpolation and coronal or sagittal ICAs rather than piecewise constant interpolation or transversal ICAs.

The first aim of the present study was to replicate a study by Eritaia et al. [4]. In that study it is described how the linear spacing of sagittal ICAs affects the validity of ICV estimates using piecewise constant interpolation. A relationship that was identical for practical purposes was found in the present study. In both studies the validity of the ICV estimates decreased and grew more uncertain with increased linear spacing. For a more detailed comparison the difference in linear spacing between the two

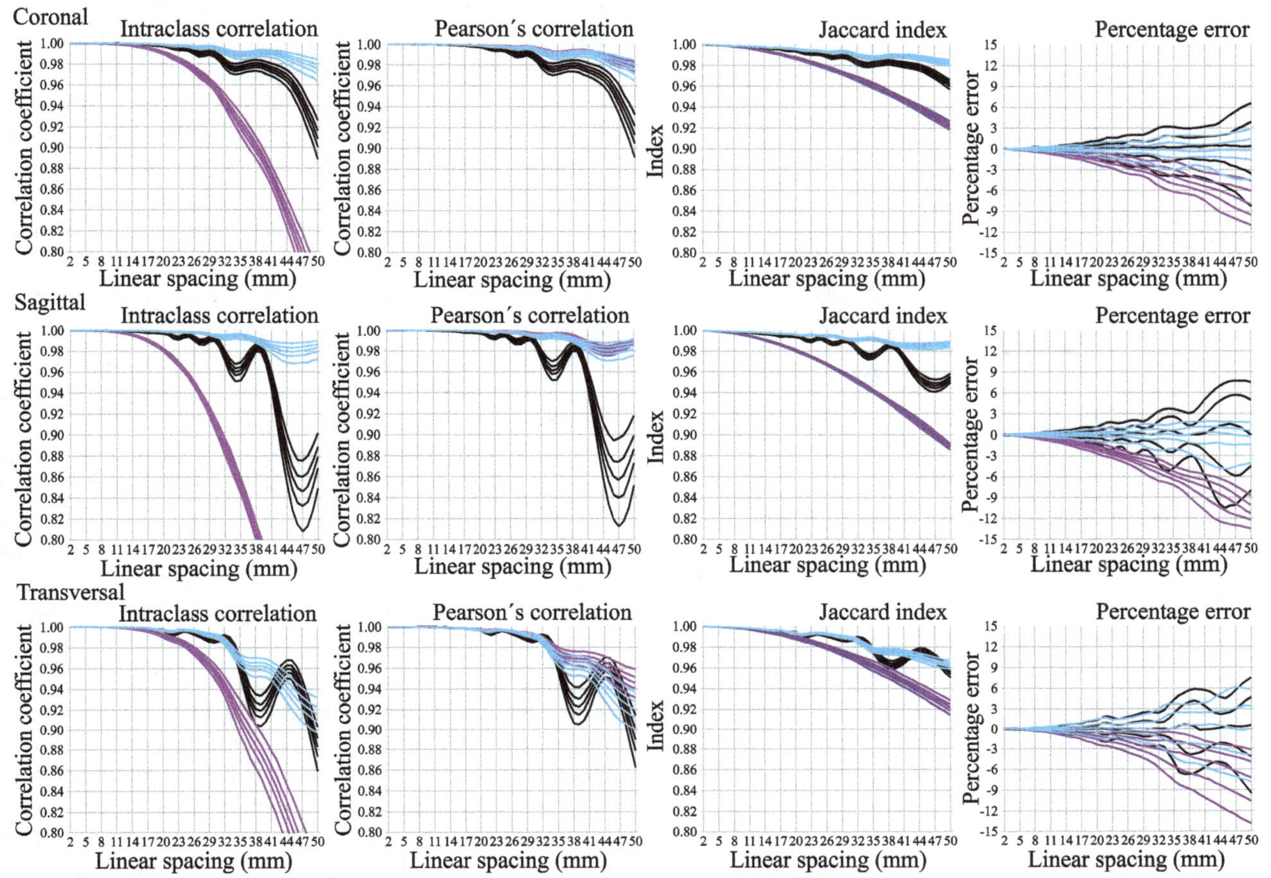

Figure 3 Validity of intracranial volume estimates. The validity of intracranial volume (ICV) estimates compared to the ICV segmentations is given by percentile curves (95th, 75th, 50th, 25th and 5th percentile) for piecewise constant interpolation (black graphs), piecewise linear interpolation (purple graphs) and cubic spline interpolation (blue graphs). The percentiles are calculated for intra-class correlation coefficients (first column), Pearson's correlation (second column), Jaccard index (third column), and percentage errors (fourth column). Besides interpolation method the validity of the estimates depends upon the linear spacing between intracranial areas (X-axis) and orientation of the intracranial areas, either coronal (first row), sagittal (second row) or transversal (third row).

studies must be taken into account. As Eritaia et al. used a spacing between slices (slice thickness plus slice gap) of 0.938 mm, a segmentation of every 25th slice equals to a linear spacing of 23.45 mm (25th slice * 0.938 mm/slice). At this linear spacing Eritaia et al. found an ICC of 0.993-0.997 between the 5th and 95th percentiles. In the present study the ICC values at a linear spacing of 24 mm were 0.993-0.996.

Unlike in the study by Eritaia et al. [4], percentiles of the percentage errors for each linear spacing were calculated instead of percentiles of their maximum at each combination. This was done mainly to reduce the influence of extremes that could bias the evaluation. Hence, the present results should be more generalizable. The already established use of sagittal ICAs with small linear spacing for ICV estimation when using piecewise constant interpolation was still supported by the current results.

The second aim of the present study was to extend our knowledge about how linear spacing affects the validity of ICV estimates to also include coronal and transversal ICAs. The piecewise constant interpolation method has been used both in transversal [1] and coronal orientation [18]. The present study shows that there is a difference in validity depending on the orientation of the ICAs. This difference is negligible at smaller linear spacings (<= 15 mm), but as the linear spacing increases the differences become more apparent. At larger linear spacings, coronal ICAs resulted in the most robust and valid ICV estimates when using piecewise constant interpolation, while both sagittal and transversal ICAs showed large shifts in validity. Most studies use small linear spacings and the validity in these studies should thus be high regardless of the orientation of the ICAs.

As the coronal and transversal ICAs used in the present study were reformatted from sagittally segmented volumes,

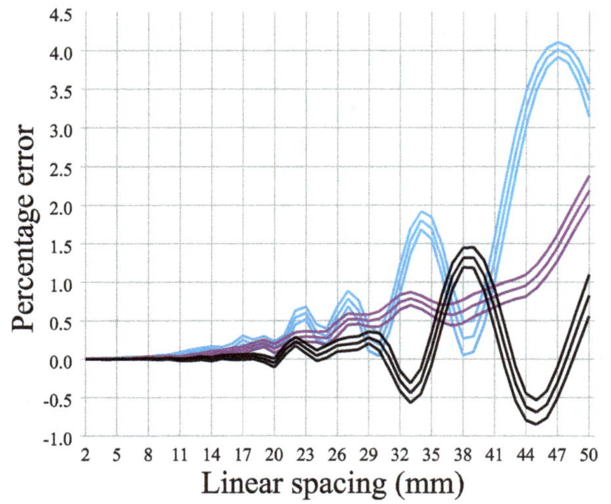

Figure 4 Differences in absolute percentage error between piecewise constant and cubic spline interpolation. T-test of the mean absolute percentage error between intracranial volume estimates calculated by piecewise constant interpolation and cubic spline interpolation using coronal (purple graphs), sagittal (blue graphs) and transversal (black graphs) intracranial areas. For each orientation the mean and 95 percent confidence intervals are illustrated. Positive percentage errors indicate the improvements when using cubic spline interpolation compared to using piecewise constant interpolation and negative percentages the opposite.

possible difficulties associated with actually segmenting in coronal or transversal orientation are not covered. Further, the MRIs were not realigned to correct for head tilt. While there was barely any lateral tilt of the heads, the coronal plane had been aligned during the MRI examinations so that it was perpendicular to the longitudinal axis of hippocampus (a slight backward tilt of the head). This alignment of the coronal plane makes the results for the transversal and coronal orientations less generalizable for studies where a similar alignment is not used. The generalizability should still be high, but less so for large linear spacings in these orientations.

The third aim of the present study was to evaluate if the validity of the ICV estimates could be improved by the use of another interpolation method than piecewise constant interpolation. Using the polynomial interpolation methods the oscillations were reduced, resulting in more robust ICV estimates. While the piecewise linear interpolation increasingly underestimated the volumes, resulting in low ICC and Jaccard index, the Pearson's correlation remained high. This was true regardless of ICA orientation. The cubic spline interpolation on the other hand resulted in improvements of ICC, Jaccard index, Pearson's correlation and absolute percentage error (Figure 4), but only for sagittal and coronal ICAs. It seems that because the cubic spline interpolation assumes a smoothly varying shape, it failed to consistently recover the lost information of the more irregular transversal ICAs. Figure 6 summarizes, by means of an example, how the different interpolation methods work at the different orientations and linear spacings.

In large studies manual estimation of ICV is seldom used. Two and a half hour per ICV might seem impossibly time-consuming. Even segmenting every 10th mm, which takes some 15 minutes per ICV, is generally considered to be too time consuming. This is the main reason why automatic ICV estimation has been preferred in these settings. Two commonly used automatic approaches, evaluated by Nordenskjöld et al. [19], are FreeSurfer [20] and SPM [21]. Nordenskjöld et al. found that FreeSurfer (version 5.1.0) had a Pearson's correlation of 0.937 to manual ICV segmentations while SPM 8 had a Pearson's correlation of 0.856 (correlations calculated by the square root of R^2 from univariate linear regression models). In a more recent study by Malone et al. FreeSurfer (version 5.3.0) had a Pearson's correlation of 0.895 to manual estimates of ICV, while SPM 8

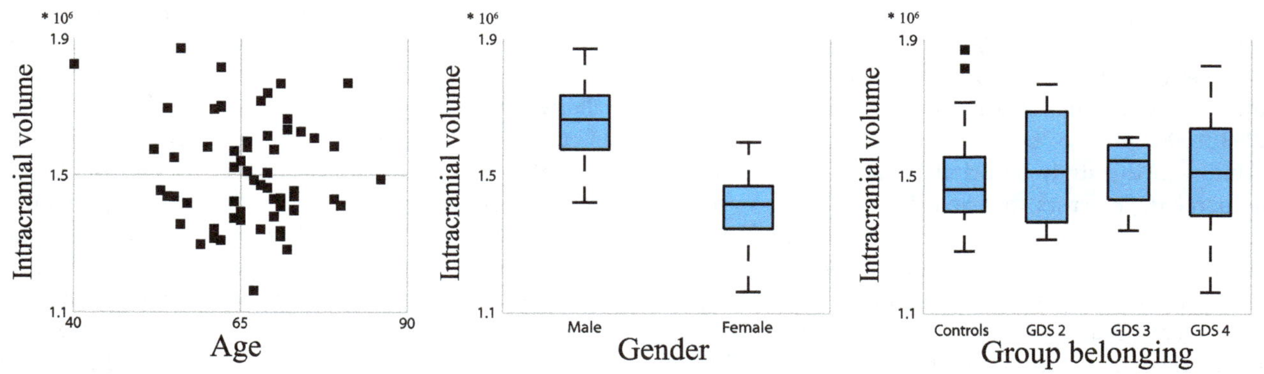

Figure 5 Relation between intracranial volume and age, gender and group belonging. Relation between the intracranial volumes and age, gender and group belonging. The groups consists of controls and patients with stage two, three or four on the global deterioration scale (GDS). Age is given in years and intracranial volume in cubic millimeter.

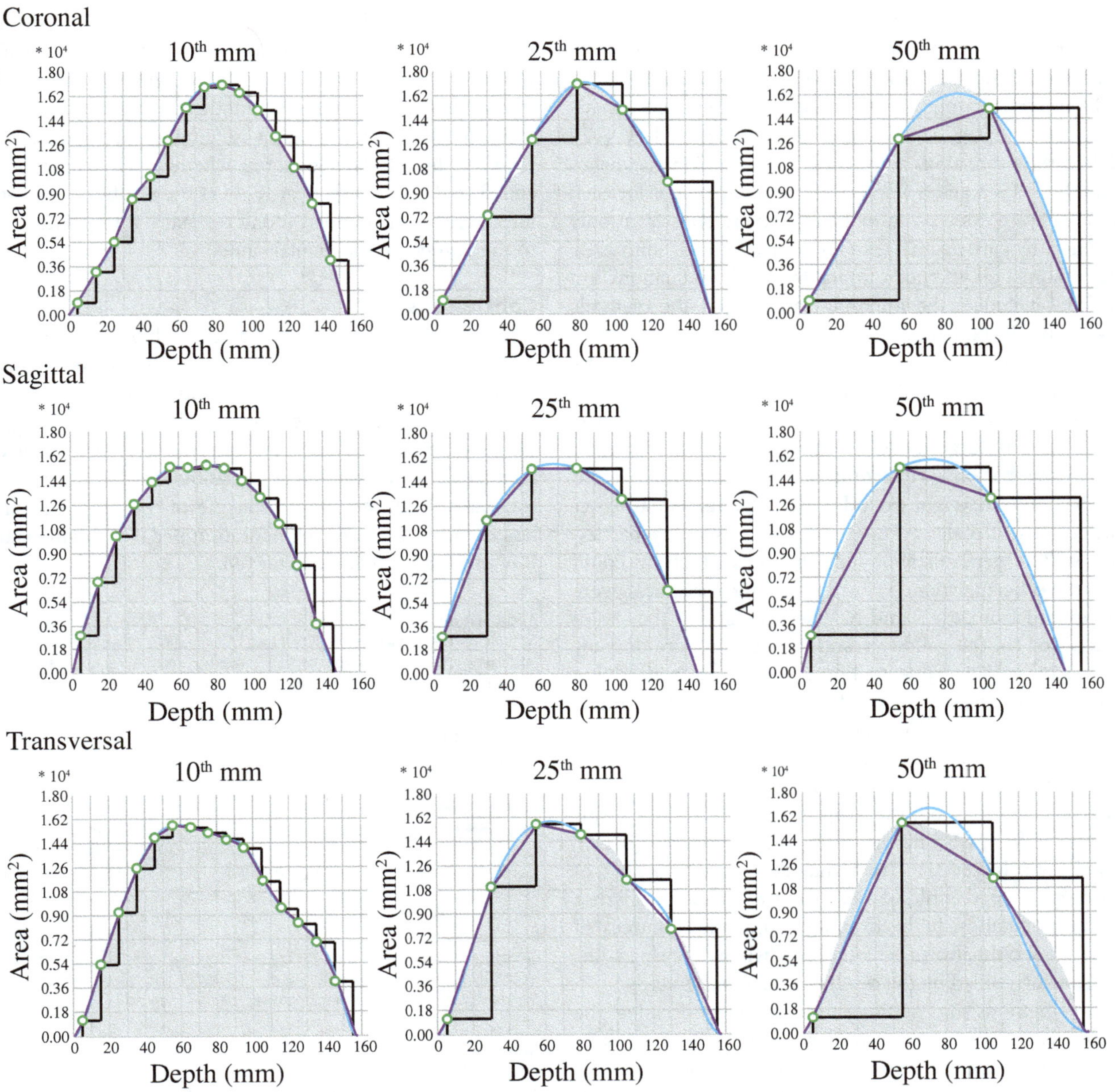

Figure 6 Estimates of an intracranial volume visualized in comparison to the actual volume. Visualization of a randomly chosen intracranial volume compared to 27 different estimates of this volume. The estimates differ with respect to interpolation method, linear spacing and orientation of the intracranial areas used to calculate the estimates. The gray areas represent the actual volume and the green dots the known intracranial areas (ICA). The estimates are visualized by black graphs (piecewise constant interpolation), purple graphs (piecewise linear interpolation) and blue graphs (cubic spline interpolation). The X-axis describes at what depths the ICAs were measured and the Y-axis the size of the areas. Coronal ICAs are ordered from anterior to posterior and transversal ICAs from superior to inferior. All estimates in the illustration were calculated beginning with the ICA at a depth of 5 mm.

and SPM 12 had Pearson's correlations of 0.760 and 0.970 respectively to such estimates [22]. Better correlations can be achieved using manual segmentations even at a linear spacing of 50 mm. In the present study the median Pearson's correlation at this linear spacing was 0.985 using sagittal ICAs and cubic spline interpolation. The time needed for such manual segmentations should be less than 5 minutes per ICV. Possible bias due to pathological brain atrophy, as might be the case with FreeSurfer (version 3.0.2) [23], or even due to age related atrophy as seen in SPM 8 [19] would also be avoided.

Beside the commonly used FreeSurfer and SPM, there might exist automatic methods for ICV assessment that perform as well as manual segmentations of every 50th mm. For example, Keihaninejad et al. showed promising results in that two out of four evaluated automatic methods had ICCs of 0.98-0.99 to manual estimates of ICV [12]. While the evaluations were done for T1-weighted images from both 1.5 T and 3 T scanners, the comparisons for each scanner were done using manual segmentations from only five healthy participants. Like for many, if not all, automatic ICV estimation methods, more thorough evaluations are needed, including the important aspect that the methods should not be biased by atrophy.

The evaluated algorithms for ICV estimation in the present study require MRI scans that include the whole intracranial vault. This requirement might exclude participants with larger heads if care is not taken during the MRI examinations. This could be the case in the present study where the eight excluded participants had a higher proportion of males compared to the remaining participants. The generalizability of the present study could therefore be questioned. Further, as the estimates were computed from the same ICV segmentations they were compared to, the validity results in Figure 3 are only affected by variance due to linear spacing. When adding other sources of variance to the measures, such as intra-rater variance, the ICCs can be expected to drop. This was also confirmed when evaluating the intra- and inter-rater effect on the sagittal segmentations. Regardless of interpolation method, the drop in ICC for sagittally estimated ICVs just due to intra-rater variance (ICC = 0.996) was larger than that due to a linear spacing of 10 mm (5th percentile of ICCs > 0.998). Thus, properties of the population to be examined and other sources of variance should always be considered when choosing a linear spacing guided by the results of the present study.

The methods and settings used for preprocessing the image data in the present study might have been suboptimal. Specifically, the reformatting of the image data was done by a linear interpolation when other interpolation methods would arguably have been better [24]. However, the error introduced by the linear interpolation is likely negligible because of the large size of the ICVs.

One of the most important aspects of measures of intracranial volume is that they should not be biased by atrophy. The ICVs in the present study were segmented following the dura mater to make sure not to include such a bias in the findings. There was no difference in ICV due to group belonging (controls, GDS 2, 3 or 4) or any correlation to age, which speaks against a possible bias in the manual segmentations. The highly similar results for the piecewise constant interpolation to those of Eritaia et al. [4], that only included normal controls, also indicate that atrophy has not affected the present results.

When reporting the use of ICV estimates calculated by linearly spaced ICAs, at least three pieces of information should be included in the specifications. These are: 1) orientation of the ICAs, 2) linear spacing, preferably in mm, and 3) interpolation method. If an interpolation method other than the piecewise constant interpolation is used, it should also be noted whether zeros have been added to the subsamples of ICAs at the positions were the intracranial vaults ended (done to assure interpolation up to the borders of the cranial vaults).

Conclusions

The present study showed that the validity of ICV estimates by linearly spaced ICAs is barely affected by the orientation of the ICAs or the choice of interpolation method at small linear spacings (<= 15 mm). At larger linear spacings cubic spline interpolation on sagittal or reconstructed coronal ICAs resulted in the most valid estimates. Even at a linear spacing of 50 mm, requiring less than five minutes segmentation per ICV, highly valid ICV estimates could be achieved.

Abbreviations

GDS: Global deterioration scale; ICA: Intracranial area; ICC: Intra-class correlation coefficient; ICV: Intracranial volume; IR/GR: Inversion recovery/gradient echo; MCI: Mild cognitive impairment; MRI: Magnetic resonance image.

Competing interests

The authors declare that they have no competing interests.

Authors' contributions

NK conceived the study and participated in its design, did manual segmentations of the intracranial volumes, performed the statistical analyses and drafted the manuscript. EO participated in the design of the study and helped to draft the manuscript. MR participated in the design of the study, helped with the statistical analyses and helped to draft the manuscript. CE helped to draft the manuscript. HM participated in the design of the study and helped to draft the manuscript. AW conceived and designed the Gothenburg MCI study, which the present study is as substudy of, and helped to draft the manuscript. All authors read and approved the final manuscript.

Acknowledgments

We thank Simon Skau for segmenting intracranial volumes used for the inter-rater statistics, colleagues at the memory clinic in Mölndal for scientific discussions and support, the radiology department in Mölndal for a solid work, and Hjalmar Svensson Foundation, Insamlingsstiftelsen för neurologisk forskning, Swedish Brain Power, and Wilhelm och Martina Lundgrens Vetenskapsfond 1 for financial contributions.

Author details

[1]Institute of Psychiatry and Neurochemistry, Department of Neuroscience and physiology, The Sahlgrenska Academy, University of Gothenburg, Box 430, SE-405 30 Göteborg, Sweden. [2]Department of Mathematical Sciences, Chalmers University of Technology and University of Gothenburg, SE-412 96 Göteborg, Sweden. [3]Department of Philosophy, Linguistics and Theory of Science, University of Gothenburg, Box 200, SE-405 30 Göteborg, Sweden.

References

1. Whitwell JL, Crum WR, Watt HC, Fox NC. Normalization of cerebral volumes by use of intracranial volume: implications for longitudinal quantitative MR imaging. AJNR Am J Neuroradiol. 2001;22:1483–9.

2. Eckerström C, Olsson E, Borga M, Ekholm S, Ribbelin S, Rolstad S, et al. Small baseline volume of left hippocampus is associated with subsequent conversion of MCI into dementia: the Goteborg MCI study. J Neurol Sci. 2008;272:48–59.
3. Olsson E, Eckerström C, Berg G, Borga M, Ekholm S, Johannsson G, et al. Hippocampal volumes in patients exposed to low-dose radiation to the basal brain. A case–control study in long-term survivors from cancer in the head and neck region. Radiat Oncol. 2012;7:202.
4. Eritaia J, Wood SJ, Stuart GW, Bridle N, Dudgeon P, Maruff P, et al. An optimized method for estimating intracranial volume from magnetic resonance images. Magn Reson Med. 2000;44:973–7.
5. Malykhin NV, Lebel RM, Coupland NJ, Wilman AH, Carter R. In vivo quantification of hippocampal subfields using 4.7 T fast spin echo imaging. Neuroimage. 2010;49:1224–30.
6. Surdhar I, Gee M, Bouchard T, Coupland N, Malykhin N, Camicioli R. Intact limbic-prefrontal connections and reduced amygdala volumes in Parkinson's disease with mild depressive symptoms. Parkinsonism Relat Disord. 2012;18:809–13.
7. Butler C, van Erp W, Bhaduri A, Hammers A, Heckemann R, Zeman A. Magnetic resonance volumetry reveals focal brain atrophy in transient epileptic amnesia. Epilepsy Behav. 2013;28:363–9.
8. Reetz K, Costa AS, Mirzazade S, Lehmann A, Juzek A, Rakowicz M, et al. Genotype-specific patterns of atrophy progression are more sensitive than clinical decline in SCA1, SCA3 and SCA6. Brain. 2013;136:905–17.
9. Travis SG, Huang Y, Fujiwara E, Radomski A, Olsen F, Carter R, et al. High field structural MRI reveals specific episodic memory correlates in the subfields of the hippocampus. Neuropsychologia. 2014;53:233–45.
10. Peters F, Villeneuve S, Belleville S. Predicting progression to dementia in elderly subjects with mild cognitive impairment using both cognitive and neuroimaging predictors. J Alzheimers Dis. 2014;38:307–18.
11. Buckner RL, Head D, Parker J, Fotenos AF, Marcus D, Morris JC, et al. A unified approach for morphometric and functional data analysis in young, old, and demented adults using automated atlas-based head size normalization: reliability and validation against manual measurement of total intracranial volume. Neuroimage. 2004;23:724–38.
12. Keihaninejad S, Heckemann RA, Fagiolo G, Symms MR, Hajnal JV, Hammers A. A robust method to estimate the intracranial volume across MRI field strengths (1.5T and 3T). Neuroimage. 2010;50:1427–37.
13. Reisberg B, Ferris SH, de Leon MJ, Crook T. Global Deterioration Scale (GDS). Psychopharmacol Bull. 1988;24:661–3.
14. Wallin A, Göthlin M, Gustavsson M, Zetterberg H, Eckerström C, Blennow K, et al. Progression from mild to pronounced MCI is not associated with cerebrospinal fluid biomarker deviations. Dement Geriatr Cogn Disord. 2011;32:193–7.
15. McGraw KO, Wong SP. Forming inferences about some intraclass correlation coefficients. Psychol Methods. 1996;1:30–46.
16. Matlab function ICC [http://www.mathworks.com/matlabcentral/fileexchange/22099-intraclass-correlation-coefficient-icc-]
17. Sepkoski Jr JJ. Quantified coefficients of association and measurement of similarity. Math Geol. 1974;6:135–52.
18. Raz N, Ghisletta P, Rodrigue KM, Kennedy KM, Lindenberger U. Trajectories of brain aging in middle-aged and older adults: regional and individual differences. Neuroimage. 2010;51:501–11.
19. Nordenskjöld R, Malmberg F, Larsson EM, Simmons A, Brooks SJ, Lind L, et al. Intracranial volume estimated with commonly used methods could introduce bias in studies including brain volume measurements. Neuroimage. 2013;83:355–60.
20. Fischl B. FreeSurfer. Neuroimage. 2012;62:774–81.
21. Ashburner J. SPM: a history. Neuroimage. 2012;62:791–800.
22. Malone IB, Leung KK, Clegg S, Barnes J, Whitwell JL, Ashburner J, et al. Accurate automatic estimation of total intracranial volume: a nuisance variable with less nuisance. Neuroimage. 2015;104:366–72.
23. Pengas G, Pereira JM, Williams GB, Nestor PJ. Comparative reliability of total intracranial volume estimation methods and the influence of atrophy in a longitudinal semantic dementia cohort. J Neuroimaging. 2009;19:37–46.
24. Lehmann TM, Gönner C, Spitzer K. Survey: interpolation methods in medical image processing. IEEE Trans Med Imaging. 1999;18:1049–75.

14

Whole-heart four-dimensional flow can be acquired with preserved quality without respiratory gating, facilitating clinical use: a head-to-head comparison

Mikael Kanski[1], Johannes Töger[1,2], Katarina Steding-Ehrenborg[1], Christos Xanthis[1,3], Karin Markenroth Bloch[4], Einar Heiberg[1,5,6], Marcus Carlsson[1] and Håkan Arheden[1*]

Abstract

Background: Respiratory gating is often used in 4D-flow acquisition to reduce motion artifacts. However, gating increases scan time. The aim of this study was to investigate if respiratory gating can be excluded from 4D flow acquisitions without affecting quantitative intracardiac parameters.

Methods: Eight volunteers underwent CMR at 1.5 T with a 5-channel coil (5ch). Imaging included 2D flow measurements and whole-heart 4D flow with and without respiratory gating (Resp(+), Resp(−)). Stroke volume (SV), particle-trace volumes, kinetic energy, and vortex-ring volume were obtained from 4D flow-data. These parameters were compared between 5ch Resp(+) and 5ch Resp(−). In addition, 20 patients with heart failure were scanned using a 32-channel coil (32ch), and particle-trace volumes were compared to planimetric SV. Paired comparisons were performed using Wilcoxon's test and correlation analysis using Pearson r. Agreement was assessed as bias ± SD.

Results: Stroke volume from 4D flow was lower compared to 2D flow both with and without respiratory gating (5ch Resp(+) 88 ± 18 vs 97 ± 24.0, $p = 0.001$; 5ch Resp(−) 86 ± 16 vs 97.1 ± 22.7, $p < 0.01$). There was a good correlation between Resp(+) and Resp(−) for particle-trace derived volumes ($R^2 = 0.82$, 0.2 ± 9.4 ml), mean kinetic energy ($R^2 = 0.86$, 0.07 ± 0.21 mJ), peak kinetic energy ($R^2 = 0.88$, 0.14 ± 0.77 mJ), and vortex-ring volume ($R^2 = 0.70$, −2.5 ± 9.4 ml). Furthermore, good correlation was found between particle-trace volume and planimetric SV in patients for 32ch Resp(−) ($R^2 = 0.62$, −4.2 ± 17.6 ml) and in healthy volunteers for 5ch Resp(+) ($R^2 = 0.89$, −11 ± 7 ml), and 5ch Resp(−) ($R^2 = 0.93$, −7.5 ± 5.4 ml), Average scan duration for Resp(−) was shorter compared to Resp(+) (27 ± 9 min vs 61 ± 19 min, $p < 0.05$).

Conclusions: Whole-heart 4D flow can be acquired with preserved quantitative results without respiratory gating, facilitating clinical use.

Keywords: Cardiac MRI, 4D flow, Respiratory gating, Kinetic energy, Particle trace, Vortex ring size

* Correspondence: hakan.arheden@med.lu.se
[1]Department of Clinical Physiology, Lund University, Lund University Hospital, Lund, Sweden
Full list of author information is available at the end of the article

Background

The use of three-dimensional, time-resolved, three-component (4D) phase-contrast cardiovascular magnetic resonance (CMR), also called 4D flow, is increasingly used to study blood flow patterns [1-6], quantify kinetic energy [4, 7-11], and for particle tracing analysis [5, 12]. Due to the possibility of off-line flow quantifications, visualization of vascular anatomy and derivation of various parameters, 4D flow is emerging as a new powerful tool in CMR, e.g. in patients with congenital vascular anomalies [13, 14]. However, 4D flow of the whole heart is limited by scan times [5], which are long even when applying acceleration techniques [15]. Respiratory gating, usually being used to reduce respiratory motion artifacts [16-19], further prolongs the acquisition time by unpredictable amounts, whereas it may be difficult in some patients. Acquisition of 4D flow without respiratory gating has the advantage of reduced and known scan time and could therefore simplify 4D flow acquisitions in the clinical setting in orthopnoeic and claustrophobic patients.

Nordmeyer et al. [20] have previously investigated the effect of respiratory gating in 4D flow and found a large reduction in scan time for 4D flow without respiratory gating compared to with respiratory gating, and no significant differences for stroke volume (SV) quantifications in greater vessels. However, intracardiac 4D flow was not investigated. Intracardiac measures, especially those based on particle tracing, may be more sensitive to respiratory motion as the diaphragm movement affects the position of the heart, and the effect of respiratory gating on intracardiac 4D flow parameters has not previously been investigated. Therefore, we aimed to investigate the effect on quantitative intracardiac flow parameters and particle tracing quality in 4D flow with and without respiratory gating.

Material and methods

Study design and CMR protocol

The study was approved by the Regional Ethical Review Board in Lund, Sweden, and all subjects provided written consent. Ten (10) healthy volunteers (4 men, 6 women, age 27 ± 2 years) underwent CMR in a 1.5 T Philips Achieva scanner (Philips Healthcare, Best, The Netherlands). The CMR protocol consisted of cardiac function cine imaging (short axis, 2–3- and 4-chamber view), 2D flow measurements (aorta and main pulmonary artery (MPA)) and 4D flow sequences with respiratory gating (Resp(+)) and without any respiratory gating (Resp(−)). The protocol was repeated twice for each subject on the same day; the first scan using a 32 channel coil (32ch), and the second scan using a 5 channel coil (5ch). In 2 of the 10 subjects, the 5ch and 32ch scans could not be performed on the same day and were performed after 7 days in one subject. The other subject was re-scanned after 36 days but the dataset was excluded from comparison between coils as it was deemed too long time between 32ch and 5ch scans. Due to artifacts seen in 4D flow Resp(+) acquisitions using the 32ch coil (unpublished observations; probably due to steady-state loss or residual breathing), the 32ch scan only included the Resp(−) 4D flow sequence. One possible explanation to why these artifacts are seen in the 32ch acquisition and not the 5ch acquisition is the fact that the 32ch coil consists of smaller coils and therefore signal from the subcutaneous fat will be more prominent compared to the 5ch coil. The 4D flow sequences were both preceded and followed by 2D flow acquisitions in order to test intrastudy variability in stroke volume (SV). The CMR protocol is summarized in Table 1.

Furthermore, 20 patients with heart failure underwent CMR using a 32ch coil including cardiac function cine imaging (short axis, 2–3- and 4-chamber view), and Resp(−) 4D flow.

CMR sequence parameters

4D flow A segmented gradient echo (TFE) sequence, 2 views per segment, with retrospective ECG-triggering and a SENSE parallel imaging factor of 2 was used. 4D flow was acquired with respiratory gating (Resp(+)) and without respiratory gating (Resp(−)) with a field of view covering the entire heart. In the Resp(+) sequence, a pencil navigator beam was positioned in the center of the right lung diaphragm with two-thirds of the navigator in the liver. The width of the navigator acceptance window was 5 mm. The acquired temporal resolution was 51–54 ms, i.e. 15–22 phases acquired, which were then reconstructed to 40 heart phases. Typical scanning parameters were TE/

Table 1 CMR protocol for healthy volunteers. Ao = Aorta, MPA = Main pulmonary artery, 2ch, 3ch, 4ch = two-chamber, three-chamber, four-chamber

Sequence	
1.	Subject placed in scanner with 32-channel cardiac coil
2.	Cine images: 2ch, 3ch, 4ch, short-axis
3.	2D flow: Ao, MPA
4.	4D flow Resp(−)
5.	2D flow: Ao, MPA
6.	Switch to 5-channel cardiac coil, short break for subject
7.	Cine images: 2ch, 3ch, 4ch, short-axis
8.	2D flow: Ao, MPA
9.	4D flow Resp(+)
10.	4D flow Resp(−)
11.	2D flow: Ao, MPA
12.	End of protocol

TR: 3.7/6.2 ms, flip angle: 8°, acquired and reconstructed voxel size: 3 × 3 × 3 mm^3, number of acquired slices 40–52, VENC 100 cm/s. Concomitant gradient terms were compensated by the CMR scanner. Phase unwrapping was performed offline using an automatic algorithm with manual corrections as needed. Phase background errors (e.g. due to eddy currents) were corrected offline by subtraction of a linear fit of velocities in stationary tissue.

2D flow A non-segmented phase-contrast gradient echo sequence with retrospective ECG-triggering during free breathing was used to measure through-plane flow. Typical scanning parameters were TE/TR: 5.3/8.6 ms, flip angle: 15°, temporal resolution: 23–35 ms (35 phases), spatial resolution: 1.2 × 1.2 × 6 mm, VENC: 200 cm/s for both aorta (Ao) and main pulmonary artery (MPA). For 2D flow scans, phase background as well as concomitant gradients were compensated by the scanner software.

Cine images Standard steady-state free precession cine images were acquired in the two-chamber, three-chamber, four-chamber and short axis views. Typical scanning parameters were: TE/TR: 1.6/3.2 ms, flip angle: 60°, spatial resolution: 1.25 × 1.25 × 8 mm, no slice gap.

Particle tracing

Particle tracing (PT) uses the measured 4D flow information to compute blood motion. The PT quality of the collected 4D flow data was evaluated as follows, based on a method previously described [5]:

1) The position of the short-axis cine images were manually adjusted to match the 4D flow data to reduce offsets due to breath-holding positions, as shown in Fig. 1.
2) The volume of the left ventricle (LV) was manually delineated at end-diastole, as seen in Fig. 1. Furthermore, the locations of the mitral valve and aortic valve at end-systole were manually delineated using long-axis (2ch, 3ch, 4ch) cine images.
3) One particle for each 4D flow voxel in the LV end-diastolic volume was traced backward in time to end-systole to find the PT inflow volume, and traced forward in time to end-systole to find the PT outflow volume.
4) Particles traced forward in time with a final position on the basal side of the aortic valve were considered as outflowing blood. Particles traced backward in time with a final position on the basal side of the mitral valve were considered as inflowing blood. Each particle contributed a volume equal to the 4D flow voxel size.
5) In healthy volunteers with normal valve function, the particle trace inflow and outflow should be equal. Therefore, the inflowing volume was compared to the outflowing volume.
6) Fig. 1 shows an illustration of the above method. Particle tracing was performed using a 4th-order Runge–Kutta method with a constant timestep of 5 ms. Linear interpolation of the 4D flow velocity data was used in space and time.

Image analysis

The freely available software Segment (http://segment.heiberg.se) was used for all image analysis [21]. Particle tracing was performed using an in-house developed code to Segment, consisting of a 4th Runge–Kutta method and linear interpolation in space and time, as previously described [12].

Stroke Volume analysis In short, the stroke volume (SV) was first measured in the 2D flow images by delineating the vessels over time using a region of interest (ROI). In the 4D flow data, a 2D plane was computed from the 2D flow images, and the ROI was copied to the computed image plane. Manual corrections of the ROI position were performed if needed.

Kinetic Energy analysis The LV was defined by manually drawing the contours of the blood volume in short-axis slices over the entire cardiac cycle. The delineations were then transferred to the 4D data set and KE was calculated as the sum of ½mv^2 for each voxel [22], where m is the mass of blood in one voxel and v is the velocity in the voxel. Manual corrections of delineations were performed when needed.

Vortex ring volume Lagrangian coherent structures (LCS) were computed as previously described [12]. Particle tracing computations required for the LCS algorithm were implemented in CUDA-C and performed on Graphical Processing Unit (GPU) cards. LCS indicative of vortex-ring formation were delineated in the long-axis views. Then, the vortex-ring volume was delineated in short-axis slices 4 mm apart, guided by the long-axis delineations. Total vortex volume was defined as the summed volume of all slices.

Particle trace visualizations

Blood flow was visualized using FourFlow v1.2.14, open source software for flow visualization (http://fourflow.heiberg.se). Particles were emitted every 25–30 ms during diastole in the left atrium to visualize diastolic inflow into the LV. Images were saved after the rapid filling phase of the LV.

Statistical analysis

Statistical analysis was performed using Graphpad for Windows (v6.04, Graphpad Software Inc, La Jolla, USA). Group values are given as mean ± SD. Measurements

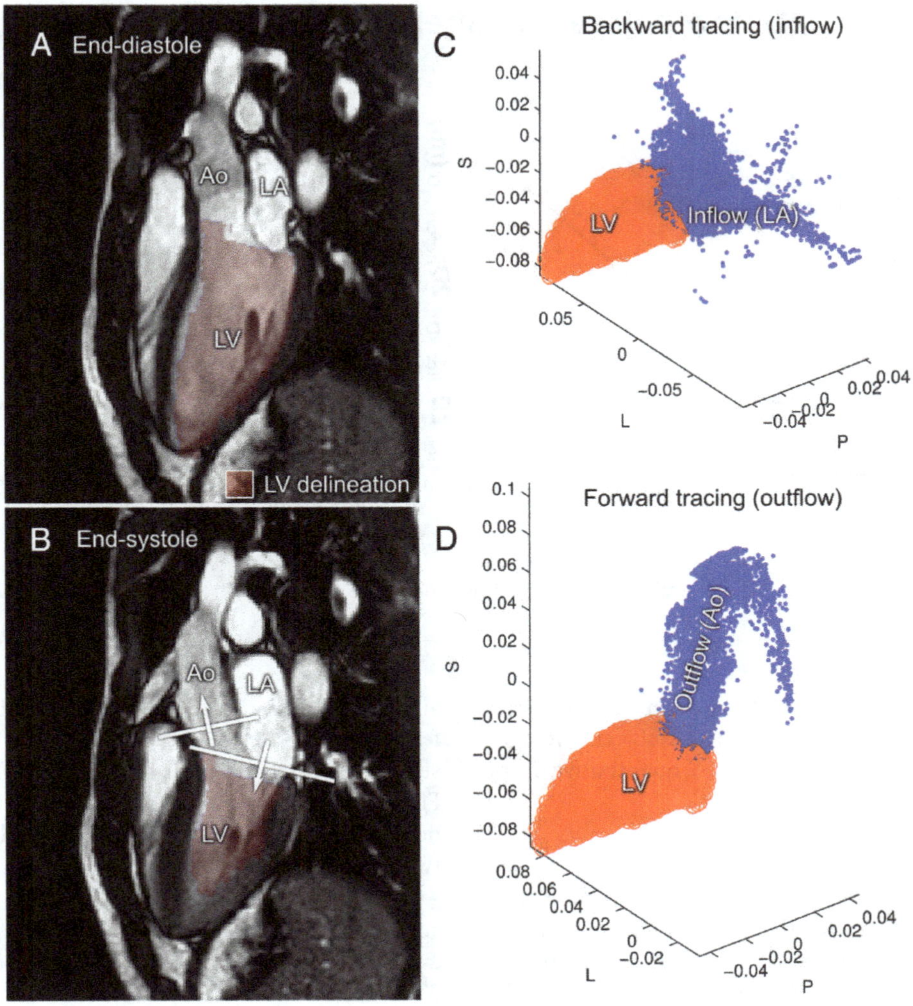

Fig. 1 Data evaluation of particle trace (PT). **a**: Using the short-axis manual delineation of the LV, all 4D flow voxels inside the LV at end-diastole were selected for particle trace analysis. Panel B shows the planes used to define inflow and outflow. Panel **c** and **d**: One particle was placed in each voxel and traced backward in time to end-systole (*inflow*, **c**), and forward to end-systole (*outflow*, **d**). For inflow analysis **c**, all particles on the basal side of the mitral valve at end-systole (**b**) were considered as inflowing blood. For outflow analysis (**d**), all particles on the basal side of the aortic valve (**b**) at end-systole were considered as inflowing blood. *L = Left-Right axis, P = Posterior-Anterior axis, S = Superior-Inferior axis*

acquired from different sequences were compared using a paired non-parametric two-tailed test (Wilcoxon) and linear regression. Correlation analysis was performed using Pearson r. Agreement was assessed as bias ± SD [23]. Differences with *P*-values <0.05 were considered statistically significant.

Results

Subject and patient characteristics are shown in Table 2.

Excluded data

In one subject, the difference in scan duration between Resp(−) and Resp(+) 4D flow acquisitions was only 2 min (5 %), suggesting inaccurate navigator triggering, and these data were therefore excluded. Another subject was excluded due to a zipper artifact through the base of

Table 2 Subject demographics and characteristics

	Healthy volunteers	Patients with heart failure
Sex (male/female, n)	5/3	16/4
Age (years)	28 ± 1	68 ± 8
Height (cm)	172 ± 11	176 ± 9
Heart rate (bpm)	66 ± 10	68 ± 16
LV-EF (%)	60 ± 4	28 ± 10
Underlying disease (%)		
- Dilated cardiomyopathy	N/A	45
- Ischemic heart disease	N/A	55

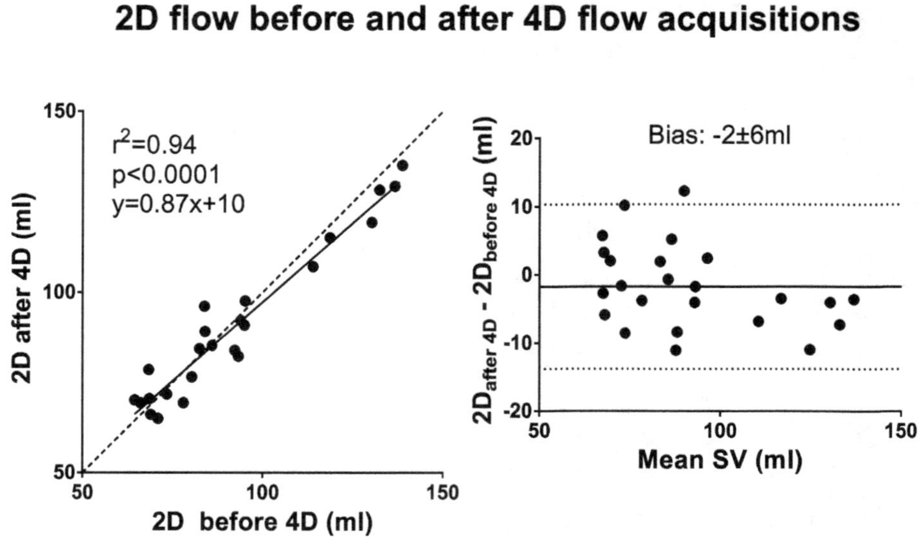

Fig. 2 Stability of stroke volume (SV) over the experiment in healthy volunteers. The scatter plot (*left*) shows SV (ml) from 2D flow acquired before and after 4D flow acquisitions. The Bland-Altman analysis (*right*) shows bias (solid line) ±1.96SD (dashed lines). The SV did not vary significantly over the experiment

left ventricle, however, the difference in scan duration was analyzed in this subject. Thus, 8 subjects were included and analyzed with respect to quantitative intracardiac measures.

4D flow and 2D flow

There was a strong correlation between 2D flow measurements before and after the 4D flow sequences, indicating stability of both physiology and measurement over the scan duration ($R^2 = 0.94$, $p < 0.0001$; −1.7 ± 6.2 ml Fig. 2). For comparison between 2D and 4D, the 2D flow acquired prior to 4D was used. Bias is presented in absolute measures and as percentage in Table 3.

Stroke volume (SV) in aorta and pulmonary artery with 4D flow was lower compared to SV from 2D flow (5ch Resp(+): 88 ± 18 ml vs 97 ± 24 ml, $p < 0.01$; 5ch Resp(−): 86 ± 16 ml vs 97 ± 24 ml, $p < 0.01$). Regression analysis showed somewhat higher correlation between SV from 4D flow and 2D flow for Resp(+) compared to the Resp(−) sequences, and Bland-Altman analyses showed similar bias between the different 4D sequences and 2D flow (Fig. 3). There was a good correlation between SV from 4D Resp(+) and 4D Resp(−) (R2 = 0.55, $p < 0.001$, bias: 2 ± 11 ml).

Particle tracing analysis in healthy volunteers and in patients

There was good correlation between PT volumes derived from Resp(+) 4D flow compared to PT volumes derived from Resp(−) 4D flow (Fig. 4). PT inflow was higher than PT outflow with 5ch Resp(−) (91.8 ± 20.0 vs 78.4 ± 21.3, $p < 0.05$) but no difference was seen with 5ch Resp(+) or 32ch Resp(−) (88.7 ± 17.9 ml vs 81.9 ± 14.1 ml, $p = 0.08$; and 92.5 ± 19.9 vs 84.9 ± 15.7, p = 0.11). There was no difference in bias between the 5ch Resp(+) and 5ch Resp(−) sequences (6.8 ± 9.3 ml vs 13.3 ± 11.7 ml; $p = 0.25$). Fig. 5 shows correlation and bias ± SD for PT inflow vs outflow. In patients, there was a good correlation between PT inflow volume and planimetric SV ($R^2 = 0.62$, −4.2 ± 17.6 ml, Fig. 6) and in healthy volunteers the correlation was good for 5ch Resp(+) ($R^2 = 0.89$, 10.7 ± 7.2 ml), 5ch Resp(−) ($R^2 = 0.93$, −7.5 ± 5.5 ml), and 32ch Resp(−) ($R^2 = 0.76$, −15.0 ± 12.3 ml). Visualization of Resp(+) and Resp(−) particle trace in one healthy volunteer is presented in Fig. 7. Particle trace visualizations for all subjects are shown in Additional file 1.

Table 3 Bias in absolute measures and percentage difference

Comparison	Absolute	Percentage
2D before and after 4D (Fig. 2)	−2 ± 6 ml	−1 ± 7 %
5ch Resp(+) 4D SV vs 2D SV (Fig. 3)	−10 ± 12 ml	−10 ± 11 %
5ch Resp(−) 4D SV vs 2D SV (Fig. 3)	−13 ± 12 ml	−14 ± 12 %
32ch Resp(−) 4D SV vs 2D SV (Fig. 3)	−12 ± 14 ml	−12 ± 13 %
PT Resp(+) vs PT Resp(−) (Fig. 4)	0 ± 9 ml	2 ± 12 %
5ch Resp(+) PT Inflow vs Outflow (Fig. 5)	7 ± 9 ml	8 ± 9 %
5ch Resp(−) PT Inflow vs Outflow (Fig. 5)	13 ± 12 ml	17 ± 16 %
32ch Resp(−) PT Inflow vs Outflow (Fig. 5)	8 ± 11 ml	8 ± 10 %
32ch Resp(−) vs planimetric SV (Fig. 6)	−4 ± 18 ml	−8 ± 23 %
5ch Resp(−) vs 5ch Resp(+) mean KE (Fig. 8)	0.1 ± 0.2 mJ	4 ± 12 %
5ch Resp(−) vs 5ch Resp(+) KE peak values (Fig. 8)	0.1 ± 0.8 mJ	1 ± 17 %
Vortex volume Resp(−) vs Resp(+) (Fig. 9)	−3 ± 9 ml	−4 ± 13 %
4D SV 32ch Resp(−) vs 5ch Resp(−) (Fig. 10)	2 ± 7 ml	2 ± 8 %

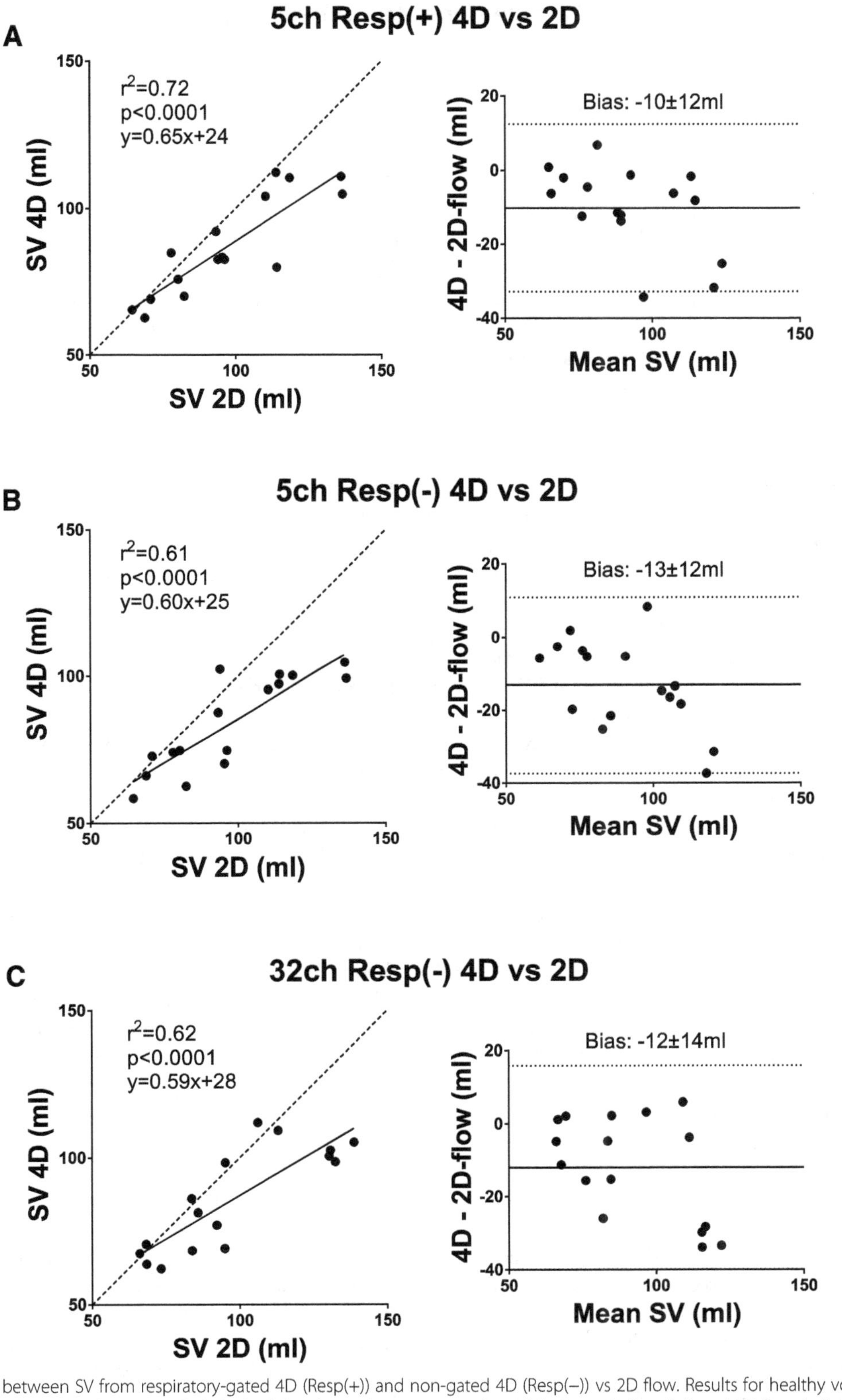

Fig. 3 Comparison between SV from respiratory-gated 4D (Resp(+)) and non-gated 4D (Resp(−)) vs 2D flow. Results for healthy volunteers. Both SV deduced from Ao and MPA flow are included. The left column shows scatter plots of SV from 4D flow (ml) and 2D flow (ml). Dashed lines show the line of identity. The right column shows the corresponding Bland Altman plots (bias ± 1.96SD). Panel **a** shows comparison between Resp(+) 4D and 2D. using a 5 channel coil. Panels **b** and **c** show the same results for SV from 4D Resp(−) acquired with a 5 channel cardiac coil and a 32 channel cardiac coil, respectively. The bias and spread were similar for all three methods

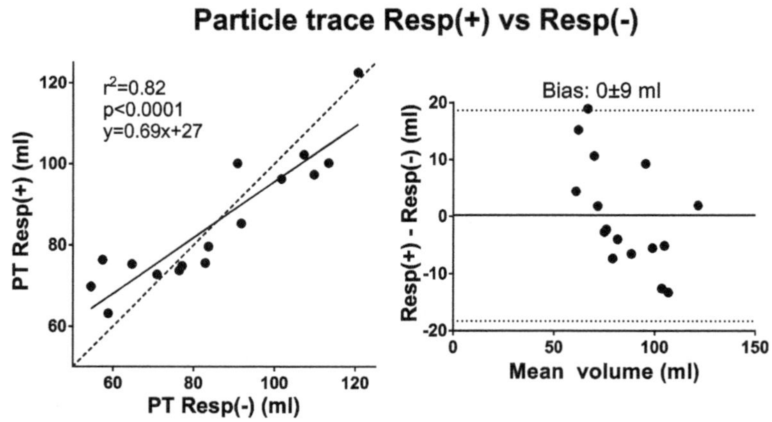

Fig. 4 Particle-trace analysis in healthy volunteers. Scatter plot with particle trace (PT) derived SV (ml) from 5ch Resp(+) vs 5ch Resp(−). Dashed line represent line of identity. Bland-Altman analysis shows the bias (bias ± 1.96SD)

Kinetic energy and vortex ring size

Kinetic energy was studied on individual basis in the healthy volunteers and the KE plots are presented subject by subject in Fig. 8. There was good correlation between Resp(+) and Resp(−) mean KE values ($R^2 = 0.86$, $p = 0.001$; bias 0.07 ± 0.21 mJ) and peak KE values ($R^2 = 0.88$, $p < 0.0001$; bias 0.14 ± 0.77 mJ) (Fig. 9). For vortex volume, there was good correlation between 5ch Resp(+) and 5ch Resp(−) ($R^2 = 0.70$, $p < 0.01$; bias −2.5 ± 9.4 ml, Fig. 10). Visualization of Resp(+) and Resp(−) vortex ring delineation in one healthy volunteer is presented in Fig. 7. Vortex ring visualizations for all subjects are shown in Additional file 1.

Comparison between coils

There was no statistically significant difference between 32ch Resp(−) and 5ch Resp(−) regarding 2D flow (96 ± 25 ml vs 97 ± 24, $p = 0.68$; bias 1.6 ± 9.5 ml), 4D SV (88 ± 18 ml vs 86 ± 16 ml, $p = 0.32$; bias 2.1 ± 6.7 ml, Fig. 11), particle trace inflow (94 ± 19 ml vs 92 ± 20 ml, $p = 0.38$; bias 2.7 ± 8.3 ml), particle trace outflow (85 ± 16 ml vs 81 ± 19 ml, p = 0.47; bias 3.6 ± 7.0 ml), mean KE (1.6 ± 0.4 mJ vs 1.5 ± 0.5 mJ, p = 0.69; bias 0.04 ± 0.25 mJ), and vortex-ring size (70 ± 14 vs 65 ± 16, $p = 0.38$; bias 4.7 ± 11.8 ml). Also, KE curves from 32ch acquisition were similar to 5ch Resp(−) and 5ch Resp(+) (Fig. 8).

Scan duration

In three healthy volunteers scan duration was not measured and could not be assessed retrospectively. Thus, scan duration was measured in seven subjects. Paired non-parametric analysis (Wilcoxon) of the 5ch data shows a consistently shorter scan duration for the Resp(−) sequence compared to Resp(+) (27 ± 9 min vs 61 ± 19 min, $p < 0.05$).

Discussion

This study shows a head-to-head comparison and validation of intracardiac flow measures using 4D-flow sequences with and without respiratory gating. Our results show that 4D flow without respiratory gating, Resp(−), yields similar quantitative results and reduced scan time compared to 4D flow with respiratory gating, Resp(+), and comparable results in patients with heart failure.

Relation to earlier studies

The results of the present study show that respiratory gating may be excluded when studying intracardiac and large vessel blood flows acquired using 4D flow at 1.5 T. This is in line with results presented by Nordmeyer et al. [20] who showed that the respiratory gating may be omitted at 3 T when studying large vessel blood flow. However, our study at 1.5 T shows a slightly higher bias which can be explained by the field-strength difference as shown in a previous study [7]. Furthermore, we performed a validation between 5ch and 32ch acquired data which shows that 32ch Resp(−) yields similar results as 5ch Resp(−). To our knowledge there is no previous head-to-head comparison between the 32ch and 5ch coil.

This study shows an underestimation of 4D flow SV compared to 2D flow, which is in line with previous results at 1.5 T and 3 T [7, 24]. In a phantom study with steady flow (as opposed to the pulsatile flow in the heart), Brix et al. showed a 10 % overestimation of 4D flow compared to 2D [25], although their in vivo results show a small underestimation (−2 ± 15 ml, computed from presented values). Furthermore, we observed an underestimation of particle trace volumes compared to 2D flow, which is in line with previous studies on particle tracing [5, 12]. This may be explained by the clinically non-significant mitral regurgitation commonly seen in healthy volunteers [26] when comparing LV planimetry to 2D aortic blood flow. Further error sources include low temporal and spatial resolution, which have been shown

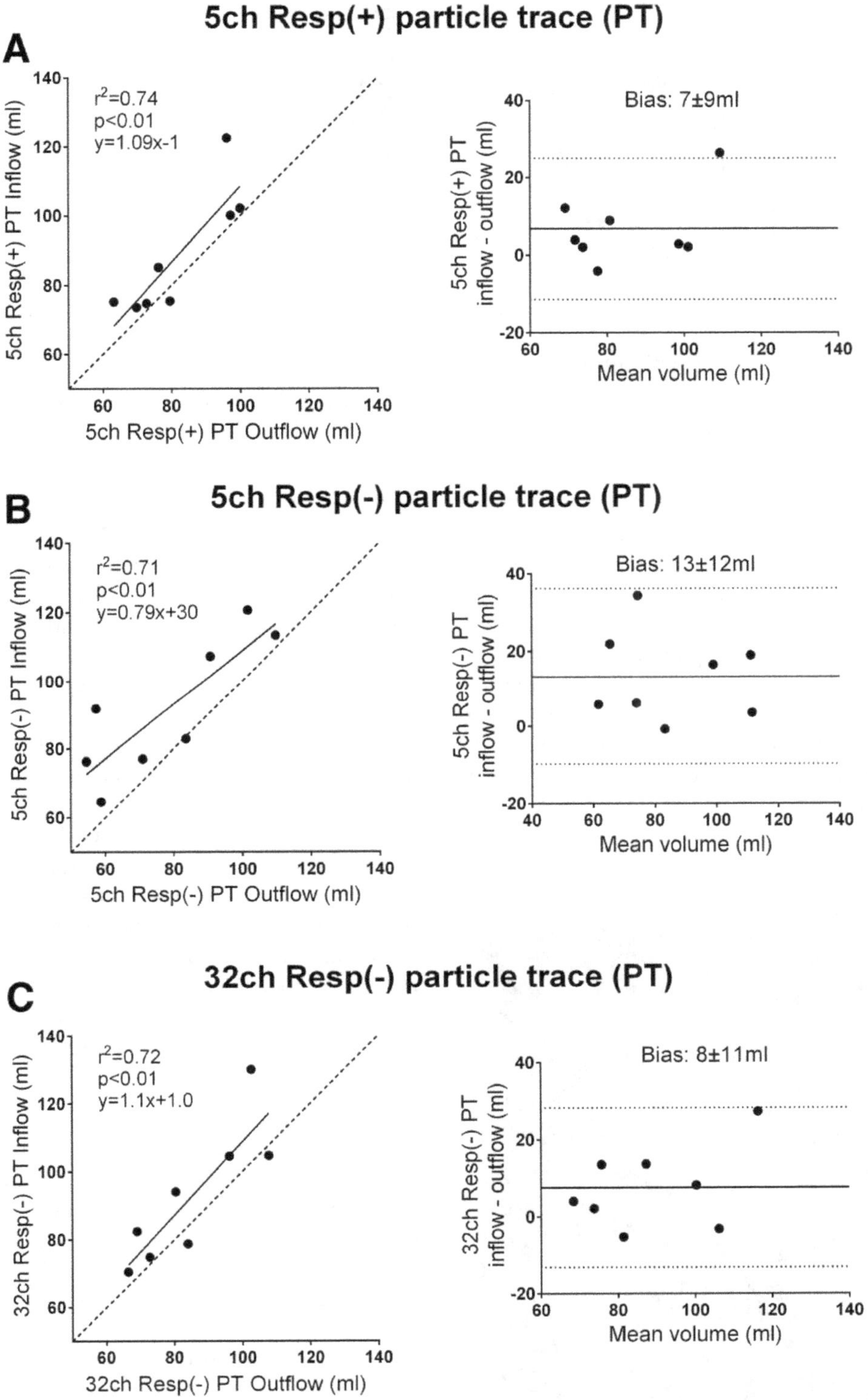

Fig. 5 Comparison between inflow vs outflow in healthy volunteers. There was a similar correlation between 5ch Resp(+) (panel **a**), 5ch Resp(−) (panel **b**), and 32ch Resp(−) (panel **c**). Bias is shown in the corresponding Bland-Altman plot (bias ± 1.96SD)

in a computational study to give lower particle tracing volumes [27]. A mild mitral insufficiency can also explain the larger particle trace inflow volume compared to particle trace outflow volume seen in this study.

In this study we observed the effect of acquiring 4D flow without respiratory navigator. When using Resp(−), scan time was reduced by 58 %. This can be compared to the 40 % reduction seen in the study by Nordmeyer et

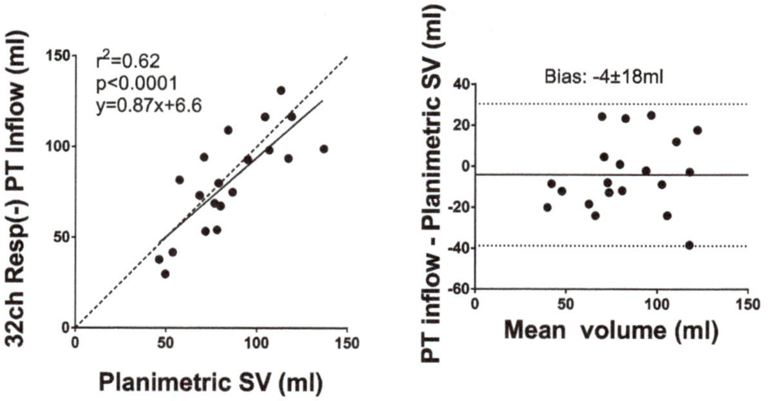

Fig. 6 Comparison between particle-trace inflowing blood to planimetric stroke volume in 20 patients with heart failure. Left: the dashed line represents line of identity. Bias is shown in the Bland-Altman plot to the right (bias ± 1.96SD)

al. [20]. The difference in scan time reduction between our study and that of Nordmeyer et al. may be explained by a multitude of factors including protocol design, differences in positioning and size of acceptance windows of the respiratory navigator, and physiological differences in e.g. heart rate and respiratory rate. The scan durations in this study are, even upon omission of the respiratory navigator, longer compared to contemporary work [10, 11, 28]. The scan time is influenced by 1) k-space readout technique (we use Cartesian in contrast to the faster spiral or radial read-outs [10, 11, 28]), 2) degree of parallel acquisition (we use 2 views per segment compared to up to 8 views per segment), and 3) size of the 3D box covering the area of interest, where we covered the entire heart and included the atria and ascending aorta, compared to others who only acquire data limited to e.g. the left ventricle.

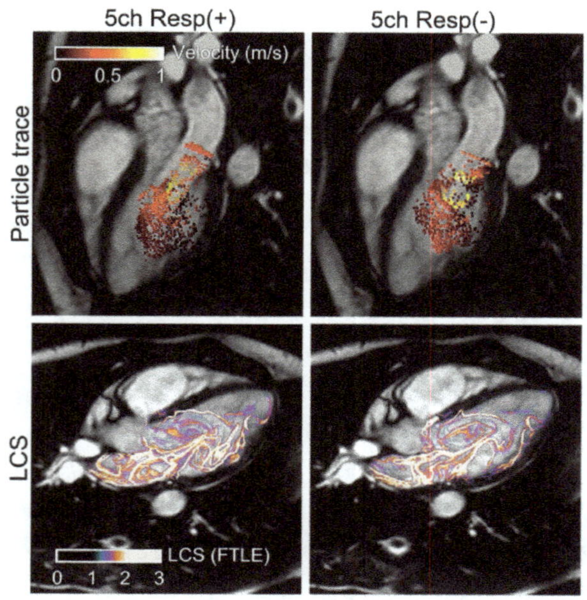

Fig. 7 Visualization of particle trace (*top* panels) and vortex volume with LCS (*bottom* panels) in one healthy volunteer using 5ch Resp(+) (*left* column) and 5ch Resp(−) (*right* column) in the 3 chamber view of the heart. For visualizations for all subjects, see Additional file 1

In the present study a VENC of 200 cm/s was used in arteries since the flow in these vessels, in absence of stenosis, often reach 150 cm/s and to avoid aliasing in routine clinical scans. Since anti-aliasing can be cumbersome in the clinical work flow, we chose a high VENC to avoid aliasing in most cases. Intracardiac velocities seldom exceed 100 cm/s, and we therefore chose a lower VENC of 100 cm/s to minimize noise since the velocity noise is proportional to VENC, as shown by Nilsson et al. [29] In the case aliasing occurs, it is possible to perform aliasing corrections in a research setting.

Clinical implications

When applying respiratory gating, the 4D flow sequence may be extensively prolonged. Gating efficiency has been reported to range from 50–70 % [20, 30], i.e. up to doubled scan duration. In this study, the mean scan duration for Resp(+) was twice as long as Resp(−), and yet the two different techniques yielded similar results for SV when comparing to 2D flow and in PT analyses, and also for whole heart 4D measurements such as KE. This suggests that the 4D flow measures considered in this study can be acquired without respiratory gating.

We chose to analyze the patients with regards to particle-trace inflow vs planimetric stroke volume, since this comparison is not influenced by the presence of mitral insufficiency commonly seen in patients with

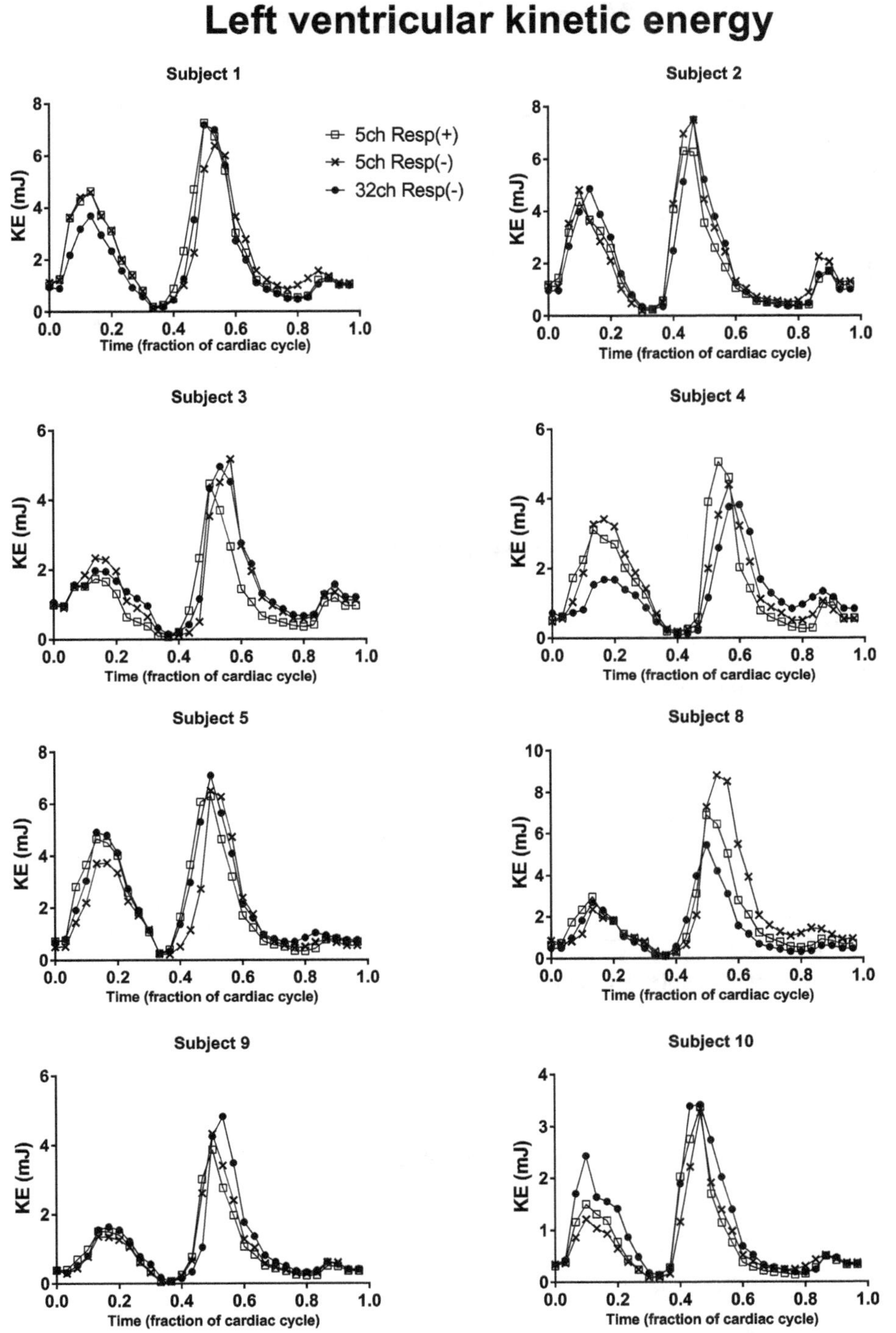

Fig. 8 LV kinetic energy (KE, mJ) presented subject by subject over the cardiac cycle as fraction of cardiac cycle in healthy volunteers. Note the similarity of the KE plots for each subject. Subject 8 performed the 32ch acquisition 36 days after the 5ch acquisition, which may affect the appearance of the KE curve

dilated ventricles. Our results show that 4D Resp(−) can be used with comparable results as in healthy volunteers, and that intracardiac diastolic blood flow can be accurately measured in patients.

Flow in the right atrium (RA) is known to be significantly affected by the respiratory cycle [31]. Therefore, gating the 4D flow acquisition to one point in the respiratory cycle may only show one aspect of RA flow. A

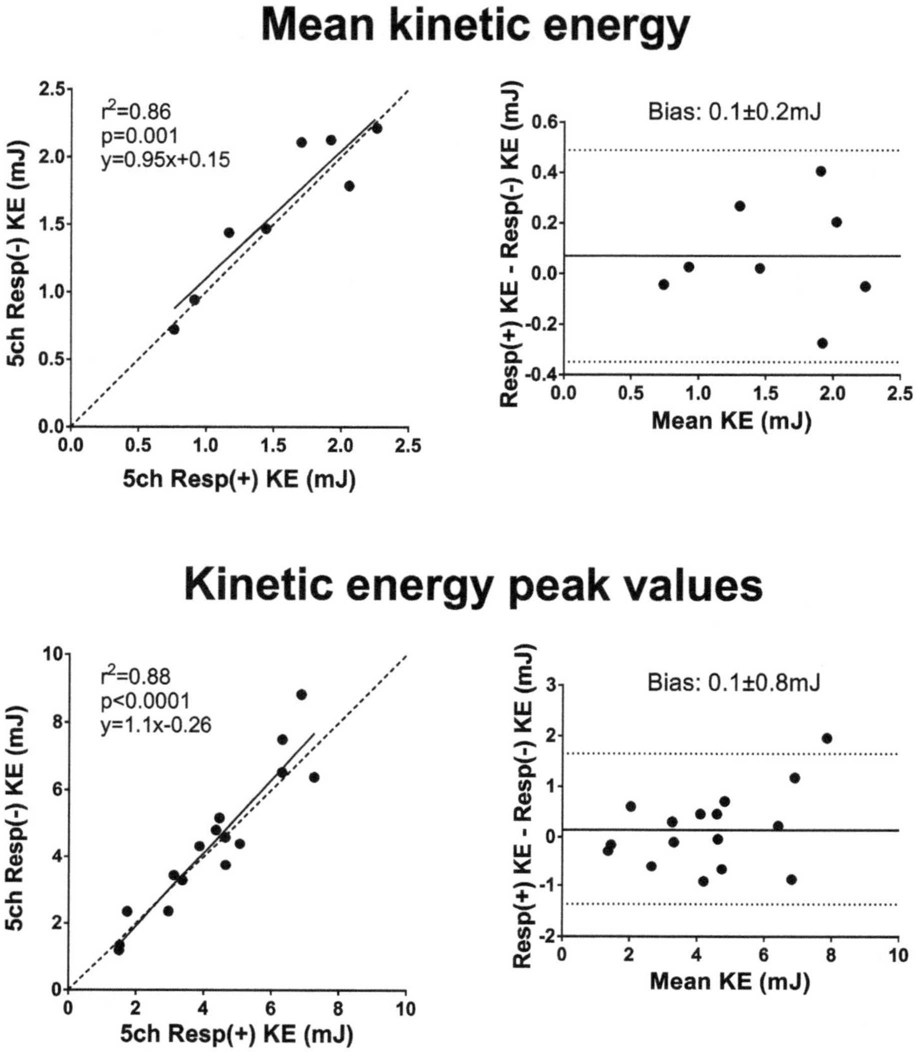

Fig. 9 Mean LV kinetic energy (KE, mJ) and peak KE values for 5ch Resp(–) vs 5ch Resp(+) in healthy volunteers. Note the significant correlation between the two sequences. Dashed lines represent line of identity. The bias is shown in the corresponding Bland-Altman plot (bias ± 1.96SD)

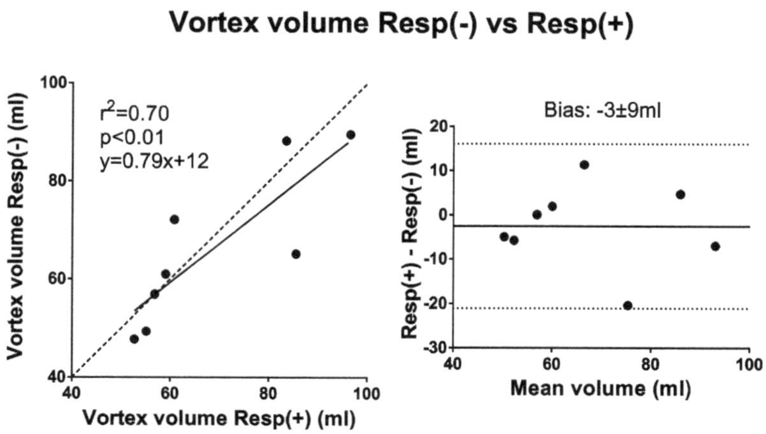

Fig. 10 Vortex-volume results for 5ch Resp(–) compared to 5ch Resp(+) in healthy volunteers. There was a statistically significant correlation. Dashed line represents line of identity. Bland-Altman analysis shows the bias (bias ± 1.96SD)

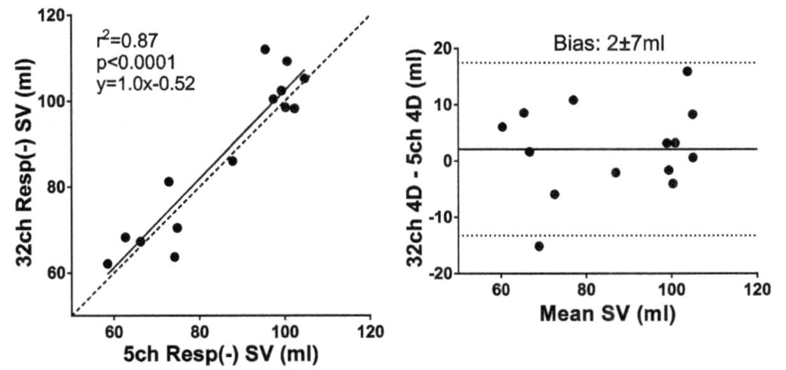

Fig. 11 Comparison between 32ch and 5ch coil in healthy volunteers. There was a strong correlation between 4D flow SV using 32ch and 5ch coil. Dashed line represents line of identity. Bland-Altman analysis shows the bias (bias ± 1.96SD)

4D flow acquisition without respiratory gating would instead show the average flow pattern in the right atrium, which may better capture physiological RA flow conditions. Our results suggest that this can be performed without affecting measurements of stroke volume and the quantitative parameters in the left ventricle presented in this study.

One subject was excluded due to a low difference in scan times between Resp(+) and Resp(−) acquisitions. This suggests that the respiratory gating accepted almost all data in the Resp(+) scan, and therefore was not effective in discriminating between respiratory phases in this subject. Thus, even when applying careful and accurate positioning of the respiratory navigator, gating may still not work as expected. However, the present results show that for the flow parameters investigated in this study, the effect of respiratory gating is of small importance.

Limitations

The sample size of the head-to-head comparison in healthy volunteers is small, and therefore non-parametric statistical tests were used. However, the results of the present study are decisive and unlikely to change significantly with a larger sample size. Two subjects underwent CMR with the 5ch and the 32ch coils on two different occasions instead of on the same day. However, this does not affect comparison of the influence of respiratory gating.

Conclusions

This study shows that 4D flow acquired without respiratory gating yields comparable quantitative measurements, both for vessel flow and for the quantitative intracardiac parameters particle tracing, kinetic energy and vortex ring formation, compared to 4D flow with respiratory gating. Therefore, whole-heart 4D flow without respiratory gating can be used for quantification of intracardiac blood flow.

Abbreviations

2ch: 2-chamber; 3ch: 3-chamber; 4ch: 4-chamber; 32ch: 32-channel coil; 5ch: 5-channel coil; 2D: Two-dimensional; 4D: Three-dimensional, time-resolved, three-component flow; Ao: Aorta; CMR: Cardiovascular magnetic resonance; CUDA: Compute unified device architecture; ECG: Electrocardiogram; GPU: Graphical processing unit; KE: Kinetic energy; LCS: Lagrangian coherent structures; LV: Left ventricle; MPA: Main pulmonary artery; PT: Particle tracing; RA: Right atrium; Resp(+): Sequence with respiratory gating; Resp(−): Sequence without respiratory gating; ROI: Region of interest; SD: Standard deviation; SV: Stroke volume; TE: Echo time; TR: Repetition time; TFE: Turbo-field echo; VENC: Velocity encoding value.

Competing interests

KMB is an employee of Philips Healthcare, Lund, Sweden. EH is the founder of Medviso AB, Lund, Sweden, that develops medical image-analysis software. The remaining authors declare that they have no competing interests.

Authors' contributions

All authors participated in conception and design of the study. MK recruited the volunteers and collected the data. MK and JT drafted the manuscript. MK, JT, and KSE performed the data analysis. CX developed the CUDA-C version of the LCS algorithm. KMB contributed with sequence programming. HA had full access to and was responsible for the integrity of the data. All authors critically revised the manuscript for important intellectual content, and all authors read and approved the final manuscript.

Authors' information

MK: MD; JT: PhD; KSE: PT, PhD; CX: PhD; KMB: PhD; EH: PhD, associate professor; MC: MD, PhD, associate professor; HA: MD, PhD, professor

Acknowledgments

The authors thank the volunteers for showing patience with the long scan durations and late evenings. This study was supported by the Swedish Research Council (2011-3916, 2012-4944); the Swedish Heart-Lung Foundation; Lund University Faculty of Medicine; Lund University Hospital, Lund, Sweden; and Region Skåne.

Author details
[1]Department of Clinical Physiology, Lund University, Lund University Hospital, Lund, Sweden. [2]Department of Numerical Analysis, Center of Mathematical Sciences, Lund University, Lund, Sweden. [3]Department of Computer Science and Biomedical informatics, University of Thessaly, Lamia, Greece. [4]Philips Healthcare, Lund, Sweden. [5]Department of Biomedical Engineering, Faculty of Engineering, Lund University, Lund, Sweden. [6]Center for Mathematics, Faculty of Engineering, Lund University, Lund, Sweden.

References

1. Kim WY, Walker PG, Pedersen EM, Poulsen JK, Oyre S, Houlind K, et al. Left ventricular blood flow patterns in normal subjects: a quantitative analysis by three-dimensional magnetic resonance velocity mapping. J Am Coll Cardiol. 1995;26:224–38.
2. Kilner PJ, Yang GZ, Wilkes a J, Mohiaddin RH, Firmin DN, Yacoub MH. Asymmetric redirection of flow through the heart. Nature. 2000;404:759–61.
3. Kozerke S, Hasenkam JM, Pedersen EM, Boesiger P. Visualization of flow patterns distal to aortic valve prostheses in humans using a fast approach for cine 3D velocity mapping. J Magn Reson Imaging. 2001;13:690–8.
4. Bolger AF, Heiberg E, Karlsson M, Wigström L, Engvall J, Sigfridsson A, et al. Transit of blood flow through the human left ventricle mapped by cardiovascular magnetic resonance. J Cardiovasc Magn Reson. 2007;9:741–7.
5. Eriksson J, Carlhäll CJ, Dyverfeldt P, Engvall J, Bolger AF, Ebbers T. Semi-automatic quantification of 4D left ventricular blood flow. J Cardiovasc Magn Reson. 2010;12:9.
6. Töger J, Carlsson M, Söderlind G, Arheden H, Heiberg E. Volume Tracking: A new method for quantitative assessment and visualization of intracardiac blood flow from three-dimensional, time-resolved, three-component magnetic resonance velocity mapping. BMC Med Imaging. 2011;11:10.
7. Carlsson M, Töger J, Kanski M, Bloch K, Ståhlberg F, Heiberg E, et al. Quantification and visualization of cardiovascular 4D velocity mapping accelerated with parallel imaging or k-t BLAST: head to head comparison and validation at 1.5 T and 3 T. J Cardiovasc Magn Reson. 2011;13:55.
8. Arvidsson PM, Töger J, Heiberg E, Carlsson M, Arheden H. Quantification of left and right atrial kinetic energy using four-dimensional intracardiac magnetic resonance imaging flow measurements. J Appl Physiol. 2013;114:1472–81.
9. Eriksson J, Dyverfeldt P, Engvall J, Bolger AF, Ebbers T, Carlhäll CJ. Quantification of presystolic blood flow organization and energetics in the human left ventricle. Am J Physiol Heart Circ Physiol. 2011;300:H2135–41.
10. Fredriksson AG, Zajac J, Eriksson J, Dyverfeldt P, Bolger AF, Ebbers T, et al. 4-D blood flow in the human right ventricle. Am J Physiol Heart Circ Physiol. 2011;301:H2344–50.
11. Zajac J, Eriksson J, Dyverfeldt P, Bolger AF, Ebbers T, Carlhäll C-J. Turbulent kinetic energy in normal and myopathic left ventricles. J Magn Reson Imaging. 2014;00:1–9.
12. Töger J, Kanski M, Carlsson M, Kovács SJ, Söderlind G, Arheden H, et al. Vortex Ring Formation in the Left Ventricle of the Heart: Analysis by 4D Flow MRI and Lagrangian Coherent Structures. Ann Biomed Eng. 2012;40:2652–62.
13. Valverde I, Nordmeyer S, Uribe S, Greil G, Berger F, Kuehne T, et al. Systemic-to-pulmonary collateral flow in patients with palliated univentricular heart physiology: measurement using cardiovascular magnetic resonance 4D velocity acquisition. J Cardiovasc Magn Reson. 2012;14:25.
14. Goubergrits L, Riesenkampff E, Yevtushenko P, Schaller J, Kertzscher U, Hennemuth A, et al. MRI-based computational fluid dynamics for diagnosis and treatment prediction: Clinical validation study in patients with coarctation of aorta. J Magn Reson Imaging. 2014;00.
15. Markl M, Chan FP, Alley MT, Wedding KL, Draney MT, Elkins CJ, et al. Time-resolved three-dimensional phase-contrast MRI. J Magn Reson Imaging. 2003;17:499–506.
16. McConnell MV, Khasgiwala VC, Savord BJ, Chen MH, Chuang ML, Edelman RR, et al. Comparison of respiratory suppression methods and navigator locations for MR coronary angiography. AJR Am J Roentgenol 1997;168:1369-1375.
17. Baltes C, Kozerke S, Atkinson D, Boesiger P. Retrospective Respiratory Motion Correction for Navigated Cine Velocity Mapping. J Cardiovasc Magn Reson. 2004;6:785–92.
18. Yi W, Rossman Phillip J, Grimm Roger C, Riederer Stepen JERL. Navigator-Echo-based Real-Time Respiratory Gating and Triggering for Reduction of Respiration Effects in Three-dimensional Coronary MR Angiography. Radiology. 1996;198:55–61.
19. Ehman RL, Felmlee JP. Adaptive technique for high-definition MR imaging of moving structures. Radiology. 1989;173:255–63.
20. Nordmeyer S, Riesenkampff E, Crelier G, Khasheei A, Schnackenburg B, Berger F, et al. Flow-sensitive four-dimensional cine magnetic resonance imaging for offline blood flow quantification in multiple vessels: a validation study. J Magn Reson Imaging. 2010;32:677–83.
21. Heiberg E, Sjögren J, Ugander M, Carlsson M, Engblom H, Arheden H. Design and validation of Segment-freely available software for cardiovascular image analysis. BMC Med Imaging. 2010;10:1.
22. Carlsson M, Heiberg E, Toger J, Arheden H. Quantification of left and right ventricular kinetic energy using four-dimensional intracardiac magnetic resonance imaging flow measurements. Am J Physiol Heart Circ Physiol. 2012;302:H893–900.
23. Bland JM, Altman DG. Statistical methods for assessing agreement between two methods of clinical measurement. Lancet. 1986;1:307–10.
24. Giese D, Wong J, Greil GF, Buehrer M, Schaeffter T, Kozerke S. Towards highly accelerated Cartesian time-resolved 3D flow cardiovascular magnetic resonance in the clinical setting. J Cardiovasc Magn Reson. 2014;16:42.
25. Brix L, Ringgaard S, Rasmusson A, Sørensen TS, Kim WY. Three dimensional three component whole heart cardiovascular magnetic resonance velocity mapping: comparison of flow measurements from 3D and 2D acquisitions. J Cardiovasc Magn Reson. 2009;11:3.
26. Enriquez-Sarano M, Akins CW, Vahanian A. Mitral regurgitation. Lancet. 2009;373:1382–94.
27. Olcay AB, Pottebaum TS, Krueger PS. Sensitivity of Lagrangian coherent structure identification to flow field resolution and random errors. Chaos. 2010;20:017506.
28. Eriksson J, Bolger AF, Ebbers T, Carlhäll CJ. Four-dimensional blood flow-specific markers of LV dysfunction in dilated cardiomyopathy. Eur Heart J Cardiovasc Imaging. 2013;14:417–24.
29. Nilsson A, Bloch KM, Carlsson M, Heiberg E, Ståhlberg F. Variable velocity encoding in a three-dimensional, three-directional phase contrast sequence: Evaluation in phantom and volunteers. J Magn Reson Imaging. 2012;36:1450–9.
30. Sigfridsson A, Petersson S, Carlhäll C-J, Ebbers T. Four-dimensional flow MRI using spiral acquisition. Magn Reson Med. 2012;68:1065–73.
31. Brecher GA, Mixter G. Effect of respiratory movements on superior cava flow under normal and abnormal conditions. Am J Physiol. 1953;172:457–61.

15

Case report of a young stroke patient showing interim normalization of the MRI diffusion-weighted imaging lesion

Ann-Christin Ostwaldt[1*], Tatiana Usnich[2], Christian H. Nolte[1,2], Kersten Villringer[1] and Jochen B. Fiebach[1]

Abstract

Background: In acute ischemic stroke, diffusion weighted imaging (DWI) shows hyperintensities and is considered to indicate irreversibly damaged tissue. We present the case of a young stroke patient with unusual variability in the development of signal intensities within the same vessel territory.

Case presentation: A 35-year-old patient presented with symptoms of global aphasia and hypesthesia of the left hand. MRI demonstrated a scattered lesion in the MCA territory. After rtPA therapy the patient received further MRI examination, three times on day 1, and once on day 2, 3, 5 and 43. The posterior part of the lesion showed the usual pattern with increasing DWI hyperintensity and decreased ADC, as well as delayed FLAIR positivity. However, the anterior part of the lesion, which was clearly visible in the first examination completely normalized on the first day and only reappeared on day 2. This was accompanied by a normalization of the ADC as well as an even further delayed FLAIR positivity.

Conclusion: We showed that interim normalization of DWI and ADC in the acute phase can not only be found in rodent models of stroke, but also in humans. We propose that DWI lesion development might be more variable during the first 24 h after stroke than previously assumed.

Keywords: Magnetic resonance imaging, Acute ischemic stroke, Time course, Normalization

Background

Acute cerebral ischemia can be visualized with MRI diffusion weighted imaging (DWI) within minutes after its onset [1]. It has been suggested that in the majority of human stroke patients DWI positive cerebral ischemia indicate irreversible tissue damage leading to infarction [2]. However, lately reversal of parts of the DWI lesion has been demonstrated in association with early recanalization [3–5]. In animal models the occurrence of interim or sustained normalization of both DWI and apparent diffusion coefficient (ADC) seem to depend on the occlusion times [6, 7]. In contrast to DWI, lesions on fluid-attenuated inversion recovery (FLAIR) are usually seen several hours after stroke onset [8] in humans.

Here we present a case of partial interim normalization of DWI and ADC visualized with serial MRI in a young stroke patient.

Case presentation

A 35 year old female patient was admitted with incomplete global aphasia and a fluctuating slight hypesthesia of the left hand. Her baseline National Institutes of Health Stroke Scale score (NIHSS) was 4 and arterial hypertension was the only vascular risk factor. The patient was repeatedly examined in the MRI 57 min as well as 3.3 h, 5.5 h and 7.6 h after symptom onset, and on the second, third, fifth and 43rd day post-stroke. These data were obtained from the prospective 1000Plus Study (NCT00715533). The patient gave written informed consent. At baseline, the anterior M2 branch of the right middle cerebral artery (MCA) was occluded. DWI showed a scattered lesion affecting the anterior and posterior part of the right MCA territory and perfusion imaging showed a corresponding deficit. Intravenous rt-PA

* Correspondence: aostwaldt@mgh.harvard.edu
[1]Center for Stroke Research Berlin (CSB), Charité Universitätsmedizin Berlin, Hindenburgdamm 30, 12200 Berlin, Germany
Full list of author information is available at the end of the article

was administered directly after the first MRI scan. The follow-up examinations showed a patent MCA branch 5.5 h after symptom onset, complete normalization of the perfusion deficit on day 2 and no signs of hemorrhagic transformation. The patient's symptoms had substantially improved, resulting in a NIHSS of 0 at discharge. Infarct size on FLAIR was 31.76 ml at day 5.

On the first examination 57 min after onset, the anterior part of the lesion was clearly hyperintense on DWI; however, on the second examination at 3.3 h it was not visible any more and did not reappear until day 2 (Fig. 1). For a more detailed analysis of this phenomenon, the image datasets for each time point were coregistered and regions-of-interest (ROIs) for both the anterior and the posterior part of the lesion were created on DWI day 5 images. Signal intensities (rSI) were determined relative to the contralateral side, as previously described [8].

As can be seen in Fig. 2, DWI and ADC rSI values of the anterior lesion normalized for the time period between 3.3 h and 25 h after symptom onset (Fig. 2a-b). Also, the fluid-attenuated inversion recovery (FLAIR) rSI values of the anterior lesion were much lower than the values of the posterior lesion and only at day 3 post-stroke did the FLAIR rSI in the anterior lesion reach values substantially different from 1 (Fig. 2c).

Conclusions

We demonstrated that the degree and time course of DWI hyperintensities can differ within one lesion in the first day after stroke. To the best of our knowledge, this is the first time that the exact time course of DWI reversal and reappearance was visualized using highly repetitive MRI examinations. Our findings resemble those in rodent models of stroke [6], where lesions normalized on the DWI and ADC after recanalization and reappeared at day 2 after stroke. In stroke patients, reversible DWI hyperintensities have been demonstrated for very small, mainly embolic lesions [9]. Also it has been shown that recanalization (either after intraarterial or intravenous thrombolysis) could evoke DWI lesion reversal in some patients, with parts of lesion showing later reappearance [3–5]. Therefore, we hypothesize, that a possible explanation for the interim normalization of a large part of the initial lesion in our case would be the fast recanalization and reperfusion of the tissue. It therefore seems that the baseline DWI lesion contains tissue with benign oligemia and only cell damage which could not

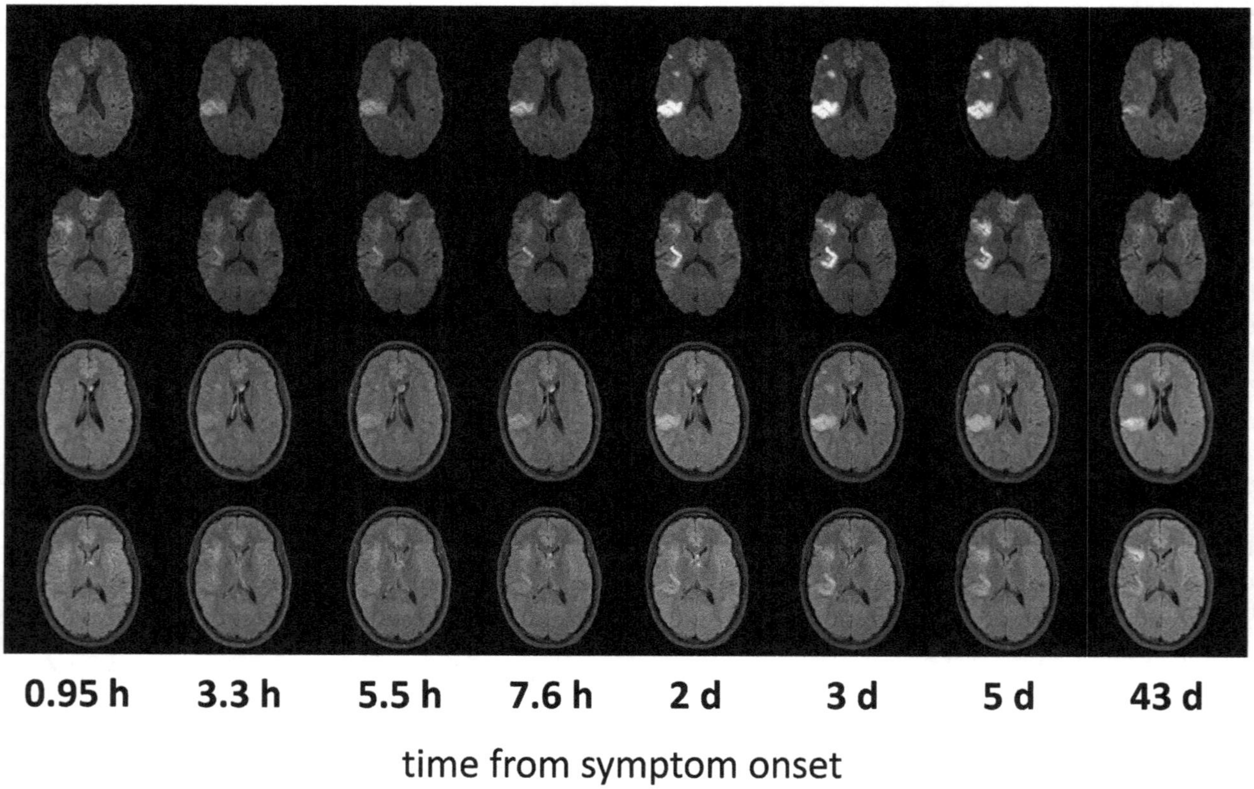

Fig. 1 Development of the anterior and the posterior lesion on serial DWI and FLAIR images. The first and second rows show the diffusion-weighted images (DWI) on two slices depicting the lesion development over time from symptom onset. The third and fourth row shows the coregistered fluid-attenuated inversion recovery (FLAIR) images corresponding to the DWI slices

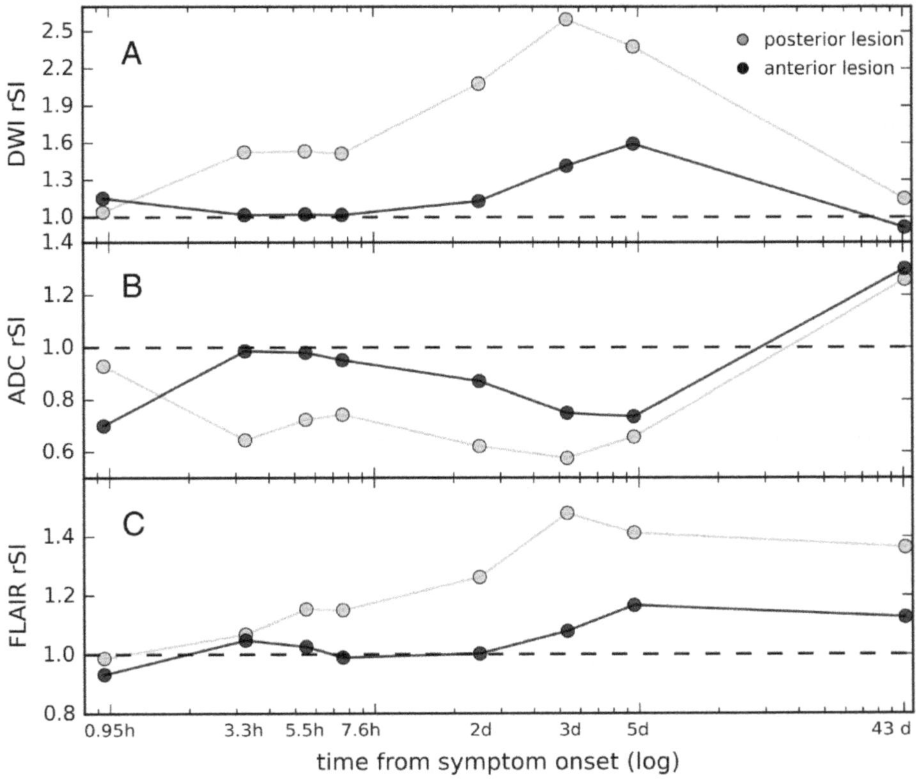

Fig. 2 Development of relative signal intensity (rSI) for the anterior and the posterior lesion separately. **a** + **b**) Diffusion-weighted imaging (DWI) and apparent diffusion coefficient (ADC) rSI show the normalization of the anterior lesion and its reappearance at day 2. **c**) The fluid attenuated inversion recovery (FLAIR) rSI shows that the anterior part of the lesion is FLAIR positive much later than the posterior part

be prevented will reveal itself on follow-up examinations. It might well be possible, that an interim normalization as observed in our case is more common in stroke patients. However, this will rarely be observed due to lack of MRI follow-ups in clinical routine.

We conclude that DWI lesion visibility might be more prone to fluctuation and variability during the first 24 h after stroke than previously assumed and baseline DWI may include tissue with benign oligemia. Therefore, during interpretation of DWI one has to keep in mind that an interim normalization can occur and which might delay lesion visualization.

Abbreviations

MRI: Magnetic resonance imaging; DWI: Diffusion-weighted imaging; ADC: Apparent diffusion coefficient; NIHSS: National Institutes of health stroke scale; MCA: Middle cerebral artery; ROI: Region-of-interest; rSI: Relative signal intensity; FLAIR: Fluid-attenuated inversion recovery.

Competing interests

The authors declare that they have no competing interests.

Authors' contributions

AO was responsible for analyzing and interpreting the imaging data. She generated the figures and drafted the manuscript. TU and CN were the responsible treating physicians of the patients. TU additionally helped analyzing the data. CN was responsible for the data collection on the clinical side and made contributions to interpretation of the results. KV participated in design and coordination of the study and substantially helped in interpreting the results and drafting the manuscript. JF was responsible for conception and design of the study and agree to be accountable for accuracy or integrity of the work. All authors read and approved the final manuscript.

Acknowledgements

This research received funding from the Federal Ministry of Education and Research via the grant Center for Stroke Research Berlin (01EO0801 and 01EO1301).

Consent

Written informed consent was obtained from the patient for publication of this case report and any accompanying images. A copy of the written consent is available for review by the editor of this journal.

Author details

[1]Center for Stroke Research Berlin (CSB), Charité Universitätsmedizin Berlin, Hindenburgdamm 30, 12200 Berlin, Germany. [2]Department of Neurology, Charité Universitätsmedizin Berlin, Hindenburgdamm 30, 12200 Berlin, Germany.

References

1. Moseley M, Cohen Y, Mintorovitch J, Chileuitt L, Shimizu H, Kucharczyk J, et al. Early detection of regional cerebral ischemia in cats: comparison of diffusion-weighted and T2-weighted MRI and spectroscopy. Magn Reson Med. 1990;14:330–46.
2. Fiehler J, Fiebach JB, Gass A, Hoehn M, Kucinski T, Neumann-Haefelin T, et al. Diffusion-weighted imaging in acute stroke – a tool of uncertain value? Cerebrovasc Dis. 2002;14:187–96.

3. Soize S, Tisserand M, Charron S, Turc G, Ben Hassen W, Labeyrie MA, et al. How sustained is 24-h diffusion-weighted imaging lesion reversal? Serial magnetic resonance imaging in a patient cohort thrombolyzed within 4.5 h of stroke onset. Stroke. 2015;46:704–10.
4. Kidwell CS, Saver JL, Starkman S, Duckwiler G, Jahan R, Vespa P, et al. Late secondary ischemic injury in patients receiving intraarterial thrombolysis. Ann Neurol. 2002;52:698–703.
5. Sakamoto Y, Kimura K, Iguchi Y, Shibazaki K, Aoki J. Dramatic changes of a DWI lesion in a patient with acute ischemic stroke treated with IV t-PA. J Neuroimaging. 2013;23:228–30.
6. Neumann-Haefelin T, Kastrup A, de Crespigny A, Yenari MA, Ringer T, Sun GH, et al. Serial MRI after transient focal cerebral ischemia in rats: dynamics of tissue injury, blood–brain barrier damage, and edema formation. Stroke. 2000;31:1965–72.
7. Li F, Liu KF, Silva MD, Omae T, Sotak CH, Fenstermacher JD, et al. Transient and Permanent Resolution of Ischemic Lesions on Diffusion-Weighted Imaging After Brief Periods of Focal Ischemia in Rats: Correlation With Histopathology. Stroke. 2000;31:946–54.
8. Cheng B, Brinkmann M, Forkert ND, Treszl A, Ebinger M, Köhrmann M, et al. Quantitative measurements of relative fluid-attenuated inversion recovery (FLAIR) signal intensities in acute stroke for the prediction of time from symptom onset. J Cereb Blood Flow Metab. 2013;33:76–84.
9. Albach FN, Brunecker P, Usnich T, Villringer K, Ebinger M, Fiebach JB, et al. Complete Early Reversal of Diffusion-Weighted Imaging Hyperintensities After Ischemic Stroke Is Mainly Limited to Small Embolic Lesions. Stroke. 2013;44:1043–8.

16

A case of intra-articular ganglion cysts of the knee joint: correlation between arthroscopic and magnetic resonance imaging

Sayaka Kodaira[1], Takahito Nakajima[1*], Ryosuke Takahashi[1], Shingo Moriya[1], Tomoyuki Nakagawa[2], Hidenori Ohtake[1] and Yoshito Tsushima[1]

Abstract

Background: Intra-articular ganglion cysts of the knee are rare. Here we report a case of an arthroscopically confirmed ganglion cyst arising from the posterior cruciate ligament (PCL) along with preoperative magnetic resonance imaging (MRI) findings.

Case presentation: A 39-year-old female admitted a hospital with left knee pain with flexion and extension. MRI revealed a cystic lesion along the PCL. The lesion exhibited slight but homogeneous hyperintensity on T1 weighted images. Thin septals were visible within the lesion. Arthroscopic examination revealed a mass lesion with a white fibrous capsule, located near the PCL. A gel-like liquid spurted from the mass upon puncture. The lesion was completely resected. Histological examination revealed loose connective tissue and fibroblasts with collagen, thus confirming the diagnosis of a ganglion cyst.

Conclusion: Many reports have suggested intra-articular ganglion cysts of the knee are rare. In our study, a cystic lesion may have been impinged between the PCL and intercondylar notch, resulting in flexion and extension difficulty in the left knee. Arthroscopic resection is the major treatment of intra-articular ganglion cyst, and preoperative MRI findings can predict the correct arthroscopic approach. We have reported a case in which an intra-articular ganglion attached to the PCL.

Keywords: Ganglion, MRI, Arthroscopy, Intra-articular, knee

Background

Intra-articular ganglion cysts are well known to occur in the dorsal wrist, palm, and shoulder but rarely to originate in the knee joint [1, 2]. Ganglion cysts of the knee arise from both the cruciate ligaments and menisci as well as from the popliteal tendon, alar folds, and subchondral bone [2–4]. Here we report a case of an arthroscopically confirmed ganglion cyst arising from the posterior cruciate ligament (PCL) along with preoperative magnetic resonance imaging (MRI) findings.

* Correspondence: sojin@gunma-u.ac.jp
[1]Department of Diagnostic Radiology and Nuclear Medicine, 3-39-22, Showa, Maebashi, Gunma, Japan
Full list of author information is available at the end of the article

Case presentation

A 39-year-old female presented with a 1-year history of gait difficulty and left knee pain with flexion and extension. She also indicated listlessness and stiffness of her left lower leg; however, she had no history of trauma to the knee. Upon examination, the active range of motion of the left knee was slightly limited to 0°–120°.

MRI revealed a well-defined cystic lesion extending along the PCL, adjacent to the lateral condyle of the femur. The lesion exhibited slight but homogeneous hyperintensity, relative to the muscles on T1 weighted images and apparent hyperintensity on T2 weighted

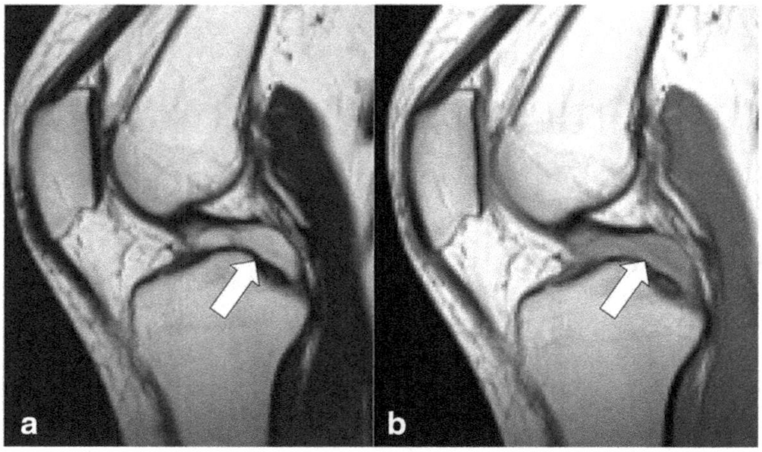

Fig. 1 Sagittal magnetic resonance images revealed a cystic lesion located between the posterior cruciate ligament and intercondylar notch. This lesion exhibited apparent hyperintensity on T2 weighted images (T2WI, **a**) and slight hyperintensity on T1WI (**b**)

images. The lesion appeared to attach broadly to the PCL (Fig. 1). Thin septals were visible within the lesion, not containing a solid component. A small amount of thin wedge-shaped synovial fluid was observed in the lateral joint space, which was continuous with the lesion (Fig. 2). The menisci, cartilages, muscles, and ligaments were normal.

Arthroscopic examination revealed a mass lesion with a white fibrous capsule, located near the PCL (Fig. 3a). A transparent dark reddish-brown viscous gel-like liquid spurted from the mass upon puncture with a probe (Fig. 3b). The lesion was completely resected in a piecemeal manner.

Histological examination revealed loose connective tissue and fibroblasts with interspersed thicker bundles of collagen, thus confirming the diagnosis of a ganglion cyst (Fig. 4a). Immunohistochemical analysis revealed scattered S-100-positive cells among the loose connective tissue (Fig. 4b).

No recurrence was detected for 6 months after successful arthroscopic excision.

Discussion

García et al. first described preoperative MRI findings of cystic masses of the knee in 1991 [5]. Although Lee et al. had used computed tomography (CT) to evaluate cystic masses of the knee in 1987 [2], the majority of the cysts observed were popliteal cysts; intra-articular ganglion cysts of the knee remain rare. Differential diagnoses of ganglion cysts may include pigmented villonodular synovitis, synovial chondromatosis, meniscal or parameniscal cysts, and synovial

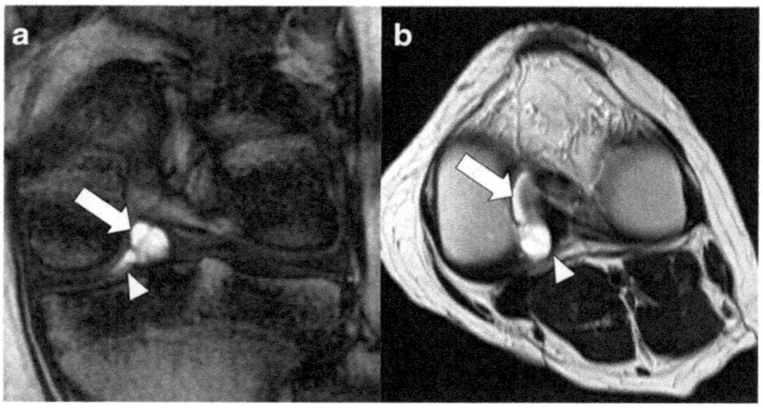

Fig. 2 A multiloculated cystic lesion (arrow) was observed to be attached to the posterior cruciate ligament adjacent to lateral condyle of the femur on T2* weighted images (T2*WI, **a**) and T2WI (**b**). A small amount of thin wedge-shaped synovial fluid (arrowhead) was visible in the lateral joint space

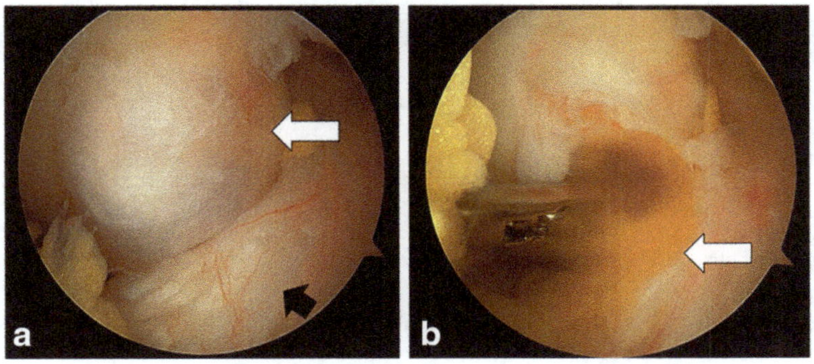

Fig. 3 a Arthroscopic examination identified a mass located anteriorly to the posterior cruciate ligament (PCL). The cyst (white arrow) was located between the anterior cruciate ligament (black arrow) and PCL, tightly attached to the PCL, and covered with a white capsule. **b** The mass was arthroscopically excised in a piecemeal manner and the exuded viscous liquid (arrow) when punctured

hemangioma [4]. Intra-articular ganglion cysts of the knee are majorly detected as incidental findings using MRI, with a reported prevalence between 0.9 [6] and 1.3 % [3].

In 1997, Liem et al. reported 23 cases of intra-articular ganglion cysts of the knee along with the classifications and frequencies of the originating sites, which included the infrapatellar fat pad, within the anterior cruciate ligament (ACL), posterior to the ACL, anterior to the PCL, posterior to the PCL, in the intercondylar notch, at the bony attachment of ACL, and even outside of the knee joint [3]. In our study, a cystic lesion located on anterior portion of the PCL may have been impinged between the PCL and intercondylar notch, resulting in flexion and extension difficulty in the left knee [1, 7].

Brown and Dandy has reported 95 % of patients they treated with arthroscopic total resection had no recurrence [8]. CT-guided aspiration has also been reported in some cases [7, 9]. However, because complete excision using ultrasound-, CT-, and arthroscopic-guided aspiration is not possible and has high rate of recurrence, arthroscopic resection should be recommended [10]. Furthermore, preoperative MRI findings can predict the correct arthroscopic approach through an anterolateral, posteromedial, or posterolateral portal [10–12].

Conclusion

We have reported a case in which an intra-articular ganglion attached to the PCL was detected using preoperative MRI. MRI is useful for depicting ganglion features, including size and location. This modality may also facilitate preoperative decisions regarding the direction of the arthroscopic approach.

Consent

Informed consent was obtained from the patient for publication of this case report and accompanying images. Availability of data and materials.

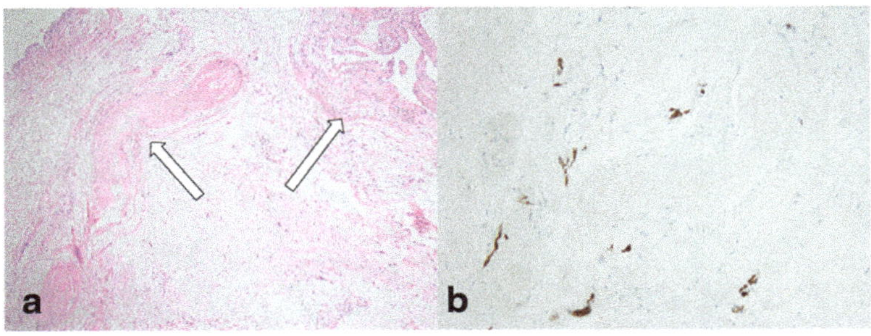

Fig. 4 a Hematoxylin–eosin staining revealed loose connective tissue and fibroblasts with interspersed thicker bundles of collagen (10× magnification). **b** Immunohistochemistry revealed scattered S-100-positive cells among the loose connective tissue (40× magnification)

Abbreviations

ACL: anterior cruciate ligament; CT: computed tomography; MRI: magnetic resonance imaging; PCL: posterior cruciate ligament.

Competing interests

The authors declare that they have no competing interests.

Authors' contributions

SK and TN organized and wrote this manuscript. DT and SM analyzed and interpreted the patient data regarding the intra-articular ganglion cyst. TN performed the surgical process and the histological examination of this ganglion cyst. YT was a major contributor in writing the manuscript. All authors have read and approved the final manuscript.

Acknowledgements

This publication was partially funded by Grant-in-Aid for Challenging Exploratory Research.

Author details

[1]Department of Diagnostic Radiology and Nuclear Medicine, 3-39-22, Showa, Maebashi, Gunma, Japan. [2]Zenshukai Hospital, 1381, Ninomiya, Maebashi, Gunma, Japan.

References

1. Seki K, Mine T, Tanaka H, Isida Y, Taguchi T. Locked knee caused by intraarticular ganglion. Knee Surg Sports Traumatol Arthrosc. 2006;14:859–61.
2. Lee KR, Cox GG, Neff JR, Arnett GR, Murphey MD. Cystic masses of the knee: arthrographic and CT evaluation. Am J Roentgenol. 1987;148:329–34.
3. Bui-Mansfield LT, Youngberg RA. Intraarticular ganglia of the knee: prevalence, presentation, etiology, and management. Am J Roentgenol. 1997;168:123–7.
4. Krudwig WK, Schulte K-K, Heinemann C. Intra-articular ganglion cysts of the knee joint: a report of 85 cases and review of the literature. Knee Surg Sports Traumatol Arthrosc. 2004;12:123–9.
5. García A, Hodler J, Vaughn L, Haghighi P, Resnick D. Case report 677. Intraarticular ganglion arising from the posterior cruciate-ligament. Skeletal Radiol. 1991;20:373–5.
6. McLaren DB, Buckwalter KA, Vahey TN. The prevalence and significance of cyst-like changes at the cruciate ligament attachments in the knee. Skeletal Radiol. 1992;21:365–9.
7. Kim R, Kim K, Lee J, Lee K. Ganglion cysts of the posterior cruciate ligament. Arthroscopy: The Journal of Arthroscopic & Related Surgery. 2003;19:41–5.
8. Brown MF, Dandy DJ. Intra-articular ganglia in the knee. Arthroscopy. 1990; 6:322–3.
9. Youngberg RA. Intraartcular gnglia of the knee: prevalence, presentation, etiology, and management. Am J Roentgenol. 1997;168:123–7.
10. Dinakar B, Khan T, Kumar AC, Kumar A. Ganglion cyst of the anterior cruciate ligament: a case report. J Orthop Surg. 2005;13:181–5.
11. Drosos GGI, Pozo JLJ. Large extrasynovial intracapsular ganglia of the knee: a report of 3 cases. J Arthrosc Relat Surg. 2005;21:1362–5.
12. Amin M, Torreggiani W, Sparkes J. Infrapatellar ganglion that developed from infrapatellar fat and had minimal intraarticular extension. Knee Surg Sport Traumatol Arthrosc. 2008;16:179–81.

Cardiovascular magnetic resonance feature tracking in small animals – a preliminary study on reproducibility and sample size calculation

Tomas Lapinskas[1,2,5*†], Jana Grune[2,3,5†], Seyedeh Mahsa Zamani[2], Sarah Jeuthe[4,5], Daniel Messroghli[2,4,5], Rolf Gebker[2,5], Heike Meyborg[2], Ulrich Kintscher[3,5], Remigijus Zaliunas[1], Burkert Pieske[2,5], Philipp Stawowy[2,5†] and Sebastian Kelle[2,5†]

Abstract

Background: Cardiovascular magnetic resonance feature tracking (CMR-FT) is a novel tissue tracking technique developed for noninvasive assessment of myocardial motion and deformation. This preliminary study aimed to evaluate the observer's reproducibility of CMR-FT in a small animal (mouse) model and define sample size calculation for future trials.

Methods: Six C57BL/6 J mice were selected from the ongoing experimental mouse model onsite and underwent CMR with a 3 Tesla small animal MRI scanner. Myocardial deformation was analyzed using dedicated software (TomTec, Germany) by two observers. Left ventricular (LV) longitudinal, circumferential and radial strain (Ell_{LAX}, Ecc_{SAX} and Err_{SAX}) were calculated. To assess intra-observer agreement data analysis was repeated after 4 weeks. The sample size required to detect a relative change in strain was calculated.

Results: In general, Ecc_{SAX} and Ell_{LAX} demonstrated highest inter-observer reproducibility (ICC 0.79 (0.46–0.91) and 0.73 (0.56–0.83) Ecc_{SAX} and Ell_{LAX} respectively). In contrast, at the intra-observer level Ell_{LAX} was more reproducible than Ecc_{SAX} (ICC 0.83 (0.73–0.90) and 0.74 (0.49–0.87) Ell_{LAX} and Ecc_{SAX} respectively). The reproducibility of Err_{SAX} was weak at both observer levels. Preliminary sample size calculation showed that a small study sample (e.g. ten animals to detect a relative 10% change in Ecc_{SAX}) could be sufficient to detect changes if parameter variability is low.

Conclusions: This pilot study demonstrates good to excellent inter- and intra-observer reproducibility of CMR-FT technique in small animal model. The most reproducible measures are global circumferential and global longitudinal strain, whereas reproducibility of radial strain is weak. Furthermore, sample size calculation demonstrates that a small number of animals could be sufficient for future trials.

Keywords: Cardiovascular magnetic resonance, Feature tracking, Myocardial strain, Small animal model, Reproducibility

* Correspondence: tomas.lapinskas@lsmuni.lt; lapinskas@dhzb.de
†Equal contributors
[1]Department of Cardiology, Medical Academy, Lithuanian University of Health Sciences, Eiveniu Street 2, LT-50161 Kaunas, Lithuania
[2]Department of Internal Medicine / Cardiology, Deutsches Herzzentrum Berlin, Augustenburger Platz 1, 13353 Berlin, Germany
Full list of author information is available at the end of the article

Background

Clinical decision making mostly relies on a quantitative assessment of cardiac structure and function with left ventricular (LV) mass, volumes and ejection fraction (EF) being as critical parameters in many more situations than just selection of appropriate treatment strategy or prediction of cardiac outcomes [1]. However, all these parameters as global quantitative measures have some important limitations [2].

The superior measure for the assessment of global and regional myocardial function is myocardial strain which represents the percentage change in dimension from the resting phase to one achieved of a force or stress [3]. Majority of imaging techniques for myocardial deformation rely on identification and tracking of specific anatomical features. The cardiovascular magnetic resonance (CMR) tissue tracking approach is comparable with speckle tracking echocardiography where myocardium typically has a speckled appearance. In general, a tissue tracking method begins by identifying a relatively small window on one image and searching for the most comparable image pattern in a window of the same size in the subsequent frame [4]. Due to the lack of intramyocardial landmarks and excellent contrast between blood pool and myocardial tissue, CMR feature tracking (CMR-FT) technique focuses on endocardial and epicardial contouring [5].

Measurement of strain using CMR imaging became possible after the introduction of myocardial tagging techniques in which created tagging patterns provide information about myocardial motion during the entire cardiac cycle [6, 7]. However, the need for additional image acquisition and time consuming post-processing makes this technique less attractive.

CMR-FT technique provides quantitative information about myocardial deformation using conventional balanced steady state free precession (bSSFP) cine images and can be used in the assessment of the myocardial mechanics of all cardiac chambers [8–10] and in various clinical scenarios [11–13]. The CMR-FT algorithm is based on optical flow technology and was commercially introduced by several vendors. Interestingly, new calculation algorithms such as non-rigid, elastic image registration has been validated recently and became available in real-life setting [14].

CMR-FT has been validated against myocardial tagging technique for the assessment of regional myocardial motion in humans [15, 16]. Furthermore, recent studies have shown that myocardial deformation parameters may predict future events [17–19] or anticipate response to treatment [20, 21]. Thereby, regional myocardial deformation parameters became a promising new biomarker to detect subtle changes in myocardial motion.

Current literature reports excellent inter- and intra-observer agreement [22–24] and high inter-study reproducibility [25] of quantitative assessment of myocardial mechanics using CMR-FT. Importantly, derived myocardial deformation parameters are similar and highly reproducible in subjects examined at different field strength MRI scanners [26]. However, there are no studies assessing reproducibility of myocardial deformation parameters in small animals.

Accordingly, we performed this preliminary study to evaluate inter- and intra-observer reproducibility of CMR-FT derived strain measurements in a small animal (mouse) model. Also, we calculated the necessary study sample size to define the number of animals required for future studies.

Methods

Six C57BL/6 J male, mice were randomly selected from the ongoing experimental mouse model onsite. Animals used in this study were maintained in accordance with Guide for the Care and Use of Laboratory Animals published by the US National Institutes of Health. The study was approved by the local authorities (G0099/14).

Cardiac magnetic resonance

All CMR measurements were performed on a 3 Tesla small animal MRI system (MR Solutions, Guildford, United Kingdom) with a quadrature birdcage cardiac volume coil. After induction of inhalative anesthesia using isoflurane-oxygen (4–5%), animals were placed on a dedicated mouse sledge and MR-compatible ECG electrodes were attached to the paws. Anesthesia was maintained with isoflurane-oxygen (1.5–2%) to adjust heart rate at 400–450 beats per minute. Images were acquired using respiratory and ECG-gated gradient-echo cine sequences in two-chamber long-axis, four-chamber long-axis and five to seven short-axis planes completely covering the LV. Relevant acquisition parameters included: 15 phases per cardiac cycle, repetition time (TR) 10 ms, echo time (TE) 3 ms, averages 4, field of view (FOV) 40 × 40 mm, pixel size 0.15 × 0.15 mm, slice thickness 1 mm. All animals underwent two CMR examinations with a four-week time interval between each study.

Left ventricular volumetric and functional analysis

Volumetric analysis was performed offline using commercially available software CMR^{42} (Circle Cardiovascular Imaging Inc., Calgary, Canada). LV end-diastolic (LV EDV) and end-systolic (LV ESV) volumes were quantified using manual planimetry of the endocardial and epicardial surface from short-axis stack and LV stroke volume (LV SV), LV EF, myocardial mass and cardiac output were calculated.

Feature tracking

The cine images were used to calculate myocardial strain and strain rate offline using dedicated software (TomTec Imaging Systems, 2D CPA, MR, Cardiac Performance Analysis, Unterschleissheim, Germany). Endocardial and epicardial contours were manually drawn in both long-axis and one mid-ventricular short-axis views at end-diastole for each mouse by two independent observers. After application of a tracking algorithm the software automatically identified endocardial borders throughout the cardiac cycle and computed mean segmental and global myocardial strain and strain rate parameters. All images were analyzed three times and derived measurements were averaged. LV global longitudinal strain and strain rate (Ell_{LAX} and $SRll_{LAX}$) were calculated by averaging the strain curves of both two-chamber and four-chamber long-axis views (three measurements in two imaging planes of two scans in six mice resulted in 72 measurements) whereas global circumferential and radial strain (Ecc_{SAX} and Err_{SAX}) and strain rate ($SRcc_{SAX}$ and $SRrr_{SAX}$) were derived using one mid-ventricular short-axis view containing both papillary muscles (three measurements in one imaging plane of two scans in six mice resulted in 36 measurements) (Fig. 1). To assess intra-observer agreement data analysis was repeated 4 weeks after initial assessment.

Statistical analysis

Reproducibility testing

Data was analyzed using Microsoft Excel and IBM SPSS Statistics version 23.0 software (SPSS Inc., Chicago, IL, USA) for Windows. Data are expressed as mean ± standard deviation (SD). The Shapiro-Wilk test was used to determine whether the data was normally distributed. Non-parametric variables were compared using the Wilcoxon test. A p value of <0.05 was considered statistically significant. Inter- and intra-observer reproducibility was quantified using intraclass correlation coefficient (ICC) and Bland-Altman analysis [27]. Agreement was considered excellent for ICC >0.74, good for ICC 0.60–0.74, fair for ICC 0.40–0.59, and poor for ICC <0.40 [28].

Sample size calculation

Study sample size required to detect a relative 5, 8 and 10% change in strain with power of 90% and significance of 5% was calculated as follows [29]:

$$n = f(\alpha, P)\cdot\sigma^2\cdot 2/\delta^2$$

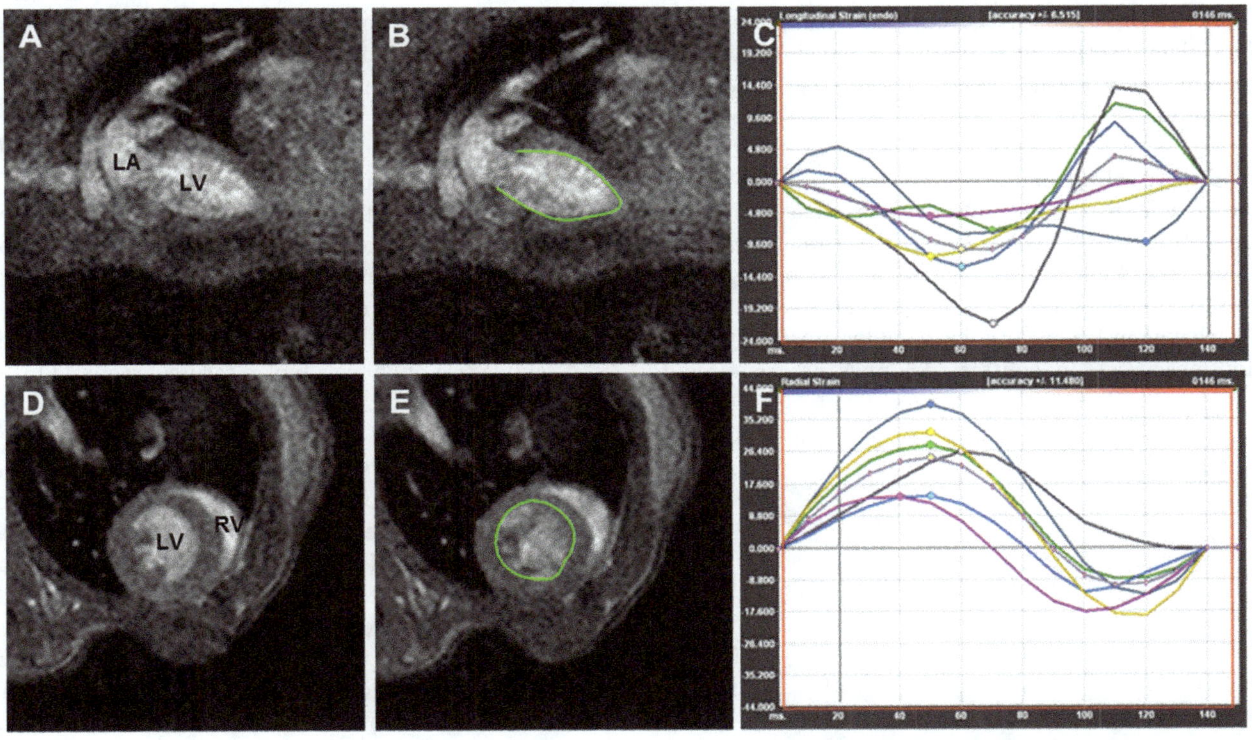

Fig. 1 Cine CMR images without and with endocardial contouring and examples of CMR-FT myocardial strain curves in mouse. A frame from cine image of the LV two-chamber view depicting LV and LA (**a**). The same LV two-chamber cine image after application of tissue tracking algorithm (**b**) and example of LV longitudinal strain curves obtained from two-chamber cine image (**c**). Cine image of LV short-axis view at mid-ventricular level before (**d**) and after (**e**) automatic endocardial border detection. An example of LV radial strain curves derived from short-axis cine image (**f**). LV = left ventricle; LA = left atrium; CMR-FT = cardiovascular magnetic resonance feature tracking

where n is the sample size, α the significance level, P the study power required and f the value of the factor for different values of α and P (f = 10.5 for α = 0.05 and p = 0.090), with σ the standard deviation of differences in measurements between two studies and δ the desired difference to be detected.

Results

Demographic characteristics, volumetric and functional parameters of study population are summarized in Table 1. All studies were completed and image quality was sufficient to perform CMR-FT analysis. Table 2 demonstrates CMR-FT derived strain parameters obtained by two observers.

Inter-observer and intra-observer reproducibility

The reproducibility for measurements was variable. Mean differences ± SD, limits of agreement and ICC for strain parameters are given in Table 3. There was excellent inter-observer reproducibility for Ecc_{SAX}: ICC 0.79 (0.46–0.91) and Ell_{LAX}: ICC 0.73 (0.56–0.83). In contrast, the level of intra-observer reproducibility was better for Ell_{LAX}: ICC 0.83 (0.73–0.90) and lower for Ecc_{SAX}: ICC 0.74 (0.49–0.87). The least reproducible measure for both observer levels was Err_{SAX}: ICC 0.68 (0.37–0.84) and ICC 0.69 (0.41–0.84) for inter-observer and intra-observer level respectively. Bland-Altman plots demonstrate inter-observer and intra-observer reproducibility for left ventricular Ell_{LAX}, Ecc_{SAX} and Err_{SAX} (Fig. 2).

Sample size calculation

The change in reproducibility has an impact on sample size required to detect significant differences in strain parameters. Table 4 lists the required sample sizes for each strain measure. For example, to show a relative 10% change in Ecc_{SAX} in mice would require ten animals (not measures). In contrast, 85 mice are required to detect a 5% change in Err_{SAX} with CMR-FT (power of 90% and α error of 0.05).

Table 1 Demographic, volumetric and functional characteristics of study subjects

Parameter	Value
Study population (n)	6
Male gender	6 (100%)
LV EDV (μl)	40.60 ± 10.15
LV ESV (μl)	18.02 ± 7.32
LV SV (μl)	22.57 ± 6.90
LV EF (%)	56.18 ± 10.70
Cardiac output (ml/min)	9.70 ± 3.27
LV Mass (mg)	58.87 ± 13.56

Results are reported as mean ± standard deviation. *LV* left ventricle / ventricular, *EDV* end-diastolic volume, *ESV* end-systolic volume, *SV* stroke volume, *EF* ejection fraction

Table 2 Comparison of CMR-FT derived strain parameters obtained by observers in six mice (72 measures for longitudinal and 36 measures for circumferential and radial strain respectively)

	Measurements obtained by two observers (inter-observer level)	
	First observer	Second observer
Ell_{LAX} (%)	−10.32 ± 5.47	−11.97 ± 6.36
Ecc_{SAX} (%)	−9.60 ± 3.68	−11.97 ± 5.97
Err_{SAX} (%)	12.59 ± 6.78	12.64 ± 7.23
	Measurements obtained by one observer (intra-observer level)	
	First measurement	Second measurement
Ell_{LAX} (%)	−10.32 ± 5.47	−11.57 ± 6.84
Ecc_{SAX} (%)	−9.60 ± 3.68	−8.48 ± 6.50
Err_{SAX} (%)	12.59 ± 6.78	10.32 ± 7.88

Results are expressed as mean ± standard deviation. Ell_{LAX} left ventricular long-axis longitudinal strain, Ecc_{SAX} left ventricular short-axis circumferential strain, Err_{SAX} left ventricular short-axis radial strain

Discussion

The current pilot study was designed to assess the inter-observer and intra-observer reproducibility of CMR-FT for the analysis of strain and strain rate in a small animal (mouse) model and to define the number of animals required for future studies. Our preliminary data analysis demonstrates very promising results:

- CMR-FT can be used for quantitative assessment of cardiac motion in small animals
- Good to excellent inter-observer and intra-observer reproducibility was found for LV circumferential and longitudinal strain, whereas radial strain is highly variable between repeated measurements
- Sample size calculation demonstrates relatively small sample size of animals (not measures) required to detect a 5, 8 and 10% change in strain parameters.

Small animal models play an important role in the understanding of cardiac mechanics in the various types of cardiovascular disease. There is growing evidence that advanced measures of myocardial deformation (strain or torsion) are better predictors of outcome compared with the routinely used ejection fraction or wall motion score index [30]. However, in the past the majority of animal experiments focused on changes in routine parameters as LV mass, volumes and/or function. The analysis of myocardial deformation offers quantitative assessment of early changes in LV diastolic function [31] and new findings in previously reported "negative" studies or studies with no obvious effect after therapy may improve our understanding of the underlying pathophysiology.

Table 3 Inter-observer and intra-observer reproducibility for LV longitudinal, circumferential and radial strain

	Parameter	Mean difference ± SD	Limits of agreement	ICC (95% CI)
Inter-observer	Ell_{LAX} (%)	−1.65 ± 5.38	−12.2 to 8.90	0.73 (0.56 to 0.83)
	Ecc_{SAX} (%)	−2.37 ± 3.71	−9.64 to 4.89	0.79 (0.46 to 0.91)
	Err_{SAX} (%)	0.05 ± 6.94	−13.55 to 13.66	0.68 (0.37 to 0.84)
Intra-observer	Ell_{LAX} (%)	−1.25 ± 4.62	−10.30 to 7.79	0.83 (0.73 to 0.90)
	Ecc_{SAX} (%)	1.11 ± 4.79	−8.27 to 10.50	0.74 (0.49 to 0.87)
	Err_{SAX} (%)	−2.27 ± 6.98	−15.95 to 11.42	0.69 (0.41 to 0.84)

Results are reported as mean ± standard deviation. *ICC* intraclass correlation coefficient, *CI* confidence interval. Other abbreviations as in Table 2

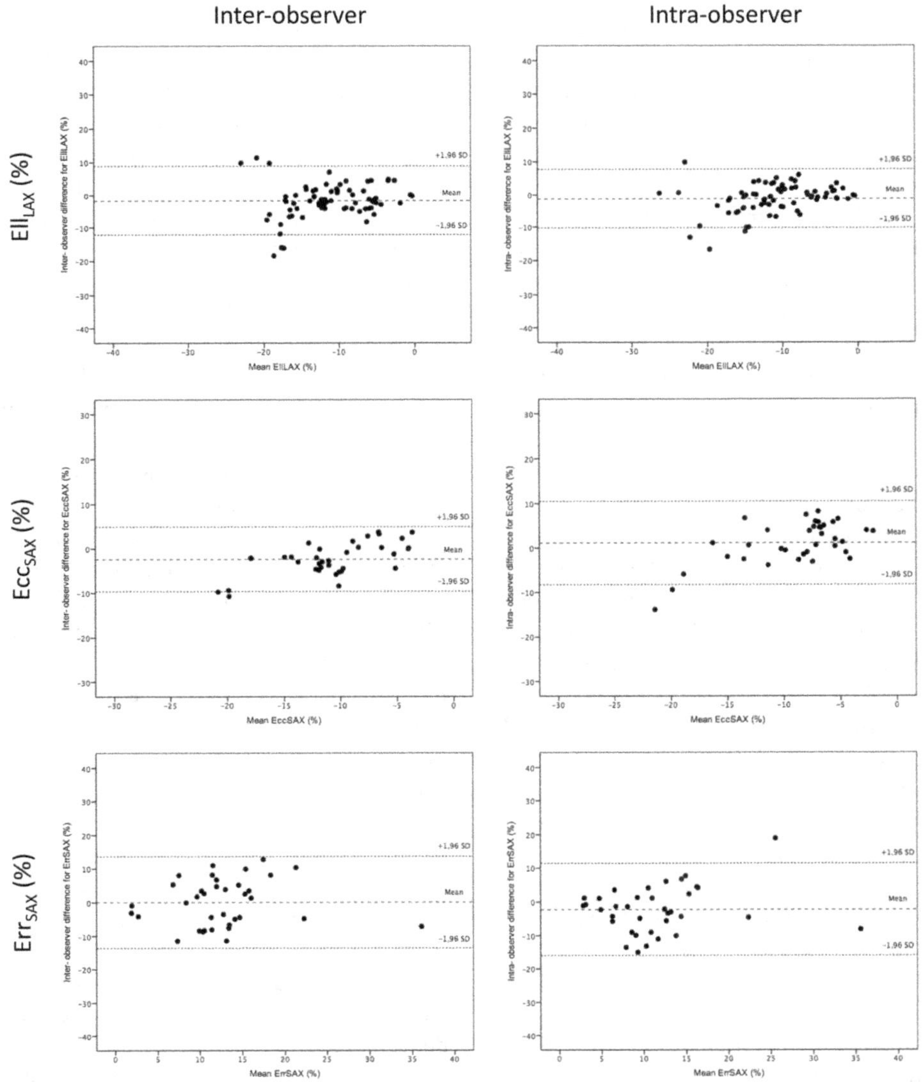

Fig. 2 Bland-Altman plots with limits of agreement (1.96 standard deviations) demonstrates the inter-observer and intra-observer reproducibility of CMR-FT for LV strain parameters. The middle-dashed line is the mean of difference of measures. The upper and lower dotted lines are ±1.96 standard deviation. Ell_{LAX} = left ventricular long-axis longitudinal strain; Ecc_{SAX} = left ventricular short-axis circumferential strain; Err_{SAX} = left ventricular short-axis radial strain

Table 4 Sample size calculation for LV longitudinal, circumferential and radial strain to detect 5, 8 and 10% relative change with 90% power and α error of 0.05

Parameter	Mean difference ± SD	Sample size (n)		
		5%	8%	10%
Ell_{LAX} (%)	−0.98 ± 7.96	53	21	13
Ecc_{SAX} (%)	−3.46 ± 6.84	39	15	10
Err_{SAX} (%)	3.48 ± 10.06	85	33	21

Abbreviations as in Table 2

Previous studies have demonstrated the feasibility of two-dimensional (2D) speckle tracking echocardiography to assess myocardial motion in small animal models. Peng et al., evaluated the feasibility of circumferential and radial strain to detect LV dysfunction in a heart failure mouse models. They demonstrated that mice subjected to transverse aortic constriction experienced an immediate and sustained decrease in circumferential and radial strain [32]. The technical challenges with 2D echocardiography as limited imaging projections, small animal hearts and lower spatial resolution still limit its widespread use.

CMR-FT as a novel tissue tracking method became available in 2009 [33] and immediately evoked great interest in the CMR community. The CMR-FT algorithm tracks the endocardial and epicardial borders over time using conventional cine images. The advantages are that CMR-FT does not require acquisition of additional sequences and helps to protect animals from prolonged anesthesia. Furthermore, quantitative assessment of myocardial deformation can be performed retrospectively as cine images are a part of routine CMR study.

CMR-FT has been validated against the traditional CMR tagging techniques and showed excellent correlation between the two methods [34]. As opposed to speckle tracking echocardiography, only a small number of studies have been done using CMR tagging technique in small animal models [35, 36] and none using CMR-FT.

The temporal resolution of the tissue tracking technique is very important to meaningful interpretation of the results. If it is too low, an effect known as image decorrelation appears and the local patterns could become less comparable [4]. Under the conscious state the normal murine heart rate ranges from 500 to 700 beats per minute (bpm) [37]. During anesthesia, we were able to adjust mice heart rate at 400–450 bpm and achieve temporal resolution of 15 phases per cardiac cycle. There are no studies reporting minimal number of cardiac phases required to assess myocardial strain using CMR-FT. However, it should be mentioned that expected average temporal resolution in human studies is 25–35 phases per cardiac cycle (e.g., 30–40 ms at a heart rate of 60 bpm) [38]. Future studies assessing the impact of temporal resolution on the myocardial tracking accuracy of CMR-FT in animals and humans are necessary.

Higher reproducibility enables smaller changes to be detected with greater reliability. Comparative studies have reported that the most consistent parameters derived from CMR-FT are global circumferential and global longitudinal strain [33, 34]. Augustine et al., reported reasonable agreement between myocardial tagging and CMR-FT for global circumferential strain but not for longitudinal or radial strain. Inter-observer variability was acceptable for circumferential, but poor for radial strain [39]. Morton et al., evaluated inter-study reproducibility in healthy volunteers and found that global circumferential strain was the most reproducible measure [22]. Studies analyzing reproducibility of myocardial deformation parameters in small animal models are lacking. Haggery et al., conducted a study to evaluate the inter-observer and intra-observer variability in mice using stimulated echo CMR (DENSE) and reported high reproducibility for LV strains and torsion with better agreement of measurements at the inter-observer level. Myocardial strains were generally more reproducible than corresponding strain rates [40].

To improve reproducibility in our study, all measurements were derived three times. This strategy has been reported to increase the reproducibility of measurements in previous studies [10, 23]. Our study also demonstrates good to excellent inter-observer agreement for global circumferential and global longitudinal strain. In contrast, the reproducibility of longitudinal strain is better at the intra-observer level. However, the reproducibility of radial strain was weak, as expected and as reported in previous human studies [35].

The variability between measurements is an important factor for determining the ability of the technique to detect relevant differences between the individuals or significant change at follow-up examinations and becomes important not only in the context of experimental studies, but also in the clinical setting [29]. Clinical practice involves measuring of different parameters for a variety of purposes, such as diagnosis of the disease or prediction of future events. Measurements are almost always prone to various types of errors which make the measured value to differ from the true value. If these measurements are performed by different observers, differences may be due to bias of the observers [41].

In our study, inter-observer reproducibility and intra-observer reproducibility of the LV global circumferential strain were excellent while global longitudinal strain demonstrated good inter-observer and intra-observer agreement. The excellent reproducibility means that parameters could be used to detect differences between individuals or focus on intra-individual changes during follow-up studies.

Sample size calculation is an important aspect of study design and enables determination of how large the study sample should be. Too small sample size can miss the real effect, whereas too large sample size leads to unnecessary waste of time and resources (animals). Estimates of required sample size depend on the variability of the population – the greater the variability, the larger the required sample size. The most favored scientific method in experiments is calculation of sample size by power analysis. In the present pilot study, we estimated the variability of the difference because the standard deviation of a difference in measurement in an animal is lower than variability of the population. Therefore, the number of animals needed to test a hypothesis could be reduced because the effect of animal-to-animal variation on the measurement is eliminated [42]. In the light of the current discussion of improving animal welfare by methodological refinements to reduce suffering, ameliorated imaging techniques are an important tool to achieve it.

Reproducibility and sample size are affected by image quality and variability of measurements. We successfully performed measurements in all animals and to decrease variability of measurements used averaged results of repeated analyses. Nevertheless, our calculations could give the impression that sample sizes required to detect relative changes in strain parameters are too low (e.g. ten animals per group are needed to detect a relative 10% change in Ecc_{SAX} or 13 animals for Ell_{LAX}). It is important to remember that the addition of a 25% dropout rate (proportion of eligible subjects who will not complete the study or provide only partial information) before planning a study will further increase the final sample size. Despite the small number of animals included in the study we could demonstrate that myocardial deformation parameters are highly reproducible. However, larger animal studies are necessary to confirm our preliminary findings.

Limitations

Our study is limited due to the small number of animals and larger sample size may be required to detect more subtle differences. In addition, CMR-FT was performed on 2D and low temporal resolution (15 phases per cardiac cycle) cine images.

Conclusions

Myocardial deformation parameters represent a new potential biomarker for the detection of early myocardial dysfunction. Cardiac mechanics parameters derived from conventional cine images using CMR-FT technique in small animal models are highly reproducible. The most reproducible measures are global circumferential and global longitudinal strain, whereas reproducibility of radial strain is weak. Relatively small study sample size could be sufficient to detect changes if parameter variability is low.

Abbreviations

CMR: Cardiovascular magnetic resonance; Ecc_{SAX}: Left ventricular short-axis circumferential strain; Ell_{LAX}: Left ventricular long-axis longitudinal strain; Err_{SAX}: Left ventricular short-axis radial strain; FT: Feature tracking; LV: Left ventricle / ventricular; $SRcc_{SAX}$: Left ventricular short-axis circumferential strain rate; $SRll_{LAX}$: Left ventricular long-axis longitudinal strain rate; $SRrr_{SAX}$: Left ventricular short-axis radial strain rate

Acknowledgements

We thank Anne Gale for editorial assistance.

Funding

This work was supported by the grant in aid of Novartis (Germany). TL received support from the Hospital of Lithuanian University of Health Sciences. SK was supported by Philips Healthcare. TL, UK, BP and SK received support from German Centre for Cardiovascular Research.

Authors' contributions

SJ carried out the animal experiments and CMR studies. JG and SMZ calculated myocardial deformation parameters. TL performed statistical analysis and drafted the manuscript. DM, HM, UK and PS participated in the design of the study. RG helped with the interpretation of data. RZ and BP made substantial contributions to concept of the study and revised the manuscript for important intellectual content. SK designed and coordinated the study, helped with interpretation of the data and to draft the manuscript. All authors have read and approved the final manuscript.

Consent for publication

Not applicable.

Competing interests

The authors declare that they have no competing interests.

Author details

[1]Department of Cardiology, Medical Academy, Lithuanian University of Health Sciences, Eiveniu Street 2, LT-50161 Kaunas, Lithuania. [2]Department of Internal Medicine / Cardiology, Deutsches Herzzentrum Berlin, Augustenburger Platz 1, 13353 Berlin, Germany. [3]Center for Cardiovascular Research, Institute of Pharmacology, Charité-Universitätsmedizin Berlin, Berlin, Germany. [4]Department of Internal Medicine / Cardiology, Charité-Universitätsmedizin Berlin, Berlin, Germany. [5]DZHK (German Centre for Cardiovascular Research), Partner Site Berlin, Berlin, Germany.

References

1. St John Sutton M, Pfeffer MA, Moye L, Plappert T, Rouleau JL, Lamas G, Rouleau J, Parker JO, Arnold MO, Sussex B, Braunwald E. Cardiovascular death and left ventricular remodeling two years after myocardial infarction: baseline predictors and impact of long-term use of captopril: information from the survival and ventricular enlargement (SAVE) trial. Circulation. 1997;96:3294–9.
2. Cikes M, Solomon SD. Beyond ejection fraction: an integrative approach for assessment of cardiac structure and function in heart failure. Eur Heart J. 2016;37:1642–50.

3. Ibrahim E-SH. Myocardial tagging by cardiovascular magnetic resonance: evolution of techniques – pulse sequences, analysis algorithms, and applications. J Cardiovasc Magn Reson. 2011;13:36.
4. Pedrizzetti G, Claus P, Kilner PJ, Nagel E. Principles of cardiovascular magnetic resonance feature tracking and echocardiographic speckle tracking for informed clinical use. J Cardiovasc Magn Reson. 2016;18(1):51.
5. Claus P, Omar AM, Pedrizzetti G, Sengupta PP, Nagel E. Tissue tracking technology for assessing cardiac mechanics: principles, normal values, and clinical applications. JACC Cardiovasc Imaging. 2015;8:1444–60.
6. Zerhouni EA, Parish DM, Rogers WJ, Yang A, Shapiro EP. Human heart: tagging with MR imaging – a method for noninvasive assessment of myocardial motion. Radiology. 1988;169:59–63.
7. Axel L, Dougherty L. MR imaging of motion with spatial modulation of magnetization. Radiology. 1989;171:841–5.
8. Wang J, Khoury DS, Thohan V, Torre-Amione G, Nagueh SF. Global diastolic strain rate for the assessment of left ventricular relaxation and filling pressures. Circulation. 2007;115:1376–83.
9. Schneeweis C, Lapinskas T, Schnackenburg B, Berger A, Hucko T, Kelle S, Fleck E, Gebker R. Comparison of myocardial tagging and feature tracking in patients with severe aortic stenosis. J Heart Valve Dis. 2014;23(4):432–40.
10. Kowallick JT, Kutty S, Edelmann F, Chiribiri A, Villa A, Steinmetz M, Sohns JM, Staab W, Bettencourt N, Unterberg-Buchwald C, Hasenfuß G, Lotz J, Schuster A. Quantification of left atrial strain and strain rate using cardiovascular magnetic resonance myocardial feature tracking: a feasibility study. J Cardiovasc Magn Reson. 2014;16:60.
11. Kempny A, Fernández-Jiménez R, Orwat S, Schuler P, Bunck AC, Maintz D, Baumgartner H, Diller GP. Quantification of biventricular myocardial function using cardiac magnetic resonance feature tracking, endocardial border delineation and echocardiographic speckle tracking in patients with repaired tetralogy of Fallot and healthy controls. J Cardiovasc Magn Reson. 2012;14:32.
12. Schneeweis C, Qiu J, Schnackenburg B, Berger A, Kelle S, Fleck E, Gebker R. Value of additional strain analysis with feature tracking in dobutamine stress cardiovascular magnetic resonance for detecting coronary artery disease. J Cardiovasc Magn Reson. 2014;16:72.
13. Meyer CG, Frick M, Lotfi S, Altiok E, Koos R, Kirschfink A, Lehrke M, Autschbach R, Hoffmann R. Regional left ventricular function after transapical vs transfemoral transcatheter aortic valve implantation analysed by cardiac magnetic resonance feature tracking. Eur Heart J Cardiovasc Imaging. 2014;15:1168–76.
14. Morais P, Marchi A, Bogaert JA, Dresselaers T, Heyde B, D'hooge J, Bogaert J. Cardiovascular magnetic resonance myocardial feature tracking using a non-rigid, elastic image registration algorithm: assessment of variability in a real-life clinical setting. J Cardiovasc Magn Reson. 2017;19(1):24.
15. Kraitchman DL, Sampath S, Castillo E, Derbyshire JA, Boston RC, Bluemke DA, Gerber BL, Prince JL, Osman NF. Quantitative ischemia detection during cardiac magnetic resonance stress testing by use of FastHARP. Circulation. 2003;107:2025–30.
16. Moody WE, Taylor RJ, Edwards NC, Chue CD, Umar F, Taylor TJ, Ferro CJ, Young AA, Townend JN, Leyva F, Steeds RP. Comparison of magnetic resonance feature tracking for systolic and diastolic strain and strain rate calculation with spatial modulation of magnetization imaging analysis. J Magn Reson Imaging. 2015;41:1000–12.
17. Nahum J, Bensaid A, Dussault C, Macron L, Clémence D, Bouhemad B, Monin JL, Rande JL, Gueret P, Lim P. Impact of longitudinal myocardial deformation on the prognosis of chronic heart failure patients. Circ Cardiovasc Imaging. 2010;3:249–56.
18. Smith BM, Dorfman AL, Yu S, Russell MW, Agarwal PP, Ghadimi Mahani M, Lu JC. Relation of strain by feature tracking and clinical outcome in children, adolescents, and young adults with hypertrophic cardiomyopathy. Am J Cardiol. 2014;114:1275–80.
19. Buss SJ, Breuninger K, Lehrke S, Voss A, Galuschky C, Lossnitzer D, Andre F, Ehlermann P, Franke J, Taeger T, Frankenstein L, Steen H, Meder B, Giannitsis E, Katus HA, Korosoglou G. Assessment of myocardial deformation with cardiac magnetic resonance strain imaging improves risk stratification in patients with dilated cardiomyopathy. Eur Heart J Cardiovasc Imaging. 2015;16:307–15.
20. Mahfoud F, Urban D, Teller D, Linz D, Stawowy P, Hassel JH, Fries P, Dreysse S, Wellnhofer E, Schneider G, Buecker A, Schneeweis C, Doltra A, Schlaich MP, Esler MD, Fleck E, Böhm M, Kelle S. Effect of renal denervation on left ventricular mass and function in patients with resistant hypertension: data from a multi-centre cardiovascular magnetic resonance imaging trial. Eur Heart J. 2014;35:2224–31b.
21. Bernard A, Donal E, Leclercq C, Schnell F, Fournet M, Reynaud A, Thebault C, Mabo P, Daubert JC, Hernandez A. Impact of cardiac resynchronization therapy on left ventricular mechanics: understanding the response through a new quantitative approach based on longitudinal strain integrals. J Am Soc Echocardiogr. 2015;28:700–8.
22. Morton G, Schuster A, Jogiya R, Kutty S, Beerbaum P, Nagel E. Inter-study reproducibility of cardiovascular magnetic resonance myocardial feature tracking. J Cardiovasc Magn Reson. 2012;14:43.
23. Schuster A, Paul M, Bettencourt N, Hussain ST, Morton G, Kutty S, Bigalke B, Chiribiri A, Perera D, Nagel E, Beerbaum P. Myocardial feature tracking reduces observer-dependance in low-dose dobutamine stress cardiovascular magnetic resonance. PLoS One. 2015;10:e0122858.
24. Lapinskas T, Bučius P, Urbonaitė L, Stabinskaitė A, Valuckienė Ž, Jankauskaitė L, Benetis R, Žaliūnas R. Left atrial mechanics in patients with acute STEMI and secondary mitral regurgitation: a prospective pilot CMR feature tracking study. Medicina (Kaunas). 2017;53(1):11–8.
25. Kowallick JT, Morton G, Lamata P, Jogiya R, Kutty S, Lotz J, Hasenfuß G, Nagel E, Chiribiri A, Schuster A. Inter-study reproducibility of left ventricular torsion and torsion rate quantification using MR myocardial feature tracking. J Magn Reson Imaging. 2016;43:128–37.
26. Schuster A, Morton G, Hussain ST, Jogiya R, Kutty S, Asrress KN, Makowski MR, Bigalke B, Perera D, Beerbaum P, Nagel E. The intra-observer reproducibility of cardiovascular magnetic resonance myocardial feature tracking strain assessment is independent of field strength. Eur J Radiol. 2013;82(2):296–301.
27. Bland JM, Altman DG. Statistical methods for assessing agreement between two methods of clinical measurement. Lancet. 1996;8476:307–10.
28. Oppo K, Leen E, Angerson WJ, Cooke TG, McArdle CS. Doppler perfusion index: an interobserver and intraobserver reproducibility study. Radiology. 1998;208:453–7.
29. Grothues F, Smith GC, Moon JC, Bellenger NG, Collins P, Klein HU, Pennell DJ. Comparison of interstudy reproducibility of cardiovascular magnetic resonance with two-dimensional echocardiography in normal subjects and in patients with heart failure or left ventricular hypertrophy. Am J Cardiol. 2002;90:29–34.
30. Stanton T, Leano R, Marwick TH. Prediction of all-cause mortality from global longitudinal speckle strain: comparison with ejection fraction and wall motion scoring. Circ Cardiovasc Imaging. 2009;2:356–64.
31. Flachskampf FA, Biering-Sørensen T, Solomon SD, Duvernoy O, Bjener T, Smiseth OA. Cardiac imaging to evaluate left ventricular diastolic function. JACC Cardiovasc Imaging. 2015;8:1071–93.
32. Peng Y, Popovic ZB, Sopko N, Drinko J, Zhang Z, Thomas JD, Penn MS. Speckle tracking echocardiography in the assessment of mouse models of cardiac dysfunction. Am J Physiol Heart Circ Physiol. 2009;297:H811–20.
33. Maret E, Todt T, Brudin L, Nylander E, Swahn E, Ohlsson JL, Engvall JE. Functional measurements based on feature tracking of cine magnetic resonance images identify left ventricular segments with myocardial scar. Cardiovasc Ultrasound. 2009;7:53.
34. Hor KN, Gottliebson WM, Carson C, Wash E, Cnota J, Fleck R, Wansapura J, Klimeczek P, Al-Khalidi HR, Chung ES, Benson DW, Mazur W. Comparison of magnetic resonance feature tracking for strain calculation with harmonic phase imaging analysis. JACC Cardiovasc Imaging. 2010;3:144–51.
35. Zhong J, Liu W, Yu X. Characterization of three-dimensional myocardial deformation in the mouse heart: an MR tagging study. J Magn Reson Imaging. 2008;27:1263–70.
36. Kramer SP, Powell DK, Haggerty CM, Binkley CM, Mattingly AC, Cassis LA, Epstein FH, Fornwalt BK. Obesity reduces left ventricular strains, torsion, and synchrony in mouse models: a cine displacement encoding with stimulated echoes (DENSE) cardiovascular magnetic resonance study. J Cardiovasc Magn Reson. 2013;15:109.
37. Ho D, Zhao X, Gao S, Hong C, Vatner DE, Vatner SF. Heart rate and electrocardiography monitoring in mice. Curr Protoc Mouse Biol. 2011;1:123–39.
38. Schuster A, Hor KN, Kowallick JT, Beerbaum P, Kutty S. Cardiovascular magnetic resonance myocardial feature tracking: concepts and clinical applications. Circ Cardiovasc Imaging. 2016;9(4):e004077.
39. Augustine D, Lewandowski AJ, Lazdam M, Rai A, Francis J, Myerson S, Noble A, Becher H, Neubauer S, Petersen SE, Leeson P. Global and regional left ventricular myocardial deformation measures by magnetic resonance feature tracking in healthy volunteers: comparison with tagging and relevance of gender. J Cardiovasc Magn Reson. 2013;15:8.

Ultra-high b-value diffusion-weighted imaging features of the prostatic leiomyoma

Yanguang Shen[1], Yan Zhong[1], Haiyi Wang[1], Lu Ma[1], Yingwei Wang[1], Jinjin Pan[1], Zhonghua Sun[2] and Huiyi Ye[1*]

Abstract

Background: Leiomyoma of the prostate is a rare benign tumor arising from smooth muscle fibers. Most cases are incidental findings observed during pathological examinations after resection of the prostate. To the best of our knowledge, only few studies have reported the conventional magnetic resonance imaging (MRI) findings of such tumors; however, no reports have described the ultra-high b-value diffusion-weighted imaging (DWI) and apparent diffusion coefficient (ADC) findings of prostatic leiomyomas.

Case presentation: We report MR imaging characteristics and surgical pathologic findings of a case of prostatic leiomyoma treated by robot-assisted transperitoneal laparoscopic approach. Typical MR features showed a homogeneous lesion with slightly hypointense signal compared to the skeletal muscle on T2-weighted images, and isointense signal relative to the muscle on T1-weighted images with fat suppression, which collectively demonstrate apparent homogeneous enhancement with a non-enhanced envelope. A slightly hyperintense signal compared to the skeletal muscle was observed on ultra-high b-value DWI, and higher ADC values were observed as compared to the prostate cancer.

Conclusions: Prostatic leiomyoma is a benign tumor. This case indicates that MRI features of prostatic leiomyoma are helpful for the differential diagnosis of prostate cancer.

Keywords: Prostate, Leiomyoma, Magnetic resonance imaging, Diffusion weighted imaging

Background

Leiomyoma of the prostate is a rare benign tumor arising from smooth muscle fibers. Most cases are incidental findings observed during anatomopathological examinations after a resection of the prostate [1]. Prostatic hyperplasia often includes leiomyomatous nodules [2]. They are most often removed surgically. To the best of our knowledge, only six reports have described the conventional MRI findings of such tumors, and no studies have presented the ultra-high b-value diffusion-weighted imaging and ADC findings of prostatic leiomyomas [3, 4]. Here, we present MRI findings of a patient with benign prostate hypertrophy and prostate cancer who was incidentally diagnosed with a prostatic leiomyoma. Ultrasound guided systematic transperineal prostatic biopsy and subsequent histological examination of biopsy samples confirmed prostatic cancer in the prostatic left zone (Gleason score 3 + 3 = 6). The patient was operated successfully by a robot-assisted laparoscopic radical prostatectomy.

* Correspondence: 13701100368@163.com; 13701100368@163.com
[1]Department of Radiology, Chinese PLA General Hospital, Fuxing Road NO.28, Box 100853, Beijing, China
Full list of author information is available at the end of the article

Case presentation

A 76-year-old man was referred to our urology department with repeated symptoms of dysuria, frequent urination, urgency, and painful micturition for one month. His past medical history showed no hypertension, diabetes, or any history of surgery.

Laboratory data on admission showed that the total prostate specific antigen level was 7.76 ng/ml, free prostate specific antigen level was 0.618 ng/ml, and white blood cell count was 10,750/mm^3; however, urinalysis and blood chemistry were all within normal range. Digital rectal examination revealed an enlarged prostate, a prominent median sulcus, a smooth rubbery consistency with no palpable nodule, and elastic enlarged prostate.

Ultrasound scan showed an enlarged prostate (38 mm in anteroposterior diameter, 43 mm in longitudinal diameter, and 51 mm in transverse diameter), prostatic hyperplasia, and a gland of 43 g.

Patient's pelvis was imaged in 3.0-T MRI (Discovery 750, GE Healthcare, Milwaukee, WI, USA) using a surface phased array coil. Conventional MRI sequences included both axial fast spin-echo T2-weighted imaging (T2WI) and DWI. T2WI of the entire prostate and seminal vesicles was performed in axial, coronal, and sagittal planes. Conventional DWI with b-values of 0 and 1000 s/mm^2 was also performed in the axial plane. The ultra-high b-value DWI was performed with b-values of 3000 s/mm^2 in the axial plane. Both axial T2WI and DWI were obtained at the same slice location. Dynamic contrast-enhanced (DCE) MRI was also performed. Fifteen ml of Gadobenate dimeglumine (MultiHance; Bracco Sine, Shanghai, China) was injected intravenously at a rate of 3 ml/s using a power injector (Spectris; MedRad, Warrendale, PA), followed by a 20 ml saline flush. DCE-MRI was performed in the transverse plane at baseline (pre-contrast) and during arterial, venous, and delayed phases. MR imaging parameters are shown in Table 1.

Conventional MRI displayed a round tumor in the prostatic bottom protruding into the bladder with an isointense signal compared to the muscle on T1-weighted images (T1WI) with fat suppression and a homogeneous lesion with slightly hypointense signal on T2WI (Fig. 1). Ultra-high b-value DWI (b = 3000 s/mm^2) features showed slightly homogeneous hyperintense signal compared to the muscle, and the mean ADC value was $0.817 \pm 0.016 \times 10^{-3}$ mm^2/s. The tumor was strongly and homogeneously enhanced during the arterial phase with continuous signal increase of mass in the venous and delayed phases (a persistent pattern). Normal prostatic glandular tissue with a non-enhanced capsule around the mass was clearly distinguished from the tumor as a homogeneous isointense signal compared to the muscle. No central necrosis was demonstrated in the tumor.

In addition, a low signal intensity area on T2WI showed significantly higher signal nodule on ultra-high b-value DWI, and the mean ADC value was $0.517 \pm 0.015 \times 10^{-3}$ mm^2/s. It was found in the left transition and peripheral zone. The tumor showed clear enhancement with an irregular boundary and without capsule on DCE (Fig. 2). At the same time, prostate benign hyperplasia nodules were also found in the middle area of right transition zone, and these features were similar to the prostatic leiomyoma observed on T2WI, T1WI and DWI. The mean ADC value was $0.710 \pm 0.049 \times 10^{-3}$ s/mm^2. The nodular was enhanced heterogeneously during the arterial phase with continuous signal increase of mass in the venous and delayed phases (a persistent pattern). There was no capsule. The preoperative MRI diagnosis revealed prostatic cancer with benign prostatic hyperplasia; however, the prostatic leiomyoma was not considered at the initial diagnosis.

Ultrasound guided systematic transperineal prostatic biopsy and subsequent histological analysis of biopsy samples confirmed prostatic cancer in the left zone (Gleason score 3 + 3 = 6).

A robot-assisted laparoscopic radical prostatectomy was performed to remove the whole prostate. In addition, histopathological examinations revealed leiomyoma based on following features: firstly, the tumor was composed primarily of hyalinized connective tissue containing spindle cells; secondly, spindle cells were arranged with a fascicular and whorled manner in foci. The cancer was found in peripheral and transitional zones of the left posterior lobe.

Discussion and conclusions

Most cases of prostatic leiomyoma are diagnosed as incidental findings related to the history of progressive prostatism. The first case report of a prostatic leiomyoma found at autopsy was published in 1876. On that report, prostatic leiomyoma was defined as a circumscribed or encapsulated mass of smooth muscle with 1 cm or more in diameter containing varying amounts of fibrous tissue

Table 1 MR imaging acquisition parameters

Protocol	Sequence	TR(msec)	TE(msec)	FA	FOV(cm)	Matrix	Section thickness	Intersection gap	NEX	Bandwidth
Axial T2WI	FR FSE	6627	115.1	90	20 × 20	288 × 288	3 cm	0.5 cm	2.0	62.5kHZ
Coronal T2WI	FR FSE	7229.6	115.1	90	18 × 18	288 × 288	3 cm	0.5 cm	2.0	62.5kHZ
Sagittal T2WI	FR FSE	12,333.1	108.9	90	22 × 22	288 × 288	3 cm	0.5 cm	1.5	83.31kHZ
DWI(b = 1000 s/mm^2)	SE-EPI	2700	76.8	90	36 × 32	130 × 128	3 cm	0.5 cm	6	250kHZ
DWI(b = 3000 s/mm^2)	SE-EPI	2700	76.8	90	32 × 32	130 × 128	3 cm	0.5 cm	6	250kHZ
Axial LAVA-Flex	3D–LAVA	3.9	1.8	15	40 × 36	288 × 192	4 cm	–2.0 cm	0.71	166.7kHZ
Contrast-enhanced imaging	3D–LAVA	2.7–4.4	1.3–2.0	15	38–40 × 30–40	288 × 256	4 cm	–0.5-0 cm	0.69–0.73	125–142.9kHZ

FR FSE fast recovery fast spin echo, *SE/EPI* spin-echo echo-planar imaging, *3D/LAVA* three-dimensional liver acquisition with volume acceleration, *TE* echo time, *TR* repetition time, *FA* flip angle, *FOV* field of view

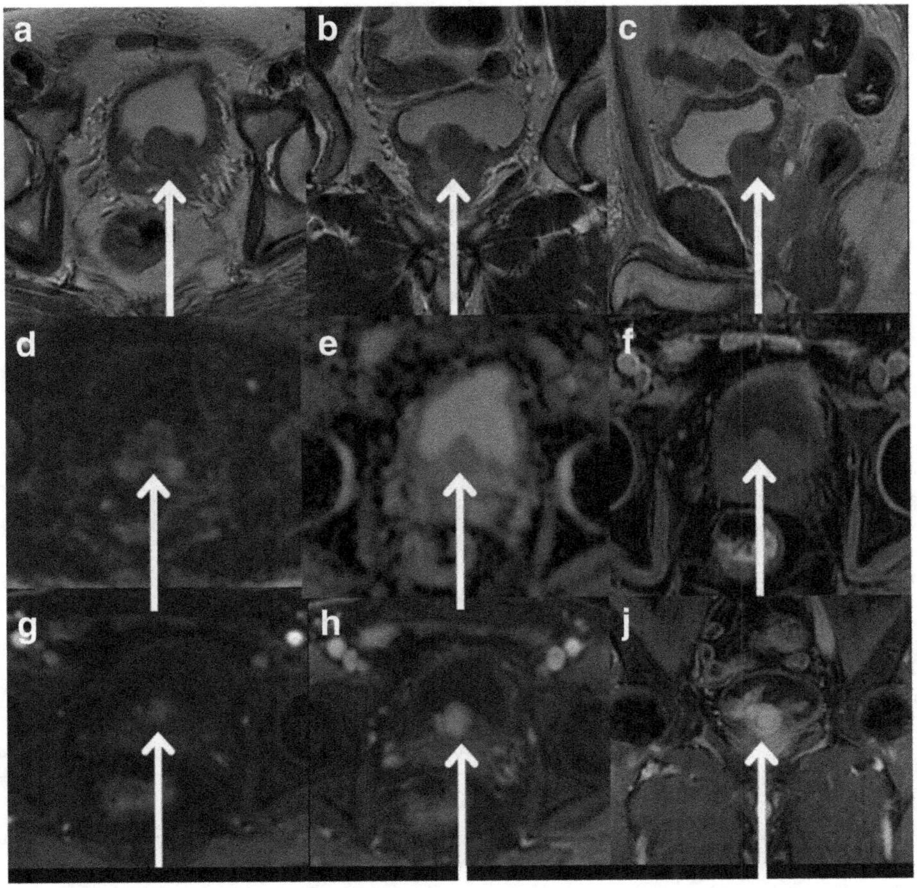

Fig. 1 MR images of prostatic leiomyoma. **a**, **b**, **c** Axial, Coronal, and Sagittal High-resolution T2WI images show a well-circumscribed nodule with a capsule (homogeneous low signal intensity) in the bottom of prostatic left inner zone as homogeneous and slightly hypointense signal compared to the muscle (arrows). **d** On ultra-high b-value DWI ($b = 3000$ s/mm^2), slightly high signal nodule compared to the muscle (arrows) was observed. **e** On ultra-high b-value DWI apparent diffusion coefficient map, ADC value was $0.817 \pm 0.016 \times 10^{-3}$ mm^2/s. **f** On T1WI MRI with fat suppression (Pre scanned imaging), the homogeneous isointense signal of nodule compared to the muscle was found. **g**, **h**, **j** On Axial contrast T1WI during the arterial phase, the tumor was strongly and homogeneously enhanced. During venous and delay phases, the tumor showed continuous signal increase (arrows). The margin of tumor was clear, and the envelope was not enhanced

but devoid of glandular elements, which was either obviously prostatic or juxtaprostatic in origin and position [5, 6]. However, the pathogenesis of such tumor remains unclear. Several theories have described that it is formed as a result of chronic inflammatory reactions or embryological ability [6, 7] and may originate from smooth muscle elements of the periglandular prostatic tissue, prostatic capsule, or Mullerian duct remnant. The main clinical symptom is urinary disturbance, as reported in case of benign prostatic hypertrophy differing in localization within the prostate. Occasionally, it may present as a large mass bulging into the rectum producing rectal symptoms [5, 8]. This disease is benign and surgical resection is recommended if present with severe clinical symptoms.

Typical imaging features of prostatic leiomyoma on contrast-enhanced CT have been reported in some cases, which show a round hypodense mass and homogeneous enlargement of the prostate with well circumscribed appearance [8–11]. Only a few studies have reported that typical MRI features of prostatic leiomyoma show an isointense and homogeneous signal mass on T1WI, slightly hyperintense or hypointense on T2WI, and homogeneous and strongly enhanced lesion on contrast-enhanced MR images [11–13], The manifestation of our case was compatible with those criteria reported in the literature. In contrast, Ringoir and colleagues have reported a heterogeneous prostatic leiomyoma with cystic and solid components in the right prostate lobe on MRI [14]. To the best of our knowledge, ultra-high b-value DWI and ADC features of the prostatic leiomyoma have not been reported in the literature till date. Only Mussi et al. have reported 3 cases with low and intermediate b-values DWI and ADC maps (b values = 50, 400 and 800) [15]. In our case report, typical features of the prostatic leiomyoma were slightly

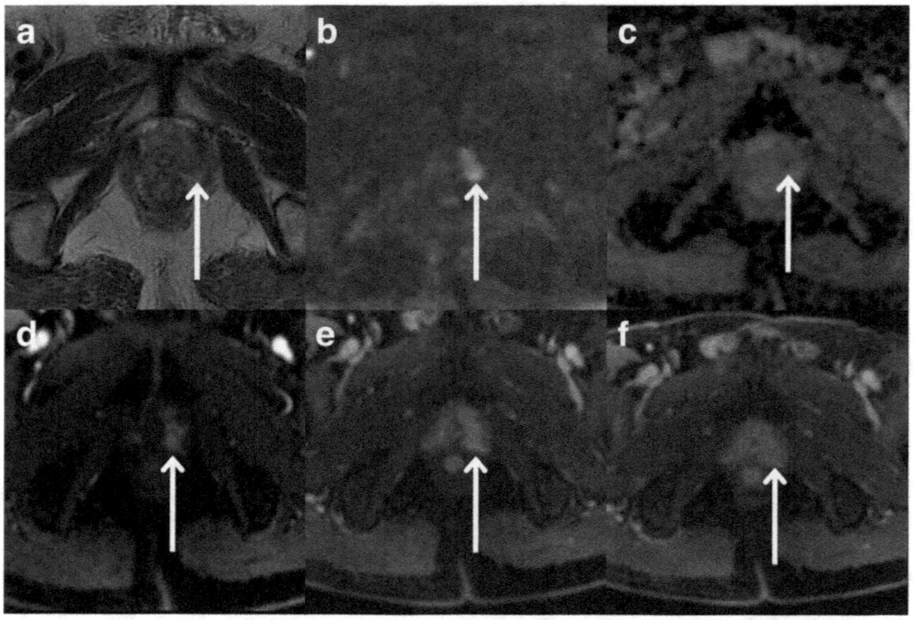

Fig. 2 MR images of prostate cancer. **a** High-resolution T2WI shows low signal intensity area in the left transition (TZ) and peripheral zone (PZ) (arrows). **b** On ultra-high b-value DWI (b = 3000 s/mm^2), left-side lesions were observed as significantly higher signal nodules (arrows). **c** On ultra-high b-value DWI (b = 3000 s/mm^2) ADC map, ADC value of the left-side lesion was 0.517 ± 0.015 × 10^{-3} mm^2/s (arrows). **d** On axial contrast T1WI during the arterial phase, the tumor was enhanced strongly and non-homogeneously (arrows). **e, f** On axial contrast T1WI during venous and delay phases, the tumor was enhanced strongly and non-homogeneously (continuous signal increase, arrows). The margin of tumor was not clear, and there was no envelope

homogeneous hyperintense signal compared to the muscle on DWI and a higher ADC value as compared to the prostate cancer, which altogether reflecting pathological characteristics of abundant muscle or fibrous tissue component.

The major differential diagnosis of prostatic leiomyoma is prostate cancer. DWI is a functional technique enabling qualitative and quantitative assessment of the prostate cancer with high diagnostic accuracy. Prostatic cancer shows a higher signal intensity on DWI and a lower ADC value as compared to normal prostatic tissue [16, 17]. The American College of Radiology and European Society of Urogenital Radiology guidelines have recommended the use of a high b-value (≥ 1400 s/mm^2) as it suppresses the signal of normal prostatic tissue effectively; thus, the contrast between cancerous and non-cancerous lesions can be emphasized better on DWI. It is difficult to differentiate prostatic leiomyoma from prostate cancer while using low and intermediate b-values DWI and ADC maps (b values = 50, 400 and 800). If the MR scanner yields an adequate signal-to-noise ratio, the use of a very high b-value (e.g. 2000 s/mm^2) is more advantageous for cancer detection [18, 19]. Zhang, et al. have reported that DWI with an ultra-high b-value of 3000 s/mm^2 is found to be the most accurate and reliable MRI modality for prostatic cancer detection and localization [20]. ADC values can be useful for the characterization of clinically significant cancer. The similar signal feature was seen in the prostatic leiomyoma and prostate cancer on T2WI in this case, but the ADC value of prostate cancer was lower than that of leiomyoma. In addition, DCE-MRI added only little information for differentiating between prostate leiomyoma and prostate cancer. Multiparametric-MRI can detect clinically significant prostate cancer with high accuracy [21]. In this case, the differentiation of leiomyoma from prostatic cancer may be easily done by MRI findings alone.

However, MRI features of stromal hyperplastic nodules of benign prostatic hyperplasia (BPH) are similar to the prostatic leiomyoma; thus, it is poorly identified because of the overlapping of conventional imaging features [22]. Patch and Rhea have pointed out that most cases with combined leiomyoma and BPH can be missed on MRI, and 25.4% of 181 consecutive patients with total prostectomy show leiomyoma in benign hyperplastic nodules [23]. Stromal hyperplastic nodules and prostatic leiomyoma are benign and non-cancerous lesions.

The final diagnosis also depends on pathological examinations. The most commonly evidenced diagnostic method is B-ultrasound guided transrectal prostate biopsy or transurethral resection of the prostate. Macroscopically, a leiomyoma relates to a well-defined nodular formation [24]. Microscopically, it is characterized by intersecting bundles not atypical, smooth muscle cells with uniform cigar-shaped, and slightly vesicular nuclei. The spindle cell population is desmin, smooth muscle actin (SMA), and androgen receptor positive [12]. To date, no reports have indicated recurrence of prostatic leiomyomas after surgical removal [8].

In conclusion, we report a relatively rare leiomyoma of the prostate gland. Upon observation of a well-circumscribed tumor with no enhanced capsule with homogeneous and almost isointense signal compared to the muscle on T1WI and slightly hypointense signal on T2WI with a strong and homogeneous enhancement by DCE-MRI in the prostatic inner zone, leiomyoma should be considered in the differential diagnosis.

Abbreviations

ADC: Apparent diffusion coefficient; BPH: Benign prostatic hyperplasia; DCE: Dynamic contrast enhancement; DWI: Diffusion weighted imaging; MRI: Magnetic resonance imaging; SH: Stromal hyperplasia; SMA: Smooth muscle actin; T1WI: T1-weighted image; T2WI: T2-weighted image

Acknowledgements

We would like to thank Haiyi Wang, Lu Ma, and Yan Zhong from PLA General Hospital for their thoughtful suggestions and technical support with this paper.

Funding

This work was supported by grants from the Health Care Special Project (14BJZ02). The funding source has estimated the feasibility of the study, but has no role in the collection, analysis, or interpretation of the data or in the decision to submit the manuscript for publication.

Authors' contributions

Conceived and designed the experiments: HY, YS, YZ, HW, LM, JP, YW. Performed the experiments: YS, YZ. Analyzed the data: YS. Manuscript written: YS, ZS. All authors read and approved the final manuscript.

Consent for publication

Permission was granted to use the de-identified patient information and images. The patient and his family have kindly provided written informed consent for the case report to be published.

Competing interests

The authors declare that they have no competing interests.

Author details

[1]Department of Radiology, Chinese PLA General Hospital, Fuxing Road NO.28, Box 100853, Beijing, China. [2]Department of Medical Radiation Sciences, Curtin University, Perth 6102, Australia.

References

1. Oderda M, Mondaini N, Bartoletti R, Vigna D, Fiorito C, Marson F, Peraldo F, Bosio A, Maletta F, Pacchioni D, Gontero P. Leiomyomata of the genitourinary tract: a case series from the "rare urological neoplasm" registry. Scand J Urol. 2013;47(2):158–62.
2. Imai S, Ayabe Y, Iiyama T, Muramatsu H, Matsuo Y, Kudo S. Leiomyoma of the prostate: CT and MR findings. Abdom Imaging. 2002;27(6):674–6.
3. Fasih N, Prasad Shanbhogue AK, Macdonald DB, Fraser-Hill MA, Papadatos D, Kielar AZ, Doherty GP, Walsh C, McInnes M, Atri M. Leiomyomas beyond the uterus: unusual locations, rare manifestations. Radiographics. 2008;28(7):1931–48.
4. Aoun F, de Saint Aubain Somerhausen N, van Velthoven R, Peltier A. Prostate sparing robot-assisted laparoscopic treatment of leiomyoma of the prostate. J Robot Surg. 2014;8(4):389–92.
5. Leonard A, Baert L, Van Praet F, Van de Voorde W, Van Poppel H, Lauweryns J. Solitary leiomyoma of the prostate. Br J Urol. 1988;62(2):184–5.
6. Kaufman JJ, Berneike RR. Leiomyoma of the prostate. J Urol. 1951;65(2):297–310.
7. Vassilakis GB. Pure leiomyoma of prostate. Urology. 1978;11(1):93–4.
8. Regan JB, Barrett DM, Wold LE. Giant leiomyoma of the prostate. Arch Pathol Lab Med. 1987;111(111):381–2.
9. Coulier B, Lens V, Mailleux P, Lefebvre Y. Prostatic leiomyoma. J Belg Radiol. 1995;78(3):182–3.
10. Laxman GG, Rao MS. Conservatively managed symptomatic leiomyoma of the prostate. JAMA. 1995;93(5):209.
11. Masuda H, Yamanaka H, Nakata S, Sato J, Ogawa A, Kosaku N. A case of pure leiomyoma of the prostate. Hinyokika Kiyo. 1999;45(4):277–80.
12. Nakamura K, Shiramizu M. Pure leiomyoma of prostate presenting with rectal symptoms: a case report. Acta Urol Jpn. 1992;38(9):1067–9.
13. Kitajima K, Kaji Y, Imanaka K, Hayashi M, Kuwata Y, Sugimura K. MR imaging findings of pure prostatic leiomyoma: a report of two cases. J Comput Assist Tomogr. 2006;30(6):910–2.
14. Ringoir A, Rappe B, Dhaene K, Schallier D. Prostatic Leiomyoma: a case report. Urol Case Rep. 2016;25(9):45–7.
15. Mussi TC, Costa YB, Obara MT, Queiroz MR, Garcia RG, Longo JA, Lemos GC, Baroni RH. Multiparametric magnetic resonance imaging findings of prostatic pure leiomyomas. Einstein (Sao Paulo). 2016;14(3):374–7.
16. Barentsz JO, Richenberg J, Clements R, Choyke P, Verma S, Villeirs G, Rouviere O, Logager V, Fütterer JJ, European Society of Urogenital Radiology. ESUR prostate MR guidelines 2012. Eur Radiol. 2012;22(4):746–57.
17. van As NJ, de Souza NM, Riches SF, Morgan VA, Sohaib SA, Dearnaley DP, Parker CC. A study of diffusion-weighted magnetic resonance imaging in men with untreated localised prostate cancer on active surveillance. Eur Urol. 2009;56(6):981–7.
18. Ueno Y, Kitajima K, Sugimura K, Kawakami F, Miyake H, Obara M, Takahashi S. Ultra-high b-value diffusion-weighted MRI for the detection of prostate cancer with 3-T MRI. J Magn Reson Imaging. 2013;38(1):154–60.
19. Katahira K, Takahara T, Kwee TC, Oda S, Suzuki Y, Morishita S, Kitani K, Hamada Y, Kitaoka M, Yamashita Y. Ultra-high-b-value diffusion-weighted MR imaging for the detection of prostate cancer: evaluation in 201 cases with histopathological correlation. Eur Radiol. 2011;21(1):188–96.
20. Zhang K, Shen Y, Zhang X, Ma L, Wang H, An N, Guo A, Ye H. Predicting prostate biopsy outcomes: a preliminary investigation on screening with ultrahigh B-value diffusion-weighted imaging as an innovative diagnostic biomarker. PLoS One. 2016;11(3):e0151176. https://doi.org/10.1371/journal.pone.0151176.
21. Ueno Y, Tamada T, Bist V, Reinhold C, Miyake H, Tanaka U, Kitajima K, Sugimura K, Takahashi S. Multiparametric magnetic resonance imaging: Current role in prostate cancer management. Int J Urol. 2016;23(7):550–7.
22. Liu X, Zhou L, Peng W, Wang C, Wang H. Differentiation of central gland prostate cancer from benign prostatic hyperplasia using monoexponential and biexponential diffusion-weighted imaging. Magn Reson Imaging. 2013;31(8):1318–24.
23. Patch FS, Rhea LJ. Leiomyoma of the prostate gland. Br J Urol. 1935;7(3):213–28.
24. Barba J, Tolosa E, Panizo AF, Berian JM. Prostatic leiomyoma. Case report. Archivos Espanoles de Urologia. 2011;64(7):631–5.

19

Improving the evaluation of cardiac function in rats at 7T with denoising filters

Benoit Tricot[1,2], Maxime Descoteaux[1,3], Matthieu Dumont[1], Frederic Chagnon[4], Luc Tremblay[1], André Carpentier[5], Olivier Lesur[1,4], Martin Lepage[1] and Alain Lalande[6*]

Abstract

Background: We investigate the use of different denoising filters on low signal-to-noise ratio cardiac images of the rat heart acquired with a birdcage volume coil at 7T. Accuracy and variability of cardiac function parameters were measured from manual segmentation of rat heart images with and without filtering.

Methods: Ten rats were studied using a 7T Varian system. End-diastolic and end-systolic volumes, ejection fraction and left ventricle mass (LVM) were calculated from manual segmentation by two experts on cine-FLASH short-axis slices covering the left ventricle. Series were denoised with an anisotropic diffusion filter, a whole variation regularization or an optimized Rician non-local means (ORNLM) filtering technique. The effect of the different filters was evaluated by the calculation of signal-to-noise (SNR) and contrast-to-noise (CNR) ratios, followed by a study of intra- and inter-expert variability of the measurement of physiological parameters. The calculated LVM was compared to the LVM obtained by weighing the heart ex vivo.

Results: The SNR and the CNR increased after application of the different filters. The performance of the ORNLM filter was superior for all the parameters of the cardiac function, as judged from the inter- and intra-observer variabilities. Moreover, this filtering technique resulted in the lowest variability in the LVM evaluation.

Conclusions: In cardiac MRI of rats, filtering is an interesting alternative that yields better contrast between myocardium and surrounding tissues and the ORNLM filter provided the largest improvements.

Keywords: Small animal, Non-local means filtering, Cine-MRI, Denoising

Background

Magnetic Resonance Imaging (MRI) is a valuable tool for the detection of cardiovascular diseases. Owing to its fair temporal and high spatial resolutions, MRI is now an established and reliable technique for the assessment of cardiac structure, function, perfusion, and it can assess myocardial viability [1]. Animal models, and particularly transgenic rats and mice, are increasingly used for the study of genes and biological mechanisms involved in heart diseases [2]. MRI has become the gold-standard for the non-invasive examination of these models. This is despite challenges imposed by an elevated heart rate (up to 600 beats per minute for the mouse) and small heart [3]. High-quality heart images of animal models are typically acquired with dedicated high-field MRI systems, respiratory and cardiac gating strategies as well as optimized pulse sequences. Dedicated multi-element cardiac coil arrays can further increase the signal-to-noise ratio (SNR) in images of the rat heart [4], and this is particularly relevant for fast and kinetic imaging. However, these coils are not widely available and their cost is relatively high. Birdcage volume coils provide a lower SNR but they have been more popular and more widely used because of their versatility and their superior radio-frequency homogeneity.

In our study, we investigated the effect of three filtering techniques applied to low-SNR cine images of the rat heart acquired with a birdcage volume coil. In particular, we assessed their effect on the accuracy and the variability of

* Correspondence: alain.lalande@u-bourgogne.fr
[6]Le2I, Faculté de Médecine, Université Bourgogne Franche-Comté, 7 Bld Jeanne d'Arc, 21079 Dijon Cedex, BP 87900, France
Full list of author information is available at the end of the article

cardiac function parameters obtained from these images. The filtering techniques investigated were an anisotropic diffusion filter routinely used in image processing, a total variation regularization filter and an optimized Rician non-local means (ORNLM) filter [5]. Intra- and inter-observer variabilities were assessed for the following parameters: end-diastolic volume (EDV), end-systolic volume (ESV), ejection fraction (EF) and left ventricle mass (LVM). The LVM obtained after image analysis was also compared to the LVM measured ex vivo [6]. The main goal was to determine whether evaluation of the cardiac function with a birdcage volume coil could be improved by applying filtering technique as post-processing.

Methods

MRI acquisition

Ten ($n = 10$) male and female Fischer rats of varying age (7–14 weeks) and varying weights (roughly from 100 to 270 g) were imaged using a 7T Varian scanner, with a 63 mm-diameter volume coil. Series of short-axis cine images covering the left ventricle were obtained with an ECG and respiratory-gated cine-FLASH sequence (TR: 80% of the R-R interval: typically around 166–180 ms; TE: 2.10 ms; flip angle: 20°; matrix size: 256 × 256; in plane resolution: 195 × 195 μm^2; 15 slices; slice thickness: 1 mm; 16 frames covering the entire cardiac cycle) [7]. The acquisition time for one short-axis plane was between 78 s and 138 s depending on heart and respiration rates. The total acquisition time was between 25 and 44 min depending on the number of slices that were required to cover the entire left ventricle. The protocol was approved by the institutional animal ethics board, which follows the guidelines issued by the Canadian Council on Animal Care. Animals were anesthetized with isoflurane during imaging (1.5% in air). After imaging, they were euthanized by CO2 inhalation and their left ventricles were excised and weighed.

Image processing

Three denoising filters were tested on the entire data set, which was split in 16 different 3D volumes (one for each phase of the cardiac cycle). Each 3D volume was made up of the totality of the short-axis slices covering the entire left ventricle for one specific phase of the cardiac cycle. The three filtering techniques were: i) anisotropic diffusion filtering [8], ii) total variation regularization [9] and iii) non-local means with optimized Rician noise bias correction (ORNLM) [5]. Anisotropic filtering is based on the anisotropic diffusion heat equation [8]. This is an edge-preserving filter in that smoothing occurs along structures and not across them, as opposed to isotropic or linear diffusion, which are equivalent to Gaussian smoothing. The total variation regularization attempts to promote the piecewise constant nature of images by enhancing edges and by smoothing across homogeneous and flat-intensity regions. It is also strongly based on the gradients of the images. Finally, due to the Rician noise nature of cardiac MR images, the last technique that we tested was the non-local means approach with Rician bias correction [10] implemented in Dipy [11]. For ORNLM, each 3D volume was processed using non-local means filtering with automatic noise standard deviation estimation of the background, search volume of 1331 neighbors and neighborhood size of 26 neighbors.

The three denoising filters were implemented in an in-house built software using third party libraries. This software was written in Python and was run on a Windows 7 platform. The ORLNM implementation was taken from Dipy (http://nipy.org/dipy/). For the anisotropic diffusion filter, the 3D implementation of the algorithm was taken from SimpleITK (http://www.simpleitk.org/). Finally the total variation regularization was taken from scikit (http://scikit-image.org/).

Image analysis

The SNR and the contrast-to-noise ratio (CNR) were calculated on a mid-ventricular short-axis slice at end-diastole for each data set. Regions of interest (ROIs) were drawn in the blood pool, in the myocardium and in the background of the image for noise estimation. The same regions of interest were used with three different filtering strategies and the background area was located outside the animal in the bottom right of the image. As the SNR is higher than 4, the Rician noise distribution can be approximated by a Gaussian distribution [12], and then the SNR of the blood and the myocardium were calculated as the ratio between the mean signal intensity in the corresponding ROI and the standard deviation of the signal in the background of the image. The CNR was calculated as the difference between the SNR of the blood and the SNR of the myocardium.

Cine images were manually segmented by two experienced observers using the Segment software (http://medviso.com/products/segment/) [13]. The segmentation was done twice by the same observer (observer 1) over a two-month period, and once by the second observer (observer 2). The first segmentation of observer 1 was considered for the comparison between the two observers. End-diastolic and end-systolic volumes (EDV, ESV), ejection fraction (EF) and left ventricle mass (LVM) were calculated (defined as the myocardial volume multiplied by 1.05 g.cm^{-3}). A two-tailed paired Student's t-test was used to determine any significant differences between measurements from different segmentations. The correlation coefficients were calculated between the two observers and between the two measurements by observer 1 for each parameter. Agreement for intra and inter-observer observations was tested by calculating the difference between the two measures, taking the first measure of observer 1 as the reference. There was a high variation in the heart weights ex vivo such that results are presented in terms of an absolute but also relative differences (%). In this latter case, for each parameter, the difference between the two measurements was normalized to their average. The results are expressed in absolute values (respectively in percentage) as mean ± standard deviation. Finally, the LVM obtained from the images was compared to the LVM calculated from the ex vivo heart weight, which was used as the gold standard. The results were calculated as a percentage difference from the ex vivo value and are displayed as mean ± standard deviation.

Results

Figure 1 shows typical results of the post-processing with the different filtering techniques on a short-axis slice. Visually, the noise is reduced in the filtered images than in the raw image. The mean total time for processing a data set is roughly equal to 0.72 min for the anisotropic filter, to 0.63 min for the total variation regularization and to 10 min for ORNLM. Table 1 shows the mean SNR of the blood and the myocardium, as well as the CNR between the blood and the myocardium for the raw images and the filtered images. The mean SNR increases at least 8-fold with all filters compared to the raw images. The total-variation filter resulted in the highest mean SNR but also in a high variability as shown by the high value of the standard deviation. The ORNLM filter yielded the second highest mean SNR with a lower standard deviation. The anisotropic diffusion filter yielded the smallest improvement in SNR and CNR but the standard deviations were also the lowest.

The mean values of the EDV and ESV measured with the different filters by observer 1 ranged from 382 μL to 888 μL and from 104 μL to 261 μL, respectively. The EF values varied between 67% and 80% and the LVM values between 453 mg and 1010 mg. Even though the rats were healthy, we selected a large range of rat size in order to test our approach on a wide range of heart size, which explain the variation in cardiac volumes and masses between rats.

The results of inter and intra-observer studies are summarized in Tables 2 and 3, and Fig. 2.

For the intra-observer variability, there was an excellent coefficient correlation ($r > 0.934$) between the two measurements by observer 1 for all the parameters, except for the EF derived from raw images ($r = 0.725$) and to a lesser degree for the EF with the total variation filter ($r = 0.870$). The agreement analysis revealed that the mean difference was less than 5% for all the parameters with the different filters, except for ESV and LVM with the anisotropic filter (−6.6% and 5.6%, respectively).

For the inter-observer variability, there was also an excellent correlation ($r > 0.904$) between the two observers for all the parameters with the exception of EF, regardless

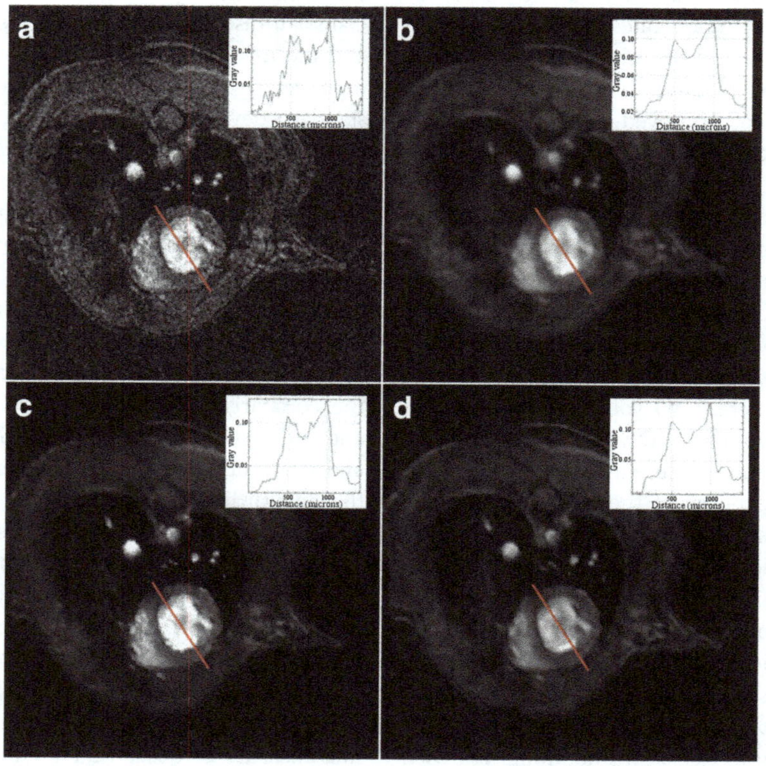

Fig. 1 Example of image filtering on a short axis slice. For each image, the plot displays the signal along the corresponding red line located at the level of the left ventricle. With FLASH sequence, the blood appears in white and the myocardium in grey. **a**) raw image (no filter), **b**) anisotropic filter, **c**) total variation filter and **d**) ORNLM filter

Table 1 Image quality with the different filtering techniques

	SNR blood	SNR myocardium	CNR
No filter	12 ± 2	5 ± 1	6 ± 2
Anisotropic filter	82 ± 15	39 ± 7	43 ± 11
Total variation filter	192 ± 133	89 ± 60	103 ± 76
Optimized Rician Non-local Means filter	110 ± 74	46 ± 35	64 ± 41

Mean signal to noise ratio (SNR) of the blood and of the myocardium and contrast to noise ratio (CNR) between the blood and the myocardium on raw and filtered images

of the filtering method used (r values ranging from 0.544 to 0.764), and of ESV with total variation filter. The ORLNM filter yielded the best correlation between the two observers for EF ($r = 0.764$). On the contrary, the unfiltered images yielded the lower correlation. The agreement analysis indicated a bias between the two observers (mean difference > 8.5%) for the evaluation of the systolic volume (ESV), regardless of the type of images being used. However, all the other parameters (EDV, EF and LVM) had a mean difference of less than 5% between the two observers only after application of the ORNLM filter. There were significant inter-observer differences ($p < 0.05$) in all parameters derived from raw images. After filtering, the differences decreased and became non-significant for some parameters, particularly for EF. For the intra-observer comparison, no significant difference was found between the two measurements, except for ESV and EF calculated after application of the ORNLM filter with p-values just below 0.05.

Table 2 Intra observer variation study for all parameters on raw and filtered images

	Difference	Difference (%)	r
No filter			
EDV (μL)	0.5 ± 16.3	0.2 ± 4.1	0.995
ESV (μL)	−2.4 ± 17.2	−2.7 ± 14.5	0.939
EF (%)	0.7 ± 3.2	0.8 ± 4.6	0.725
LVM (mg)	13.2 ± 28.7	1.5 ± 4.0	0.994
Anisotropic filter			
EDV (μL)	7.6 ± 22.0	2.2 ± 4.3	0.995
ESV (μL)	8.4 ± 13.2	6.6 ± 7.5	0.977
EF (%)	−1.3 ± 1.6	−1.4 ± 2.8	0.950
LVM (mg)	−35.1 ± 49.9	−5.6 ± 7.9	0.972
Total variation filter			
EDV (μL)	0.8 ± 22.2	0.1 ± 3.7	0.991
ESV (μL)	−4.7 ± 16.3	−3.0 ± 12.5	0.955
EF (%)	1.0 ± 3.1	1.6 ± 4.4	0.870
LVM (mg)	−0.4 ± 31.2	−0.6 ± 4.1	0.986
Optimized Rician non-Local Means filter			
EDV (μL)	−0.3 ± 7.7	−0.5 ± 1.9	0.999
ESV (μL)	−4.8 ± 6.9*	−4.8 ± 5.9*	0.989
EF (%)	1.1 ± 1.5*	1.6 ± 2.0*	0.934
LVM (mg)	12.6 ± 30.5	3.3 ± 6.0	0.983

Correlation coefficient (r) and evaluation of the absolute and relative mean difference (%). EDV: End diastolic volume; ESV: End systolic volume; EF: Ejection fraction; LVM: Left ventricular mass. $^{*}p \leqslant 0.05$

Table 3 Inter observer variation study for all parameters on raw and filtered images

	Difference	Difference (%)	r
No filter			
EDV (μL)	31.7 ± 13.0	6.2 ± 3.5***	0.998
ESV (μL)	23.5 ± 21.6	14.4 ± 14.0**	0.926
EF (%)	−2.3 ± 3.9	−3.3 ± 5.6*	0.544
LVM (mg)	−32.8 ± 23.8	−5.2 ± 3.9**	0.993
Anisotropic filter			
EDV (μL)	21.3 ± 16.1	4.3 ± 3.6**	0.996
ESV (μL)	13.3 ± 22.1	9.9 ± 14.9	0.909
EF (%)	−1.7 ± 4.9	−2.4 ± 7.6	0.692
LVM (mg)	−81.8 ± 48.9	−12.5 ± 8.4***	0.971
Total variation filter			
EDV (μL)	28.7 ± 19.2	5.8 ± 4.3**	0.994
ESV (μL)	11.4 ± 24.6	8.6 ± 18.1	0.856
EF (%)	−0.9 ± 4.4	−1.3 ± 6.4	0.706
LVM (mg)	−63.3 ± 30.1	−10.0 ± 5.5***	0.987
Optimized Rician non-Local Means filter			
EDV (μL)	26.9 ± 19.1	4.7 ± 3.2**	0.997
ESV (μL)	19.5 ± 20.2	13.5 ± 13.9*	0.904
EF (%)	−2.4 ± 3.7	−3.2 ± 6.3	0.764
LVM (mg)	−29.2 ± 27.0	−4.6 ± 3.9**	0.991

Correlation coefficient (r) and evaluation of the absolute and relative mean difference (%). EDV: End diastolic volume; ESV: End systolic volume; EF: Ejection fraction; LVM: Left ventricular mass. $^{*}p \leqslant 0.05$, $^{**}p \leqslant 0.01$, $^{***}p \leqslant 0.001$

The LVM values obtained from the images and the LVM obtained by weighing the left ventricle ex vivo are reported in Table 4 and displayed in Fig. 3. The correlation coefficient was excellent in all cases ($r > 0.943$). The mean percentage error was lower than 5% for observer 2 regardless of the type of images, whereas it became higher than 5% for observer 1 when analyzing the images filtered with the anisotropic diffusion filter and the total variation filter (8.3% and 8.8% respectively). The lowest variability (i.e. standard deviation) was obtained with the ORNLM filter for both observers (5.1% for observer 1 and 3.8% for observer 2).

Discussion

Dedicated multi-element cardiac radio-frequency coils can provide high quality images of the rat heart. When this type of coil is not available, an alternative is to use a birdcage volume coil and to increase the number of

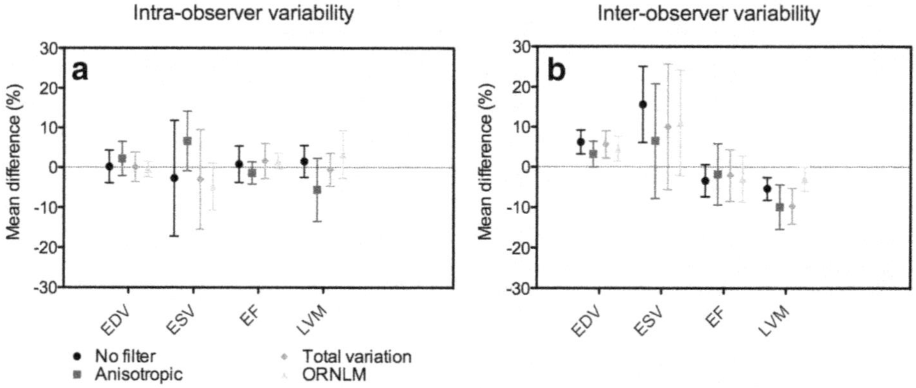

Fig. 2 a) Intra and **b**) inter-observer variabilities for the calculation of the different parameters. The graphics display the relative mean difference ± standard deviation

acquisitions (averages) in order to increase the SNR. This solution is limited as it increases the acquisition time and the duration of anesthesia.

Our results suggest that ORNLM filtering is a reliable tool to compensate for the low SNR of cardiac images acquired with a birdcage volume coil. Although the processing time is a little longer than with the other filtering methods, it remains relatively fast. All filters tested in this study were found to improve significantly the SNR and the CNR. The total variation regularization filter yielded the largest improvement. However, the contours of the cardiac tissue were better delineated with the ORLNM filter, especially at the interface between the myocardium and the chest cavity wall. This visual observation is confirmed by the inter-observer study, where the differences in the LVM found by the two observers were lower than with the raw images, whereas these differences increased with the anisotropic filter and total variation regularization. In addition, the error and the variability in the evaluation of the cardiac function was minimized with the ORLNM filter. Moreover, the agreement between the LVM determined from ORNLM-filtered images and the LVM calculated from the ex vivo heart weight was the highest (according to the lowest values of difference in the Table 4). The higher standard deviation in SNR with filtering was due to differences in signal intensity between acquisitions and sometimes the presence of artefacts in the background areas, and these two effects were amplified with filtering.

Table 4 Correlation coefficient (r) and agreement (mean of difference) studies between in-vivo (from raw or filtered images) ex-vivo left ventricular weight estimation

	Observer 1		Observer 2	
	Difference (%)	r	Difference (%)	r
No filter	2.4 ± 5.4	0.961	−2.9 ± 6.7	0.947
Anisotropic filter	8.3 ± 6.4	0.960	−2.5 ± 5.3	0.951
Total variation filter	8.8 ± 6.2	0.960	−1.6 ± 7.5	0.943
Optimized Rician Non-Local Means filter	2.3 ± 5.1	0.960	−0.2 ± 3.8	0.986

The differences between the two observers for the end-systolic volume were higher than for any other parameter. This could be explained by the contraction of the papillary muscles, as well as the relatively high EF of healthy rats, which makes it harder to distinguish the left ventricle cavity at end systole. Despite this, the differences in EF between the two observers were non-significant after filtering the images. This is an important observation as EF is arguably the most important parameter when evaluating cardiac function. ORLNM filtering also provided convincing results in the intra-observer study, reducing the variability in the measurements made by the same observer. However, the differences between the two measurements by the same observer were found to be significant for EF and ESV with this filter, despite low mean differences and standard deviations. We note that the coefficient of correlation is relatively low for EF, due to the low number of rats, and we expect that these values would increase if the number of rats increased. However, in our opinion, the ranking will stay the same and then the ORNLM filter should provide the best results even with more data.

It should be noted that unfiltered images perform reasonably well with respect to the cardiac function measurements as well as for the left ventricular weight estimation. However, the important increase of SNR and CNR using filtering and the significant differences between observers without filtering for the calculation of the EF (with low correlation coefficient) demonstrate the necessity to perform filtering (and in particular ORLNM filtering).

A limitation of this study concerns the comparison between in vivo and ex vivo data for the measurement of LVM. Although weighing the left ventricle ex vivo is the best way to have absolute comparison, the different physiological conditions (between in vivo and ex vivo) and the excision of the heart can induce errors in measurements which could decrease the correlation and the agreement between ex vivo

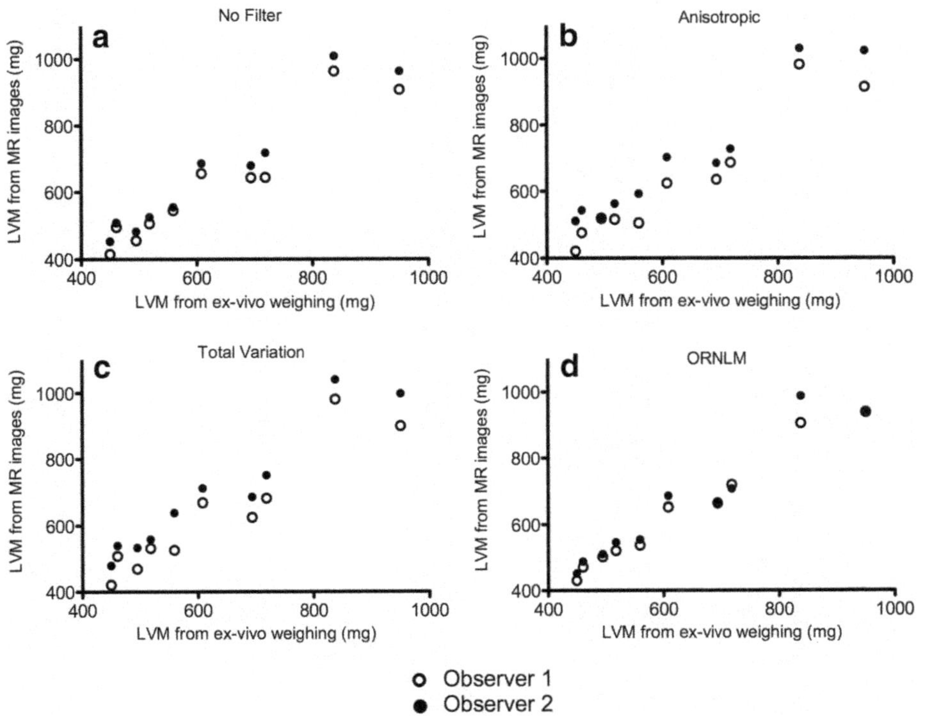

Fig. 3 LVM obtained from the images and by weighing the LV ex-vivo for the different approaches. Comparison of the values obtained by weighing the LV ex-vivo (Fischer rats, weights from roughly 100 to 270 g) and from images with the different following approaches: **a**) no filter, **b**) anisotropic filter, **c**) total variation filter and **d**) ORNLM filter

and in vivo results. Moreover, the choice of acquiring 16 phases of the cardiac cycle was made as a trade-off between image quality and acquisition time, and this sample rate may not be high enough to capture cleanly the systolic motion. However, it is unclear whether more phases would have improved the quality of the manual segmentation. A limitation of the results is that reproducibility was evaluated on only one set of in vivo image acquisition, thus evaluating the influence of filtering on the variation due to segmentation only. Future studies are needed to fully evaluate reproducibility on two different sets of in vivo image acquisitions. Finally, this study should be extended to other small animals such as mice.

Conclusion

In conclusion, multi-element cardiac coil arrays are not always available for cardiac MRI in small animals. Filtering images after acquisition could be an alternative to the use of these coils. ORNLM filtering was superior to an anisotropic filter and to a total variation filter and could potentially also improve images acquired with a phased array coil.

Abbreviations

CNR: Contrast-to-noise ratio; ECG: Electrocardiogram; EDV: End-diastolic volume; EF: Ejection fraction; ESV: End-systolic volume; FLASH: Fast low angle shot; LVM: Left ventricle mass; MRI: Magnetic Resonance Imaging; ORNLM: Optimized Rician non-local means filter; ROI: Region of interest; SNR: Signal-to-noise ratio; TE: Echo time; TR: Repetition time

Acknowledgments

Martin Lepage, Olivier Lesur and André Carpentier are members of the FRQS funded CRCHUS. None of the authors have any competing interests.

Funding

Grant support from the « Programme d'aide financière interne » of the Research Centre of the Sherbrooke University Hospital Centre (CRCHUS).
This work was also partially funded by a CFQCU (Conseil Franco-Québécois de Coopération Universitaire) grant (grant number 2014–134/SCAC).
The fundings (CRCHUS and CFQCU) do not played any role in the design of the study and in collection, analysis, and interpretation of data and in writing the manuscript.

Authors' contributions

Study conception: BT, MD1, LT, AL. Acquisition of data: BT, MD2, FC, OL, ML. Analysis, conception of the post-processing tools and post-processing of the data: BT, MD1, AL. Draft of the manuscript: BT, MD1, AL. Critical review: AC, FC, LT, OL, ML. All authors read and approved the final manuscript.

Consent for publication

Not applicable.

Competing interests

The authors declare that they have no competing interests.

Author details

[1]Centre d'Imagerie Moléculaire de Sherbrooke, CHUS - Hôpital Fleurimont, Sherbrooke, Canada. [2]Center for Systems Biology, Massachusetts General Hospital and Harvard Medical School, Boston, USA. [3]Département d'Informatique, Université de Sherbrooke, Sherbrooke, Canada. [4]Soins Intensifs Médicaux, CHUS - Hôpital Fleurimont, Sherbrooke, Canada. [5]Département de Médecine, CHUS - Hôpital Fleurimont, Sherbrooke, Canada.

[6]Le2I, Faculté de Médecine, Université Bourgogne Franche-Comté, 7 Bld Jeanne d'Arc, 21079 Dijon Cedex, BP 87900, France.

References

1. Lima JA, Desai MY. Cardiovascular magnetic resonance imaging: current and emerging applications. J Am Coll Cardiol. 2004;44(6):1164–71.
2. Bader M. Rat models of cardiovascular diseases. Methods Mol Biol. 2010;597:403–14.
3. Price AN, Cheung KK, Cleary JO, Campbell AE, Riegler J, Lythgoe MF. Cardiovascular Magnetic Resonance Imaging in Experimental Models. Open Cardiovasc Med J. 2010;4:278–92.
4. Riegler J, Cheung KK, Man YF, Cleary JO, Price AN, Lythgoe MF. Comparison of segmentation methods for MRI measurement of cardiac function in rats. J Magn Reson Imaging. 2010;32(4):869–77.
5. Coupé P, Yger P, Prima S, Hellier P, Kervrann C, Barillot C. An optimized blockwise nonlocal means denoising filter for 3-D magnetic resonance images. IEEE Trans Med Imaging. 2008;27(4):425–41.
6. Siri FM, Leinwand LA, Jelicks LA, Gardin JM. Gated magnetic resonance and hypertrophied murine imaging hearts of normal. Am J Phys. 1997;272: H2394–402.
7. Schneider JE, Cassidy PJ, Lygate C, Tyler DJ, Wiesmann F, Grieve SM, Hulbert K, Clarke K, Neubauer S. Fast, high-resolution in vivo cine magnetic resonance imaging in normal and failing mouse hearts on a vertical 11.7 T system. J Magn Reson Imaging. 2003;18(6):691–701.
8. Perona P, Malik J. Scale-space and edge detection using anisotropic diffusion. IEEE Trans Pattern Anal Machine Intell. 1990;12(7):629–39.
9. Rudin LI, Osher S, Fatemi E. Nonlinear total variation based noise removal algorithms. Physica D. 1992;60:259–68.
10. Coupé P, Manjon JV, Gedamu E, Arnold D, Robles M, Collins DL. Robust Rician noise estimation for MR images. Med Image Anal. 2010;14(4):483–93.
11. Garyfallidis E, Brett M, Amirbekian B, Rokem A, van der Walt S, Descoteaux M, Nimmo-Smith I, Contributors D. Dipy, a library for the analysis of diffusion MRI data. Front Neuroinform. 2014; https://doi.org/10.3389/fninf.2014.00008.
12. Gudbjartsson H, Patz S. The Rician distribution of noisy MRI data. Magn Reson Med. 1995;34(6):910–4.
13. Heiberg E, Sjögren J, Ugander M, Carlsson M, Engblom H, Arheden H. Design and Validation of Segment – a Freely Available Software for Cardiovascular Image Analysis. BMC Med Imaging. 2010;10:1.

20

Structural and functional brain changes in perimenopausal women who are susceptible to migraine: a study protocol of multi-modal MRI trial

Bo Hu[1†], Xu Wang[2†], Jie-bing He[2], Yu-jie Dai[3], Jin Zhang[1], Ying Yu[1], Qian Sun[1], Lin-FengYan[1], Yu-Chuan Hu[1], Hai-Yan Nan[1], Yang Yang[1], Alan D. Kaye[4], Guang-Bin Cui[1*] and Wen Wang[1*]

Abstract

Background: As a common clinical symptom that often bothers midlife females, migraine is closely associated with perimenopause. Previous studies suggest that one of the most prominent triggers is the sudden decline of estrogen during perimenopausal period. Hormone replacement therapy (HRT) is widely used to prevent this suffering in perimenopausal women, but effective diagnostic system is lacked for quantifying the severity of the diseaase. To avoid the abuse and overuse of HRT, we propose to conduct a diagnostic trial using multimodal MRI techniques to quantify the severity of these perimenopausal migraineurs who are susceptible to the decline of estrogen.

Methods: Perimenopausal women suffering from migraine will be recruited from the pain clinic of our hospital. Perimenopausal women not suffering from any kind of headache will be recruited from the local community. Clinical assessment and multi-modal MR imaging examination will be conducted. A follow up will be conducted once half year within 3 years. Pain behavior, neuropsychology scores, fMRI analysis combined with suitable statistical software will be used to reveal the potential association between these above traits and the susceptibility of migraine.

Discussion: Multi-modal imaging features of both healthy controls and perimenopausal women who are susceptible to estrogen decline will be acquired. Imaging features will include volumetric characteristics, white matter integrity, functional characteristics, topological properties, and perfusion properties. Clinical information, such as basic information, blood estrogen level, information of migraine, and a bunch of neurological scale will also be used for statistic assessment. This clinical trial would help to build an effective screen system for quantifying the severity of illness of those susceptible women during the perimenopausal period.

Keywords: Perimenopausal, Migraine, Multi-modal, Voxel-based morphology (VBM), Functional connectivity (FC), Diffusional kurtosis imaging (DKI), Artery spin labeling (ASL)

* Correspondence: cgbtd@126.com; wangwen@fmmu.edu.cn
[†]Bo Hu and Xu Wang contributed equally to this work.
[1]Department of Radiology & Functional and Molecular Imaging Key Lab of Shaanxi Province, Tangdu Hospital, Fourth Military Medical University (Air Force Medical University), 569 Xinsi Road, Xi'an 710038, Shaanxi, China
Full list of author information is available at the end of the article

Background

As a common headache disorder, migraine is characterized by recurrent headache attacks accompanied with symptoms including nausea and vomiting [1]. According to the World Health Organization (WHO), migraine is considered as one of the most disabling and burdensome diseases [2, 3]. In general, adult females experience migraine attacks twice more than males, and although men and women reported similar headache severity and frequency, women reported more migraine related symptoms [4, 5].

This gender difference is mainly caused by the difference in sex hormone. Estrogen quantities are relatively stable in men and undergo a much more gradual decline with age as compared with women [6]. For example, previous studies revealed that migraine is closely linked to the menopausal period of women, and one of the most prominent triggers is the sudden decline of estrogen [7–9]. Estrogen can bind to its receptors of nucleus or cytoplasm in the brain, and then exert its function of pain transmission by gene transcription and protein synthesis [10]. However, this procedure would be disturbed by the sudden drop of estrogen in perimenopausal period, which would furtherly result in the susceptibility to migraine [6].

Since the decline of estrogen begins in perimenopausal period, giving hormone replacement therapy (HRT) in this period is considered as an effective method to treat migraine [11, 12]. To avoid the abuse and overuse of HRT which could cause some severe unpleasant complications, those women should be given the lowest effective dose of medication [13, 14]. However, headache is a subjective feeling, and effective diagnostic system is still lacked for quantifying the degree of migraine, which could result in the abuse and overuse of HRT in treating this disease.

In the past two decades, functional magnetic resonance imaging (fMRI) technique has become an indispensable tool in migraine research and has greatly contributed to our understanding of migraine pathophysiology [15–17]. It could show anatomic and functional cerebral transformations associated with the clinical evolution and could be applied to most individuals without adverse effects. Maleki et al. found that female migraineurs have thicker posterior insula and precuneus cortices as compared with both male migraineurs and healthy controls of both sexes [18]. Compared to healthy controls, Kim and colleagues revealed a reduction of gray matter (GM) density in migraineurs, including insula, motor/premotor, prefrontal, cingulate, posterior parietal, and orbitofrontal cortex [19]. Huang et al. found reduced fractional anisotropy (FA) in the right frontal of migraine patients by using a tract-based spatial statistics (TBSS) method, which means the microstructure of white matter (WM) in that region is impaired [20]. Liu et al. found that the resting-state functional connectivity (FC) was disrupted in patients with long-term migraine through the method of graph theory [21]. However, these researches are all focused on both male and female patients at all ages, which contributes little to quantify the degree of migraine in perimenopausal women. According to our knowledge, no previous studies had researched the imaging abnormality of perimenopausal women who are susceptible to the decline of estrogen. Since estrogen plays a pivotal role in pain transmission in our brain [10], we thus raised the current hypothesis that brain structure and function of these women who are susceptible to estrogen drop exhibit unique characteristic changes in multi-modal images.

Consequently, we would like to conduct a prospective clinical trial to investigate the imaging abnormalities in these susceptible perimenopausal women. At the beginning, perimenopausal women around who had migraine will be recruited from the pain clinic of our hospital. Perimenopausal women around who did not have migraine will be recruited as healthy controls (HC) from the local community. Then, these subjects will undergo a series of multi-modal MRI brain scans and neuropsychology scales to assess the mental and physical state of these subjects. Multi-modal MR images of these two groups of subjects will be compared to find significant features as objective biomarkers.

Methods

The flowchart of the current trial is described in Fig. 1.

Subject

All subjects will be provided informed, written consents after the study procedure has been fully explained in detail. Females who match the following criteria would be included in the migraine group: (1) age ranges from 40 to 55 years old; (2) irregular menstrual cycle; (3) suffered from migraine; (4) normal neurological examination. Females who match the following criteria would be included in the HC group: (1) age ranges from 40 to 55 years old; (2) irregular menstrual cycle; (3) not suffered from any kinds of headache; (4) normal neurological examination. Exclusion criteria will be as follows: (1) severe psychiatric disorders, such as dementia, episode, epilepsy, major depression; (2) significant neurological illness, such as significant head trauma, tumor, meningitis or central nervous system (CNS) inflammatory lesions and vascular complications clues; (3) any MRI contraindications; (4) alcohol, nicotine or drug abuse.

Sample size have been estimated by referring to other studies [22, 23]. A sample size of 40 patients per group will be suitable for a power of 0.8 and an alpha significance level of 0.05 (two-side). Considering the drop-out

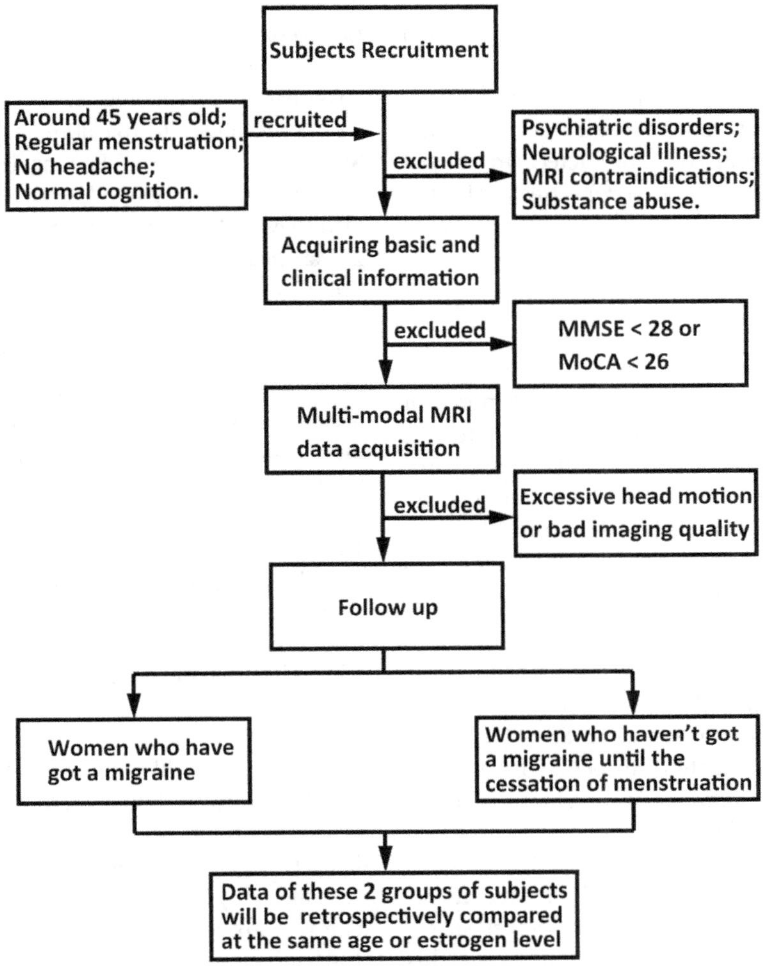

Fig. 1 The flowchart of the current trial

ratio (25%) and unqualified images of included subjects, the total sample size is 55 in each group.

Clinical assessments

Demographic and clinical features of all subjects will be collected and recorded, such as age, education level, body mass index (BMI), occupation and menstrual cycle. All participants will receive the following battery of neuropsychological tests: Montreal Cognitive Assessment (MoCA) and Mini-mental State Examination (MMSE) will be used to assess the mental state of subjects. The Short Form health survey (SF-36) will be applied to evaluate the quality of life, and Self-rating Depression Scale (SDS) and Self-rating Anxiety Scale (SAS) will be performed to measure the severity of self-reported depression and anxiety. Migraine will be diagnosed according to the International Headache Society (IHS) criteria of the International Classification of Headache Disorders (ICHD-3 beta version) [1]. The following data will be collected from migraine participants: (1) type of migraine (migraine with aura, migraine without aura, etc.), (2) frequency of migraine attacks, (3) duration of migraine attacks, (4) headache location (unilateral or bilateral), (5) Migraine Disability Assessment Scale (MIDAS) score (the score is divided into 4 grades, higher grade means more severer disability). Blood samples were drawn at the screening centers and processed within 2 h according to a standardized protocol to assess the hormone level [24].

Follow up

A follow up will be conducted within three years after individual's first visit. Individuals will come back to the medical center once half year for countercheck, and all the protocols and evaluations will be the same as that they get at the first time. In addition, medication type and dose will also be recorded.

Multi-modal MRI examination

Multi-modal imaging examination will be performed with a 3.0-T MRI system (MR750; GE Healthcare, Milwaukee, WI, USA) using an 8-channel head coil array with foam padding to restrict head motion. Multi-modal scans including high-resolution three-dimensional brain volume T1-weighted imaging (T1WI), diffusion kurtosis imaging (DKI), resting-state blood oxygenation level-dependent (RS-BOLD) imaging and three-dimensional pseudo-continuous arterial spin labeling (3D-pCASL) imaging will be conducted to detect microstructural and functional properties. All the sequences we mentioned will use the isotropic spatial resolution.

High-resolution T1WI

Sagittal three-dimensional brain volume (3D-BRAVO) sequence will be used for the acquisition of high-resolution T1-weighted images, according to the following parameters: echo time (TE) = 3.2 ms, repetition time (TR) = 8.2 ms, TI = 450 ms, flip angle (FA) = 12°, field of view (FOV) =256 × 256 mm^2, matrix = 256 × 192, slice thickness = 1.0 mm, slice number = 166. The whole procedure will cost 4 min 43 s.

DKI

DKI datasets will be collected using a douple-spin-echo diffusion tensor echo planar imaging (SE-SS-DT-EPI) sequence with a clinically oriented protocol. The acquisition parameters are as follows: six-b-values of 0,500, 1000,1500, 2000, and 2500 s/mm^2, 10 b_0 images, 30 diffusion gradient directions, TR = 6500, TE = 108 ms, FOV =256 × 256 mm^2, matrix = 128 × 128, slice thickness = 3 mm, FA = 90°, slice number = 50, voxel size = 2 mm × 2 mm × 5 mm. The acquisition time for this protocol will be 6 min.

RS-bold

RS-BOLD images will be collected using a gradient-recalled echo-planar imaging (GRE-EPI) sequence with the following parameters: TR = 2000 ms, TE = 40 ms, FA = 90°, slice number = 36, inter slice gaps = 0 mm, FOV = 240 × 240 mm^2, matrix = 64 × 64, slice thickness = 3 mm, in-plane spatial resolution = 3 × 3 mm^2. Participants will be reminded to lie quietly in the scanner with their eyes closed and thinking nothing during data acquisition. The whole procedure will cost 6 min 10 s.

3D-pCASL

Resting-state perfusion imaging was performed using pCASL sequence with a 3D fast spin-echo acquisition and background suppression: TR = 5046, 11.1 ms, FOV = 128 × 128 mm2, matrix = 128 × 128 mm2, slice thickness = 3 mm, FA = 111°, number of excitation = 3, no gap; 40 axial slices; number of excitation = 3. The whole procedure will cost 4 min 53 s.

Imaging data processing

High-resolution T1WI data

All T1 imaging data will be processed and examined for voxel-based morphological (VBM) analyses using the VBM8 toolbox (http://dbm.neuro.uni-jena.de/vbm/) in Statistical Parametric Mapping (SPM) (SPM8, Wellcome Department of Imaging Neuroscience Group, London, UK; http://www.fil.ion.ucl.ac.uk/spm) running in MATLAB 2014a platform. We will perform an optimized VBM protocol in which a brain-tissue-only template will be used other than a whole-brain template. Brain Extraction Tool (integrated in MRIcro; http://www.mricro.com) was used to remove non-brain region images [25]. After removal of nonbrain regions, images will be segmented into GM, white matter (WM), and cerebrospinal fluid (CSF) by using the Diffeomorphic Anatomical Registration Through Exponentiated Lie algebra (DARTEL) algorithm [26]. Afterward, the normalized images would be averaged by using SPM mean function. To create the final template, all average images would be smoothed using an isotropic Gaussian kernel with a full width at half maximum (FWHM) of 8 mm.

DKI data

All DKI images will be processed using a combination of FMRIB's Software Library (FSL) [27] and in-house image processing tools developed in MATLAB. The diffusion dataset will be modulated to get potential 3D head motion and eddy current distortion using FSL eddy correct. The toolbox implement in MTALAB will be applied to deal with diffusional kurtosis tensors. Region of interest (ROI) of headache will be drawn by hand. DKI parameters of migraine pain-ROIs, such as mean kurtosis (MK), mean diffusivity (MD) and fractional anisotropy (FA), will be measured. All feature maps will be spatially normalized to the standard MNI space by using the transformation fields derived from tissue segmentation of structural images and resampled to 3 mm isotropic voxels.

BOLD data

RS-BOLD data will be preprocessed in the toolbox of MATLAB (Data Processing Assistant for Resting-State fMRI, DPARSF; http://www.restfmri.net/forum/DPARSF). SPM8, RS-fMRI data analysis toolkit (REST1.6; http://www.restfmri.net) and graph-theoretical network analysis (GRATNA; https://www.nitrc.org/projects/gretna) will also be selected to deal with the images. The first 10 time points will be discarded to ensure stable magnetization and allow the participants to adapt to the EPI scanning environment. After that, slice timing and head motion will be conducted, and scans with head motion of translation > 3.0 mm or rotation > 3° will be excluded. The functional images will then be spatially normalized to Montreal

Neurological Institute (MNI) space using the transformation fields derived from tissue segmentation of individual structural images and resampled to $3 \times 3 \times 3$ mm^3. The resulting images will be smoothed with 8 mm FWHM isotropic Gaussian kernel. Linear trends will be removed from the image time series, and data will be band-pass filtered at 0.01–0.08 Hz. Finally, nuisance signals such as 24-parameter head motion profiles, white matter, and cerebrospinal fluid signals will be regressed out from each voxel's time series to exclude non-neuronal sources [28].

Amplitude of low frequency fluctuation (ALFF), regional homogeneity (ReHo) and functional connectivity (FC) values will be estimated in the DPARSFA software that is developed to extract abnormal regions between two groups. Small-world properties and network efficiency will be calculated in the GRETNA software to compare the topological characteristics between two groups.

3D-pCASL data

For the ASL fMRI data, corresponding CBF images were obtained using an automated image postprocessing tool embedded in the GE healthcare MR-750 system. Subsequently, the CBF images will be spatially normalized to the standard MNI space by using the transformation fields derived from tissue segmentation of structural images and resampled to 3 mm isotropic voxels. The resulting images will be transformed to z scores using Fisher's transformation approach and then will be smoothed with 8 mm FWHM isotropic Gaussian kernel.

Statistical analysis

Statistical Package for the Social Sciences (SPSS) 18.0 (SPSS, Chicago, IL, USA) will be used to analyze the socio-demographic and clinical data. SPM8 and REST 1.8 will be used to analyze the imaging data. All statistical tests were conducted with a significance level of 5%.

Socio-demographic and clinical data

We will use 2-sample Student-t test for discrete quantitative data (age, body mass index, educational level, migraine history, frequency of migraine attacks, duration of migraine attacks, SAS score, SDS score, MMSE score, MoCA score and MIDAS scores), and the chi-square ($\chi 2$) test for nominal qualitative data (gender, type and location of migraine).

Structural parameters

Both voxel-based and ROI-based 2-sample Student-t test will be applied to compare global gray matter (GMV) MK, MD and FA between susceptible group and healthy control group with age, sex, education and BMI as covariance. Moreover, non-parametric Spearman correlation will be performed to delineate a possible relationship between local morphologic alterations and clinical data as well as diffusional alterations and clinical data. Significance threshold, which is corrected for comparison using Family Wise Error (FWE) method, will be set at $P < 0.05$. For each design matrix, significant effects both in the negative and positive directions are considered.

Functional and perfusion parameters

Both voxel-based and ROI-based 2-sample Student-t test will be applied to compare global ReHo, ALFF/fALFF, CBF between susceptible group and healthy control group with age, sex, education and BMI as covariance. The reference time series for headache-related seed regions will be acquired by averaging the time series for all voxels within them. Correlations of this time-series will be calculated to measure FCs among these regions in each participant. To evaluate group differences in the resting-state topological properties, nonparametric permutation tests were applied [29]. Initially, we will calculate the between-group differences of the mean values for each topological property. Next, an empirical distribution of the difference will be obtained by randomly reallocating every property value into two groups and recomputing the mean differences between the two randomized groups (5,000 permutations) to test the null hypothesis that the observed group differences only occurred by chance. The 95th percentile points of each distribution will be used as critical values for a two-tailed test to determine whether the observed group differences could occur by chance. Non-parametric Spearman correlation will also be performed to delineate a possible relationship between functional alterations and clinical data as well as perfusion alterations and clinical data. Significance threshold will be set at $P < 0.05$ (FWE corrected).

Correlation analysis

Linear regression analysis will be performed across the migraine groups to assess relationships between imaging properties and cognitive testing scores and clinical information. When the most sensitive parameters are found, a receiver operating characteristic (ROC) curve will be plotted to testify the sensitivity and specificity of the certain parameter for quantifying the degree of migraine and screening the accompanied cognitive decline.

Outcomes measure

Primary outcomes measure

White matter integrity (e.g. MD, MK and FA changes),

Secondary outcomes measure

Headache level (1–10, VAS), volumetric characteristics (e.g. GMV atrophy), functional characteristics (e.g. ReHo, ALFF/fALFF and FC and abnormalities), topological properties (e.g. small-world properties and network efficiency) and perfusion properties (e.g. CBF changes).

Discussion

Multi-modal imaging features of perimenopausal women who are susceptible to estrogen decline will be acquired. Imaging sequences will include 3D-BRAVO, DKI, RS-BOLD and 3D-pCASL. Imaging features for assessment will include volumetric characteristics, white matter integrity, functional characteristics, topological properties and perfusion properties. Clinical information, such as information of migraine, headache level, MIDAS score, SAS, SDS, MMSE, MoCA and SF-36 will also be acquired for assessment.

The structural imaging could reflect the long-term impact of migraine on the brain structure, including GM volume and WM integrity. VBM has been pervasively used to investigate structural changes in migraine in the last decade. Some of them observed significant GM abnormalities in several brain regions of migraine patients [30–32], including right superior temporal gyrus, right inferior frontal gyrus and left precentral gyrus etc., but the result in other studies were not significant [33–35]. Two recent meta-analysis considered that migraine could cause GMV changes, and these changes were related to gender [36]. The integrity of WM is usually measured by calculating several parameters of its diffusional ability, such as MD, MK and FA. Several previous studies had compared these parameters between migraine patients and healthy controls, and they found significant increases or decreases in brain regions like thalami, corpus callosum and internal capsule [37–40]. Previous studies had also investigated the difference of WM integrity between migraine patients with and without aura and between ictal and interictal period [37, 41]. In addition, imaging researches about WM integrity in children or adolescent who have migraine had also been conducted [42, 43]. In the current study, we hope that the long-term impact of the susceptibility of estrogen drop on brain structure could also be reflected in structural imaging.

The functional imaging could reflect the impact of migraine on the brain activity, including neural activity and perfusion condition. RS-BOLD signal had attracted considerable attention in migraine patient to examine potential alterations of brain induced by recurrent migraine attacks. In migraine patients, previous studies have detected various alterations regarding functional connectivity in pain related regions including the periaqueductal gray area (an important region involved in nociceptive processing) [44], as well as insular which is stronger functionally coupled to the dorsal caudal pons and periaqueductal gray area than healthy controls [45]. Other recent studies have reported changed ReHo, ALFF/fALFF or FC in the executive control network [46, 47], and the default mode network [35]. In addition, the functional topologic properties of migraineurs were also observed in precentral gyrus, anterior cingulate gyrus, thalamus and etc. [21, 48]. Previous researches had identified CBF abnormalities as an imaging biomarker in migraineurs, but these CBF studies were all based on single-photon emission computed tomography (SPECT), which is invasive and difficult to generalize in clinical trial [49, 50]. Recently, ASL is an emerging MRI sequence that can be easily performed without contrast injection or any side effects. Some recent studies stressed the significant abnormalities in somatosensory cortex or other brain regions of migraineurs [51, 52], while one study declared that they didn't see and significant changes [53]. We hope that the impact of the susceptibility of estrogen drop on brain activity could also be reflected in functional imaging.

Trial status

This is the first version of the study protocol, and the recruitment had begun in July 2016, and it will be completed in around 2020.

Abbreviations

3D-pCASL: three-dimensional pseudo-Continuous Arterial Spin Labeling; ALFF: Amplitude of Low Frequency Fluctuation; DKI: Diffusion Kurtosis Imaging; FA: Fractional Anisotropy; FA: Fractional Anisotropy; FC: Functional Connectivity; fMRI: functional Magnetic Resonance Imaging; GM: Gray Matter; HRT: Hormone Replacement Therapy; MD: Mean Diffusivity; MK: Mean Kurtosis; MMSE: Mini-Mental State Examination; MoCA: Montreal Cognitive Assessment; ReHo: Regional Homogeneity; ROI: Region Of Interest; RS-BOLD: Resting-State Blood Oxygenation Level-Dependent; SAS: Self-rating Anxiety Scale; SDS: Self-rating Depression Scale; SF-36: Short Form health survey; T1WI: T1-Weighted Imaging; TBSS: Tract-Based Spatial Statistics; WM: White Matter

Acknowledgements

We would like to thank Shang Lei for the insightful discussions on the sample size calculation and Liu Xu-Feng for the help with neuropsychological assessments selection.

Funding

This study is financially supported with the Natural Science Foundation of China (No. 81571656 to Dr. Wen Wang) and Key Project for Science Research and Development of Shaanxi Province (No. 2017SF-012 to Dr. Hai-Yan Nan) but not commercial organization. The funding source has estimated the feasibility of the study, but has no role in the collection, analysis, or interpretation of the data or in the decision to submit the manuscript for publication.

Authors' contributions

All listed authors contributed to this project. BH and XW contributed equally to this project in preparing the protocol, informed consent and trial registration. JBH and YJD drafted the manuscript. JZ, YY, QS, LFY, HYN, YCH, and ADK made critical revision of the manuscript for important intellectual content. CGB and WW are corresponded equally to this study. All authors read and approved the final manuscript.

Consent for publication
Not applicable.

Competing interests
The authors declare that they have no competing interests.

Author details
[1]Department of Radiology & Functional and Molecular Imaging Key Lab of Shaanxi Province, Tangdu Hospital, Fourth Military Medical University (Air Force Medical University), 569 Xinsi Road, Xi'an 710038, Shaanxi, China. [2]Student Brigade, Fourth Military Medical University (Air Force Medical University), 169 West Changle Road, Xi'an 710032, Shaanxi Province, China. [3]Department of Clinical Nutrition, Xijing Hospital, The Fourth Military Medical University, Xi'an, China. [4]Departments of Anesthesiology and Pharmacology, Louisiana State University School of Medicine, New Orleans, Louisiana, USA.

References
1. Headache Classification Committee of the International Headache S: the international classification of headache disorders, 3rd edition (beta version). Cephalalgia 2013, 33(9):629–808.
2. Leonardi M, Steiner TJ, Scher AT, Lipton RB. The global burden of migraine: measuring disability in headache disorders with WHO's classification of functioning, disability and health (ICF). J Headache Pain. 2005;6(6):429–40.
3. Buse DC, Lipton RB. Global perspectives on the burden of episodic and chronic migraine. Cephalalgia. 2013;33(11):885–90.
4. Burch RC, Loder S, Loder E, Smitherman TA. The prevalence and burden of migraine and severe headache in the United States: updated statistics from government health surveillance studies. Headache. 2015;55(1):21–34.
5. Buse DC, Loder EW, Gorman JA, Stewart WF, Reed ML, Fanning KM, Serrano D, Lipton RB. Sex differences in the prevalence, symptoms, and associated features of migraine, probable migraine and other severe headache: results of the American migraine prevalence and prevention (AMPP) study. Headache. 2013;53(8):1278–99.
6. Chai NC, Peterlin BL, Calhoun AH. Migraine and estrogen. Curr Opin Neurol. 2014;27(3):315–24.
7. MacGregor EA. Migraine, the menopause and hormone replacement therapy: a clinical review. J Fam Plann Reprod Health Care. 2007;33(4):245–9.
8. Martin VT. Migraine and the menopausal transition. Neurol Sci. 2014;35(Suppl 1):65–9.
9. Martin VT, Pavlovic J, Fanning KM, Buse DC, Reed ML, Lipton RB. Perimenopause and menopause are associated with high frequency headache in women with migraine: results of the American migraine prevalence and prevention study. Headache. 2016;56(2):292–305.
10. Amandusson A, Blomqvist A. Estrogenic influences in pain processing. Front Neuroendocrinol. 2013;34(4):329–49.
11. Ibrahimi K, Couturier EG, MaassenVanDenBrink A. Migraine and perimenopause. Maturitas. 2014;78(4):277–80.
12. Macgregor EA. Perimenopausal migraine in women with vasomotor symptoms. Maturitas. 2012;71(1):79–82.
13. MacGregor EA. Estrogen replacement and migraine. Maturitas. 2009;63(1):51–5.
14. Shuster LT, Faubion SS, Sood R, Casey PM. Hormonal manipulation strategies in the management of menstrual migraine and other hormonally related headaches. Curr Neurol Neurosci Rep. 2011;11(2):131–8.
15. Colombo B, Rocca MA, Messina R, Guerrieri S, Filippi M. Resting-state fMRI functional connectivity: a new perspective to evaluate pain modulation in migraine? Neurol Sci. 2015;36(Suppl 1):41–5.
16. Chen Z, Chen X, Liu M, Liu S, Shu S, Ma L, Yu S. Altered functional connectivity of the marginal division in migraine: a resting-state fMRI study. J Headache Pain. 2016;17(1):89.
17. Huang J, DeLano M, Cao Y. Visual cortical inhibitory function in migraine is not generally impaired: evidence from a combined psychophysical test with an fMRI study. Cephalalgia. 2006;26(5):554–60.
18. Maleki N, Linnman C, Brawn J, Burstein R, Becerra L, Borsook D. Her versus his migraine: multiple sex differences in brain function and structure. Brain. 2012;135(Pt 8):2546–59.
19. Kim JH, Suh SI, Seol HY, Oh K, Seo WK, Yu SW, Park KW, Koh SB. Regional grey matter changes in patients with migraine: a voxel-based morphometry study. Cephalalgia. 2008;28(6):598–604.
20. Huang Q, Lv X, He Y, Wei X, Ma M, Liao Y, Qin C, Wu Y. Structural differences in interictal migraine attack after epilepsy: a diffusion tensor imaging analysis. Epilepsy Behav. 2017;77:8–12.
21. Liu J, Zhao L, Lei F, Zhang Y, Yuan K, Gong Q, Liang F, Tian J. Disrupted resting-state functional connectivity and its changing trend in migraine suffers. Hum Brain Mapp. 2015;36(5):1892–907.
22. Alsop DC, Detre JA, Golay X, Gunther M, Hendrikse J, Hernandez-Garcia L, Lu H, MacIntosh BJ, Parkes LM, Smits M, et al. Recommended implementation of arterial spin-labeled perfusion MRI for clinical applications: a consensus of the ISMRM perfusion study group and the European consortium for ASL in dementia. Magn Reson Med. 2015;73(1):102–16.
23. Rusinek H, Ha J, Yau PL, Storey P, Tirsi A, Tsui WH, Frosch O, Azova S, Convit A. Cerebral perfusion in insulin resistance and type 2 diabetes. J Cereb Blood Flow Metab. 2015;35(1):95–102.
24. Hayes RB, Sigurdson A, Moore L, Peters U, Huang WY, Pinsky P, Reding D, Gelmann EP, Rothman N, Pfeiffer RM, et al. Methods for etiologic and early marker investigations in the PLCO trial. Mutat Res. 2005;592(1–2):147–54.
25. Smith SM. Fast robust automated brain extraction. Hum Brain Mapp. 2002;17(3):143–55.
26. Ashburner J. A fast diffeomorphic image registration algorithm. NeuroImage. 2007;38(1):95.
27. NeuroImage. Advances in functional and structural MR image analysis and implementation as FSL. NeuroImage. 2004;23(Suppl 1):S208–19.
28. Friston KJ, Williams S, Howard R, Frackowiak RS, Turner R. Movement-related effects in fMRI time-series. Magn Reson Med. 1996;35(3):346–55.
29. Bullmore ET, Suckling J, Overmeyer S, Rabe-Hesketh S, Taylor E, Brammer MJ. Global, voxel, and cluster tests, by theory and permutation, for a difference between two groups of structural MR images of the brain. IEEE Trans Med Imaging. 2002;18(1):32–42.
30. Valfrè W, Rainero I, Bergui M, Pinessi L. Voxel-based morphometry reveals gray matter abnormalities in migraine. Headache the J Head & Face Pain. 2010;48(1):109–17.
31. Jin C, Yuan K, Zhao L, Zhao L, Yu D, Deneen KMV, Zhang M, Qin W, Sun W, Tian J. Structural and functional abnormalities in migraine patients without aura. NMR Biomed. 2013;26(1):58–64.
32. Obermann M, Wurthmann S, Steinberg BS, Theysohn N, Diener HC, Naegel S. Central vestibular system modulation in vestibular migraine. Cephalalgia. 2014;34(13):1053–61.
33. Schmidtwilcke T, Gänssbauer S, Neuner T, Bogdahn U, May A. Subtle grey matter changes between migraine patients and healthy controls. Cephalalgia. 2008;28(1):1–4.
34. Russo A, Tessitore A, Giordano A, Corbo D, Marcuccio L, De SM, Salemi F, Conforti R, Esposito F, Tedeschi G. Executive resting-state network connectivity in migraine without aura. Cephalalgia. 2012;32(14):1041.
35. Tessitore A, Russo A, Giordano A, Conte F, Corbo D, Stefano MD, Cirillo S, Cirillo M, Esposito F, Tedeschi G. Disrupted default mode network connectivity in migraine without aura. J Headache & Pain. 2013;14(1):1–7.
36. Dai Z, Zhong J, Xiao P, Zhu Y, Chen F, Pan P, Shi H. Gray matter correlates of migraine and gender effect: a meta-analysis of voxel-based morphometry studies. Neuroscience. 2015;299:88–96.
37. Coppola G, Tinelli E, Lepre C, Iacovelli E, Di LC, Di LG, Serrao M, Pauri F, Fiermonte G, Bianco F. Dynamic changes in thalamic microstructure of migraine without aura patients: a diffusion tensor magnetic resonance imaging study. Eur J Neurol. 2014;21(2):287–e213.
38. Kara B, Kiyat AA, Onat L, Ulusoy L, Mutlu A, Sirvanci M. DTI findings during spontaneous migraine attacks. Clin Neuroradiol. 2013;23(1):31.
39. Yu D, Yuan K, Zhao L, Dong M, Liu P, Yang X, Liu J, Sun J, Zhou G, Xue T. White matter integrity affected by depressive symptoms in migraine without aura: a tract-based spatial statistics study. NMR Biomed. 2013;26(9):1103–12.
40. Kai Y, Wei Q, Peng L, Ling Z, Yu D, Zhao L, Dong M, Liu J, Yang X, Deneen KMV. Reduced fractional anisotropy of Corpus callosum modulates inter-hemispheric resting state functional connectivity in migraine patients without Aura. PLoS One. 2012;7(9):e45476.

41. Rocca MA, Pagani E, Colombo B, Tortorella P, Falini A, Comi G, Filippi M. Selective diffusion changes of the visual pathways in patients with migraine: a 3-T tractography study. Cephalalgia. 2008;28(10):1061–8.
42. Eidlitz-Markus T, Zeharia A, Haimi-Cohen Y, Konen O. MRI white matter lesions in pediatric migraine. Cephalalgia. 2013;33(11):906–13.
43. Candee MS, McCandless RT, Moore KR, Arrington CB, Minich LL, Bale JF, Jr.: White matter lesions in children and adolescents with migraine. Pediatr Neurol 2013, 49(6):393–396.
44. Mainero C, Boshyan J, Hadjikhani N. Altered functional magnetic resonance imaging resting-state connectivity in periaqueductal gray networks in migraine. Ann Neurol. 2011;70(5):838–45.
45. Tso AR, Trujillo A, Guo CC, Goadsby PJ, Seeley WW. The anterior insula shows heightened interictal intrinsic connectivity in migraine without aura. Neurology. 2015;84(10):1043–50.
46. Tessitore A, Russo A, Conte F, Giordano A, De Stefano M, Lavorgna L, Corbo D, Caiazzo G, Esposito F, Tedeschi G. Abnormal connectivity within executive resting-state network in migraine with Aura. Headache. 2015;55(6):794–805.
47. Russo A, Marcelli V, Esposito F, Corvino V, Marcuccio L, Giannone A, Conforti R, Marciano E, Tedeschi G, Tessitore A. Abnormal thalamic function in patients with vestibular migraine. Neurology. 2014;82(23):2120–6.
48. Liu J, Zhao L, Li G, Xiong S, Nan J, Li J, Yuan K, von Deneen KM, Liang F, Qin W, et al. Hierarchical alteration of brain structural and functional networks in female migraine sufferers. PLoS One. 2012;7(12):e51250.
49. Nishimiya M, Matsuda H, Imabayashi E, Kuji I, Sato N. Comparison of SPM and NEUROSTAT in voxelwise statistical analysis of brain SPECT and MRI at the early stage of Alzheimer's disease. Ann Nucl Med. 2008;22(10):921–7.
50. Ansar MA, Osaki Y, Kazui H, Oku N, Takasawa M, Kimura Y, Begum NN, Ikejiri Y, Takeda M, Hatazawa J. Effect of linearization correction on statistical parametric mapping (SPM): a 99mTc-HMPAO brain perfusion SPECT study in mild Alzheimer's disease. Ann Nucl Med. 2006;20(8):511–7.
51. Youssef AM, Ludwick A, Wilcox SL, Lebel A, Peng K, Colon E, Danehy A, Burstein R, Becerra L, Borsook D. In child and adult migraineurs the somatosensory cortex stands out ... Again: an arterial spin labeling investigation. Hum Brain Mapp. 2017;38(8):4078–87.
52. Cadiot D, Longuet R, Bruneau B, Treguier C, Carsin-Vu A, Corouge I, Gomes C, Proisy M. Magnetic resonance imaging in children presenting migraine with aura: association of hypoperfusion detected by arterial spin labelling and vasospasm on MR angiography findings. Cephalalgia. 2018;38(5):949–58.
53. Gil-Gouveia R, Pinto J, Figueiredo P, Vilela PF, Martins IP. An arterial spin labeling MRI perfusion study of migraine without Aura attacks. Front Neurol. 2017;8:280.

21

Gadoxetic acid-enhanced magnetic resonance imaging significantly influences the clinical course in patients with colorectal liver metastases

B. G. Sibinga Mulder[1], K. Visser[1], S. Feshtali[2], A. L. Vahrmeijer[1], R. J. Swijnenburg[1], H. H. Hartgrink[1], R. van den Boom[2], M. C. Burgmans[2] and J. S. D. Mieog[1*]

Abstract

Background: Gadoxetic acid (Primovist™)-enhanced magnetic resonance imaging (P-MRI) scans have higher accuracy and increased detection of small colorectal liver metastases (CRLM) compared to CT scans or conventional MRI scans. But, P-MRI scans are still inconsistently acquired in the diagnostic work up of patients with CRLM. The aim of this study was to determine the influence of P-MRI scans on treatment plan proposition and subsequently the clinical course of the patient.

Methods: Eighty-three consecutive patients with potentially resectable CRLM based on a conventional CT scan underwent P-MRI scanning prior to treatment. Treatment plans proposed by the multidisciplinary team were compared before and after P-MRI scanning and related to the final treatment and diagnosis, the accuracy for the CT scan and P-MRI scan was calculated.

Results: P-MRI scans led to a change of treatment in 15 patients (18%) and alteration of extensiveness of local therapy in another 17 patients (20%). All changes were justified leading to an accuracy of 93% for treatment proposition based on P-MRI scan, compared to an accuracy of 75% for the CT scan.

Conclusions: P-MRI scans provide additional information that can aid in proposing the most suitable treatment for patients with CRLM and might prevent short-term reintervention.

Keywords: Colorectal liver metastases, Primovist MRI, Treatment proposition

Background

Liver metastases arise in 50–65% of patients with colorectal cancer [1, 2]. Long-term survival can be achieved with surgical resection or local ablation therapy in patients with resectable colorectal liver metastases (CRLM).

Imaging plays a principal role in staging of CRLM. Nowadays, the most used imaging modalities are contrast-enhanced computed tomography (CT) or multi-detector row CT (MDCT). Both are limited in the detection of nodal involvement and characterization of small liver lesions compared to magnetic resonance imaging (MRI) scans [3]. A CT scan has a sensitivity and specificity of 68 and 94%, respectively, and a gadolinium contrast-enhanced MRI scan of 90 and 87%, respectively [4]. Different contrast agents can be administered for contrast-enhanced hepatic MRI scans, like gadoxetic acid, also called Primovist™ (P-MRI) (Bayer AG, Germany) [5, 6]. The reported sensitivity of P-MRI for the detection of CRLM is 87–100% and the specificity is approximately 95% [7–9]. However, CT is still the most frequently used to assess liver involvement and plan surgical resection (Dutch Oncoline guidelines: CRC). P-MRI is not routinely acquired prior to liver resection in most centers [8, 10]. In addition, literature is lacking about the direct effect on treatment strategy in a clinical setting, including local therapy, systemic therapy or conservative treatment in a larger

* Correspondence: j.s.d.mieog@lumc.nl
[1]Department of Surgery, Leiden University Medical Center, P.O. Box 9600, Leiden 2300 RC, The Netherlands
Full list of author information is available at the end of the article

patient cohort. Therefore, there is still no convincing evidence whether P-MRI scans should play a more prominent role in the diagnostic process of patients with potential treatable CRLM and should be standardly acquired. The aim of this study was to determine the impact of P-MRI scans on treatment plan proposition and subsequently the clinical course of patients with potentially treatable CRLM, based on preoperative CT scans.

Methods

The study was designed as a retrospective cohort study in which consecutive patients were included. The study was approved by the scientific review board of the Department of Radiology of the Leiden University Medical Center (LUMC) in 2017. Patient confidentiality was guaranteed using anonymized data and radiologic images, and all data was entered into an encrypted and secured database.

Patients

All patients with potential CRLM were discussed by a multidisciplinary team (MDT) of hepatobiliary surgeons, medical oncologists and (interventional) radiologists. In Fig. 1 a flowchart is presented illustrating the standard operation procedure concerning the loco regional treatment of CRLM in the LUMC. Patients presented at the MDT meeting between July 2014 and August 2017 with primary resectable or primary irresectable (but potentially resectable after conversion therapy) CRLM based on the contrast enhanced (CE)-CT scan, of whom a P-MRI was obtained, were included in this study. Patients with permanent irresectable CRLM were not included. Patients who were previously treated for their CRLM with local therapy or systemic chemotherapy were also included. Patients in whom the time interval between acquirement of the CT scan and P-MRI or P-MRI and treatment was >2 months were excluded. Age, sex, localization of CRC, number of comorbidities, previous surgery and/or systemic therapy for CRC, and previous local therapy and/or systemic therapy for CRLM were noted.

CT scan

All CT scans included an arterial phase scan and a portal venous phase scan, using slices of 5 mm or less for reconstructive images. Contrast-enhance CT scans obtained in the LUMC were performed on a 16-slice spiral CT (Aquillion-16, Toshiba, Tokyo, Japan) using the following scanning parameters: 16 × 1 mm scanning, 120 KV, rotation 0.5 s, contrast Ultravist 370 (dose weight depended: for a standard patient (75 kg) 120 ml was injected. Based on weight categories 46–60 kg, 60–80 kg, 80–100 kg, 100+ kg 20% more or less of the dose was administered) with a delay of 75 s for portal venous phase. Further parameters of CT scanning: the current modulation for the tube varying is from 10 to 500 mA. The pitch factor is 0.8125. Noise index with standard deviation of 10 is used. An Adaptive Iterative Dose Reduction (AIDR) 3D is used as reconstruction algorithm. The reconstruction kernel is FC 18 (soft tissue filter). The CT scans were scored for the presence, the number, location and size of all liver metastases. All scans were evaluated by one of four radiologists from the LUMC, all with at least 5 years of experience in liver imaging.

P-MRI scan

All P-MRI scans were performed in the LUMC on a Philips Ingenia 1.5 or 3.0 T. Gadoxetic acid was the intravenously administered contrast medium (10 ml Primovist). MRI sequences included transveral and coronal T2 TSE (TE 80

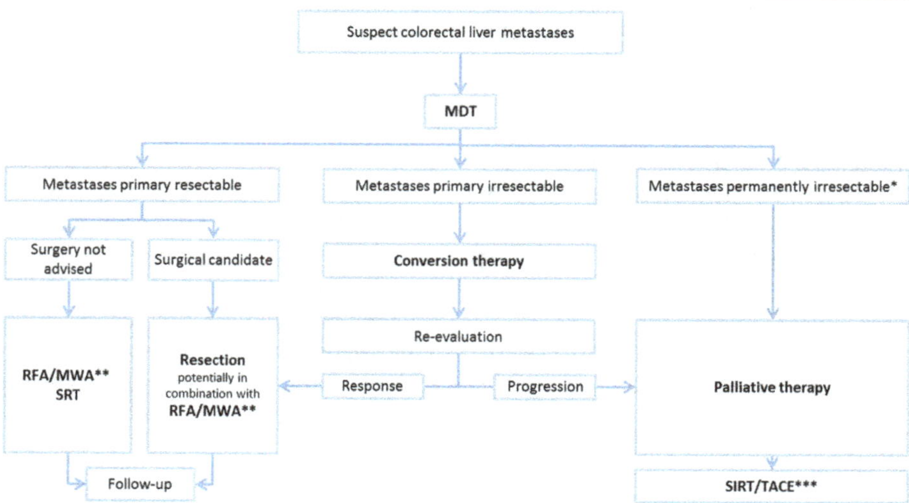

Fig. 1 Standard operation procedure concerning the loco regional treatment of CRLM in the Leiden University Medical Center

and 250), transversal T1FFE mDIXON, diffusion weighted imaging at b0–10–500–1000, dynamic multiphase contrast-enhanced T1FFE images, including 20 min post-contrast images. See Additional file 1: Table S1 for additional information about the used sequences. P-MRIs were read by one of four dedicated abdominal radiologist, each with at least x years of experience after board certification in radiology. Readers were not blinded for clinical information or prior medical imaging.

Study design

All patients were discussed by the MDT, which is a weekly meeting during which all patients who are potentially operable are discussed. As stated before, Fig. 1 gives an overview of all possible treatment options in the LUMC. During the first MDT meeting a treatment plan was proposed based on the CT scan and classified as [1]: local therapy, consisting of either resection, percutaneous ablation or resection + ablation by radiofrequency ablation or microwave ablation [2], conversion therapy with intent of local therapy or [3] follow-up in case of suspicion of benign lesion(s). Of note, patient with irresectable disease were excluded. Subsequently, an P-MRI scan was made and a treatment plan was proposed during the second MDT meeting, potentially changing the previously proposed treatment plan [1]: local therapy [2], adjustment of the local therapy, in case the extensiveness of the local therapy was altered [3], conversion therapy [4], palliation, in case of diffuse disseminated disease resulting in less than 20% of healthy liver parenchyma, or extrahepatic disease (EHD) or [5] follow-up.

Finally, the proposed treatment plan based on the P-MRI scan was compared to the actual performed treatment.

For clarification, 'conversion therapy' is administered with the purpose of reverting the disease from irresectable to resectable. Conversion therapy was mostly a combination of capecitabine with oxaliplatin (CAPOX) usually given in 3 week cycles with a maximum of eight cycles total. 'Palliation' is applied if resection is not considered a (future) option.

In case the patients underwent surgery, the liver was assessed with intra-operative ultrasound by a radiologist. Additionally, in some patients near-infrared fluorescence (NIRF) imaging, using indocyanine green, was performed for the detection of occult liver metastases [11].

Follow-up

In case the liver lesions were resected, standard pathological assessment of the lesions was performed. The pathological assessment was used as reference. Follow-up of the liver occurred every 4 months with CE-CT scan and CEA serum level measurements. In case new intrahepatic lesions were identified during the first follow-up visit, these lesions were probably already present during the procedure and were therefore missed on the P-MRI scan. During the follow-up process of the patients whose lesions were defined as benign, it became clear if these lesions were indeed not CRLM. A minority of patients were referred back to the external hospital for follow-up.

Statistical analysis

Data were analyzed using a statistical software program (SPSS, version 23.0). The change in treatment proposition between MDT meeting 1 and 2 was evaluated using an independent samples *t*-test with standard error and 95% confidence interval. Furthermore, an independent samples *t*-test was performed for 1) comparison of the interval between the date of P-MRI scan and date of actual treatment between the patients who underwent local therapy without adjustment of the local therapy and with adjustment, and 2) for the change in treatment proposition between the group with CT-scan acquired in an external hospital and in the LUMC. The statistical results were considered to indicate significance if the P-value was less than 0.05.

Results

Patients

In total, 83 patients were included in the study cohort. Patient and treatment characteristics are summed in Table 1.

Treatment proposition

The type of treatment was changed in 15 patients (18%) due to the P-MRI scans, all these changes were in concordance with the actual treatment performed.

Table 1 Patient and treatment characteristics

	$N = 83$
Age at time of CT scan; mean ± SD	64.8 ± 10.7
Sex, male; n (%)	56 (68)
Synchronous CRLM; n (%)	44 (53)
Comorbidities; n (%)	
0	36 (43)
1	28 (34)
≥ 2	19 (23)
Previous CRLM surgery, n (%)	18 (22)
CT scan made in LUMC, n (%)	32 (39)
Days between; mean ± SD	
CT and P-MRI	29.0 ± 17.1
Days between P-MRI and treatment	28.0 ± 15.8
Actual treatment; n (%)	
Local	50 (60)
Neo-adjuvant chemotherapy	15 (18)
Palliation	10 (12)
Follow-up	8 (10)

The intended extensiveness of the local therapy was altered in another 17 patients (20%) due to the P-MRI scan: in 11 patients more malignant lesions were identified with P-MRI (mean number additional lesions: 1.6 range; 1–3) (mean size additional lesions: 6.7 mm; range 2–16 mm), the additional identified lesions were located peripheral, superficial and central in the liver. In six patients less lesions were defined as malignant (mean number: 2.0 range; 1–6). These lesions were either considered as cysts ($n = 3$), haemangiomas ($n = 5$), steatosis ($n = 2$) or could not be retrieved ($n = 2$) on the P-MRI scan.

Together the treatment plan proposition was altered in 32 patients (38%; standard error of the mean: 5%; 95% confidence interval: 28–49%). The treatment plan of the remaining 51 patients (61%) was not altered. Table 2 gives an overview of the changes in treatment plan.

Actual treatment

In 56 patients the intended treatment based on the P-MRI scan was local therapy and the extensiveness of the local therapy was altered during the treatment in 10 patients, either more lesions (in six patients) or less lesions (in 4 four patients) were detected and resected during surgery. For detection of lesions ultrasound and NIRF imaging could be used. The additional lesions were biopsied for histological confirmation. The patients with lesions that could not be retrieved did not develop CRLM during the follow-up period, so these lesions were considered false-positive.

In five patients, who were deemed resectable on both CT and MRI, no resection or ablation was performed because a too diffuse disease ($n = 3$) or too extensive tumour burden ($n = 2$) was encountered during surgical exploration. They were palliated instead.

In one patient the proposed treatment based on the CT-scan and P-MRI was local therapy but eventually this patient was not fit for surgery, therefore, he was palliated.

The extensiveness of local therapy of the other 40 patients was not altered, they were treated within a mean of 29.0 days (SD 12.6 days) after the P-MRI scan was obtained, which was not significantly different from the 15 patients with adjusted local therapy (28.3 days (SD 20.7 days)) (P-value = 0.904).

In addition, there was no significant difference in change of treatment plan between patients whose CT scans were from external hospitals (31% change of treatment) and patients whose CT scans were from the LUMC (41% change of treatment) (p-value = 0.48).

An overview of the changes in treatment plan proposition during MDT meeting 1 and 2, and the actual treatment performed is given in Fig. 2.

Follow-up

All patients had a follow-up period of at least 3 months, median follow-up period was 14.4 months (1.38–41.7). Fifteen (18%) patients developed new intrahepatic CRLM within a median time of 5.3 months (0.8–14.0) after local treatment, in three of these patients the new intrahepatic CRLM occurred within 4 months after local therapy. Of the eight patients with lesions deemed benign, the median follow-up period was 22.0 months (4.1–41.2). One patient developed diffuse CRLM within 6 months. This patient presented with one lesion that couldn't be characterized on the CT scan and was assessed as a hemorrhagic-cyst on the P-MRI, but eventually turned out to be a metastasis.

Accuracy

The treatment plan proposition based on the P-MRI was accurate in 77 patients (93%). In five patients an too extensive disease was encountered during surgery and in one patient a CRLM was characterized as a hemorrhagic-cyst on the P-MRI scan. The treatment plan proposition based on the CT scan of these six patients was the same as the P-MRI. The 15 changes of treatment type due to P-MRI findings were all correct, so the accuracy of the CT scan for treatment plan proposition was accurate in 62 patients (75%).

Discussion

Our study focusses on the effect of the P-MRI on the treatment plan proposition and clinical course in patient with potential resectable CRLM based on CT scans. The initial treatment plan proposal based on the CT scan was changed in 38% of the patients due to the findings on P-MRI scans. Compared to the final treatment, the proposition based on the P-MRI scan was accurate in

Table 2 Comparison of the treatment plans proposed during MDT 1 and MDT 2

	MDT 2						
MDT 1		Local	Local therapy adjustment	Neoadjuvant	Palliation	Follow-up	Total
	Local	39	*17*	**5**	**3**	**4**	68
	Neoadjuvant	0	0	9	**1**	**1**	11
	Follow-up	**1**	0	0	0	3	4
	Total	40	17	14	4	8	83

Changes in treatment plan are shown in bold. Extensiveness adjustment of local therapy in italic

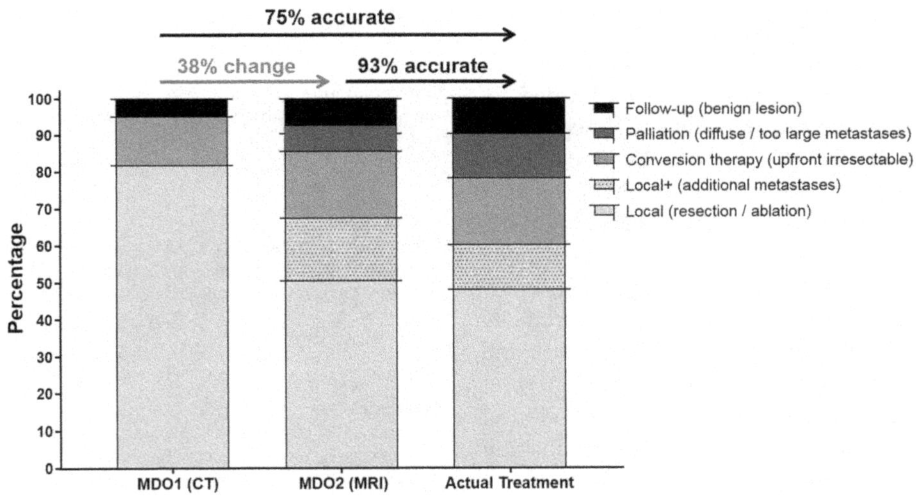

Fig. 2 Changes in treatment plan and actual treatment in percentages

93% of the patients, compared to 75% of the propositions based on CT scans.

The diagnostic accuracy of the P-MRI scans in patients with CRLM and also the impact on surgical strategy has been previously described: in a study of Sofue et al., the surgical strategy changed in 33% of the patients due to the P-MRI [12]. The recent study of Jhaveri et al. describes changes in surgical strategy due to P-MRI scans in 45% of the patients receiving neoadjuvant therapy [13]. In contrast, Kang et al. also investigated the changes in surgical strategy, but only changed the surgery in 3% of the patients [14]. Only Vreugdenburg et al. also determined the impact of P-MRI scans on patient management, but only four of the 13 included studies investigated patient outcome, mainly focusing on surgical strategy instead of treatment strategy [9].

Our single center study emphasizes not only the impact of P-MRI scans on surgical strategy but on the entire treatment plan proposition. The implementation of obtaining a P-MRI scan in the diagnostic work-up of patients has several positive effects on the clinical course of the patients. The most important consequence is the prevention of unnecessary surgeries due to better differentiation between malignancies and benign lesions on P-MRI scans. A second advantage, which is also nicely demonstrated by the study of Knowles et al. is the more accurate staging based on P-MRI scans prior to conversion chemotherapy, thereby reducing intra-hepatic recurrence and avoid repeated hepatectomy [15]. In our study more patients were treated with conversion therapy prior to surgery due to new findings on the P-MRI scan. Furthermore, in other patients the intended local therapy was extended due to the additional identification of small lesions with P-MRI, resulting in the prevention of short-term reinterventions for new intrahepatic lesion development after treatment. P-MRI scanning aids in surgical planning, surgeons and/or interventional radiologist are preoperatively better prepared in comparison to CT scan alone, which might result in more curative resections and less new intrahepatic CRLM formation quickly after surgery. However, these lesions might be detected during local treatment anyway with ultrasound or other additional techniques as NIRF-guided surgery, which has the potential to detect additional small superficial lesion in approximately 15% of the patients [11, 16]. All current studies still advocate repeated therapy or resection to treat all CRLM, including recurrent CRLM, to improve survival rate [17, 18]. In addition, liver parenchyma sparing therapy improves 5-year survival rates, because repeated therapy can be applied if desired [19]. Therefore, accurate imaging can aid in proposing the most suitable treatment strategy, prevent reinterventions and treat as liver parenchyma sparing as possible. In combination with supplementary techniques, as NIRF guided surgery and intraoperative ultrasound, not only detection of CRLM will increase, also radical resection rates will improve and reinterventions can be prevented, all resulting in improved patient outcome. Therefore, future studies should also focus on the bundling of all pre- and intra-operative techniques.

Our study has several limitations. Due to the retrospective study design, decision making was retrospectively collected, however, consecutive patients were included and image and treatment plan evaluation during the MDT meetings was performed in real time and well-documented in the electronic patient charts. This resulted also a non-standardized assessment of the scans by four different radiologists. Differences between CT and MRI scan could be explained due to the differences between readers. Furthermore, readers were not blinded for the CT scans during P-MRI assessment. However, this resulted in a realistic representation of the "everyday practice". Additionally, the follow-up scans were CT scans and not P-MRI scans because this is performed according to the current national guidelines. Time-interval between obtaining the P-MRI scan and the actual treatment might be of influence. But, we found no significant differences for both the origin of acquirement of CT scans or for the time-interval. Sensitivity and specificity could not be calculated based on our study results without introducing bias. Moreover, sensitivity and specificity have been examined extensively in multiple studies, and will be of no additional value. Finally, we can interpret our results only by looking at the patient's clinical course, based on which the treatment plan proposition using P-MRI had an accuracy of 93%. However, we have no proof that these treatment propositions were superior to the treatment propositions based on the CT scans, especially, those in whom the patients were administered conversion therapy instead of upfront local therapy, as described above.

To conclude and most importantly, our study is a display of the clinical decision making in a Dutch academic center, underlining the added value of a P-MRI scan in the entire treatment process of CRLM, improving cancer care and clinical outcome for these patients. In which we showed that P-MRI scans provide additional information that can aid in proposing the most suitable treatment and might prevent short-term reintervention of patients with CRLM. Incorporating an P-MRI scan in the work-up of CRLM patients can improve treatment proposition and clinical outcome compared to CT scanning alone.

Abbreviations

CE-CT: Contrast enhanced CT; CRLM: Colorectal liver metastases; CT: Computed tomography; EHD: Extrahepatic disease; MDCT: Multi-detector row CT; MDT: Multidisciplinary team; MRI: Magnetic resonance imaging; NIRF: Near-infrared fluorescence; P-MRI: Primovist MRI

Acknowledgements

Not applicable.

Funding

This work was supported by the Bas Mulder Award (grant UL2015-7665) from the Dutch Cancer Society. This study has been performed in the scope of this Grant all data collection and analysis was supported from this funding.

Authors' contributions

All authors meet the author requirements according to ICMJE guidelines: Substantial contributions to the conception or design of the work: BS, KV, AV, MB, JM; the acquisition of data: SF, ALV, RJS, HH, RB, MB, JM; analysis of data: BM, KV; interpretation of data: BM, KV, HH, MB, JM. Drafting the work or revising it critically for important intellectual content: all. Final approval of the version to be published: all. Agreement to be accountable for all aspects of the work in ensuring that questions related to the accuracy or integrity of any part of the work are appropriately investigated and resolved: all.

Consent for publication

Not applicable.

Competing interests

The authors declare that they have no competing interests.

Author details

[1]Department of Surgery, Leiden University Medical Center, P.O. Box 9600, Leiden 2300 RC, The Netherlands. [2]Department of Radiology, Leiden University Medical Center, P.O. Box 9600, Leiden 2300 RC, The Netherlands.

References

1. Haddad AJ, Bani Hani M, Pawlik TM, Cunningham SC. Colorectal liver metastases. Int J Surg Oncol. 2011;2011:285840.
2. Alberts SR, Poston GJ. Treatment advances in liver-limited metastatic colorectal cancer. Clin Colorectal Cancer. 2011;10(4):258–65.
3. Koh FHX, Tan KK, Teo LLS, Ang BWL, Thian YL. Prospective comparison between magnetic resonance imaging and computed tomography in colorectal cancer staging. ANZ J Surg. 2018;88(6):E498–E502.
4. Schulz A, Viktil E, Godt JC, Johansen CK, Dormagen JB, Holtedahl JE, et al. Diagnostic performance of CT, MRI and PET/CT in patients with suspected colorectal liver metastases: the superiority of MRI. Acta Radiol. 2016;57(9): 1040–8.
5. Weinmann HJ, Schuhmann-Giampieri G, Schmitt-Willich H, Vogler H, Frenzel T, Gries H. A new lipophilic gadolinium chelate as a tissue-specific contrast medium for MRI. Magn Reson Med. 1991;22(2):233–7 discussion 42.
6. Ba-Ssalamah A, Bastati N, Wibmer A, Fragner R, Hodge JC, Trauner M, et al. Hepatic gadoxetic acid uptake as a measure of diffuse liver disease: where are we? J Magn Reson Imaging. 2017;45(3):646–59.
7. Colagrande S, Castellani A, Nardi C, Lorini C, Calistri L, Filippone A. The role of diffusion-weighted imaging in the detection of hepatic metastases from colorectal cancer: a comparison with unenhanced and Gd-EOB-DTPA enhanced MRI. Eur J Radiol. 2016;85(5):1027–34.
8. Kim HJ, Lee SS, Byun JH, Kim JC, Yu CS, Park SH, et al. Incremental value of liver MR imaging in patients with potentially curable colorectal hepatic metastasis detected at CT: a prospective comparison of diffusion-weighted imaging, gadoxetic acid-enhanced MR imaging, and a combination of both MR techniques. Radiology. 2015;274(3):712–22.
9. Vreugdenburg TD, Ma N, Duncan JK, Riitano D, Cameron AL, Maddern GJ. Comparative diagnostic accuracy of hepatocyte-specific gadoxetic acid (Gd-EOB-DTPA) enhanced MR imaging and contrast enhanced CT for the detection of liver metastases: a systematic review and meta-analysis. Int J Color Dis. 2016;31(11):1739–49.
10. Cho JY, Lee YJ, Han HS, Yoon YS, Kim J, Choi Y, et al. Role of gadoxetic acid-enhanced magnetic resonance imaging in the preoperative evaluation of small hepatic lesions in patients with colorectal cancer. World J Surg. 2015; 39(5):1161–6.
11. van der Vorst JR, Schaafsma BE, Hutteman M, Verbeek FP, Liefers GJ, Hartgrink HH, et al. Near-infrared fluorescence-guided resection of colorectal liver metastases. Cancer. 2013;119(18):3411–8.
12. Sofue K, Tsurusaki M, Murakami T, Onoe S, Tokue H, Shibamoto K, et al. Does Gadoxetic acid-enhanced 3.0T MRI in addition to 64-detector-row contrast-enhanced CT provide better diagnostic performance and change the therapeutic strategy for the preoperative evaluation of colorectal liver metastases? Eur Radiol. 2014;24(10):2532–9.
13. Jhaveri KS, Fischer SE, Hosseini-Nik H, Sreeharsha B, Menezes RJ, Gallinger S, et al. Prospective comparison of gadoxetic acid-enhanced liver MRI and contrast-enhanced CT with histopathological correlation for preoperative detection of colorectal liver metastases following chemotherapy and potential impact on surgical plan. HPB (Oxford). 2017;19(11):992–1000.
14. Kang SI, Kim DW, Cho JY, Park J, Lee KH, Son IT, et al. Is MRI of the liver needed during routine preoperative workup for colorectal Cancer? Dis Colon Rectum. 2017;60(9):936–44.

22

MRI assessment of aortic flow in patients with pulmonary arterial hypertension in response to exercise

Jacob A. Macdonald[1*], Christopher J. François[2], Omid Forouzan[3], Naomi C. Chesler[3] and Oliver Wieben[1,2,3]

Abstract

Background: While primarily a right heart disease, pulmonary arterial hypertension (PAH) can impact left heart function and aortic flow through a shifted interventricular septum from right ventricular pressure overload and reduced left ventricular preload, among other mechanisms. In this study, we used phase contrast (PC) MRI and a modest exercise challenge to examine the effects of PAH on systemic circulation. While exercise challenges are typically performed with ultrasound in the clinic, MRI exercise studies allow for more reproducible image alignment, more accurate flow quantification, and improved tissue contrast.

Methods: Six PAH patients and fifteen healthy controls (8 older age-matched, 7 younger) exercised in the magnet bore with an MRI-compatible exercise device that allowed for scanning immediately following cessation of exercise. PC scans were performed in the ascending aorta during a breath hold immediately after modest exercise to non-invasively measure stroke volume (SV), cardiac output (CO), aortic peak systolic flow (PSF), and aortic wall stiffness via relative area change (RAC).

Results: Images following exercise showed mild blurring, but were high enough quality to allow for segmentation of the aorta. While SV was approximately 30% lower in PAH patients ($SV_{PAH,rest} = 67 \pm 16$ mL; $SV_{PAH,stress} = 90 \pm 42$ mL) than age-matched controls ($SV_{older,rest} = 93 \pm 16$ mL; $SV_{older,stress} = 133 \pm 40$ mL) at both rest and following exercise, CO was similar for both groups following exercise ($CO_{PAH,stress} = 10.8 \pm 5.7$ L/min; $CO_{older,stress} = 11.8 \pm 5.0$ L/min). This was achieved through a compensatory increase in heart rate in the PAH subjects (74% increase as compared to 29% in age-matched controls). The PAH subjects also demonstrated reduced aortic peak systolic flow relative to the healthy controls ($PSF_{PAH,rest} = 309 \pm 52$ mL/s; $PSF_{older,rest} = 416 \pm 114$ mL/s; $PSF_{PAH,stress} = 388 \pm 113$ mL/s; $PSF_{older,stress} = 462 \pm 176$ mL/s). PAH patients and older controls demonstrated stiffer aortic walls when compared to younger controls ($RAC_{PAH,rest} = 0.15 \pm 0.05$; $RAC_{older,rest} = 0.17 \pm 0.05$; $RAC_{young,rest} = 0.28 \pm 0.08$).

Conclusions: PC MRI following a modest exercise challenge was capable of detecting differences in left heart dynamics likely induced from PAH. These results demonstrated that PAH can have a significant influence on systemic flow, even when the patient has no prior left heart disease. Image quantification following exercise could likely be improved in future studies through the implementation of free-breathing or real-time MRI acquisitions.

Keywords: Exercise, Pulmonary arterial hypertension, Stress test, Flow, MRI

* Correspondence: jamacdonald@wisc.edu
[1]Department of Medical Physics, University of Wisconsin, 1111 Highland Avenue, Room 1005, Madison, WI 53705, USA
Full list of author information is available at the end of the article

Background

It is well established that stress tests can reveal important diagnostic information beyond that seen with tests performed at a resting heart rate [1–4], such as ischemia, increased ventricular pressures, valvular regurgitation, and deficiencies in recovery to a resting state. In clinical settings, exercise tests are commonly performed with an exercise paradigm on a treadmill or stationary bicycle followed by echocardiography [3] or single photon emission computed tomography (SPECT) image acquisitions [5].

Cardiopulmonary exercise testing is increasingly used to assess disease progression in patients with pulmonary hypertension (PH) [6–8]. PH is characterized by an increase in blood pressure in the pulmonary vasculature, which can be caused by or result in vascular remodeling and stiffening of the pulmonary artery [9, 10]. While some cases of PH are the end result of left-sided heart disease that directly influence systemic circulation (World Health Organization (WHO) functional group 2) [11], pulmonary arterial hypertension (PAH; WHO functional group 1) is the result of conditions, such as connective tissue diseases, acting directly on the pulmonary vasculature [12]. In these cases, although there is no initial left heart dysfunction, right ventricular pressure overload induced by PAH can lead to a shift or distortion of the interventricular septum [13–15]. Left heart dynamics in these patients may also be altered by reduced left ventricular (LV) preload as a result of inhibited right heart flow [16], increased vascular impedance from stiffening of the aorta [17], and co-existing systemic hypertension [18]. These factors may lead to a reduced LV volume in PAH patients relative to a healthy population, which in turn may lead to diminished stroke volume and cardiac output.

PH screening and assessment is clinically performed with echocardiography, which is limited in its capabilities due to its short penetration depth [19] and difficulty in properly aligning the acoustic window with the arterial flow [20]. In addition, Doppler ultrasound does not directly measure flow, but instead produces estimates from velocity measurements and pre-established vessel area models, which can introduce systematic errors into flow estimates [21].

Magnetic resonance imaging (MRI) provides the opportunity for more accurate visualization and quantification of flow via phase contrast (PC) acquisitions. MRI allows for less dependency on the skill of the operator as a result of improved spatial resolution, larger imaging windows, and higher tissue contrast. Recent work has also demonstrated that non-invasive measures of arterial stiffness are possible with PC MRI through metrics such as pulse wave velocity (PWV) and the relative area change (RAC) of the artery between diastole and systole [22].

Despite the advantages MRI could offer over existing exercise imaging modalities in assessing pulmonary hypertension, exercise MRI is challenging because of the relatively slow acquisition speed and the narrow confinements of the magnet bore. Instead, pharmacological stress agents, such as Dobutamine, Adenosine, and Regadenoson [23–25], are used in clinical practice. The drawback of such techniques is that pharmacological stress is not physiologic and, therefore, is not the preferred method of stress for assessing pulmonary hypertension [1, 26]. In response to these shortcomings, recent advances have seen the development of MRI-compatible exercise devices that allow for exercise in the MRI room adjacent to the table [27] or in a supine position on the scanner bed inside the magnet bore [28–30].

Overall, while it is likely that a patient diagnosed with PAH will experience diminished left heart function due to factors such as right ventricular pressure overload or reduced LV preload during the progression of the disease, such effects have not been investigated in detail with exercise MRI. Previous work has performed straightforward comparisons of blood flow in the aorta of PAH patients with controls using PC MRI [31], but has not correlated these measurements with metrics of vessel stiffness or investigated the value of exercise studies for these comparisons. The goal of this study was to use a custom-made, MRI-compatible exercise device to examine the effects of pulmonary arterial hypertension on aortic flow and stiffness in response to exercise with PC MRI. We hypothesize that PH subjects will show reduced left heart efficiency (lower stroke volume, higher heart rate) relative to healthy controls and these differences will be more pronounced following exercise stress.

Methods

Subject population

This study was approved by the local Institutional Review Board and was compliant with the Health Insurance Portability and Accountability Act. Twenty-one subjects were recruited, provided written informed consent, and were screened via an MRI safety questionnaire. The 21 subjects were divided into 3 cohorts: 7 young, healthy controls (28 ± 4 years; 3 male, 4 female), 8 older, healthy controls (58 ± 10 years; 1 male, 7 female), and 6 pulmonary hypertension patients (WHO Group 1 (PAH) from systemic sclerosis, 60 ± 9 years; 1 male, 5 female). All control subjects were free of overt cardiovascular, pulmonary, and renal disease. The recruited PH subjects had no recent syncope and, like the controls, had no history of unassociated lung or cardiovascular disease. Exclusion criteria for this study included classification as New York Heart Association functional class IV (symptoms of limited cardiac capacity apparent at rest) and skeletal or muscle abnormalities which could prohibit exercise. The older, healthy control group was age-matched to the PH group. The younger control group was included to provide insight regarding loss of cardiac function via disease versus natural loss due to aging. Subjects were excluded from the final statistical analysis if image quality was too poor to delineate the aortic wall or if the subject moved out of the prescribed scanning planes during exercise.

MRI-compatible exercise device

Exercise was conducted with a custom-built, low-cost MRI-compatible stepping device which allowed subjects to exercise in a supine position in the scanner bore (Fig. 1) [28]. This permitted localizers and pre-scans to be performed prior to exercise, allowing for immediate image acquisition following the cessation of exercise. Imaging was performed following exercise rather than during exercise due to the challenging nature of breath holds during exercise, specifically in the PH population. Subjects exercised via a dynamic stepping motion to the beat of a metronome at the target exercise frequency. The exercise resistance was controlled by removable weights at the end of each lever arm. Optical displacement sensors on each lever arm provided the actual frequency of the stepping motion, allowing for real-time monitoring of the actual stepping frequency and power achieved by the subject relative to the targeted power level. To minimize axial displacement of the subject from the stepper as well as minimize chest motion during exercise, the subject was connected to the exercise equipment via a backpack harness and had hand-grips to hold on to for stabilization.

Data acquisition

Imaging was performed on one of two clinical 1.5 T MRI systems (HDxt or Discovery 450w, GE Healthcare, Waukesha, WI) using an 8 channel cardiac coil and vector electrocardiographic (ECG) gating. Flow measurements were acquired with a prospectively ECG-gated two-dimensional (2D) cine phase contrast (PC) sequence performed across a 15 s breath hold. The imaging plane was prescribed orthogonal to the ascending aorta. Imaging parameters for the PC sequence were: field of view = 35 × 35 cm, matrix size = 128 × 256 (reconstructed to 256 × 256), slice thickness = 8 mm; TR/TE = 6.1/3.7 ms, flip angle = 30°, velocity encode (VENC) = 150 cm/s, parallel-imaging (ASSET) acceleration factor = 2, temporal resolution = 25 ms, and cardiac phases = 20.

All subjects exercised at a low exercise power to guarantee the PH subjects would be able to complete the same exercise paradigm as the control groups. This exercise and imaging paradigm was designed to induce mild-to-moderate exercise stress in all subject groups (Fig. 2). A PC acquisition was performed at rest prior to exercise. Subjects then exercised at a target power of 30 W for 3 min. Immediately following the end of exercise, subjects held their breath for a second PC MRI acquisition in the ascending aorta. Total examination time was less than an hour, including set-up and take-down of the exercise equipment. Subjects typically spent less than 30 min in the scanner bore.

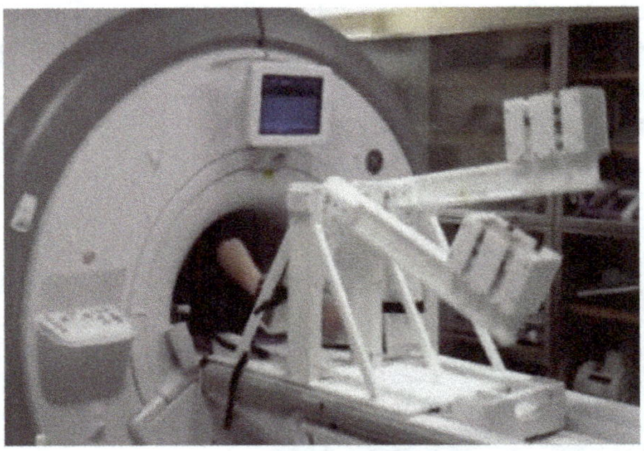

Fig. 1 MRI-compatible exercise device. The subject exercises in the magnet bore via a dynamic stepping motion to the beat of a metronome. Resistance is controlled by removable weights at the end of each lever

Data analysis

Aortic flow measurements were performed with CV Flow (Version 3.3, Medis, Leiden, Netherlands) on a GE Advantage workstation. The following parameters were calculated from the flow measurements: stroke volume (SV), cardiac output (CO), peak systolic flow (PSF), peak systolic velocity (PSV), and the relative area change (RAC) of the ascending aorta between diastole and systole. Aortic stiffness was estimated with relative area change rather than pulse wave velocity due to the limited temporal resolution of the PC sequence.

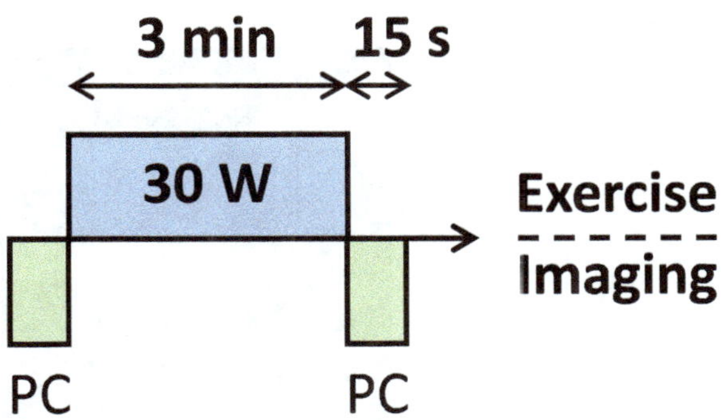

Fig. 2 Exercise and imaging paradigm for all three groups. PC imaging was performed in the ascending aorta at rest prior to exercise. This was followed by 3 min of exercise at a power of 30 W. An identical PC scan to that performed at rest immediately followed the end of exercise

Statistical methods

All statistical analysis was performed with R (Version 3.2.3, R Foundation for Statistical Computing, Vienna, Austria). Results are presented as the mean value plus or minus one standard deviation of the sampled group. To determine the statistical significance of any intragroup changes between parameters measured at rest and stress, a paired student's t-test was performed for each cohort. A one-way ANOVA test with a post-hoc Tukey's honestly significant difference (HSD) test was used to determine statistically significant intergroup differences for each parameter at rest and stress. Levene's test was used in conjunction with the ANOVA test to ensure that the assumption of equal variances between groups was valid. For all statistical tests, a threshold of $\alpha = 0.05$ was chosen for statistical significance.

Results

MRI exercise stress tests were successfully performed in 19/21 subjects. Two of the older, healthy controls shifted their body position during exercise such that the prescribed scan planes were not usable. Thus, they were omitted from the analysis. All subjects successfully completed the 15 s breath hold following exercise. Although the target exercise power for each group was 30 W, the actual exercise power achieved for the remaining young controls, older controls, and PH subjects was 38 ± 12 W, 32 ± 8 W, and 30 ± 10 W respectively. There was no statistically significant difference in the achieved exercise power between these groups ($p = 0.29$). These exercise powers resulted in an average heart rate increase of 46% for the young controls, 29% for the older controls, and 74% for the PH subjects.

Figure 3 shows a representative comparison of image quality in magnitude PC images before and immediately following exercise. For most subjects, only minimal motion artifacts were present following exercise, allowing for good segmentation of the aorta. Minor blurring was observed in the post-exercise images and reduced blood signal was seen in some areas of the aorta. Increased blurring was observed in the PH subjects relative to the control groups.

Table 1 presents the average values plus/minus one standard deviation for each hemodynamic parameter measured from the PC scans. The data distributions for SV, CO, PSV, and PSF are visualized at rest and following stress for all cohorts in Fig. 4. Statistically significant increases in heart rate, stroke volume, and cardiac output following exercise, indicated that the mild exercise paradigm was able to induce a cardiac response in all cohorts. On average, stroke volumes in the PH subjects were 30% lower than the young controls and 28% lower than the older controls at rest, and 23% lower than the younger controls and 32% lower than the older controls following exercise. Interestingly, however, PH subjects demonstrated a resting cardiac output approximately 30% lower than their healthy counterparts, while mean cardiac output measurements were comparable amongst all groups following exercise (Fig. 4b).

Measurements of peak systolic flow and peak systolic velocity showed no meaningful response to exercise in the young control groups. In contrast, the older controls showed a 19% increase in velocity and an 11% increase in flow in response to exercise. Likewise, the PH subjects demonstrated a larger 39% increase in velocity and 26% increase in flow. At both rest and exercise, the PH subjects demonstrated lower overall average values of these parameters when compared to both control groups (Fig. 4c, d).

The distribution of aortic wall stiffness measurements for each cohort is presented in Fig. 5. Significantly lower values of RAC in the older controls and PH subjects relative to the young controls at rest indicated stiffer aortic walls in these groups. Furthermore, the PH subjects had the lowest mean RAC of all groups, suggesting the stiffest vessel walls amongst the three cohorts. Although not significant, exercise showed increased vessel compliance of the older controls and PH subjects to the level of the young

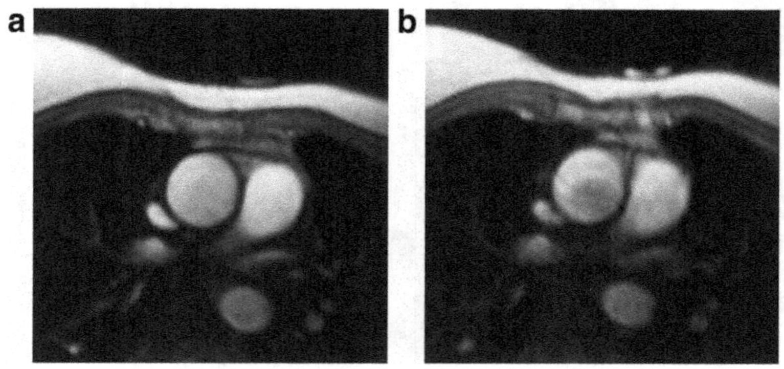

Fig. 3 Representative magnitude PC image quality in the ascending aorta (**a**) at rest and (**b**) immediately following exercise. Mild blurring was observed in images following exercise alongside some darkening of the blood, but image quality was still sufficient to delineate relevant vasculature

Table 1 Hemodynamic parameters measured in the ascending aorta at rest and immediately following exercise stress from phase contrast acquisitions. Results are presented as the mean value plus or minus one standard deviation of the samples

Variable	Rest			Stress		
	Young	Older	PAH	Young	Older	PAH
Heart rate [bpm]	66 ± 11	67 ± 9	69 ± 19	97 ± 19*	87 ± 12*	116 ± 19*
Stroke volume [mL]	96 ± 15	93 ± 16	67 ± 16	116 ± 23*	133 ± 40*	90 ± 42
Cardiac output [L/min]	6.3 ± 1.1	6.3 ± 1.6	4.5 ± 1.4	11 ± 2*	11.8 ± 5*	10.8 ± 5.7*
Peak systolic velocity [cm/s]	77 ± 21	58 ± 15	49 ± 14	78 ± 22	69 ± 27	68 ± 29*
Peak systolic flow [mL/s]	445 ± 85	416 ± 114	309 ± 52	446 ± 118	462 ± 176	388 ± 113
Relative area change	0.28 ± 0.08	0.17 ± 0.05	0.15 ± 0.05	0.28 ± 0.10	0.27 ± 0.14	0.25 ± 0.18

*Denotes statistical significance ($p < 0.05$) relative to the same cohort at rest

controls. Overall, measurements for all hemodynamic parameters following exercise usually showed more variance amongst each cohort than at rest.

Discussion

As hypothesized, PH patients demonstrated reduced LV stroke volume at rest and during stress when compared to control groups. These reduced stroke volumes may suggest the presence of a shifted interventricular septum induced by right ventricular pressure overload, reduced LV preload, or a co-existing condition, such as systemic hypertension. Future studies with imaging sequences dedicated to ventricular imaging (e.g. balanced steady-state free precession MRI) and ventricular pressure measurements could prove valuable to elucidate the relative contributions of these factors to the reduced left heart SV in these patients. Despite low stroke volumes, however, the PH patients presented a preserved cardiac output following exercise as a result of a compensatory increase in heart rate (74% increase in PH subjects as compared to 29% in age-matched controls). Therefore, while PH patients may be able to match exercise capabilities of age-matched controls in the short-term, the more rapid increase in heart rate will result in PH patients reaching a clinically-defined maximum heart rate sooner, yielding reduced exercise endurance. This behavior in the left ventricle is consistent with right

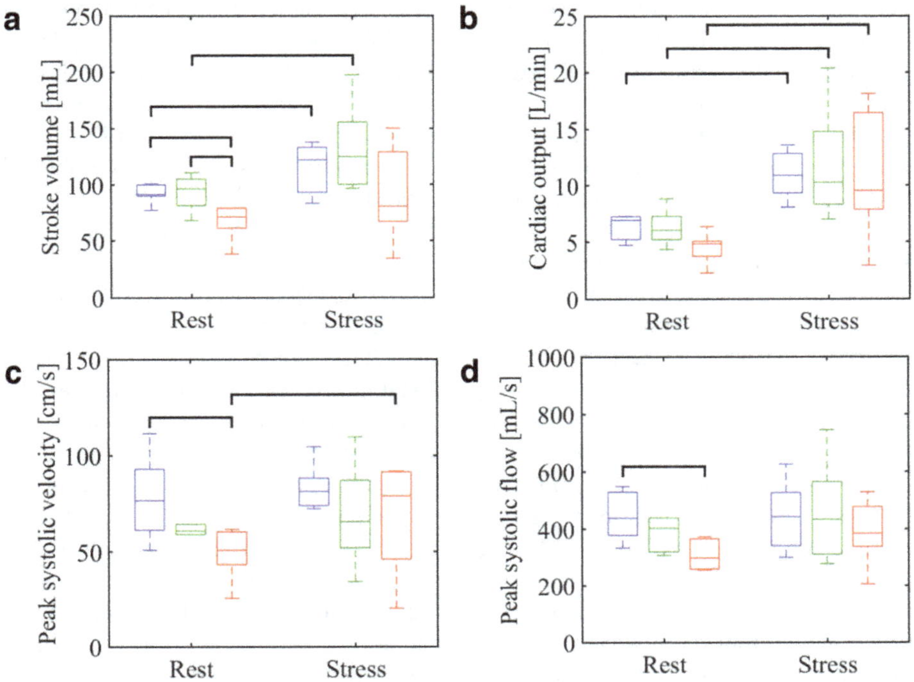

Fig. 4 Boxplots displaying the distribution of key aortic flow variables as measured with PC MRI in the ascending aorta: (**a**) stroke volume, (**b**) cardiac output, (**c**) peak systolic velocity, and (**d**) peak systolic flow. Blue indicates young controls, green indicates older controls, and red represents PH subjects. A bracket between two boxplots indicates a statistically significant ($p < 0.05$) difference between the two groups of measurements

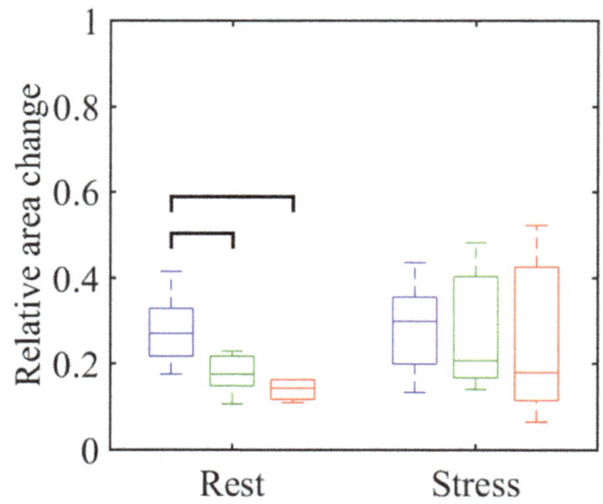

Fig. 5 Distribution of aortic wall stiffness as calculated with the relative area change method in the ascending aorta. Blue indicates young controls, green indicates older controls, and red represents PH subjects. A bracket between two boxplots indicates a statistically significant ($p < 0.05$) difference between the two groups of measurements

heart dynamics previously reported following exercise in patients with PH [32].

Although the exercise stress induced comparable levels of cardiac output in the PH population and both control groups, the PH subjects demonstrated reduced peak systolic velocity and peak systolic flow – further evidence of altered left heart hemodynamics induced by right heart changes from PAH. It is worth noting, however, that for these parameters the older control group showed decreased mean values relative to the younger group as well, suggesting the reduced capacity shown in the PH subjects may be a more complex dynamic between natural age-related loss of cardiovascular function and disease progression.

The relative area change of the aorta proved to be capable of assessing vessel stiffness, demonstrating reduced aortic compliance in the PH subjects relative to the controls. This result was consistent with the fact that the recruited patients developed PAH as a result of ongoing systemic sclerosis [33] and may have contributed to the reduced stroke volume and exercise capacity in this group. There is great value in future investigations to perform non-invasive measures in the pulmonary artery of the PH subjects to examine the extent of stiffening relative to the aorta.

The modest increase in heart rate observed across all three subject cohorts validated that the relatively low exercise power used in this study was still effective at inducing observable exercise stress in each cohort, although the cardiac response was diminished in the control groups. This demonstrated that mild exercise paradigms can be an effective method for stress imaging in subjects with reduced cardiac capacity. The drawback of using low exercise powers was observed in the younger controls, however, who were not as challenged by the paradigm and, on average, exercised at a power 25% above the targeted level. Since the resistance could be adjusted in real-time during exercise with the exercise equipment used for this study, in this case, where the young controls exercised faster than this metronome beat, there was no way to compensate and reduce their exercise power.

The potential value of performing exercise studies in a PH population was apparent, as the PH cohort showed larger relative responses to exercise than the healthy controls in all measured hemodynamic parameters except stroke volume, which is known to have a reduced response to exercise in PH subjects [32]. Performing studies with increased exercise power may induce greater differences between these cohorts than observed with the mild exercise powers used in this study. The increased cardiac response to higher exercise powers in all cohorts would also likely result in statistically significant differences between rest and stress in many of the parameters that showed non-significant increases with exercise, such as peak systolic velocity and flow. Given the disparity in exercise abilities between these cohorts, in future studies, it would be valuable to standardize our comparisons on more physiologic measures of exercise, such as a common heart rate or maximal oxygen uptake ($VO_{2,max}$), rather than a common exercise power.

While the breath held PC acquisitions were successfully completed in all subjects following exercise, some of the subjects with more limited cardiac output, expressed a greater perceived difficulty in accomplishing these breath holds. Body motion from discomfort during these breath holds may have contributed to the larger degree of blurring observed in these subjects' images. Although more challenging for these subjects, it was essential to begin imaging immediately following exercise due to the rapid recovery of heart rate back to a resting state. The potential heart rate recovery across the 15 s of imaging following cessation of exercise was not deemed to be a concern, however, as a previous study showed that even in young athletes, heart rate will only decrease an average of 5% in this time period [34]. In future studies, the implementation of free-breathing or real-time acquisitions could eliminate the need for a breath hold altogether and allow for imaging during exercise, resulting in a more comfortable exercise paradigm for subjects and a possible improvement in image quality.

There were a few limitations to this study beyond those already mentioned. The harness used to reduce chest motion was not entirely effective at preventing subject movement, as demonstrated with the two subjects who moved out of their prescribed scan planes. Motion such as this possibly led to shifts or rotations in scan planes in the other subjects, which could impact the accuracy of flow and vessel cross-sectional area measurements. In addition, the statistical power of our observations was limited by the relatively small sample size of each cohort. These factors likely contributed to increased variance and lack of statistical significance in some of the measurements.

Conclusion

In conclusion, we investigated the impact of pulmonary arterial hypertension on aortic flow with PC MRI following a modest exercise challenge. Custom-made, MR-compatible exercise equipment permitted subjects to exercise in a supine position fully in the bore of the scanner, allowing for imaging immediately following the cessation of exercise. As we hypothesized, the PH subjects showed reduced LV stroke volume and decreased cardiac efficiency relative to the healthy controls. The PH subjects demonstrated a different mechanism for increasing cardiac output in response to exercise, relying on large increases in heart rate rather than the balanced increase in heart rate and stroke volume observed in healthy controls. Cardiac output, peak systolic velocity, and peak systolic flow showed increased sensitivity to exercise-induced changes in the PH population, as well. Future studies will compare these metrics to those obtained from pulmonary flow in the same subject populations.

Abbreviations

CO: Cardiac output; LV: Left ventricle; MRI: Magnetic resonance imaging; PAH: Pulmonary arterial hypertension; PC: Phase contrast; PH: Pulmonary hypertension; PSF: Peak systolic flow; PSV: Peak systolic velocity; PWV: Pulse wave velocity; RAC: Relative area change; SPECT: Single photon emission computer tomography; SV: Stroke volume; VENC: Velocity encoding; WHO: World Health Organization

Acknowledgements

We gratefully acknowledge funding from the NIH and GE Healthcare for their research support and assistance.

Funding

Funding for this work was provided by the NIH (R01HL105598). The funding body had no role in the design of the study, the collection, analysis, and interpretation of data, or in writing the manuscript.

Authors' contributions

JAM analyzed and interpreted the MRI data and wrote the manuscript. CJF provided clinical perspective and guidance when designing the study, helped design the MRI scanning protocol, and helped interpret results. OF worked on stepper implementation and oversaw exercise challenges. NCC conceived the initial study design and obtained the grant funding this project. OW provided guidance on study design and helped design the MRI scanning protocol. All authors read and approved the final manuscript.

Ethics approval and consent to participate

All procedures performed in studies involving human participants were in accordance with the ethical standards of the institutional and/or national research committee and with the 1964 Helsinki declaration and its later amendments or comparable ethical standards. Before participation in the study, written informed consent was obtained from all individual subjects to participate in study activities and use their data in a research capacity. This study was approved by the University of Wisconsin-Madison Health Sciences Institutional Review Board (IRB 2011–0980; PI: Francois).

Consent for publication

Not applicable.

Competing interests

The University of Wisconsin receives research support from GE Healthcare. The authors declare that they have no other potential competing interests.

Author details

[1]Department of Medical Physics, University of Wisconsin, 1111 Highland Avenue, Room 1005, Madison, WI 53705, USA. [2]Department of Radiology, University of Wisconsin, Madison, USA. [3]Department of Biomedical Engineering, University of Wisconsin, Madison, USA.

References

1. Picano E, Pibarot P, Lancellotti P, Monin JL, Bonow RO. The emerging role of exercise testing and stress echocardiography in Valvular heart disease. JAC. 2009;54:2251–60. https://doi.org/10.1016/j.jacc.2009.07.046.
2. Miller TD. The exercise treadmill test: estimating cardiovascular prognosis. Cleve Clin J Med. 2008;75:424–30. https://doi.org/10.3949/ccjm.75.6.424.
3. Pina IL, Balady GJ, Hanson P, Labovitz AJ, Madonna DW, Myers J. Guidelines for clinical exercise testing laboratories : a statement for healthcare professionals from the committee on exercise and cardiac rehabilitation. Am Heart Assoc Circ. 1995;91:912–21. https://doi.org/10.1161/01.CIR.91.3.912.
4. Fletcher GF, Balady GJ, Amsterdam EA, Chaitman B, Eckel R, Fleg J, et al. Exercise standards for testing and training: a statement for healthcare professionals from the American Heart Association. Circulation. 2001;104: 1694–740. https://doi.org/10.1161/hc3901.095960.
5. Bailey IK, Griffith LS, Rouleau J, Strauss HW, Pitt B. Thallium-201 myocardial perfusion imaging at rest and during exercise: comparative sensitivity to electrocardiography in coronary artery disease. Circulation. 1977;55:79–87. https://doi.org/10.1161/01.CIR.55.1.79.
6. Arena R, Lavie CJ, Milani RV, Myers J, Guazzi M. Cardiopulmonary exercise testing in patients with pulmonary arterial hypertension: an evidence-based review. J Heart Lung Transplant. 2010;29:159–73. https://doi.org/10.1016/j.healun.2009.09.003.
7. Argiento P, Chesler N, Mule M, D'Alto M, Bossone E, Unger P, et al. Exercise stress echocardiography for the study of the pulmonary circulation. Eur Respir J. 2010;35:1273–8. https://doi.org/10.1183/09031936.00076009.
8. Naeije R, Chesler N. Pulmonary circulation at exercise. Compr Physiol. 2012; 2:711–41. https://doi.org/10.1002/cphy.c100091
9. Galie N, Hoeper MM, Humbert M, Torbicki A, Vachiery JL, Barbera JA, et al. Guidelines for the diagnosis and treatment of pulmonary hypertension. Eur Respir J. 2009;34:1219–63. https://doi.org/10.1183/09031936.00139009.
10. Reuben SR. Compliance of the human pulmonary arterial system in disease. Circ Res. 1971;29:40–50. https://doi.org/10.1161/01.res.29.1.40.
11. Kiefer TL, Bashore TM. Pulmonary hypertension related to left-sided cardiac pathology. Pulm Med. 2011. https://doi.org/10.1155/2011/381787.
12. Ungerer RG, Tashkin DP, Furst D, Clements PJ, Gong H, Bein M, et al. Prevalence and clinical correlates of pulmonary arterial hypertension in progressive systemic sclerosis. Am J Med. 1983;75:65–74. https://doi.org/10.1016/0002-9343(83)91169-5.
13. King ME, Braun H, Goldblatt a, Liberthson R, Weyman a E. Interventricular septal configuration as a predictor of right ventricular systolic hypertension in children: a cross-sectional echocardiographic study. Circulation. 1983;68: 68–75. https://doi.org/10.1161/01.CIR.68.1.68.
14. Jessup M, Sutton MS, Weber KT, Janicki JS. The effect of chronic pulmonary hypertension on left ventricular size, function, and interventricular septal motion. Am Heart J. 1987;113:1114–22. https://doi.org/10.1016/0002-8703(87)90921-5.

15. Roeleveld RJ, Marcus JT, Faes TJC, Gan T-J, Boonstra A, Postmus PE, et al. Interventricular septal configuration at MR imaging and pulmonary arterial pressure in pulmonary hypertension. Radiology. 2005;234:710–7. https://doi.org/10.1148/radiol.2343040151.
16. Gorter TM, Willems TP, Van Melle JP. Ventricular interdependence in pulmonary arterial hypertension: providing small pieces of a complex puzzle. Eur J Heart Fail. 2015;17:1–2. https://doi.org/10.1002/ejhf.195
17. Schäfer M, Ivy DD, Abman SH, Barker AJ, Browne LP, Fonseca B, et al. Apparent aortic stiffness in children with pulmonary arterial hypertension. Circ Cardiovasc Imaging. 2017;10:1–9. https://doi.org/10.1161/CIRCIMAGING.116.005817.
18. Demir N, Şahin A, Küçükşahin O, Kayacan O, Dinçer R, Sayin T, et al. Pulmonary arterial hypertension and systemic sclerosis relation: a single Centre experience. Hear Lung Circ. 2014;23:667–73. https://doi.org/10.1016/j.hlc.2014.02.002.
19. Peng H-H, Chung H-W, Yu H-Y, Tseng W-Y I. Estimation of pulse wave velocity in main pulmonary artery with phase contrast MRI: preliminary investigation. J Magn Reson Imaging. 2006;24:1303–10. https://doi.org/10.1002/jmri.20782.
20. Paz R, Mohiaddin RH, Longmore DB. Magnetic resonance assessment of the pulmonary arterial trunk anatomy, flow, pulsatility and distensibility. Eur Heart J. 1993;14:1524–30. https://doi.org/10.1093/eurheartj/14.11.1524.
21. Gill R. Measurement of blood flow by ultrasound: accuracy and sources of error. Ultrasound Med Biol. 1985;11:625–41. https://doi.org/10.1016/0301-5629(85)90035-3.
22. Forouzan O, Warczytowa J, Wieben O, François CJ, Chesler NC. Non-invasive measurement using cardiovascular magnetic resonance of changes in pulmonary artery stiffness with exercise. J Cardiovasc Magn Reson. 2015;17:109. https://doi.org/10.1186/s12968-015-0213-2.
23. Charoenpanichkit C, Hundley WG. The 20 year evolution of dobutamine stress cardiovascular magnetic resonance. J Cardiovasc Magn Reson. 2010;12:59.https://doi.org/10.1186/1532-429X-12-59.
24. Chotenimitkhun R, Gregory Hundley W. Pharmacological Stress Cardiovascular Magnetic Resonance. Postgrad Med. 2011;123:162–70. https://doi.org/10.3810/pgm.2011.05.2295.
25. Botvinick EH. Current methods of pharmacologic stress testing and the potential advantages of new agents. J Nucl Med Technol. 2009;37:14–25. https://doi.org/10.2967/jnmt.108.057802.
26. Armstrong WF, Zoghbi WA. Stress echocardiography: current methodology and clinical applications. J Am Coll Cardiol. 2005;45:1739–47. https://doi.org/10.1016/j.jacc.2004.12.078.
27. Foster EL, Arnold JW, Jekic M, Bender J, Balasubramanian V, Thavendiranathan P, et al. An MR-compatible treadmill for exercise stress cardiac magnetic resonance imaging. Magn Reson Med. 2013;67:880–9. https://doi.org/10.1002/mrm.23059
28. Forouzan O, Flink E, Warczytowa J, Thate N, Hanske A, Lee T, et al. Low cost magnetic resonance imaging-compatible stepper exercise device for use in cardiac stress tests. J Med Device. 2014;8:21–8. https://doi.org/10.1115/1.4027343.
29. Gusso S, Salvador C, Hofman P, Cutfield W, Baldi JC, Taberner A, et al. Design and testing of an MRI-compatible cycle ergometer for non-invasive cardiac assessments during exercise. Biomed Eng Online. 2012;11:13. https://doi.org/10.1186/1475-925X-11-13.
30. Von Knobelsdorff-Brenkenhoff F, Dieringer MA, Fuchs K, Hezel F, Niendorf T, Schulz-Menger J. Isometric handgrip exercise during cardiovascular magnetic resonance imaging: set-up and cardiovascular effects. J Magn Reson Imaging. 2013;37:1342–50. https://doi.org/10.1002/jmri.23924.
31. Ley S, Mereles D, Puderbach M, Gruenig E, Schöck H, Eichinger M, et al. Value of MR phase-contrast flow measurements for functional assessment of pulmonary arterial hypertension. Eur Radiol. 2007;17:1892–7. https://doi.org/10.1007/s00330-006-0559-9.
32. Laskey WK, Ferrari VA, Palevsky HI, Kussmaul WG. Pulmonary artery hemodynamics in primary pulmonary hypertension. J Am Coll Cardiol. 1993;21:406–12. https://doi.org/10.1016/0735-1097(93)90682-Q.
33. Szekanecz Z, Szücs G. Systemic sclerosis increased arterial stiffness as the marker of vascular involvement in systemic sclerosis. J Rheumatol. 2008;35:1329–33. http://www.jrheum.org/content/35/7/1329.long.
34. Darr KC, Paul DR, Morgan BJ, Thomas DP. Effects of age and training status on heart rate recovery after peak exercise. Am J Physiol - Hear Circ Physiol. 1988;254:340–3. https://doi.org/10.1152/ajpheart.1988.254.2.H340.

23

Myocardial strains from 3D displacement encoded magnetic resonance imaging

Katarina Kindberg[1,2†], Henrik Haraldsson[1,2,3*†], Andreas Sigfridsson[2,3], Jan Engvall[3], Neil B Ingels Jr[4,5], Tino Ebbers[1,2,3,6] and Matts Karlsson[1,2]

Abstract

Background: The ability to measure and quantify myocardial motion and deformation provides a useful tool to assist in the diagnosis, prognosis and management of heart disease. The recent development of magnetic resonance imaging methods, such as harmonic phase analysis of tagging and displacement encoding with stimulated echoes (DENSE), make detailed non-invasive 3D kinematic analyses of human myocardium possible in the clinic and for research purposes. A robust analysis method is required, however.

Methods: We propose to estimate strain using a polynomial function which produces local models of the displacement field obtained with DENSE. Given a specific polynomial order, the model is obtained as the least squares fit of the acquired displacement field. These local models are subsequently used to produce estimates of the full strain tensor.

Results: The proposed method is evaluated on a numerical phantom as well as *in vivo* on a healthy human heart. The evaluation showed that the proposed method produced accurate results and showed low sensitivity to noise in the numerical phantom. The method was also demonstrated *in vivo* by assessment of the full strain tensor and to resolve transmural strain variations.

Conclusions: Strain estimation within a 3D myocardial volume based on polynomial functions yields accurate and robust results when validated on an analytical model. The polynomial field is capable of resolving the measured material positions from the *in vivo* data, and the obtained *in vivo* strains values agree with previously reported myocardial strains in normal human hearts.

Background

The pumping behavior of the heart consists of complex sequences that constitute cardiac contraction and relaxation. The kinematic behavior of the heart has been analyzed extensively in order to understand the mechanisms that impair the contractile function of the heart during disease. Until recently, the only method with high enough spatial resolution of three-dimensional (3D) myocardial displacements to resolve transmural behaviors was invasive marker technology [1,2]. However, the recent development of magnetic resonance imaging (MRI) methods such as harmonic phase (HARP) analysis of tagging [3] and displacement encoding with stimulated echoes (DENSE) [4], make detailed non-invasive 3D transmural kinematic analyses of human myocardium possible for clinical and research purposes [5].

A previously presented polynomial method for cardiac strain quantification from surgically implanted markers and beads enables straightforward 3D strain computation within the myocardium [6]. For the marker and bead data, this method was shown to yield accurate and robust results, with errors smaller or comparable to a previously presented finite element method tailored for the same type of data, and has been applied to bead displacements for analyses of systolic and diastolic myocardial strains [7-9]. The method is simple in nature which aids to bridge a possible gap in understanding between different disciplines and has specifically been shown to be well suited for sparse arrays of displacement data [6]. The present work applies this polynomial method to 3D

* Correspondence: Henrik.Haraldsson@liu.se
† Contributed equally
[1]Department of Management and Engineering, Linköping University, SE-581 83 Linköping, Sweden
Full list of author information is available at the end of the article

MRI displacement data as it: 1) allows for quantification of the full 3D strain tensor; 2) resolves transmural strain variations within the myocardium, and 3) provide robustness to noise. Displacement measurements were acquired within a 3D myocardial slab at the left ventricular (LV) equator. The 3D volume was divided into segments where the polynomial method was applied to quantify the Lagrangian strain tensor. The method was evaluated on a numerical phantom as well as *in vivo* on a healthy human heart.

Methods

Strain analysis

Displacement-encoded MRI acquire displacements **u** at time t_n of timeframe n relative to a reference configuration of the myocardium, at the spatial coordinates $\mathbf{s} = (s_x, s_y, s_z)$. Lower-case letters are used to denote the coordinates of the deformed myocardium. The spatial coordinates $\mathbf{S} = (S_X, S_Y, S_Z)$ of the myocardium in the reference configuration were derived by subtracting the displacements from the spatial coordinates at the current configuration; $\mathbf{S}(t_1) = \mathbf{s} - \mathbf{u}(\mathbf{s}, t_1)$. The upper-case letters are used to denote the coordinates of the reference configuration.

$\mathbf{X} = \mathbf{X}(\mathbf{S})$ is the coordinate of a material point, defined as an infinitesimal volume of myocardial tissue, in the reference configuration and $\mathbf{x} = \mathbf{x}(\mathbf{s})$ is the coordinate after a deformation of the body. The mapping from reference to deformed configuration was modeled by a polynomial function $\mathbf{g}(\mathbf{X})$ of the coordinate of the material point in the reference configuration [6]. This polynomial position field gives an estimate $\hat{\mathbf{x}}$ of the measured coordinate **x** and can be of different order in the different reference coordinate directions, radial (X_R), circumferential (X_C), and longitudinal (X_L), depending on the number of material points along each dimension, and can thus be described as

$$\hat{\mathbf{x}} = \mathbf{g}(\mathbf{X}) = \mathbf{f}_R(X_R)\mathbf{f}_C(X_C)\mathbf{f}_L(X_L), \tag{1}$$

where $\mathbf{f}_R$, $\mathbf{f}_C$ and $\mathbf{f}_L$ are polynomial functions of X_R, X_C and X_L, respectively. The Lagrangian strain tensor **E** is a measure of deformation and is connected to the deformation gradient tensor **F** via the definition

$$\mathbf{E} = 0.5(\mathbf{F}^T\mathbf{F} - \mathbf{I}), \tag{2}$$

where **I** is the identity tensor. The deformation gradient tensor is given by differentiation, with respect to reference position, of the mapping from reference to deformed configuration, $\mathbf{F} = \partial\mathbf{x}/\partial\mathbf{X}$.

The principal strains E_1, E_2 and E_3 are obtained by diagonalization of the strain tensor, and their magnitudes are independent of any reference coordinate system. Principal strain E_1 represents maximum lengthening and E_3 represents maximum shortening.

In the subsequent analytical and *in vivo* evaluation, the 3D volumes were divided into 80 overlapping segments covering the circumference. Each of the segments was 7.5 mm thick and π/6 radians wide between the endo- and epicardial border. Within each segment the material points were transformed to local Cartesian cardiac coordinates with X_C defined as tangential to the surface of the volume and parallel with the short axis planes, X_L defined as orthogonal to the short axis planes and oriented apex-to-base, and X_R defined parallel with the short axis planes, orthogonal to X_C and oriented outwards from the volume.

Four orders of the polynomial function $\mathbf{g}(\mathbf{X})$ were analyzed. 1) A bilinear-quadratic polynomial (BLQ) was bilinear within the X_C-X_L plane and quadratic in X_R, 2) a bilinear-cubic polynomial (BLC) was bilinear within the X_C-X_L plane and cubic in X_R, 3) a linear-quadratic-cubic polynomial (LQC) was cubic in X_R, quadratic in X_C and linear in X_L and 4) a biquadratic-cubic polynomial (BQC) was biquadratic within the X_C-X_L plane and cubic in X_R. For example, for the LQC polynomial field, the estimated coordinates were given by

$$\hat{x}_i = \left(a_{1i}X_R^3 + a_{2i}X_R^2 + a_{3i}X_R + a_{4i}\right)\left(a_{5i}X_C^2 + a_{6i}X_C + a_{7i}\right)\left(a_{8i}X_L + a_{9i}\right)$$

$$= \left[X_R^3 X_C^2 X_L, \ldots, 1\right] \cdot \begin{bmatrix} c_{1i} \\ \vdots \\ c_{24i} \end{bmatrix} \tag{3}$$

where a_{ki} and c_{li} are sets of constants, $i = R, C, L$, and k and l are serial numbers for the indices. The polynomial field for each segment was determined by minimizing the squared difference between the measured and the estimated coordinates of the material points belonging to the segmentation.

$$\min_{\mathbf{c}_i} \sum_{j=1}^{m} \left(x_{ij} - \hat{x}_{ij}(\mathbf{c}_i)\right)^2, \tag{4}$$

where m is the total number of points within the segment and $\mathbf{c}_i$ are all the constants c_{li}. The polynomial was evaluated and the Lagrangian strain tensor quantified at material positions along the radial centerline within each segment. The accuracy of the polynomial function was evaluated by the residual of the polynomial mapping, determined as the root-mean-squared difference (RMS) between the measured (**x**) and estimated ($\hat{\mathbf{x}}$) coordinates within each segment. The strain analysis was performed off line using Matlab 7.6.0 (The MathWorks, Inc.).

Analytical evaluation

A previously presented analytical model [6,10] was used to evaluate the strain computation. Briefly, the model was a thick-walled cylinder that deforms to resemble the LV during systole. The cylinder was adapted to the systolic *in vivo* data with inner radius of 28.5 mm and outer radius of 42.4 mm at the reference configuration, and inner radius of 23.6 mm at the deformed configuration. Material points were sampled through the cylinder wall within ten short axis planes with 2.5 mm separation between the planes and 2.5 × 2.5 mm separation between sampled points within each plane.

Strains were computed throughout the model using the method described above. For all polynomial orders, the estimated strains were compared with the analytical strains ($\boxtimes_{IJ}$, where $I,J = R,C,L$). To mimic the acquisition of *in vivo* data, noise was added to the analytical model to investigate the noise sensitivity of the analysis method.

Three normalized distributions of noise were analyzed, each with a mean value of zero and with the standard deviations 0.05 mm, 0.10 mm and 0.30 mm, respectively. The noise levels evaluated were chosen to represent practical measurement errors in DENSE displacement measurements corresponding to SNR in the order of 35, 17 and 6.

In vivo evaluation

In vivo evaluation was performed by applying the strain quantification method to displacements acquired by DENSE MRI in a normal human heart, and comparing the results with strains obtained for normal human hearts from other studies.

Anatomical images and displacement data were acquired in a 31-year old healthy volunteer on a 1.5 T MR scanner (Philips Achieva, Philips Medical Systems, Best, The Netherlands). Displacement data were acquired, using an in-house DENSE implementation, in three cardiac phases as illustrated in Figure 1; one in systole, and two during diastole related to early and late filling. The cardiac phases were defined from balanced steady state free precession acquisition in a standard 3 chamber view with a temporal resolution of 13 ms. These images were used to define mitral valve opening (MVO) and end systole (ES), defined as aortic valve closure (AVC). These two events were used to time the measurement of displacement in systole and diastole, acquired in 3D short axis slab in two separate 3D DENSE acquisitions. For the systolic measurement, the initial reference position was encoded at end diastole (ED), defined by the ECG R-wave peak, and the displacement was read out at ES, as shown in Figure 1. For the displacement in diastole, the initial reference position was encoded at MVO and read out at both MVO + 75 ms and at MVO + 213 ms, which corresponds to approximately 22% and 62%, respectively, of the LV filling interval. The 3D DENSE acquisitions were performed with an ECG triggered, respiratory navigator gated acquisition with the following parameters: acquisition voxel size 2.5 × 2.5 × 2.5 mm, field of view 350 × 350 × 25 mm, *k*-space segmentation factor 3, EPI factor 7, parallel imaging (SENSE) with reduction factor 2, echo time 5.7 ms, repetition time 12.2 ms, balanced multi-point displacement encoding 0.35 cycles per pixel [11], 3-SPAMM [12] displacement encoding with optimized flip angle [13]. The sequence requires data acquisition of 346 heart beats. Including navigator gating, the scan time is in the order of 10-15 minutes, depending on heart rate and navigator efficiency. For this DENSE sequence, a noise level of about 0.05 mm can be expected for a typical in-vivo measurement.

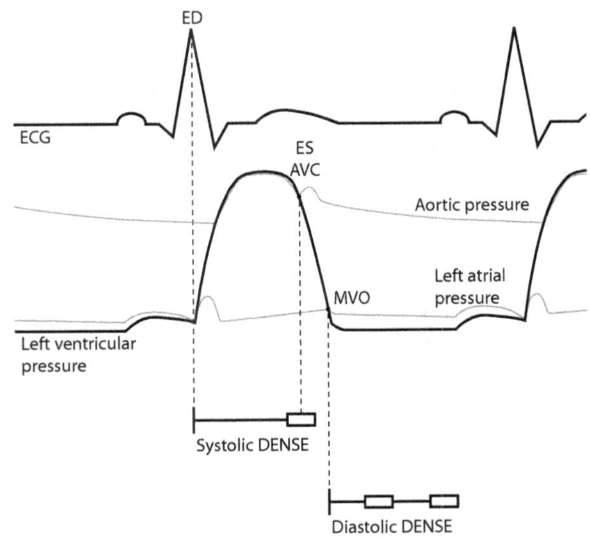

Figure 1 Timing of acquisition. Definitions of the time frames of end diastole (ED), end systole (ES), mitral valve opening (MVO) and the two time frames during diastolic filling (75 ms and 213 ms after MVO, respectively). ED is defined at the ECG R-wave peak and ES at aortic valve closure (AVC).

Segmentation of the myocardium was performed using the freely available software Segment [14]. To avoid that non-myocardial tissue could affect the myocardial strain estimates, the segmentation was conservative, excluding uncertain areas or voxels. The phase of the DENSE MRI is proportional to the myocardial displacement, but can be an arithmetic modulo 2π, which can be represented by wrapping the phase into the interval -π to π. Using the segmentation to outline the myocardium, the MRI phase was unwrapped [15] using a multigrid solver to the Poisson equations [16].

Systolic Lagrangian strains were analyzed at ES, with reference configuration at ED. Diastolic Lagrangian strains were analyzed during LV filling with reference configuration at MVO.

The research has been performed with informed consent, approved by the Regional Ethical Review Board in Linköping and carried out in compliance with the Helsinki Declaration.

Results

Analytical evaluation

The size of the errors of estimated strains is dependent on the spatial resolution of the sampled displacements [6]. Given the analytical strain components E_{IJ} of the model, the absolute errors of the estimated strains in the analytical model, $\varepsilon_{IJ} = |\boxtimes_{IJ}-E_{IJ}|$, were computed for each polynomial configuration order, integrated throughout each plane and averaged over the planes. For the noise free case, the mean ± SD error for the strain components of each polynomial order were BLQ: 0.0098 ± 0.0067, BLC: 0.0125 ± 0.0092, LQC: 0.0068 ± 0.0016, BQC: 0.0070 ± 0.0017. The errors for each component, respectively, from the linear-quadratic-cubic polynomial, for which the smallest mean errors were obtained, were ε_{RR} = 0.0081 for the radial strain, ε_{CC} = 0.0054, ε_{LL} = 0.0089, ε_{RC} = 0.0072, ε_{RL} = 0.0048 and ε_{CL} = 0.0067. The LQC RMS differences, i.e. the residual of the polynomial mapping, averaged within the analytical model, were $RMSx_R$ = 0.030 mm in the radial direction, $RMSx_C$ = 0.017 mm in the circumferential direction, and $RMSx_L$ = 0.0004 mm in the longitudinal direction. The sensitivities to noise for each polynomial are plotted in Figure 2. The LQC polynomial yielded the smallest mean errors in the ideal situation and for a simulated noise with a standard deviation of 0.05 mm while the BLQ polynomial yielded the smallest mean error for the cases with 0.10 and 0.30 mm standard deviation of noise.

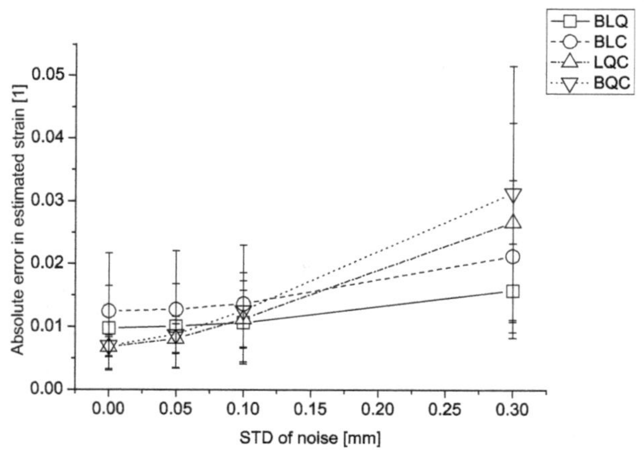

Figure 2 Sensitivities to noise. The mean ± SD absolute error in estimated strain of each polynomial for different extents of noise on the analytical model. BLQ: bilinear-quadratic polynomial, BLC: bilinear-cubic polynomial, LQC: linear-quadratic-cubic polynomial, BQC: biquadratic-cubic polynomial.

In vivo evaluation

The LQC and the BQC polynomials yielded the smallest maximum RMS differences in both systole and diastole. The results from the LQC polynomial are analyzed in further detail below. A mid-section (comprised of the short axis slices 5-7) is shown in Figure 3, 4, 5 and 6.

Systole

The systolic strain components estimated using the polynomial method are shown in Figure 3. For comparison, Figure 4 shows the corresponding components estimated using a finite element method [17].

Maximum lengthening (up to 0.74) was found in the subendocardium in the septum and lateral free wall. Maximum shortening (down to -0.35) was found in the subendocardium and was essentially evenly distributed throughout the plane.

For all three directions, the lowest RMS values were found in septum and the highest values in the posterior wall. $RMSx_R$ was within the range 0.13 - 0.40 mm, $RMSx_C$ 0.09 - 0.21 mm, and $RMSx_L$ 0.09 - 0.24 mm.

Diastole

All diastolic strain components at 75 ms (22% of the filling interval) and 213 ms (62%) after MVO at the mid-section of the 3D volume are shown in Figure 5.

The diastolic principal strains at 213 ms after MVO at the mid-section of the 3D volume are shown in Figure 6. Maximum lengthening (up to 0.35) was found in the postero-lateral wall while maximum shortening was essentially evenly distributed over the plane.

The highest RMS values were found in the posterior wall at 75 ms after MVO and in the anterior and posterior walls at 213 ms after MVO. The RMS values ranged from 0.07 mm to 0.40 mm for all directions at both diastolic times, except $RMSx_R$ at 75 ms after MVO which approached 0.50 mm in a small region in the posterior wall.

Discussion

The proposed myocardial strain quantification method was initially developed for strain computation on data from a surgically implanted transmural bead array. However, this work shows that the method can be extended to be used with displacement data from displacement-encoded MRI.

This work uses a polynomial function to find a differentiable expression from the discrete displacement field. This polynomial function assumes continuous displacement in the myocardium, which reflects the connective properties of the myocardial tissue. This a priori

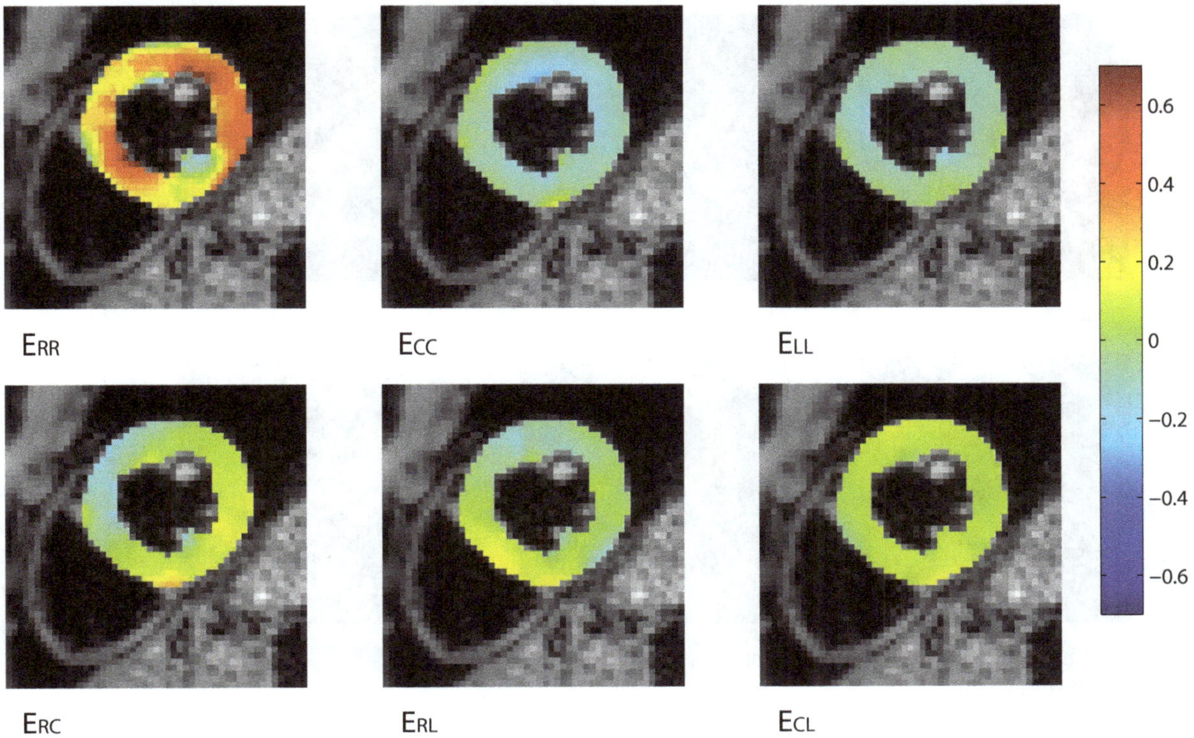

Figure 3 Systolic strains. All components of the end-systolic strain tensor at the mid-section of the 3D volume in a healthy volunteer estimated using the polynomial method.

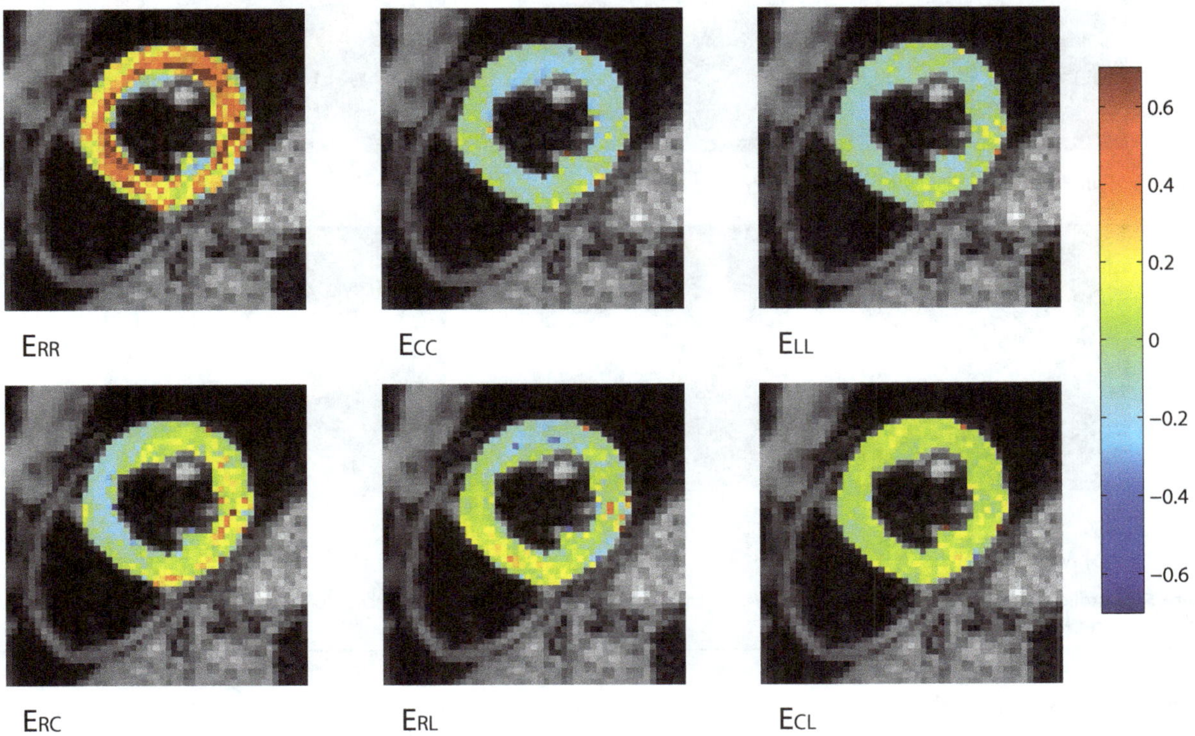

Figure 4 Systolic strains. All components of the end-systolic strain tensor at the mid-section of the 3D volume in a healthy volunteer estimated using a finite element method.

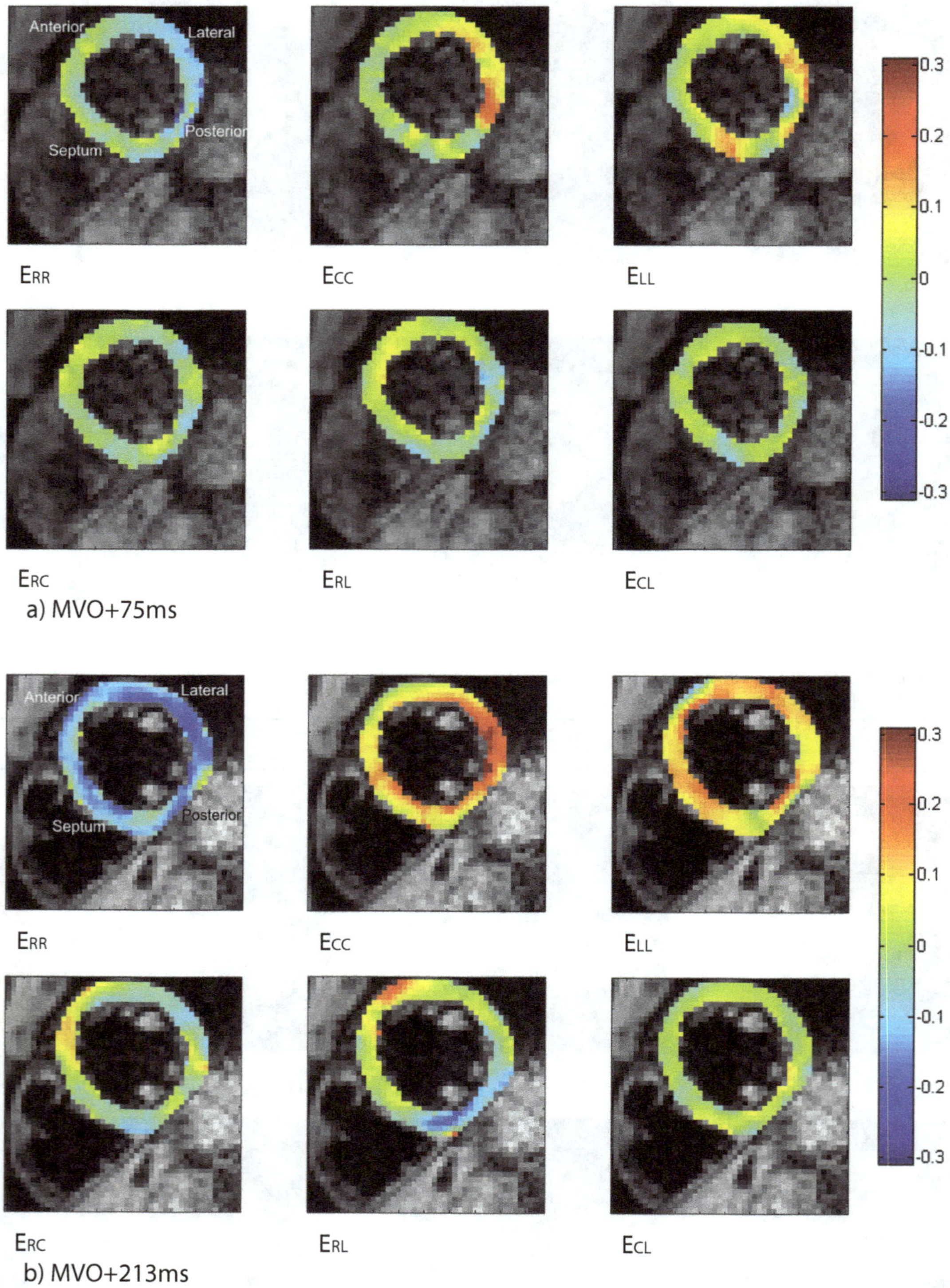

Figure 5 Diastolic strains. All components of the diastolic Lagrangian strain tensor at the mid-section of the 3D volume in a healthy volunteer. a) At 75 ms after MVO; b) At 213 ms after MVO.

information helps making the estimation more robust to noise.

The optimal order of the polynomial functions in equation (1) depends on the number of material points along each dimension, which in turn depends on the spatial resolution of the data, wall thickness and the sizes of the finite segments. Generally, the number of unknown constants in the polynomial should be less

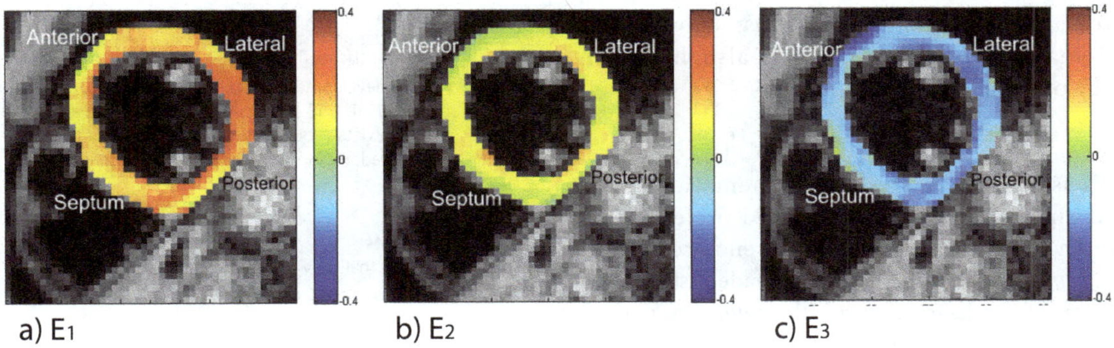

Figure 6 Diastolic principal strains. Diastolic principal strains at the mid-section of the 3D volume in a healthy volunteer, at 213 ms after MVO. a) E1; b) E2; c) E3.

than the number of measured points along each dimension, which implies that a third order polynomial requires at least five measured material points along the corresponding dimension, a second order polynomial requires at least four points and a first order polynomial requires at least three points. Furthermore, to avoid an undetermined problem, the number of data points must be equal or greater than the number of coefficients in the minimization. This implies that the minimum number of required data points depends on the polynomial orders; BLQ requires 12 data point, BLC 16, LQC 24, and BQC 36. Hence, the polynomial order is limited by the number of included data points. This requirement was fulfilled for the *in vivo* evaluation; however, the margin for the BQC polynomial was small at some locations of the myocardium.

Four different polynomial orders were evaluated. The smallest absolute errors of the estimated strains in the analytical model in the presence of low noise were obtained with a linear-quadratic-cubic polynomial. In the subsequent *in vivo* validation, the *in vivo* results of the linear-quadratic-cubic polynomial were analyzed in detail. Given the incumbent spatial resolution, the restriction on $\mathbf{f}_R(X_R)$ was the wall thickness at the late diastolic time frame and the restrictions on $\mathbf{f}_C(X_C)$ and $\mathbf{f}_L(X_L)$ were the width and height of each segment, respectively. The width ($\pi/6$ radians) and height (7.5 mm) of each segment were kept small in order to resolve local variations of deformation.

The RMS differences between the acquired *in vivo* coordinates and the coordinates estimated using the polynomial fitting method reflect the accuracy of the polynomial fitting, giving a comprehension of the extent to which the coordinates estimated by the polynomial fit to the acquired *in vivo* coordinates. For both systolic and diastolic data, the RMS differences of the LQC polynomial were highest in the posterior wall. For the systolic data the region of highest RMS differences was close to the posterior papillary muscle, which might have caused locally irregular displacements. The RMS differences may furthermore be affected by the spatially varying signal-to-noise ratio in the DENSE measurement [18]. For the diastolic data, the region of highest RMS differences coincided with the region of thinnest wall. The present implementation of the method used the same polynomial order for each segment within the 3D volume. If a data set with large variations in wall thickness is considered, e.g. a 3D slab comprising an infarct with thin wall near the infarcted myocardium, the highest accuracy could be obtained by local adjustment of the size of the segments to the size of the infarcted region and adapting the polynomial order to wall thickness and segment width.

Systolic radial, circumferential and longitudinal strains, as well as systolic circumferential-longitudinal shear, show agreement with systolic strains previously reported for human myocardium [19,20]. E_{RC}: We observed somewhat higher magnitudes of radial-circumferential shear strain than the results of Moore et al. [19], and we observed the lowest values in the anterior region of the myocardium while Moore et al. reported the lowest values in septum. E_{RL}: The observed radial-longitudinal shear values fits within mean ± 2SD of the values reported by Moore et al. [19].

Diastolic function of the LV is determined by a complex sequence of many interrelated events and parameters including active relaxation, elastic recoil, passive filling characteristics, heart rate and inotropic state. Diastolic LV filling is a highly dynamic process with early and late transmitral inflows. Thus a detailed analysis of myocardial strain during diastole requires resolving the temporal process of diastolic filling.

The highest values of circumferential strain during the first 213 ms of diastolic filling were observed in the postero-lateral wall. The same quantitative behavior has been reported in previous studies of early diastolic strains in normal human hearts [21,22]. Radial strain, interpreted as wall thinning during diastole, was most apparent in the lateral wall, which also has been reported by others [21].

Limitations

This work is limited to study the kinematics of the heart, focusing on strain. Strain should preferably be related to an unloaded, stress free reference configuration. Using *in vivo* data, there is no unloaded, stress free configuration of the heart. Instead, the reference configurations correspond to defined time points in the cardiac cycle. The strain presented in this, and similar articles within the field, therefore disregards the residual strain needed to study cardiac kinetics as opposed to kinematics.

In vivo validation of strain is challenging, which is why an analytical model was included in the validation. The analytical model can however never fully describe the cardiac kinematics. For *in vivo* estimation, the quality of the strain measurements is highly dependent on the quality of the underlying displacement data. While the polynomial fit reduces sensitivity-to-noise in the measurements, image artifacts or errors in the displacement measurements can deteriorate the strain estimates. Improving the DENSE acquisitions is an active field in the MRI research community, and strain analysis methods like the one presented in this paper will benefit directly from such improvements.

Conclusions

In conclusion, the proposed method for strain estimation within a 3D myocardial volume yields accurate results when validated on an analytical model. The polynomial field is capable of resolving the measured material positions from the *in vivo* data, and the obtained *in vivo* strains agree with previously reported myocardial strains in normal human hearts.

Acknowledgements

The study was supported by grants from Swedish Heart-Lung Foundation and Swedish Research Council.

Author details

[1]Department of Management and Engineering, Linköping University, SE-581 83 Linköping, Sweden. [2]Center for Medical Image Science and Visualization (CMIV), Linköping University, SE-581 85 Linköping, Sweden. [3]Department of Medical and Health Sciences, Linköping University, SE-581 85 Linköping, Sweden. [4]Department of Cardiothoracic Surgery, School of Medicine, Stanford University, Stanford, CA 94305, USA. [5]Research Institute of the Palo Alto Medical Foundation, Palo Alto, CA 94305, USA. [6]Department of Science and Technology, Linköping University, SE-581 83 Linköping, Sweden.

Authors' contributions

KK developed the analysis method, participated in the study design, carried out the analysis of the data, participated and coordinated the writing of the manuscript. HH participated in the study design, participated in the design of the data acquisition, participated in writing the manuscript. AS participated in the design of the data acquisition, participated in writing the manuscript. JE participated in the design of the data acquisition. NBI participated in the development of the analysis method, participated in the writing of the manuscript. TE participated in the study design, participated in the design of the data acquisition. MK participated in the design of the study. All authors read and approved the final manuscript.

Competing interests

The authors declare that they have no competing interests.

References

1. Ingels NB Jr: **Daughters GT, 2nd, Stinson EB, Alderman EL: measurement of midwall myocardial dynamics in intact man by radiography of surgically implanted markers.** *Circulation* 1975, **52(5)**:859-867.
2. Cheng A, Langer F, Rodriguez F, Criscione JC, Daughters GT, Miller DC, Ingels NB Jr: **Transmural cardiac strains in the lateral wall of the ovine left ventricle.** *Am J Physiol Heart Circ Physiol* 2005, **288(4)**:H1546-1556.
3. Osman NF, Kerwin WS, McVeigh ER, Prince JL: **Cardiac motion tracking using CINE harmonic phase (HARP) magnetic resonance imaging.** *Magn Reson Med* 1999, **42(6)**:1048-1060.
4. Aletras AH, Ding S, Balaban RS, Wen H: **DENSE: displacement encoding with stimulated echoes in cardiac functional MRI.** *J Magn Reson* 1999, **137(1)**:247-252.
5. Zhong X, Spottiswoode BS, Meyer CH, Kramer CM, Epstein FH: **Imaging three-dimensional myocardial mechanics using navigator-gated volumetric spiral cine DENSE MRI.** *Magn Reson Med* 2010, **64(4)**:1089-1097.
6. Kindberg K, Karlsson M, Ingels NB Jr, Criscione JC: **Nonhomogeneous strain from sparse marker arrays for analysis of transmural myocardial mechanics.** *J Biomech Eng* 2007, **129(4)**:603-610.
7. Carlhall CJ, Nguyen TC, Itoh A, Ennis DB, Bothe W, Liang D, Ingels NB, Miller DC: **Alterations in transmural myocardial strain: an early marker of left ventricular dysfunction in mitral regurgitation?** *Circulation* 2008, **118(14 Suppl)**:S256-262.
8. Coppola BA, Omens JH: **Role of tissue structure on ventricular wall mechanics.** *Mol Cell Biomech* 2008, **5(3)**:183-196.
9. Kindberg K, Carlhall C, Karlsson M, Nguyen TC, Cheng A, Langer F, Rodriguez F, Daughters GT, Miller DC, Ingels NB Jr: **Transmural strains in the ovine left ventricular lateral wall during diastolic filling.** *J Biomech Eng* 2009, **131(6)**:061004.
10. McCulloch AD, Omens JH: **Non-homogeneous analysis of three-dimensional transmural finite deformation in canine ventricular myocardium.** *J Biomech* 1991, **24(7)**:539-548.
11. Zhong X, Helm PA, Epstein FH: **Balanced multipoint displacement encoding for DENSE MRI.** *Magn Reson Med* 2009, **61(4)**:981-988.
12. Tsao J, Laurent D: **N-SPAMM for Efficient Displacement-Encoded Acquisition in Myocardial Tagging.** *Proceedings of the 13th Annual Meeting of ISMRM: 2005* Miami Beach, FL, USA; 2005.
13. Stuber M, Spiegel MA, Fischer SE, Scheidegger MB, Danias PG, Pedersen EM, Boesiger P: **Single breath-hold slice-following CSPAMM myocardial tagging.** *MAGMA* 1999, **9(1-2)**:85-91.
14. Heiberg E, Sjogren J, Ugander M, Carlsson M, Engblom H, Arheden H: **Design and validation of Segment-freely available software for cardiovascular image analysis.** *BMC Med Imaging* 2010, **10**:1.
15. Moon-Ho Song S, Napel S, Pelc NJ, Glover GH: **Phase unwrapping of MR phase images using Poisson equation.** *IEEE Trans Image Process* 1995, **4(5)**:667-676.
16. Farnebäck G, Rydell J, Ebbers T, Andersson M, Knutsson H: **Efficient Computation of the Inverse Gradient on Irregular Domains.** *Computer Vision, 2007 ICCV 2007 IEEE 11th International Conference on: 2007* 2007, 1-8, IEEE.
17. Waldman LK, Fung YC, Covell JW: **Transmural myocardial deformation in the canine left ventricle. Normal in vivo three-dimensional finite strains.** *Circ Res* 1985, **57(1)**:152-163.
18. Sigfridsson A, Haraldsson H, Ebbers T, Knutsson H, Sakuma H: **In vivo SNR in DENSE MRI; temporal and regional effects of field strength, receiver**

coil sensitivity and flip angle strategies. *Magn Reson Imaging* 2011, **29(2)**:202-208.

19. Moore CC, Lugo-Olivieri CH, McVeigh ER, Zerhouni EA: **Three-dimensional systolic strain patterns in the normal human left ventricle: characterization with tagged MR imaging.** *Radiology* 2000, **214(2)**:453-466.
20. Hess AT, Zhong X, Spottiswoode BS, Epstein FH, Meintjes EM: **Myocardial 3D strain calculation by combining cine displacement encoding with stimulated echoes (DENSE) and cine strain encoding (SENC) imaging.** *Magn Reson Med* 2009, **62(1)**:77-84.
21. Kuijer JP, Marcus JT, Gotte MJ, van Rossum AC, Heethaar RM: **Three-dimensional myocardial strains at end-systole and during diastole in the left ventricle of normal humans.** *J Cardiovasc Magn Reson* 2002, **4(3)**:341-351.
22. Ennis DB, Epstein FH, Kellman P, Fananapazir L, McVeigh ER, Arai AE: **Assessment of regional systolic and diastolic dysfunction in familial hypertrophic cardiomyopathy using MR tagging.** *Magn Reson Med* 2003, **50(3)**:638-642.

Volumetric BOLD fMRI simulation: from neurovascular coupling to multivoxel imaging

Zikuan Chen[1*] and Vince Calhoun[1,2]

Abstract

Background: The blood oxygenation-level dependent (BOLD) functional magnetic resonance imaging (fMRI) modality has been numerically simulated by calculating single voxel signals. However, the observation on single voxel signals cannot provide information regarding the spatial distribution of the signals. Specifically, a single BOLD voxel signal simulation cannot answer the fundamental question: is the magnetic resonance (MR) image a replica of its underling magnetic susceptibility source? In this paper, we address this problem by proposing a multivoxel volumetric BOLD fMRI simulation model and a susceptibility expression formula for linear neurovascular coupling process, that allow us to examine the BOLD fMRI procedure from neurovascular coupling to MR image formation.

Methods: Since MRI technology only senses the magnetism property, we represent a linear neurovascular-coupled BOLD state by a magnetic susceptibility expression formula, which accounts for the parameters of cortical vasculature, intravascular blood oxygenation level, and local neuroactivity. Upon the susceptibility expression of a BOLD state, we carry out volumetric BOLD fMRI simulation by calculating the fieldmap (established by susceptibility magnetization) and the complex multivoxel MR image (by intravoxel dephasing). Given the predefined susceptibility source and the calculated complex MR image, we compare the MR magnitude (phase, respectively) image with the predefined susceptibility source (the calculated fieldmap) by spatial correlation.

Results: The spatial correlation between the MR magnitude image and the magnetic susceptibility source is about 0.90 for the settings of T_E = 30 ms, B_0 = 3 T, voxel size = 100 micron, vessel radius = 3 micron, and blood volume fraction = 2%. Using these parameters value, the spatial correlation between the MR phase image and the susceptibility-induced fieldmap is close to 1.00.

Conclusion: Our simulation results show that the MR magnitude image is not an exact replica of the magnetic susceptibility source (spatial correlation ≈ 0.90), and that the MR phase image conforms closely with the susceptibility-induced fieldmap (spatial correlation ≈ 1.00).

Keywords: Bold fMRI, Neurovascular coupling, Neuroactive blob (NAB), Blood magnetism, Intravoxel dephasing, Voxelization, Magnetic fieldmap, Spatial correlation

Background

Blood oxygenation-level dependent (BOLD) functional magnetic resonance imaging (fMRI) has been widely accepted for brain functional mapping and neuroimaging [1-6]. The imaging principle of BOLD fMRI is that: a neuroactivity incurs cerebral vascular blood magnetism perturbation that can be detected by magnetic resonance imaging (MRI). In neurophysiology, the BOLD fMRI can be described by a neurovascular coupling model as follows [7-11]: a neuronal activity incurs a vascular response in terms of changes in cerebral blood flow (CBF), cerebral blood volume (CBV), and cerebral metabolic rate of oxygen ($CMRO_2$). The neuroactivity-induced biomagnetic susceptibility perturbation can be detected by T2*-weighted MRI (T2*MRI) [12]. An overall BOLD fMRI model can be decomposed into a cascade of two modules [13]. One is a neurophysiology module that addresses the vascular response to a neuroactivity in context of neurovascular coupling [7-11]; The neurovascular coupling process produces an intravascular blood biomagnetism perturbation that is

* Correspondence: zchen@mrn.org
[1]The Mind Research Network and LBERI, Albuquerque 87106, NM, USA
Full list of author information is available at the end of the article

detectable by T2*MRI [12]. Another is a MRI technology module dedicated to imaging the susceptibility-expressed neurovascular coupling states. Despite its wide acceptance for neuroimaging and brain mapping, the BOLD fMRI mechanism is not fully understood [5,14,15]. Specifically, the complicated neurovascular-coupled BOLD process is not fully understood, and the imaging performance of T2*MRI detection on a BOLD state has never been quantitatively examined in a multi-voxel simulation.

In past decades, there have been many published reports on numerical simulations of BOLD mechanism [1,6,16-18]. To our knowledge, previous BOLD simulations were carried out for investigating single voxel signals and did not address multiple voxels. This may be partially due to the computational burden and the implementation difficulty in manipulating a large 3D image matrix (e.g. 2048 × 2048 × 2048 in our simulation). In practice, a BOLD fMRI experiment produces a 4D dataset that consists of a time series of 3D image matrices (typically in size of 64 × 64 × 32 voxels) captured by T2*MRI at a discrete time point (snapshot). A multivoxel image offers many spatial features, such as "contrast and texture", "geometry: edge/shape/pattern", "topography", "topology", and so on. Furthermore, given an input source and its corresponding output image, we can assess its overall imaging performance in terms of point spread function, spatial invariance/variance, and linearity/nonlinearity of a digital imaging system.

Since T2*MRI is designed to sense an inhomogeneous fieldmap that is established via magnetization of an inhomogeneous susceptibility distribution, the underlying source of fMRI is the susceptibility-expressed distribution of a neurovascular coupling state. Therefore, for numerical BOLD fMRI simulation, we need numerically characterize the neurovascular coupling process in terms of biomagnetism susceptibility perturbation for the purpose of T2*MRI detectibility. Given a susceptibility map (representing a snapshot of dynamic BOLD susceptibility perturbation), we can carry out T2*MRI simulation in a way similar to BOLD voxel signal simulations [19-21]. Intuitively, a multivoxel BOLD fMRI simulation may be implemented by spatially arranging individual voxel signal values. In the implementation, nonetheless, we need account for the electromagnetic interaction among the voxels (due to the nonlocal effect of vascular blood magnetization [22]), especially for the magnetic influence from vasculatures in surrounding voxels that may influence the BOLD voxel signal by 10% [23].

In this paper, we propose a volumetric BOLD fMRI model that deals with a cortical field of view (FOV), as a whole matrix (without dividing into submatrices), in which the magnetic influence among the intra-FOV vasculatures are accounted for during the fieldmap calculation using a Fourier technique [16,23-25]. After calculation of the fieldmap over the FOV, we proceed to calculate the output image of T2*MRI based on intra-voxel dephasing. Upon the forward BOLD fMRI simulation, we obtain a complex-valued image (consisting of a pair of magnitude and phase parts) at each snapshot time. By comparing the MR magnitude image with the susceptibility source in a measure of spatial correlation, thereby evaluating how well the susceptibility source can be reproduced in the MR magnitude image. Meanwhile, we may compare the MR phase image with the fieldmap, thereby justifying the practice of fieldmap measurement by MR phase imaging. It is noted that the fieldmap is spatially different from the susceptibility source by a 3D convolution [13,22,26], therefore, we do not expect a morphological match between the susceptibility map and either the fieldmap or the phasemap.

The neurovascular coupling process is a complicated neurophysiological process. Experiments have shown that the BOLD activity in response to a neuroactivity may be described as a linear response model [7,8,27-32]. For the implementation of numerical simulation, we propose a linear neurovascular coupling formula to account for the biomagnetic susceptibility contributions from various neurovascular coupling aspects, such as neuroactivity (NAB: neuroactivity blob), vasculature (CBV: cerebral blood volume), blood physiology (CBF: cerebral blood flow), and blood metabolism ($CMRO_2$: cerebral metabolism rate of oxygen).

A BOLD fMRI study produces a 4D MR dataset, of which each 3D volume at a time point is interpreted as a snapshot of a dynamic BOLD state. The 4D BOLD fMRI data acquisition can be numerically simulated by a train of 3D T2*MRI snapshots provided the dynamic susceptibility perturbation is numerically specified for each snapshot time. In this report, we will only focus on the snapshot capture of a susceptibility-expressed BOLD physiological state at a specific time point. Our approach is general and we can implement a dynamic 4D BOLD fMRI simulation by repeating the snapshot imaging at a series of time points at more computation cost.

Methods

We motivate our approach by looking at a typical neuroimage as shown in Figure 1, which can be modeled as a population of local neuroactivity blobs (NAB). A spatially localized NAB is inferred from an fMRI dataset and is interpreted as (or related to) the underlying neuronal activity (neuronal origin). Because this inference is based on MR magnitude images, it is important to evaluate how well a MR magnitude image can represent a snapshot of the neuronal origin. Since the T2*MRI detection is a typical noninvasive 3D imaging modality, it is possible (virtually necessary) to quantitatively assess

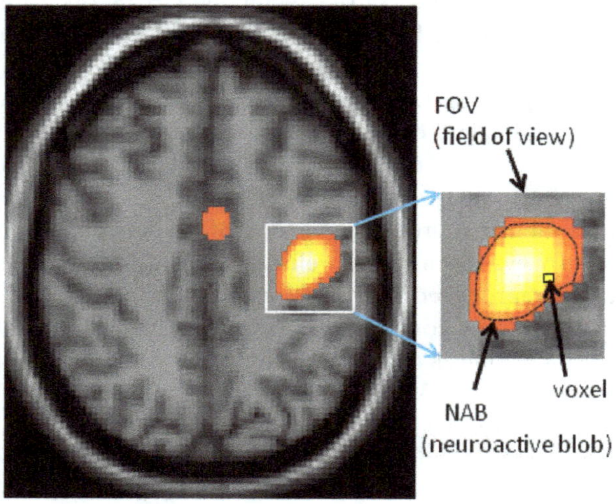

Figure 1 Illustration of a local neuroactive blob (NAB) observed at cerebral cortex by fMRI experiment. Conventionally, a NAB is inferred from an fMRI data and is considered as a local neuronal activity. However this convention has not been numerically verified from fMRI physics. This paper proposes a volumetric BOLD fMRI computation model to quantitatively examine the multivoxel fMRI formation of a magnetic susceptibility expressed BOLD state under a linear NAB-modulated neurovascular coupling assumption. Simulations are rendered over a 3D cortical FOV that contains a NAB with adequate margins in an array of vasculature-laden voxels. (The image shown in Figure 1 was taken with the written consent of the subject for a separate study in our group. The image acquisition protocol was approved by the Mind Research Network review board).

the neuronal origin inference from MR images by following the medical imaging principle: predefining an input source, predicting its output image by numerical simulation (or phantom experimental verification when applicable), and then comparing the obtained output image with the predefined input source. Accordingly, we address the NAB inference issue in Figure 1 by numerically simulating the neurovascular coupling process and the BOLD fMRI detection technology by the following steps: 1) delineating a cortical FOV that is ample enough to enclose a NAB, as demonstrated in Figure 1; 2) defining a susceptibility-expressed BOLD state under the NAB-modulated neurovascular coupling; and 3) carrying out the multivoxel BOLD fMRI simulation for a predefined susceptibility source. Upon the completion of BOLD fMRI simulation, we compare the MR magnitude image with the predefined susceptibility source in a measure of spatial correlation. A key benefit of our approach is we produce a full 3D image in form of a multivoxel matrix, in contrast to the many previous studies which focused only on one or a few voxels.

The overall diagram for the computational model of neurovascular coupling and BOLD fMRI is shown in Figure 2, which consists of two cascaded modules: 1) the "neurophysiology" module for the neurovascular coupling process from a neuronal origin to its vascular response, which should be phenotypically expressed in terms of biomagnetic susceptibility distribution for the purpose of MRI detection, and 2) the "MRI technology" module for imaging a susceptibility-expressed BOLD state by T2*MRI. According to this two-module BOLD fMRI model, the neuronal origin is a NAB-expressed neuroactivity (in response to an external stimulus, not shown), and the vascular response is a result of neurovascular coupling (numerically expressed in form of $\Delta\chi$), which in turn serves as the vascular origin of T2*MRI detection. Conventionally, the goal of brain mapping and neuroimaging is to depict the neuroactivity origin from MR magnitude images, as diagrammed by a grey double-directed arrow for the backward mapping as designated by "A ~ NAB". Based on the two-module model in Figure 2, the overall backward mapping of "A ~ NAB" can be decomposed into two steps: the first step is from the MR magnitude image to the vascular origin, as denoted by a black double-directed arrow and designated by "A~$\Delta\chi$", the second step is from the vascular origin to the neuronal origin (not shown in Figure 2). In this paper, we will look into the first step backward mapping of "A~$\Delta\chi$" by numerical T2*MRI simulation, and simplify the second step backward mapping by a linear neurovascular coupling model. Meanwhile, we also show another backward mapping: from a MR phase image to fieldmap as diagrammed by a black double-directed arrow as designated by "P~ΔB" in Figure 2.

Neurovascular coupling formulation

It is known in neurobiology and neurophysiology that a neuroactivity is accompanied by a complicated process of cellular, metabolic, and vascular processes. For simplification of computational implementation, we express the spatial distribution for the functional parcellation of a neuroactivity by a 3D Gaussian-shaped NAB embedded in a cortical FOV (with size $D_0 \times D_0 \times D_0$) by

$$NAB(x,y,z) = c\exp\left(-\frac{(x-x_0)^2}{\sigma_x^2} - \frac{(y-y_0)^2}{\sigma_y^2} - \frac{(z-z_0)^2}{\sigma_z^2}\right), \quad |x-x_0| \le \frac{D_0}{2},\ |y-y_0| \le \frac{D_0}{2},\ |z-z_0| \le \frac{D_0}{2} \tag{1}$$

where $(\sigma_x, \sigma_y, \sigma_z)$delineates an ellipsoidal profile ($\sigma_x = \sigma_y = \sigma_z$) for sphere, $\sigma_x = \sigma_y << \sigma_z$ for long ellipsoid or cylinder, $\sigma_x \neq \sigma_y \neq \sigma_z$ for general ellipsoid), (x_0, y_0, z_0) denotes the location of the NAB in the FOV, and c = max(NAB) represents the maximum activity at the NAB center (the activity strength is scaled by $0 < c < 1$). We should mention that a non-spherical blob like the one in Figure 1 can be formulated by a combination of several regular Gaussian-shaped NAB primitives that are

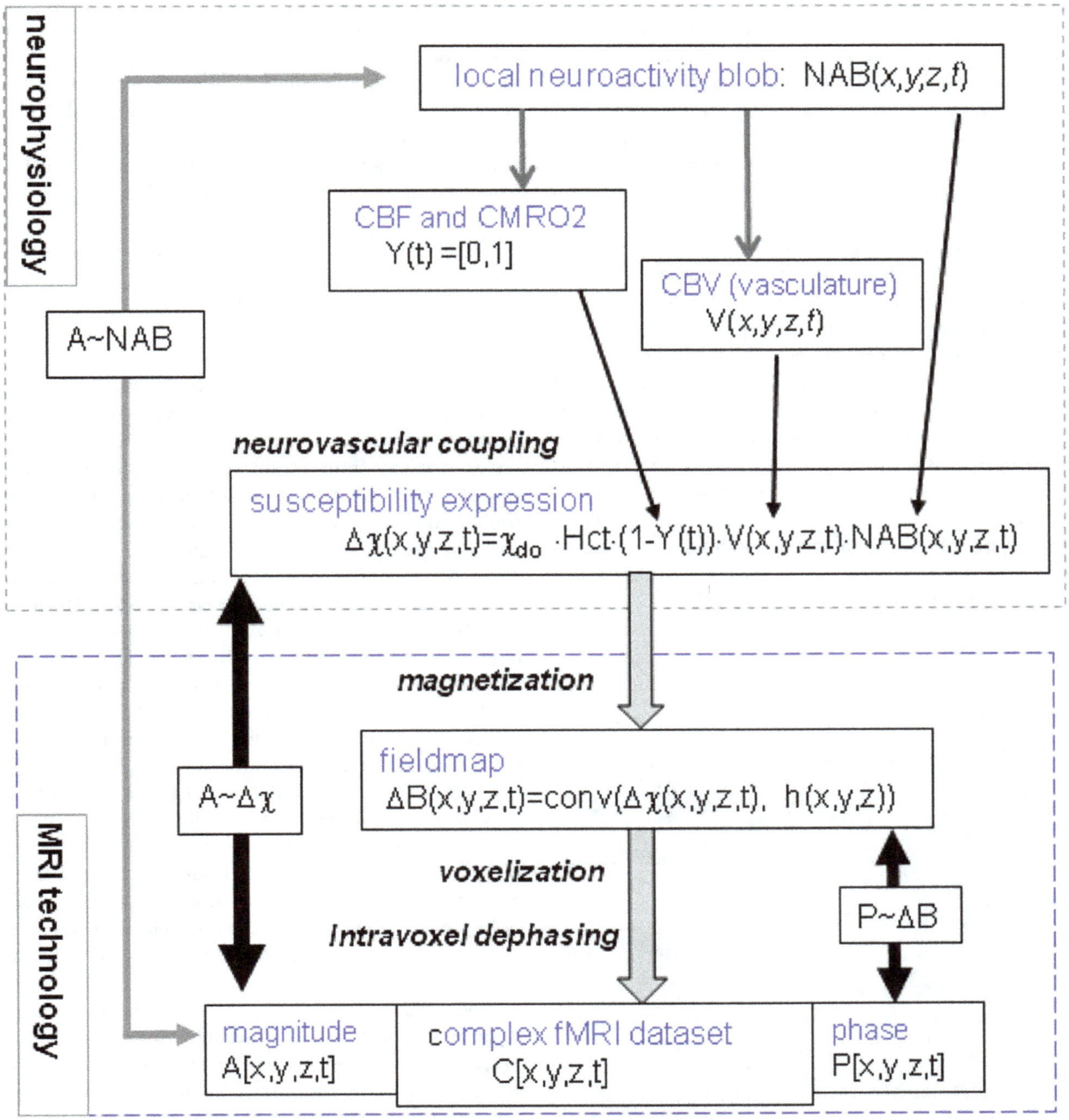

Figure 2 Overall diagram of the computational model for neurovascular coupling and BOLD fMRI. It is decomposed into a neurophysiology module (upper dashed box) and a MRI technology module (down dashed box). The linear neurovascular coupling model accounts for the local neuroactivity, blood oxygenation, and cortical vasculature by a spatiotemporal modulation. The complex fMRI dataset is resulted from susceptibility magnetization and intravoxel dephasing (T2* imaging). The complex fMRI dataset can be used for backward mappings as diagrammed by double-directed arrows. It is noted the conventional neuroimaging is diagrammed by an overall backward mapping as diagrammed by a grey double-directed arrow of A ~ NAB on the left-hand side. In this paper, we focus on the mapping from the MR magnitude image to the susceptibility source (as diagrammed by the black double-directed arrow of $A\sim\Delta\chi$), and that from the MR phase image to the fieldmap ($P\sim\Delta B$).

different in (x_0, y_0, z_0) and $(\sigma_x, \sigma_y, \sigma_z)$. The graded local neuroactivity strength over the FOV is reflected in the spatially distributed multivalues in the range of [0, c] (maximum activity strength at the NAB center, moderate strength at the NAB boundary, and zero strength outside the NAB).

In response to the neuroactivity in a NAB, the neurovascular unit regulates the cerebral microcirculation by vasodilation (increase in CBV) and a burst of blood inflow (increase in CBF). The intravascular blood oxygenation level is subject to change due to neuromodulation in the NAB, primarily occurring in the capillaries and venules. Figure 3 illustrates a neurovascular coupled blood oxygen delivery in capillary bed confined in a NAB. It is shown that the BOLD activity is spatially localized in a cortex region (NAB confinement) where the central region undergoes the maximal activity, and there is no neuronal activity outside NAB. The blood biomagnetic susceptibility perturbation is determined by the spatial modulation between the NAB distribution and the vasculature geometry. The intravascular blood volume (CBV) is determined by the vasculature geometry at a snapshot pose, and the dynamic intravascular blood flow (CBF) is determined by the intracranial blood pressure, vasculature geometry and blood fluid mechanics. All in all, for numerical simulation purpose, all these neurovascular parameters should be numerically expressed in terms of magnetic susceptibility responses (detectable by MRI technology).

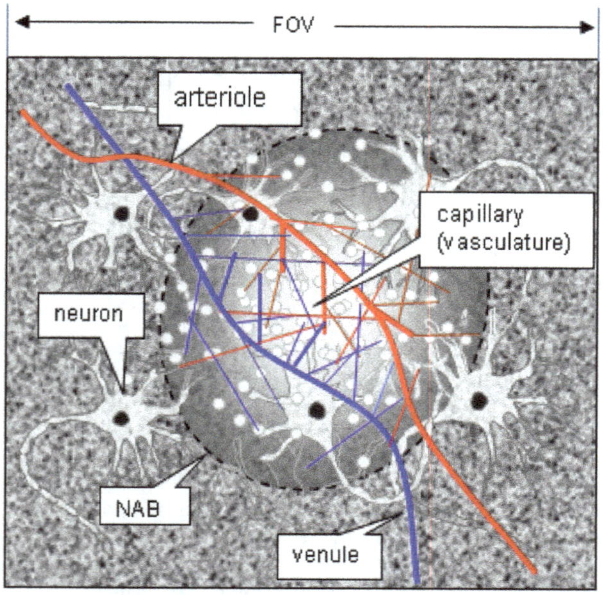

Figure 3 A 2D illustration of a localized neurovascular coupling model. The local neuroactivity is represented by a ball-shaped neuroactive blob (NAB), which confines the locality and the graded strength in a cortical FOV. The red and blue lines illustrate the oxygen-rich arterioles and oxygen-poor venules. Due to spatial weighting by NAB, the cortical regions outside the NAB has no contribution to the BOLD state. (In numerical BOLD fMRI simulation, the neuron-glial clusters are considered as the extravascular parenchyma, thus being omitted).

At a snapshot time, the cortical vasculature geometry determines the intravascular blood volume, that only takes up a fractional space of the cortical FOV, as described by blood volume fraction (*bfrac*). For human cerebral cortex, *bfrac* ≈ 2% [33]. For numerical simulation of 3D vasculature-laden FOV, we express the vasculature configuration by a binary volume that is randomly generated under the control of *bfrac*. That is,

$$V(x,y,z,t) = \begin{cases} 1, & (x,y,z) \in \text{vessel} \\ 0, & \text{otherwise} \end{cases}, \text{ with } dom(V) = FOV$$
$$\text{and } bfrac(t) = \frac{\sum_{(x,y,z)} V(x,y,z,t)}{|V|} \quad (2)$$

where $dom(V)$ denotes the space domain of the selected cortical vasculature, and $bfrac(t)$ the dynamic blood volume fraction, and |V| the volume of FOV. It is noted that the time parameter t is explicitly used to indicate the variation in vasculature geometry. We should point out that we can use *bfrac*(t) to numerically characterize the blood physiological parameters: CBV and CBF. Specifically, a vasodilation associated with CBV manifests as a slight increase in *bfrac*(t), that is $bfrac(t+\Delta t) > bfrac(t)$ for $\Delta t > 0$; and an accelerated blood flow can be equivalent to an increase in *bfrac*(t) as well. Since *bfrac* plays a control parameter during random vasculature generation (in Eq. (2)), its effect on intravascular blood physiology is exerted through the vasculature configuration geometry.

It is also known that only the red blood cells in blood stream convey oxygen that contribute to intravascular blood susceptibility perturbation. The total volume of red blood cells in normal blood is about 40%, as described in terms of hematocrit (Hct≈0.4). Blood physiology also shows that a red blood cell can carry up to 4 oxygen molecules (via attachment to 4 heme groups in a hemoglobin). Due to the oxygen detachment during microcirculation, the deoxygenated blood reveals more paramagnetism than the oxygenated blood, that is $\chi_{deoxy} > \chi_{oxy}$. Let Y(t) represent the dynamic blood oxygenation level, then (1-Y(t)) represents the dynamic deoxygenation level, that is a parameter to reflect the cerebral metabolism of oxygen ($CMRO_2$). It is noted that Y(t) = [0,1], with Y = 1 for the fully oxygenated blood in artery and Y = 0 for the fully deoxygenated blood in vein.

Based on the neurovascular-coupled blood biomagnetic perturbation mechanism, we propose a biomagnetic susceptibility expression formula for a linear neurovascular coupling model by

$$\begin{aligned} \chi_{total}(x,y,z,t) &= [\chi_{deoxy}\cdot(1-Y(t)) + \chi_{oxy}\cdot Y(t)]\cdot Hct\cdot NAB(x,y,z) \\ &\quad \cdot V(x,y,z,t) + \chi_{tissue}(x,y,z) \\ \chi_{base}(x,y,z) &\equiv \chi_{oxy}\cdot Hct\cdot NAB(x,y,z)\cdot V(x,y,z) + \chi_{tissue}(x,y,z) \\ \Delta\chi(x,y,z,t) &\equiv \chi_{total}(x,y,z,t) - \chi_{base}(x,y,z) \end{aligned} \quad (3)$$

where $\chi_{do} = \chi_{deoxy}$-χ_{oxy} = 0.27 × 4πppm (SI unit) represents the magnetic susceptibility change between deoxyhemoglobin and oxyhemoglobin, which has been used for BOLD signal simulation [17,23]. The total susceptibility χ_{total} includes contributions from both intravascular blood and extravascular tissue parenchyma. The susceptibility distribution of a selected baseline state is denoted by χ_{base}. In reference to χ_{base}, we can characterize a BOLD susceptibility perturbation state by $\Delta\chi$ in Eq. (3). Suppose the BOLD fMRI system is a linear digital imaging system, then the behavior of MR image change in reference to its baseline state can represent the intravascular susceptibility perturbation $\Delta\chi$(x, y, z, t). In other words, the linear BOLD fMRI model allows us to infer the intravascular BOLD susceptibility perturbation by observing the corresponding MR image change (in reference to their respective baselines). From Eq. (3), we can express the NAB-modulated BOLD susceptibility perturbation state by

$$\Delta\chi(x, y, z, t) = \chi_{do} \cdot (1 - Y(t)) \cdot NAB(x, y, z) \cdot V(x, y, z, t) \cdot Hct \quad (4)$$

This is a computational model for linear neurovascular coupling, which provides a mathematical formula for numerically expressing the NAB-modulated BOLD response process in a vasculature-filled FOV. Specifically, $CMRO_2$ is accounted for by Y(t), CBF and CBV by *bfrac*(t) that is implicitly embodied in V(x, y, z, t) via vasculature configuration (during vasculature geometry generation under the condition of *bfrac*(t) in Eq. (2)), and the local neuroactivity by NAB(x, y, z) which confines the neuroactivity extent and defines a graded neuroactivity strength. Usually, the blood magnetism parameter χ_{do} and the blood physiology parameter Hct assume for normal blood, which are experimentally determined constants (see Table 1).

For the neurovascular coupling formula in Eq. (4), we need to point out following aspects:

1. It is a linear neurovascular coupling formula that accounts for different neurovascular parameters by a spatiotemporal modulation. For simplicity, we do not consider the hemodynamic time lag, spatial displacement, or spatial response spread in this work, though our model will support it.

2. The BOLD susceptibility perturbation is due to the temporal modulation by the blood deoxygenation level (1-Y(t)), which is an embodiment of $CMRO_2$. The interplay among CBF, CBV and vasculature are numerically characterized by a single parameter *bfrac*(t) that reflects the blood dynamic through vasculature configuration (V (x, y, z, t)).

3. Only intravascular blood deoxyhemoglobin contributes to the BOLD susceptibility perturbation; no contribution from extravascular tissue (due to V(x, y, z) = 0 for extravascular region), nor from oxyhemoglobin (due to 1-Y = 0 for Y = 1), nor from neuronal inactive regions (due to NAB = 0).

4. The volumetric computational model can be considered as a generalization of the single voxel neurovascular coupling model ($\Delta\chi = \chi_{do}$·Hct·(1-Y)) that has been accepted for single voxel BOLD signal simulation [1,3,17,23].

Overall, a multivoxel BOLD fMRI simulation requires a predefined magnetic susceptibility distribution as the input source of T2*MRI. The susceptibility expression for a neurovascular coupling process plays a bridge between the neuroscience and MRI technology.

Table 1 Parameters and settings for numerical simulations

Parameters	Settings	Remarks
B_0	3 Tesla	Main static magnetic field
Hct	0.4 (dimensionless ratio)	Blood hematocrit
Y	0.6 (dimensionless ratio)	Oxygenation level = [0,1]
χ_{do}	0.27 × 4π ppm (SI metrics)	= χ_{dexoy} - χ_{oxy}
NAB	NAB(x, y, z) Gaussian ellipsoid	Neuroactive blob (Eq(1))
V(x, y, z)	Binary volume (radii = [2,10] μm)	Cortical vasculature (Eq(2))
FOV: $D_0 \times D_0 \times D_0$	2 × 2 × 2 mm^3	Cortical field of view
FOV support matrix	2048 × 2048 × 2048	Digital geometry (1 μm grid)
voxel: $d_0 \times d_0 \times d_0$	32 × 32 × 32, 64 × 64 × 64, 128 × 128 × 128	Three voxel sizes (1 μm grid)
$C[x_n, y_n, z_n; T_E]$	64 × 64 × 64, 32 × 32 × 32, 16 × 16 × 16	Complex multivoxel image
$A[x_n, y_n, z_n; T_E]$	Assuming non-negative	MR magnitude image(Eq(9))
$P[x_n, y_n, z_n; T_E]$	Assuming positive/zero/negative	MR phase image (Eq(9))
corrA	In a range of [0, 1]	Magnitude mapping (Eq(10)
corrP	In a range of [0, 1]	Phase mapping (Eq(11))
T_E	In a range of [0, 60] ms	Gradient echo time

Although the neurovascular coupling process is not fully understood so far, we propose a linear spatiotemporal modulation model (in Eq. (4)) that allows us to look into the effects of CBF, CBV, $CMRO_2$, and NAB on the BOLD susceptibility perturbation (which is detected by T2*MRI). In Figure 4, we illustrate a dynamic susceptibility perturbation by susceptibility timecourses of 3 voxels in a NAB, which shows that the susceptibility perturbation strength is spatially weighted by the NAB (maximum at the center and reduced toward boundary). According to Eq. (4), the numerical characterization of neurovascular-coupled 4D dynamic susceptibility perturbation $\Delta\chi(x, y, z, t)$ involves the following conditions: defining a local neuroactivity (a numerical NAB that is not necessarily in an analytic formula), generating a cortical vasculature (V(x, y, z, t)) under the control of *bfrac* (t), and assigning a value to the blood oxygenation level Y(t) (= [0, 1]). It is mentioned that if the digitization of $\Delta\chi(x, y, z, t)$ are experimentally or empirically available for a train of discrete time points (such as at the ticks t_0 through t_5 in Figure 4), it is not necessary to seek the analytic formula in Eq. (4). In the following, we will implement the numerical T2*MRI simulation for acquiring a complex MR image from a given susceptibility distribution at a snapshot time, denoted by $\Delta\chi(x, y, z)$, thus omitting the time variable t.

Forward BOLD fMRI simulation

From magnetism perturbation to fieldmap establishment

Given a snapshot of neurovascular-coupled BOLD state, $\Delta\chi(x, y, z)$, we can calculate its magnetization field distribution (resulting from the blood magnetization in a main field B_0), called the fieldmap henceforth, by [24,25,34]

$$\begin{aligned}\Delta B(x,y,z) &= IFT\left\{\left(\frac{k_z^2}{k_x^2+k_y^2+k_z^2}-\frac{1}{3}\right)\cdot FT[\Delta\chi(x,y,z)]\right\}B_0 \\ &= B_0\cdot conv(\Delta\chi(x,y,z),h(x,y,z)) \\ \text{with } h(x,y,z) &= \frac{3z^2-(x^2+y^2+z^2)}{4\pi(x^2+y^2+z^2)^{5/2}} \quad \text{(point dipole field kernel)}\end{aligned} \tag{5}$$

where *FT* and *IFT* stand for Fourier transform and inverse Fourier transform respectively, (k_x, k_y, k_z) coordinates in the Fourier domain, conv the convolution, and *h(x, y, z)* the kernel of magnetic point dipole field.

Multivoxel partition of FOV

We simulate the cortical FOV by filling it with vasculature. Figure 5 shows a 3D FOV of size $D_0 \times D_0 \times D_0$, which is filled with random vascular networks (the cortical vasculature generation technique has been reported previously [20,23]). The FOV is partitioned into voxels (voxel size = $d_0 \times d_0 \times d_0$), thereby we can represent the FOV in a small array of voxels, in which each voxel can be assigned a value by intravoxel average. The process of spatial partition into voxels and intravoxel average is called voxelization. For the vasculature V(x, y, z) in the FOV, the voxelization is expressed by

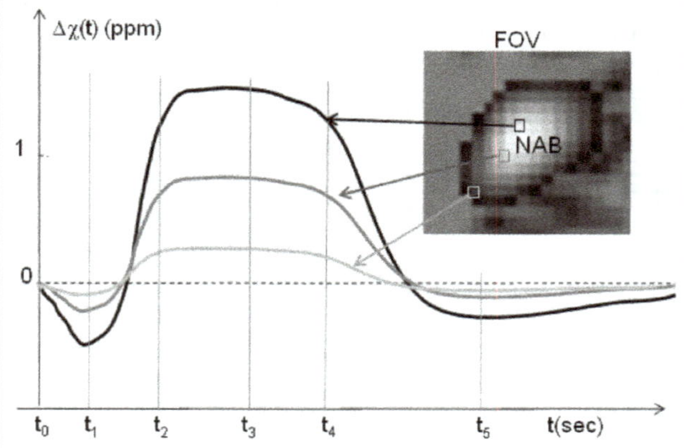

Figure 4 Illustration of dynamic magnetic susceptibility perturbation in a NAB-weighted cortical region. It is shown that the voxel at the central NAB region produces the maximum susceptibility perturbation (in comparison with the voxels outside the central NAB), and the dynamic susceptibility perturbation may assume a pres-stimulus transient initial dip (at t_1) and small post-stimulus undershoot (at t_5) in addition to the prevailing response mode (between t_2 and t_4). For dynamic BOLD fMRI simulation, the neurovascular coupling process should be numerically characterized by a dynamic magnetic susceptibility perturbation in a cortical region. It is noted that the voxel susceptibility timecourses are not necessarily mathematically tractable for numerical representations.

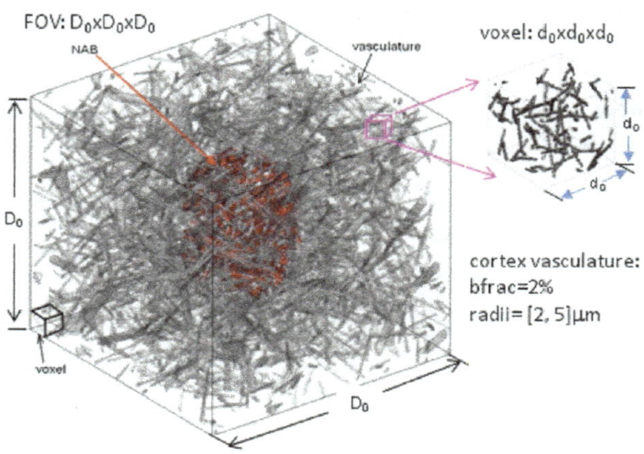

Figure 5 A typical geometry of cortical FOV that is filled with vasculature and encloses a local neuroactivity blob (NAB in red). The fMRI-detectable neurovascular coupling state is expressed as a NAB-weighted intravascular blood magnetic susceptibility perturbation distribution. The vasculature-laden FOV in size of $D_0xD_0xD_0$ is voxelized by a voxel size of $d_0xd_0xd_0$, thus producing a reduced matrix in size of $[D_0/d_0, D_0/d_0, D_0/d_0]$. The vasculature is randomly generated under a control of blood volume fraction (*bfrac*(t)), that is a parameter we use to numerically characterize CBF and CBV.

$$V[x_n, y_n, z_n] = V(x,y,z) * rect(\frac{x-x_n}{d_0}, \frac{y-y_n}{d_0}, \frac{z-z_n}{d_0}), -x| \le \frac{D_0}{2}, -y| \le \frac{D_0}{2}, -z| \le \frac{D_0}{2}$$
$$with\ rect(x,y,z) = \begin{cases} 1, -x| < 1/2, -y| < 1/2, -y| < 1/2 \\ 0, \quad \text{otherwise} \end{cases} \quad (6)$$

where * denotes the convolution, and V $[x_n, y_n, z_n]$ connotes the voxelization of V(x, y, z). It is shown that the voxelization operation (denoted by squared brackets "[ ]") suppresses the intravoxel details and produces a digital image representation of the vasculature configuration in the FOV. By applying voxelization to the 3D distributions of NAB(x, y, z), $\Delta\chi$(x, y, z), ΔB(x, y, z), we obtain the corresponding 3D matrices of NAB$[x_n, y_n, z_n]$, $\Delta\chi[x_n, y_n, z_n]$, and $\Delta B[x_n, y_n, z_n]$, respectively. For example, in our simulation (see later), the fieldmap is originally represented as a large matrix in size of 2048 × 2048 × 2048 (with a fine grid resolution as used for the digital FOV representation), which can be reduced a smaller matrix in size of 32 × 32 × 32 by voxelization with voxel size of 64 × 64 × 64.

Voxel signal calculation by intravoxel dephasing integration

Exposed to an inhomogeneous fieldmap, a proton precesses with a phase angle $\Delta\varphi(x, y, z, T_E) = \gamma \cdot \Delta B(x, y, z) \cdot T_E$, where γ is the gyromagnetic ratio. It is noted that the phase angle is different from the field value by a constant factor γT_E (Larmor law). Due to the finite dimension of a voxel (for example, d_0 = 128 micron in our simulation), its voxel signal is formed by a vector sum of all spin packets (or isochromats) inside the voxel, called intravoxel dephasing integration [19]. For a $d_0 \times d_0 \times d_0$ voxel at discrete position $[x_n, y_n, z_n]$, its BOLD signal is formed by

$$S[x_n, y_n, z_n; T_E] = \iiint_{|x-x_n|,|y-y_n|,|z-z_n|<d_0} e^{i\gamma \cdot \Delta B(x,y,z) \cdot T_E} dxdydz \quad (7)$$

where the echo time T_E is explicitly retained to remind of the T_E dependence of voxel signal (as will be demonstrated in our simulation later).

From voxel signal values to a multivoxel image

After calculating the voxel signals for all voxels in the FOV (with a specific T_E), we assemble the voxel signal values into a 3D MR matrix according to the voxelization scheme in Eq. (6) by

$$C[x_n, y_n, z_n; T_E] = \begin{cases} S[x_n, y_n, z_n; T_E], |x-x_n| < d_0, |y-y_n| < d_0, |z-z_n| < d_0 \\ void, \quad \text{otherwise} \end{cases} \quad (8)$$

which is complex-valued and explicitly T_E-dependent. Since the MR magnitude image contrast is due to a spatial distribution of voxel signal decay, we are concerned with the magnitude loss. For the phase image, we are concerned with the phase angle accumulation during the period of T_E. The magnitude loss map and phase accumulation map for a given T_E are calculated by

$$\begin{cases} A[x_n, y_n, z_n; T_E] = 1 - |C[x_n, y_n, z_n; T_E]|/|C[x_n, y_n, z_n; T_E = 0]| \\ P[x_n, y_n, z_n; T_E] = \angle C[x_n, y_n, z_n; T_E] - \angle C[x_n, y_n, z_n; T_E = 0] \end{cases} \quad (9)$$

Where $|C[x_n, y_n, z_n; T_E = 0]|$denotes the non-decay initial magnitude image and $\angle C[x_n, y_n, z_n; T_E = 0]$ the initial phase image. Henceforth, we will denote the MR magnitude and phase images as $A[x_n, y_n, z_n; T_E]$ and P $[x_n, y_n, z_n; T_E]$, respectively.

Backward mappings

In the forward BOLD fMRI calculation, we obtain a pair of MR magnitude image and phase image by Eq. (9). Considering the NAB$[x_n, y_n, z_n]$ (the voxelized version of the NAB(x, y, z) in Eq. (6)) as the neuronal origin, the conventional neuroimaging effort consists in establishing a backward mapping from the MR magnitude images to the neuronal origin, as designated by "A ~ NAB" in Figure 2. Under a linear neuruovascular coupling model, we simplify the mapping between the vascular response ($\Delta\chi$[x, y, z]) and the neuronal origin (NAB[x, y, z]) by a linear mapping in Eq. (4). On one hand, $\Delta\chi$ represents the vascular response to the neuronal origin under a neurovascular coupling process; on the other hand, it plays a vascular origin for the T2*MRI detection. In this paper, we will focus on the backward mapping from the MR magnitude image to its vascular origin as designated by "A~$\Delta\chi$" in Figure 2.

It is known that the underlying source of BOLD fMRI is the susceptibility-expressed BOLD state, which is highly dependent upon the vasculature configuration in the FOV. To reduce the effect of vessel randomness on our numerical simulation, we propose to measure the similarity of the MR magnitude image $A[x_n, y_n, z_n]$ and the predefined BOLD susceptibility map $\Delta\chi[x_n, y_n, z_n]$ by a spatial correlation coefficient as defined by

$$corrA(T_E) = \frac{\text{cov}\ (A[:; T_E], \Delta\chi[:])}{std(A[:; T_E])std(\Delta\chi[:])} \quad (10)$$

Where cov(x, y) denotes the covariance between vector x and y, std(x) the standard deviation, and ":" a nD-to-1D operator (as used by Matlab language) that reorders a high-dimensional array entries into one dimensional vector. The correlation coefficient defined in Eq. (10) gives rise to corrA ∈ [0, 1] with corrA = 1 for a perfect match (linear mapping) and corrA ≠1 for mismatch (nonlinear mapping). Since there is little decay for a short relaxation time ($A[x_n, y_n, z_n; T_E] \to 0$ for $T_E \to 0$), a meaningful corrA(T_E) should be evaluated at a relative long T_E (T_E > 0). However, a long T_E will also introduce a diffusion smearing effect, which is not addressed herein. It is noted that corrA defined in Eq. (10) is a numerical measure of the backward mapping "A~$\Delta\chi$" in Figure 2, which connotes the magnitude-vs-susceptibility correlation.

Likewise, we can measure the spatial correlation between the MR phase image $P[x_n, y_n, z_n; T_E]$ and the fieldmap $\Delta B[x_n, y_n, z_n]$ by

$$corrP(T_E) = \frac{\text{cov}\ (P[:; T_E], \Delta B[:])}{std(P[:; T_E])std(\Delta B[:])} \tag{11}$$

Likely, corrP is a numerical measure of the phase-vs-fieldmap correlation, a backward mapping designated by "P~ΔB" in Figure 2.

In summary, our computational BOLD fMRI model can be used for backward mappings: magnitude-vs-susceptibility correlation (corrA) and phase-vs-fieldmap correlation (corrP) by Eqs. (10) and (11), respectively. The goal of conventional neuroimaging and brain mapping is to render a backward mapping from MR magnitude image to neuronal origin, which consist of two steps: from the MR magnitude image to its vascular origin (as designated by "A~Δχ" and numerically measured by corrA) and then from the vascular response to its neuronal origin. In this paper, we are concerned with the mapping of "A~Δχ", with which we show the effect of MRI technology on the imaging performance of BOLD fMRI.

Results

The main parameters and their settings for the simulations we performed are listed in table 1.

The overall numerical simulation scheme is described by a flowchart in Figure 2. It starts with defining a NAB in a cortical FOV (Eq. (1)) and filling the FOV with randomly generated vascular networks (Eq. (2)). For digital geometry depiction of small vessels, the FOV is finely gridded and represented in a large support matrix in size of 2048 × 2048 × 2048 (grid resolution = 1 micron). Then the magnetic susceptibility expression of a neurovascular-coupled BOLD state is analytically described by a linear spatiotemporal modulation formula in Eq. (4). At a snapshot time, we predefine a 3D susceptibility distribution based on the following parameter settings: a Gaussian-shaped NAB, a vasculature-laden FOV (under control of *bfrac*(t) = 2%) and Y(t) = 0.6. Let B_0 = 3 T, we calculate the fieldmap from a 3D susceptibility perturbation in size of 2048 × 2048 × 2048 (assuming the same support matrix as FOV) by Eq. (5). By spatially partitioning the FOV into voxels, we calculate the voxel signals for a T_E by using the intravoxel dephasing integration in Eq. (7). At last, we assemble the voxel signal values into a 3D image matrix by Eq. (8). By repeating the multivoxel BOLD fMRI simulations for a range of T_E setting (T_E = 0:2:60 ms with an increment of 2 ms), for the different voxel sizes (128 × 128 × 128, 64 × 64 × 64, 32 × 32 × 32 micron^3), and for different vessel sizes (radii = 2 and 4 micron), we obtain a collection of MR magnitude images and phase images; from which we may observe the effect of MRI technology on the imaging performance of BOLD fMRI with respect to the echo time T_E, the image resolution, and the vessel size. In particular, we are concerned with the magnitude-vs-susceptibility correlation (corrA in Eq. (10)) and the phase-vs-fieldmap correlation (corrP in Eq. (11)). In what follows, we present the simulation results via figures.

Figure 5 shows a 3D geometry for a NAB embedded in a cortical FOV, in which the cortical vasculature is simulated with a mixture of randomly populated cylinders (radii = {2,4,8}micron). In order to show the effect of different vessel sizes, we carry out the simulations for monosized cortical vasculatures (with radii = 2 and 4 micron separately, under the condition of *bfrac* = 2%). Using monosized vasculature allows us to address the vessel-size effect on the BOLD fMRI signals (the BOLD fMRI nonlinearity due to large vessels [35]).

With 1-micron digital grid resolution, we originally represent a FOV with large support matrix in size of 2048 × 2048 × 2048. After the fieldmap calculation, we partition the fieldmap into multivoxel image arrays for three voxel sizes: 16 × 16 × 16 matrix (voxel size: 128 × 128 × 128 micron^3), 32 × 32 × 32 matrix (voxel size: 64 × 64 × 64 micron^3), and 64 × 64 × 64 matrix (voxel size 32 × 32 × 32 micron^3). With these three voxel sizes, we demonstrate the effect of image resolution on BOLD fMRI.

Figure 6 shows the NAB-profiled susceptibility perturbation map (calculated by Eq. (4)) and the subsequent fieldmap (calculated by Eq. (5)). Figure 7 shows the MR magnitude and phase images (displayed with z-slices from FOV surface to the center surface) calculated at T_E = 30 ms for voxel size = 64 × 64 × 64 micron^3. It is

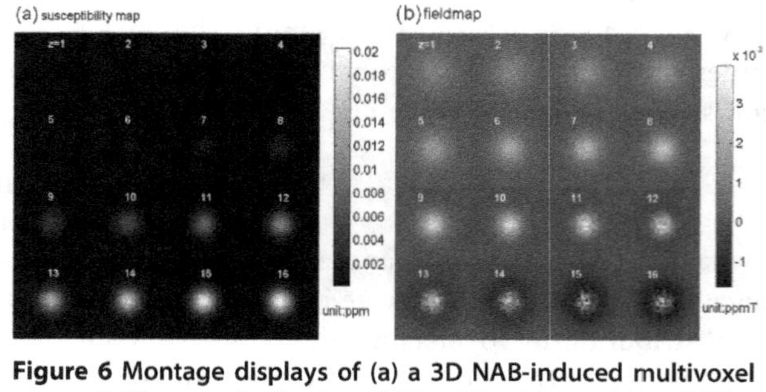

Figure 6 Montage displays of (a) a 3D NAB-induced multivoxel susceptibility map Δχ (in size of 32 × 32 × 32 matrix) and (b) the corresponding multivoxel fieldmap ΔB (calculated for B_0 = 3 T) for z-slices of z = [1,2,...,16] (z = 1 at FOV surface and z = 16 through FOV center). The 32 × 32 × 32 multivoxel matrix is calculated from a 2048 × 2048 × 2048 fine grid matrix (grid resolution = 1 micron), by voxelization with the voxel size of 64 × 64 × 64 micron^3. The 3D NAB is a Gaussian-shaped blob embedded in the cortical FOV.

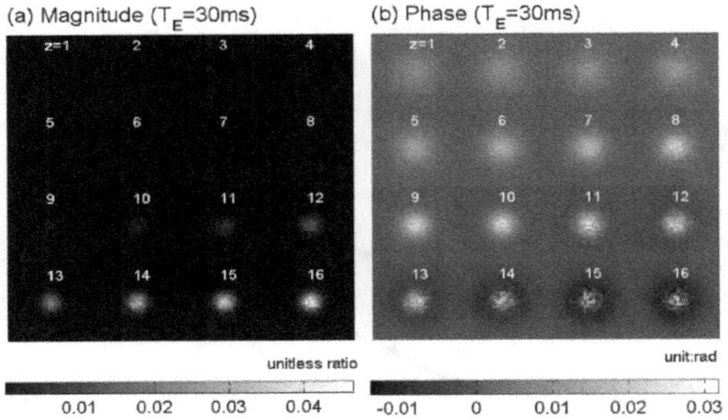

Figure 7 Montage displays of (a) the 3D multivoxel magnitude image A[x, y, z] for z = 1:1:16 and (b) the multivoxel phase image P[x, y, z] (calculated with T_E = 30 ms voxel size = 64 × 64 × 64 micron^3 and B_0 = 3 T). Note that the central z-slice of the multivoxel image is at z = 16.

noted that the magnitude image resembles the susceptibility map to a great extent, and the phase image replicates the fieldmap very well. Figure 8 shows the T_E dependence of the MR magnitude and phase images (with the central z-slice).

With the MR magnitude and phase images generated for a variety of parameter settings, we calculate the magnitude-vs-susceptibility correlation and the phase-vs-fieldmap correlation by Eqs. (10) and (11), respectively. The results are shown in Figure 9 for T_E in a range of 0 to 60 ms and three different image resolutions (see the legend). From Figure 9 we can see that the magnitude-vs-susceptibility correlation increases with respect to T_E and voxel size; on contrary, the phase-vs-fieldmap correlation decreases with respect to T_E and voxel size.

In Table 2 we present the correlation coefficients for two vasculatures (radii = 2 and 4 micron), three image resolutions (voxel size = 128 × 128 × 128, 64 × 64 × 64, and 32 × 32 × 32 micron^3), and two selected echo times (T_E = 1 ms and 30 ms).

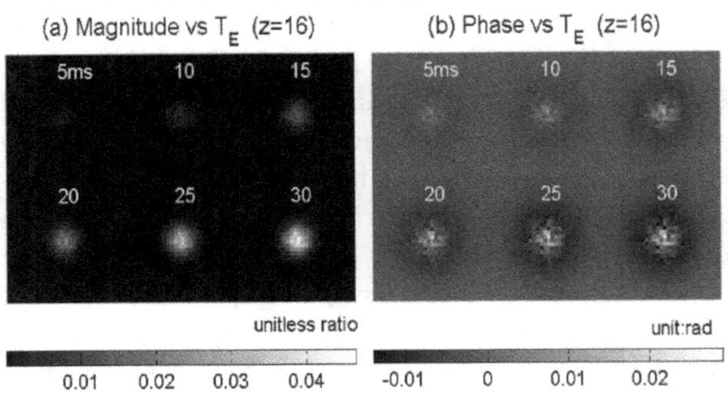

Figure 8 Montage displays of the T_E dependence of MR magnitude image at the central z-slice A[x, y, z_0; T_E] (in(a)) and the corresponding MR phase image P[x, y, z_0; T_E] (in (b)) for T_E = [5,10,15,20,25,30]**ms.**

Discussion

In this paper, we propose a magnetic susceptibility expression formula for a linear neurovascular coupling model (accounting for the neurovascular aspects: CBF, CBV, $CMRO_2$, FOV, and NAB) and a computational model for volumetric BOLD fMRI simulation. Overall, our goal is to numerically examine the principles of MRI-based neuroimaging: implementing the forward imaging from a neuronal origin (a numerical NAB), to vascular response (a numerical susceptibility distribution $\Delta\chi$, which also serves as the vascular origin of T2*MRI), to complex multivoxel MR image formation (MR magnitude images), and then rendering the backward mappings (as designated by "A ~ NAB", "A~$\Delta\chi$" and "P~ΔB" in Figure 2). In this paper, we focus on the mapping between the MR magnitude image and its vascular origin. Meanwhile, we also show the mapping between the MR phase image and the fieldmap.

We decompose the overall BOLD fMRI model into two modules in Figure 2: "neurophysiology" and "MRI technology". Due to the complexity of biophysiology and neurology, the neurovascular-coupled BOLD process is not completely understood. In contrast, the MRI technology is well understood and developed. We propose a linear neurovascular coupling formula to express a BOLD state in terms of susceptibility perturbation in Eq. (4), which accounts for the main aspects of BOLD process as parameterized by CBV, CBF, $CMRO_2$, and NAB. It should be mentioned that the linear model neurovascular coupling model has the experimental supports [27,28,31,32]. For numerical simulation, we need to express the dynamics of neurovascular coupling process and BOLD fMRI through the digitization of the involved parameters at discrete time points (snapshots). It is straightforward to extend our snapshot simulation method to dynamic BOLD fMRI simulation by repeating the snapshot imaging at a series of time points.

The cortical vasculature mainly consists of capillaries with radii in a range from 2 to 10 micron. Voxelization may suppress the intravoxel vasculature details (due to voxel size > > vessel size), consequently, we cannot discern the vascular structures in Figures 1, 6 through 8. Our simulation results show that, the magnitude-vs-susceptibility correlation decreases for larger vessel sizes, which may in part explain the experimentally observed BOLD nonlinearity due to large vessel effect [35]. In general, the magnitude-vs-susceptibility correlation takes on a correlation coefficient of 0.90 for an image resolution about 100-micron. The discrepancy between the MR magnitude and the BOLD susceptibility map (corrA≠1) may be partially understood from the nonlinearity of BOLD fMRI [13,35]. We also demonstrate the phase-vs-fieldmap correlation. The results show that,

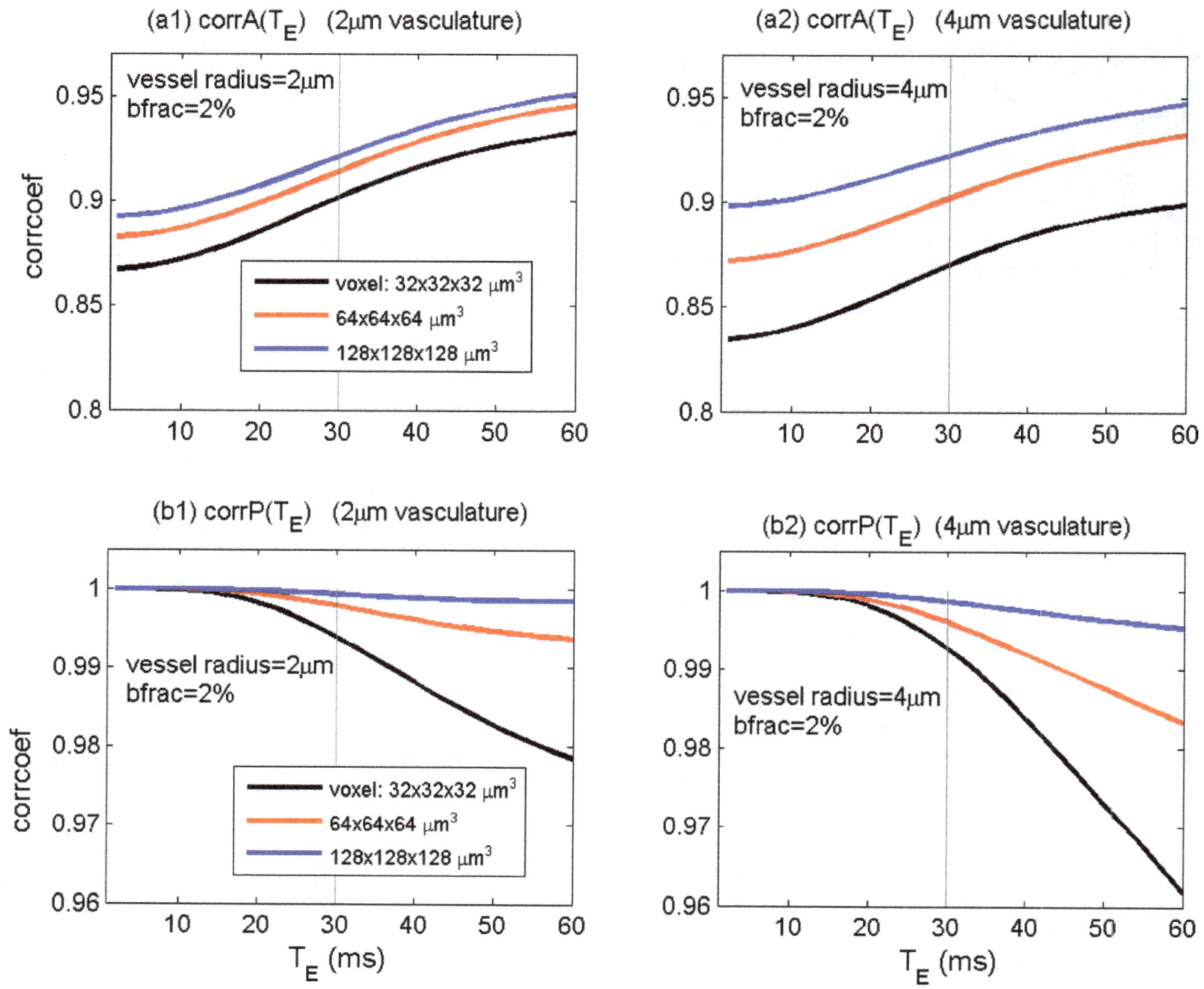

Figure 9 (a1) and (a2) corrA for the magnitude-vs-susceptibility correlations with respect to T_E = [0, 60] ms, two vasculatures of radii = 2 and 4 micron, and three voxel sizes (see legend); (b1) and (b2) corrP for the corresponding phase-vs-fieldmap correlations. It is shown that a long T_E may increase corrA but decrease corrP, and that both corrA and corrP decrease as image resolution refines. It is reminded that corrA≠1 implies mismatch and nonlinearity of the mapping.

Table 2 Spatial matching results in terms of spatial correlation coefficients corrA and corrP calculated by Eqs.(10) and (11) with the setting of B_0 = 3 T, *bfrac* = 2%, radii = 2 and 4 μm, T_E = 1 and 30 ms for three image resolutions (voxel sizes)

	2- μm-radius vessels				4- μm-radius vessels			
	T_E = 1 ms		T_E = 30 ms		T_E = 1 ms		T_E = 30 ms	
Voxel size (μm^3)	corrA	corrP	corrA	corrP	corrA	corrP	corrA	corrP
32 × 32 × 32	0.867	1.000	0.885	0.998	0.834	1.000	0.854	0.998
64 × 64 × 64	0.883	1.000	0.899	0.999	0.871	1.000	0.887	0.999
128 × 128 × 128	0.892	1.000	0.907	0.999	0.898	1.000	0.910	0.999

the corrP is close to the maximum 1.00 with respect to T_E (< 30 ms). However the corrP tends to drop for long T_E and high resolution (see Figure 9(b) and Table 2 and refer to [20] for more relevant results and explanations).

In our simulation implementation, the cortex FOV is represented by a large 3D support matrix in size of 2048 × 2048 × 2048 (with 1-micron grid resolution) in order to depict small capillaries (digital geometry requirement). The output MR images are represented in much smaller multivoxel matrices (via voxelization): 16 × 16 × 16, 32 × 32 × 32, and 64 × 64 × 64 for three image resolutions. It is reminded that the fieldmap should be calculated from the finely-gridded susceptibility map (in the large support matrix) as a whole by a FT technique (in Eq. (5)), rather than trying to divide the large matrix into smaller submatrices. The 3D FFT on a large matrix (that is too large to be processed as a whole in computer memory) is implemented by a scheme of 2D + 1D decomposition [36]. By performing the 3D FFT on the large matrix, we can account for long-distance magnetic influence of susceptibility magnetization [22,23]. Indeed the multivoxel BOLD fMRI simulation demands a proliferated computation load in comparison with the single BOLD voxel signal simulation. Specifically, the volumetric simulation on an image matrix of 32 × 32 × 32 with voxel size of 64 × 64 × 64 (necessary for digital geometrical depiction of intravascular structure) requires a large matrix of 2048 × 2048 × 2048 (with 2048 = 64 × 32). Considering that the volumetric BOLD fMRI simulation may provide the spatial features among voxels that is not available from individual voxel signals, our simulation effort is worthwhile.

The simulation results for magnitude-based and phase-based backward mappings are graphically shown in Figure 9, from which we can observe the following phenomenon: 1) The magnitude-vs-susceptibility correlation (corrA) increases with respect to T_E (shown in a range from 0 to 60 ms), whereas the phase-vs-fieldmap correlation (corrP) decreases for $T_E > 30$ ms; 2) Large voxel size (or low image resolution) cause both corrA and corrP decrease (noticeable corrP decrease for $T_E > 30$ ms); 3) Large vessels cause both corrA and corrP drop.

In addition to the study on the backward mapping between the MR magnitude image and its vascular origin, we also provide the backward mapping between the MR phase image and the fieldmap in a measure of corrP. Our simulation results show that corrP ≈ 1.00, which indicates that the MR phase image conforms very well with the fieldmap. This suggests the possibility of susceptibility reconstruction by computed inverse MRI [13,26], which is an active ongoing research topic.

Numerical simulation provides a powerful tool to look into a digital imaging system as long as all the involved parameters can be numerically characterized. In light of numerical method, a parameter must be digitized for computation. The parameter digitization does not necessarily require an analytic formula, it may be fulfilled in any way. For example, the BOLD susceptibility perturbation over a FOV in Figure 4 can be assigned a NAB-modulated spatial distribution at a snapshot time, and the dynamics can be numerically characterized by an empirical timecourse in a lookup table with respect to a discrete time (the voxel timecourses in Figure 4 are not necessarily analytically describable). Therefore, our computational model can be extended to accommodate a nonlinear neurovascular-coupled BOLD fMRI process over a broad physiological range provided that all the involved parameters can be numerically determined.

Conclusions

In this report we propose a computational model for numerically simulating volumetric BOLD MRI with a magnetic susceptibility expression for a linear neurovascular coupling state. The forward procedure for this model includes: 1) defining a neuronal origin (a numerical NAB) in a cortex region(FOV); 2) expressing the NAB-modulated vascular response by a spatial distribution of intravascular blood biomagnetic susceptibility perturbation; and 3) calculating the susceptibility-induced fieldmap by accounting for the magnetization of all vascular blood in the FOV; 4) calculating the multivoxel MR image by intravoxel dephasing integration. Upon the completion of the forward simulation, we compare the output MR magnitude image with the predefined susceptibility map in a numerical measure of magnitude-vs-susceptibility correlation, thereby quantitatively examining the reproducibility of the vascular origin by the MR magnitude image. Meanwhile, we can also compare the output MR phase image with the precomputed fieldmap in terms of phase-vs-fieldmap correlation, showing that the MR phase image conforms with the fieldmap very well.

Based on our simulation results, we conclude that, 1) the magnitude image of BOLD fMRI can approximately, but not exactly, represent the vascular origin; and 2) the phase image conforms very well with the fieldmap. Considering that the vascular response to the neuronal origin is subject to a neurovascular coupling process, we can infer that the mapping between the MR magnitude image and neuronal origin suffers more mismatch than that between the MR magnitude image and the vascular origin, even if under a linear neurovascular coupling model (because the vasculature exerts a spatial modulation that imposes additional mismatch). The volumetric computational model provides a general framework for simulating many neurovascular, physiological, and biophysical aspects. It can be extended to accommodate a nonlinear neurovascular coupling process over a broad physiological range if the magnetic susceptibility expression is numerically available (not necessarily formulable). Our simulation results pose a caveat to the MRI-based neuroimaging and brain mapping study: the MR magnitude image is not an exact reproduction which may in part explain the nonlinearity of BOLD fMRI. In future research we plan to to look into the overall nonlinearity of BOLD fMRI by incorporating the intrinsic nonlinear neurovascular coupling process.

Abbreviations

BOLD: Blood oxygenation level dependent; MR: Magnetic resonance; MRI: Magnetic resonance imaging; fMRI: Functional magnetic resonance imaging; FOV: Field of view; NAB: Neuroactive blob; CBV: Cerebral blood volume; CBF:

Cerebral blood flow; $CMRO_2$: Cerebral metabolic rate of oxygen; *bfrac*: Blood volume fraction.

Acknowledgements
This research was supported by the NIH (1R01EB006841, 1R01EB005846), NSF (0612076), and the MRN internal grant 6003-154.

Author details
[1]The Mind Research Network and LBERI, Albuquerque 87106, NM, USA.
[2]Department of Electrical and Computer Engineering, Albuquerque 87131, NM, USA.

Authors' contributions
Zikuan Chen conceived the computational model, implemented the algorithm by program, and drafted the manuscript. Vince Calhoun analyzed the model, algorithm, data, and edited the manuscript. All authors have approved the content of the manuscript.

Competing interests
The authors declare that they have no competing interests.

References

1. Boxerman JL, Bandettini PA, Kwong KK, Baker JR, Davis TL, Rosen BR, Weisskoff RM: **The intravascular contribution to fMRI signal change: Monte Carlo modeling and diffusion-weighted studies in vivo.** *Magn Reson Med* 1995, **34(1)**:4-10.
2. Boxerman JL, Hamberg LM, Rosen BR, Weisskoff RM: **MR contrast due to intravascular magnetic susceptibility perturbations.** *Magn Reson Med* 1995, **34(4)**:555-566.
3. Ogawa S, Menon RS, Tank DW, Kim SG, Merkle H, Ellermann JM, Ugurbil K: **Functional brain mapping by blood oxygenation level-dependent contrast magnetic resonance imaging. A comparison of signal characteristics with a biophysical model.** *Biophys J* 1993, **64(3)**:803-812.
4. Weisskoff RM, Zuo CS, Boxerman JL, Rosen BR: **Microscopic susceptibility variation and transverse relaxation: theory and experiment.** *Magn Reson Med* 1994, **31(6)**:601-610.
5. Yablonskiy DA, Haacke EM: **Theory of NMR signal behavior in magnetically inhomogeneous tissues: the static dephasing regime.** *Magn Reson Med* 1994, **32(6)**:749-763.
6. Pathak AP, Ward BD, Schmainda KM: **A novel technique for modeling susceptibility-based contrast mechanisms for arbitrary microvascular geometries: the finite perturber method.** *Neuroimage* 2008, **40(3)**:1130-1143.
7. Arthurs OJ, Boniface S: **How well do we understand the neural origins of the fMRI BOLD signal?** *Trends Neurosci* 2002, **25(1)**:27-31.
8. Attwell D, Iadecola C: **The neural basis of functional brain imaging signals.** *Trends Neurosci* 2002, **25(12)**:621-625.
9. Buxton RB: **Interpreting oxygenation-based neuroimaging signals: the importance and the challenge of understanding brain oxygen metabolism.** *Front Neuroenergetics* 2010, **2**:8.
10. Buxton RB, Frank LR: **A model for the coupling between cerebral blood flow and oxygen metabolism during neural stimulation.** *J Cereb Blood Flow Metab* 1997, **17(1)**:64-72.
11. Zhang N, Liu Z, He B, Chen W: **Noninvasive study of neurovascular coupling during graded neuronal suppression.** *Journal of cerebral blood flow and metabolism: official journal of the International Society of Cerebral Blood Flow and Metabolism* 2008, **28(2)**:280-290.
12. Chavhan GB, Babyn PS, Thomas B, Shroff MM, Haacke EM: **Principles, techniques, and applications of T2*-based MR imaging and its special applications.** *Radiographics: a review publication of the Radiological Society of North America, Inc* 2009, **29(5)**:1433-1449.
13. Chen Z, Calhoun VD: **Two pitfalls of BOLD fMRI magnitude-based neuroimage analysis: non-negativity and edge effect.** *J Neurosci Methods* 2011, **199(2)**:363-369.
14. Howseman AM, Bowtell RW: **Functional magnetic resonance imaging: imaging techniques and contrast mechanisms.** *Philos Trans R Soc Lond B Biol Sci* 1999, **354(1387)**:1179-1194.
15. Moon CH, Fukuda M, Park SH, Kim SG: **Neural interpretation of blood oxygenation level-dependent fMRI maps at submillimeter columnar resolution.** *J Neurosci* 2007, **27(26)**:6892-6902.
16. Marques JP, Bowtell RW: **Using forward calculations of the magnetic field perturbation due to a realistic vascular model to explore the BOLD effect.** *NMR Biomed* 2008, **21(6)**:553-565.
17. Martindale J, Kennerley AJ, Johnston D, Zheng Y, Mayhew JE: **Theory and generalization of Monte Carlo models of the BOLD signal source.** *Magn Reson Med* 2008, **59(3)**:607-618.
18. Menon RS: **Simulation of BOLD phase and magnitude changes in a voxel.** *Proc Intl Soc Mag Reson Med* 2003, **11**:1719.
19. Chen Z, Calhoun V: **A computational multiresolution BOLD fMRI model.** *IEEE Trans BioMed Eng* 2011, **58(10)**:2995-2999.
20. Chen Z, Calhoun VD: **Magnitude and Phase Behavior of Multiresolution BOLD signal.** *Concepts Magn Reson* 2010, **37B(3)**:129-135.
21. Chen Z, Chen Z, Calhoun VD: *Multiresolution voxel decomposition of complex-valued BOLD signals reveals phasor turbulence* Orlando: In: SPIE Medical Imaging;:1-11. 16 March 79613y; Orlando, FL: SPIE; 79613y.
22. Chen Z, Chen Z, Calhoun VD: *Voxel magnetic field disturbance from remote vasculature in BOLD* fMRI.In:. Orlando: SPIE Medical Imaging; 1-12. 16 March 79613x; Orlando, FL: SPIE; 79613x.
23. Chen Z, Caprihan A, Calhoun VD: **Effect of surrounding vasculature on intravoxel BOLD signal.** *Med Phys* 2010, **37(4)**:1778-1787.
24. Koch KM, Papademetris X, Rothman DL, de Graaf RA: **Rapid calculations of susceptibility-induced magnetostatic field perturbations for in vivo magnetic resonance.** *Phys Med Biol* 2006, **51(24)**:6381-6402.
25. Salomir R, de Senneville BD, Moonen CTW: **A fast calculation method for magnetic field inhomogeneity due to an arbitrary distribution of bulk susceptibility.** *Concepts Magn Reson* 2003, **B19**:26-34.
26. Chen Z, Calhoun V: **Computed inverse MRI for magnetic susceptibility map reconstruction.** *J Comp Assit Tomography* 2012, **36(2)**:265-274, March/April 2012.
27. Arthurs OJ, Williams EJ, Carpenter TA, Pickard JD, Boniface SJ: **Linear coupling between functional magnetic resonance imaging and evoked potential amplitude in human somatosensory cortex.** *Neuroscience* 2000, **101(4)**:803-806.
28. Hoge RD, Atkinson J, Gill B, Crelier GR, Marrett S, Pike GB: **Linear coupling between cerebral blood flow and oxygen consumption in activated human cortex.** *Proc Natl Acad Sci USA* 1999, **96(16)**:9403-9408.
29. Logothetis NK: **The neural basis of the blood-oxygen-level-dependent functional magnetic resonance imaging signal.** *Philos Trans R Soc Lond B Biol Sci* 2002, **357(1424)**:1003-1037.
30. Ugurbil K, Toth L, Kim DS: **How accurate is magnetic resonance imaging of brain function?** *Trends Neurosci* 2003, **26(2)**:108-114.
31. Zhang N, Yacoub E, Zhu XH, Ugurbil K, Chen W: **Linearity of blood-oxygenation-level dependent signal at microvasculature.** *Neuroimage* 2009, **48(2)**:313-318.
32. Norris DG: **Principles of magnetic resonance assessment of brain function.** *Journal of magnetic resonance imaging: JMRI* 2006, **23(6)**:794-807.
33. Uludag K, Muller-Bierl B, Ugurbil K: **An integrative model for neuronal activity-induced signal changes for gradient and spin echo functional imaging.** *Neuroimage* 2009, **48(1)**:150-165.
34. Marques JP, Bowtell R: **Application of a fourier-based method for rapid calculation of field inhomogeneity due to spatial variation of magnetic susceptibility.** *Concepts Magn Reson* 2005, , **B25**:: 65-78.
35. Zhang N, Zhu XH, Chen W: **Investigating the source of BOLD nonlinearity in human visual cortex in response to paired visual stimuli.** *Neuroimage* 2008, **43(2)**:204-212.
36. Chen Z, Ning R: **Breast volume denoising and noise characterization by 3D wavelet transform.** *Comput Med Imaging Graph* 2004, **28(5)**:235-246.

25

Herlyn-werner-wunderlich syndrome: MRI findings, radiological guide (two cases and literature review), and differential diagnosis

Riccardo Del Vescovo*, Sofia Battisti, Valerio Di Paola, Claudia L Piccolo, Roberto L Cazzato, Ilaria Sansoni, Rosario F Grasso and Bruno Beomonte Zobel

Abstract

Background: Herlyn-Werner-Wunderlich (HWW) syndrome is a very rare congenital anomaly of the urogenital tract involving Müllerian ducts and Wolffian structures, and it is characterized by the triad of didelphys uterus, obstructed hemivagina and ipsilateral renal agenesis. It generally occurs at puberty and exhibits non-specific and variable symptoms with acute or pelvic pain shortly following menarche, causing a delay in the diagnosis. Moreover, the diagnosis is complicated by the infrequency of this syndrome, because Müllerian duct anomalies (MDA) are infrequently encountered in a routine clinical setting.

Cases presentation: two cases of HWW syndrome in adolescents and a differential diagnosis for one case of a different MDA, and the impact of magnetic resonance (MR) imaging technology to achieve the correct diagnosis.

Conclusions: MR imaging is a very suitable diagnostic tool in order to perform the correct diagnosis of HWW syndrome.

Background

The association of renal agenesis with ipsilateral blind hemivagina and didelphys uterus is reported as Herlyn-Werner-Wunderlich (HWW) syndrome; this triad was initially disclosed in an English report published in 2006 [1].

The incidence of didelphys uterus, related to HWW, is approximately 1/2,000 to 1/28,000, and it is accompanied by unilateral renal agenesis in 43% of cases. The incidence of unilateral renal agenesis is 1/1,100, and 25-50% of affected women exhibits associated genital abnormalities [2].

HWW syndrome represents a type of Müllerian duct anomalies (MDA) associated with mesonephric duct anomalies. MDA are congenital entities resulting from non-development (agenesia or hypoplasia), defective vertical or lateral fusion, or resorption failure of the Müllerian (paramesonephric) ducts [3].

MDA are estimated to have an overall prevalence of 2% to 3% among all women, with an incidence of 1/200-600 among fertile women. Hypoplasia, as well as agenesis of the uterus and proximal vagina, accounts for 5%-10% of Müllerian duct anomalies, whereas didelphys uterus accounts for approximately 11% of Müllerian duct anomalies. Renal tract anomalies are associated with MDA in as many as 30% of cases [4].

A complete or partial vaginal septum is present in 75% of women with didelphys uterus [5].

The exact cause, pathogenesis and embryologic origin of HWW syndrome are unclear and remain a subject of discussion [6].

HWW syndrome is usually discovered at puberty with non-specific symptoms, like increasing pelvic pain, dysmenorrhea and palpable mass due to the associated haematocolpos or hematometra, which result from retained, longstanding menstrual flow in the obstrucucted vagina.

It rarely occurs with primary infertility in early adulthood when the vaginal septum is incomplete [7].

It is really difficult to achieve to an accurate diagnosis because menstruation is often regular and when patient complains symptoms of cyclic dysmenorrhea, they are usually given anti-inflammatory drugs and

* Correspondence: r.delvescovo@unicampus.it
Department of Radiology, Campus Bio-Medico Univeristy of Rome, Italy

oral-contraceptives, thus causing a delay in the diagnosis because they reduce or eliminate menses; ultimately, HWW is an uncommon syndrome, not often thought of as a diagnostic possibility [8].

The potential complications of this syndrome are distinct in acute complications, such as pyohematocolpos, pyosalpinx, or pelviperitonitis, and long-term complications, such as endometriosis, pelvic adhesions and increased risk of abortion or infertility [9,10].

The American Society for Reproductive Medicine (ASRM) established a classification of Müllerian duct anomalies in 1988 in order to group them in entirety (Table 1) [11].

According to this classification, HWW syndrome appears to include the addition of III uterine anomaly to Ia vaginal anomaly and renal agenesis (Table 2).

Case presentation

Patient 1

A 16-years-old female presented with a history of severe abdomino-pelvic pain, which increased lasting 2 to 7 days with each of her menstrual cycles, hindering her daily activities.

Gynecologic history indicated menarche at 13 years of age, followed by 3 years of irregular menses.

The patient denied any recent abdominal trauma, abnormal vaginal bleeding, nausea, vomiting or diarrhea.

A bimanual physical examination indicated a right-sided cystic and tender pelvic mass, movable, mildly tender to palpation. The medical staff recommended further evaluation such as US, which showed the absence of right kidney and the possibility of uterine anomaly; so Magnetic Resonance Imaging (MRI) was performed in order to evaluate the possible genito-urinary anomaly.

The MRI examination was performed on a 1.5 Tesla MR clinical scanner (Siemens, Avanto Erlangen Germany). The patient's mother gave her informed consent for MRI exam. Images were acquired on multiple planes with T1-weighted (TR 714 ms; TE 12 ms) and T2-weighted Turbo Spin Echo (TR 5530 ms; TE 150 ms) sequences; fat-suppressed T2-weighted TSE images (TR 6810 ms; TE 150 ms), Flash3D T1-weighted (TR 5.2; TE 2.5) and HASTE sequences (TR 700; TE 89). A contrast agent was not used as it was not considered necessary.

MRI imaging showed a uterine-vaginal anomaly consisting of didelphys uterus and double vagina, one of which was obstructed (Figure 1); consequently, there was accumulation of fluid exhibiting a signal intensity similar to methaemoglobin in the right uterus (slightly dilated, 14 mm diameter of the lumen) and in the right obstructed vagina (which appeared to be considerably dilated, 43 × 34 × 35 mm).

In the right ovary an expanding mass of 31 mm was hyperintense on T1-weighted images and mildly hypointense or hyperintense on T2-weighted images (Figure 2A). The mass was characterized by a typical "shading" sign (Figure 2B) and exhibited features compatible with an endometriosic cyst; there was mild fluid in the pouch of Douglas.

Table 1 Classification of müllerian duct anomalies

MULLERIAN AGENESIS OR HYPOLPLASIA	a) vagina b) cervix c) fundus d) fallopian tube e) combined agenesis or hypoplasia (two or more findings from classes I-A through I-D)
UNICORNUATE UTERUS (Agenesis or hypoplasia of one of the two Mullerian ducts)	• rudimentary horn with an endometrial cavity that communicates with the (single-horned) uterus; • rudimentary horn with an endometrial cavity that does not communicate with the uterus; • rudimentary horn with no endometrial cavity; no rudimentary horn
UTERUS DYDELPHYS (Failure of lateral fusion between vagina and two Mullerian ducts)	
BICORNUATE UTERUS (Incomplete fusion of uterine horns at the level of the fundus)	a) complete (septum extends to the internal or external os); b) partial (septum is confined to the fundal region)
SEPTATE UTERUS (Incomplete or absent resorption of uterovaginal septum)	a) complete (septum extends to the internal os); b) partial (septum does not reach the internal os)
ARCHUATE UTERUS (Light indent of the fundus of the uterus due to almost complete resorption of the uterovaginal septum)	
UTERUS EXPOSED TO DIETHYILSTILBESTROL-RELATED UTERINE ANOMALIES	a) T-shaped uterus; b) T-shaped uterus with dilated horns; c) Uterine hypoplasia

Table 2 Hww syndrome: mr findings

HWW SYNDROME	MR FINDINGS
Uterus didelphys	It is characterized by two symmetric, widely divergent uterine horns and two cervixes, with an enlarged cavity filled by bloody/ proteinaceous fluid due to haematocolpos. It appears hyperintense signal on T1 fat saturated sequences.
Hemivagina	It is an obstructed vagina due to a longitudinal septum which occludes one cervix and isolates it with consequent hematometra.
Renal aplasya	It is tipically omolateral to the vaginal anomaly (right side prevalence), with possible controlateral renal hypertrophy due to compensation but in site.
Ovaries	Possible presence of endometriosic cysts with hyperintense signal on T1 fat sat sequences and with "shading sign" on T2-weighted images and a gradual variation of signal intensity due to chronic bleeding with accumulation of high concentration of iron and protein in the endometrioma (endometriotic lesions appear hyperintense on T1-weighted images and mildly hypointense or hyperintense on T2-weighted images). Possible presence of functional cysts with no clinical significance, which appear hyperintense on T2 sequences and hypo/ isointense on T1 sequences.

There was no evidence of an expansive process in the left ovary. The extension of examination to the upper abdomen revealed right renal agenesis and apparent compensatory hypertrophy of the left kidney (Figure 3).

Patient 2

A 15-years-old woman presented with severe abdominal pain that occurred since the patient achieved menarche at 14 years of age; the patient also had irregular menstruation with severe dysmenorrhea and she reported that the pain worsened immediately prior to menstruation and improved with menstrual flow.

Upon physical examination, the findings were non-specific, with the exception of lower abdominal tenderness, arising from the pelvis, mildly tender to palpation. A gynecologic examination did not reveal any anomalies of her external genitalia or hymen.

So, MRI was then performed, using the same sequences protocol employed for Patient 1.

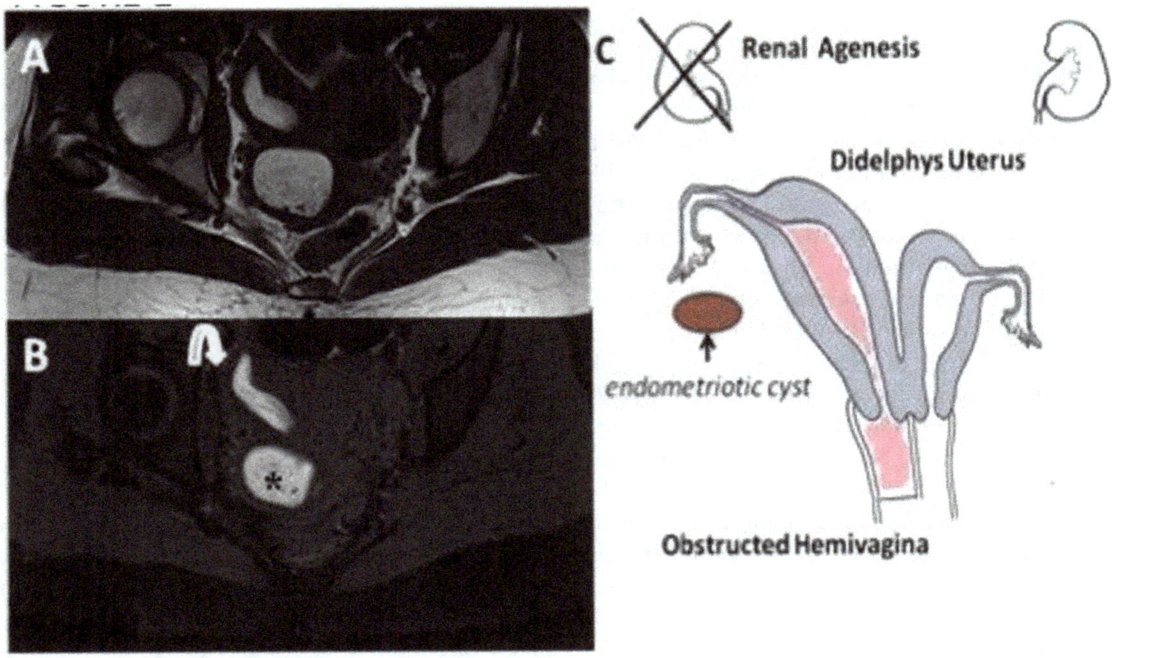

Figure 1 Herlyn-Werner-Wunderlich syndrome (C) Drawing illustrates the triad (renal agenesis, didelphys uterus, and obstructed hemivagina and in this case the presence of an endometriosic cyst. A 16-years-old girl presenting the triad of didelphys uterus (class III MDA), an obstructed right hemivagina (class I MDA), and ipsilateral renal agenesis. (A) Axial turbo spin-echo T2 weighted (B) Axial turbo spin-echo T1 fat-saturated weighted MR image showing centrally a hematocolpos (asterisk), a finding corresponding to the obstructed right hemivagina. Mild dilation of the right endometrial cavity (curved arrow) with fluid exhibiting a signal intensity similar to methaemoglobin due to haematometra.

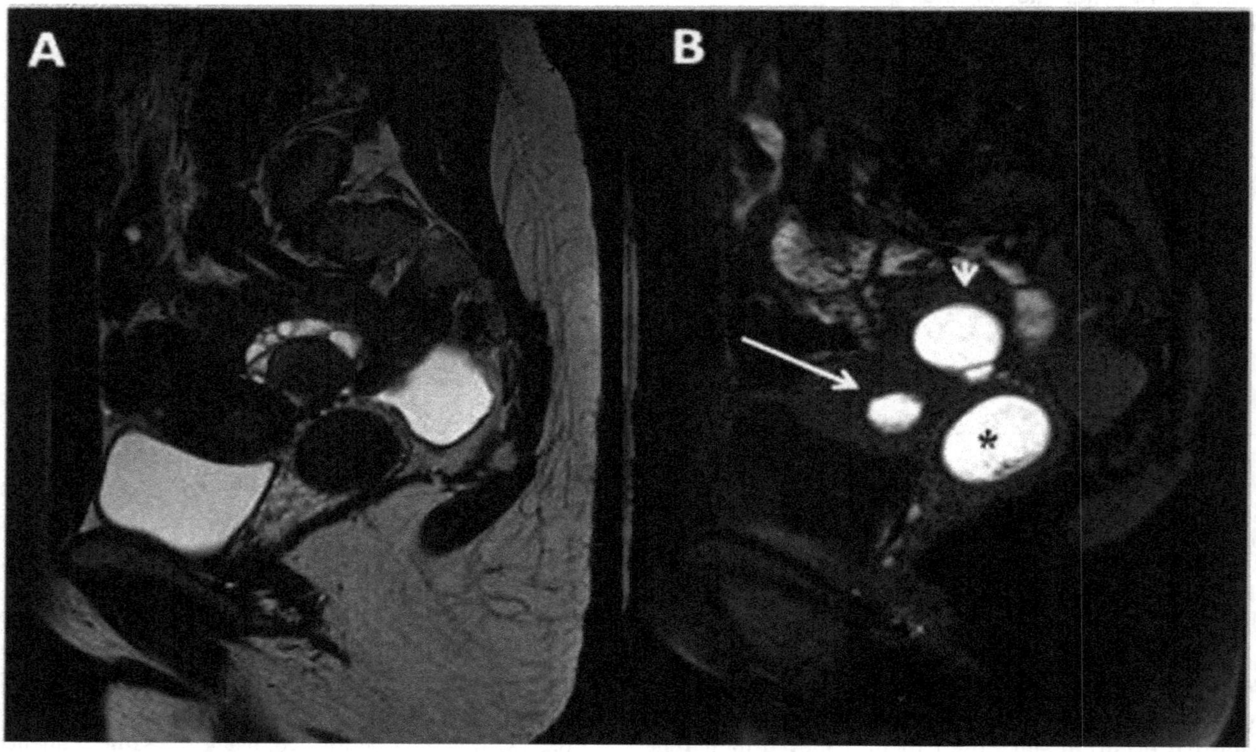

Figure 2 A) Sagittal T2 TSE weighted image showing a mild fluid in the pouch of Douglas. (B) Sagittal T1 TSE fat-suppressed weighted image showing distention of the right endometrial cavity (long straight arrow) with high-signal-intensity material distending the right endometrial cavity and cervix (asterisk), a finding indicative of right hematometrocolpos; on the right ovary presence of an endometriosic cysts appearing hyperintense on T1 fat-saturated image (short straight arrow).

Contrast agent was not given and the patient's mother provided informed consent to perform MRI exam.

MRI indicated a uterine-vaginal malformation consisting of didelphys uterus communicating with a double vagina, of which the right vagina was obstructed (Figure 4). Consequently, there was a collection of fluid that exhibited a high signal intensity on T1 fat-saturated sequences, referred to as methaemoglobin, both in the right uterus (slightly enlarged: 18 mm diameter), and in the right obstructed vagina (which appears to be highly dilated and thus compressing the bladder, 60 × 65 × 76 mm) referred to hematocolpos (Figure 5).

There was no evidence of an expansive process in the ovaries, but the extension of the examination to the upper abdomen showed right renal agenesis and apparent compensatory hypertrophy of the left kidney (Figure 6).

Patient 3: an example of differential diagnosis

A 13-years-old female presented with severe abdominal pain. She reported that the pain had begun a few months earlier and had subsequently worsened over the past several weeks. The pain worsened immediately prior to menstruation and then improved once menstrual flow began. The patient also reported worsening constipation and denied problems with urination, nausea, vomiting or diarrhea.

The patient underwent menarche 2 months prior with menses exhibiting 3 to 4 days of very light flow. Physical examination did not reveal any alteration of her external genitalia. A previous sonography revealed a solitary left kidney as well as probable unicornuate uterus.

MRI examination confirmed an unicornuate uterus with a left single horn open into a normal vagina and a controlateral non-communicating rudimentary horn that contained material with a signal intensity similar to methaemoglobin (Figure 7).

The ipsilateral Fallopian tube was characterized by fluid sero-mucinous distension (Figure 8). In the right paramedian side, at the level of the Douglas, posterior to the ideal point of continuity between uterus and rudimentary horn, there were some adjacent nodules most likely of endometrial etiology (14 mm, 38 mm in total) (Figure 9). In addition, a moderate rate of pelvic fluid was present.

The extension of the examination to the upper abdomen showed agenesis of the right kidney with compensatory hypertrophy of the left one and a left renal

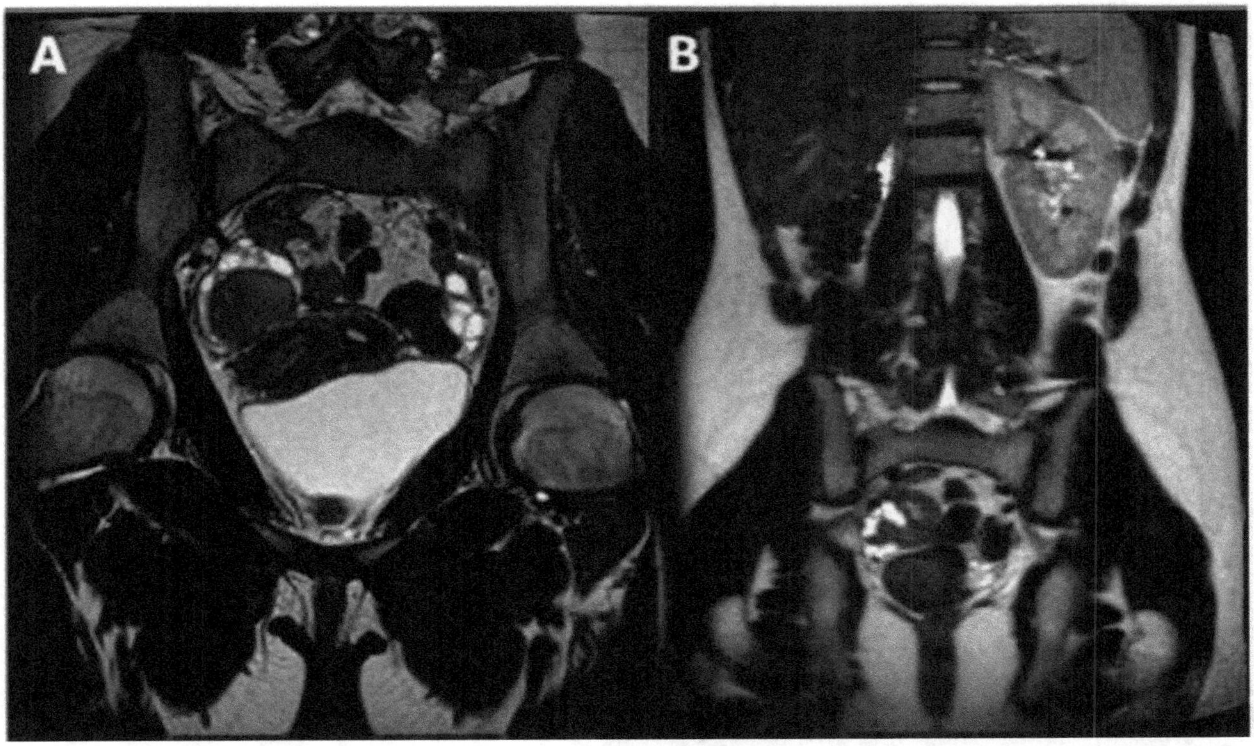

Figure 3 A) Oblique coronal TSE T2-weighted MR image shows a complete view of the anatomical defects. B) Coronal T2 Trufi MR image showing the omolateral renal aplasia with respect to the pelvic abnormalities and a solitary left kidney with a mild hypertrophy.

artery with a larger lumen, most likely of functional significance.

This is, evidently, another kind of MDA, different from the HWW syndrome, showing an association with uterine anomaly type IIb with renal aplasia, whereas HWW syndrome displays an association with Ia vaginal anomaly with a III uterine anomaly and renal aplasia.

Conclusions

It could be desirable to achieve to an early diagnosis and treatment of HWW syndrome, in order to relieve acute symptoms, preserve normal fertility and prevent several medical complications. The correct diagnosis can be difficult due to the absence of specific findings upon physical examination and to non specific symptoms which delay the diagnosis.

Ultrasonography (US) is a very helpful tool in the diagnosis of Müllerian duct anomalies, infact the detection of haematocolpos, which appears as a fluid collection with low-level echoes, can make the diagnosis of genitor-urinary tract anomaly (didelphic uterus) easier, although it cannot identify the type of Müllerian ducts anomaly (MDA), whereas MRI, in cases when the differentiation of the uterine anomaly is not easily achievable by means of previous examination (physical examination, US, hysterosalpingography), is a suitable technique for the non-invasive evaluation of female pelvic anatomy because it provides more detailed information regarding uterine morphology, the continuity with each vaginal (obstructed and non-obstructed) lumen, and fluid content nature [12].

When a high suspicion of MDA exists, US should be performed initially to delineate any abnormalities in the genital tract, however, in order to obtain an accurate MDA classification, magnetic resonance imaging must be performed.

Although US, CT scan, and hysterosalpingography are commonly used for diagnosis because of their low cost, MRI is the most accurate method for diagnosis and it could help patients in maintaining fertility by allowing the most appropriate treatment option to be used [13].

In fact, in comparison to the other modalities, MRI is more sensitive in detecting the uterine contour, the shape of the intrauterine cavity, the character of the septum, as well as associated aspects such as endometriosis, pelvic inflammation and adhesions.

However, laparoscopy should now be considered the gold standard for the evaluation of female reproductive tract anomaly, although it could be reserved when the diagnosis is not clear after imaging or when MRI is not available and not performed as a routine procedure [7].

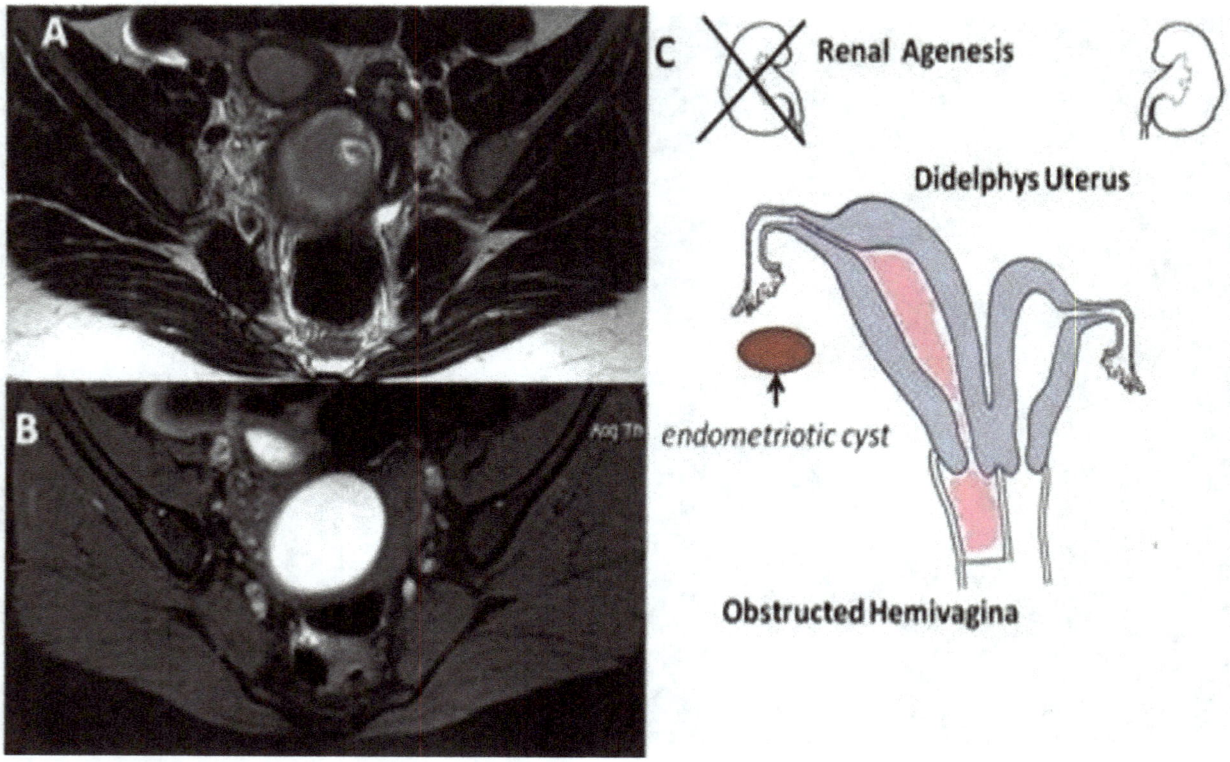

Figure 4 Herlyn-Werner-Wunderlich syndrome (C) Drawing illustrates the triad. A 15-years-old girl presenting the triad of didelphys uterus (class III MDA), an obstructed right hemivagina (class I MDA), and ipsilateral renal agenesis. (A) Axial turbo spin-echo T2 weighted MR image (B) Axial turbo spin-echo T1 fat-saturated weighted MR image showing centrally a wide hematocolpos (asterisk), corresponding to the obstructed right hemivagina. On the left side the uterus normally communicating with non-obstructed hemivagina.

The decision to perform a laparoscopy is based on the following:

- the interval between menarche and diagnosis;
- the severity of the symptoms;
- the presence of a hematometra or pyometra.

Laparoscopy can be also therapeutic in some selected cases such as: drainage of hematocolpos/hematometrocolpos, septectomy, or marsupialization of the blind hemivagina. It is considered very helpful in order to reduce pelvic pain and lower the risk of infection and of further hematometra [1].

The outcome of pregnancy in these patients reveals that 87% go on to have a successful pregnancy, while abortions occur in 23% of the patients, 15% have preterm births, and 62% have full-term pregnancies and uncomplicated deliveries.

If surgery is not an immediate option for patients with HWW syndrome, menstrual suppression with combined oral contraceptive pills is advised to prevent further accumulation of hematocolpos and further hematometra [14,15].

The consequences that potentially occur due to the failure of treatment include urinary retention, hematosalpinx (blood in the fallopian tube), endometriosis and rupture of a tubo-ovarian abscess [16].

With each diagnosis of didelphys uterus in association with obstructed hemivagina on the lower abdomen MRI, HWW syndrome should be excluded and the exam should be extended to the upper abdomen to check for the presence of ipsilateral kidney.

Renal tract anomalies are associated with MDA in up to 30% of cases due to the close embryologic relationship between the paramesonephric and mesonephric ducts.

The most common renal tract anomaly associated with MDA is renal agenesis with right side prevalence [1,17,18]. Therefore, in all patients who present an MDA, it is imperative to investigate the urinary tract.

If renal agenesia is diagnosed, patients should have continuous follow-up to check for renal functioning as the risk of renal failure is very high [19]. Another very common condition in HWW syndrome patients is associated endometriosis.

The underlying pathophysiological mechanism is potentially the increased risk of retrograde menstruation: because of the obstructed vaginal outflow, the risk

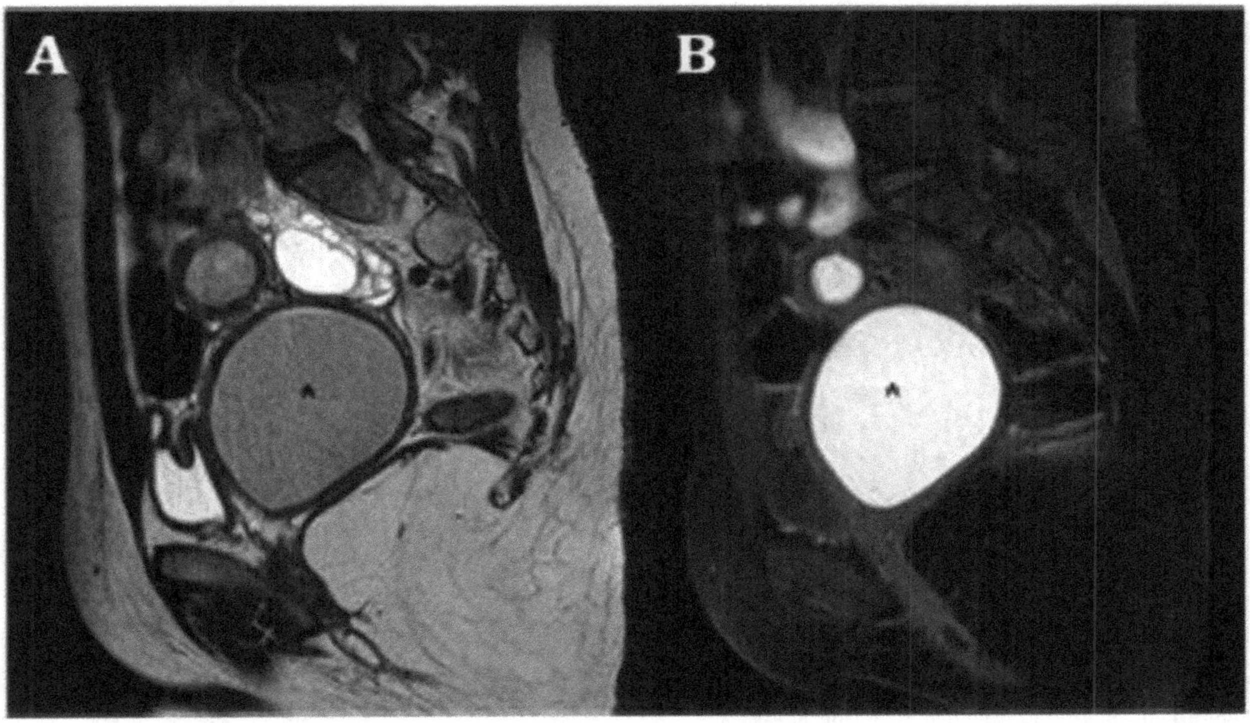

Figure 5 A) Sagittal T2-weighted MR image demonstrates an enormously dilated hemivagina (asterisk) due to the presence of the transverse septum causing the obstruction and low T2-signal-intensity contents corresponding to a high T1-signal intensity; B) consistent with blood product due to the presence of haemoglobin.

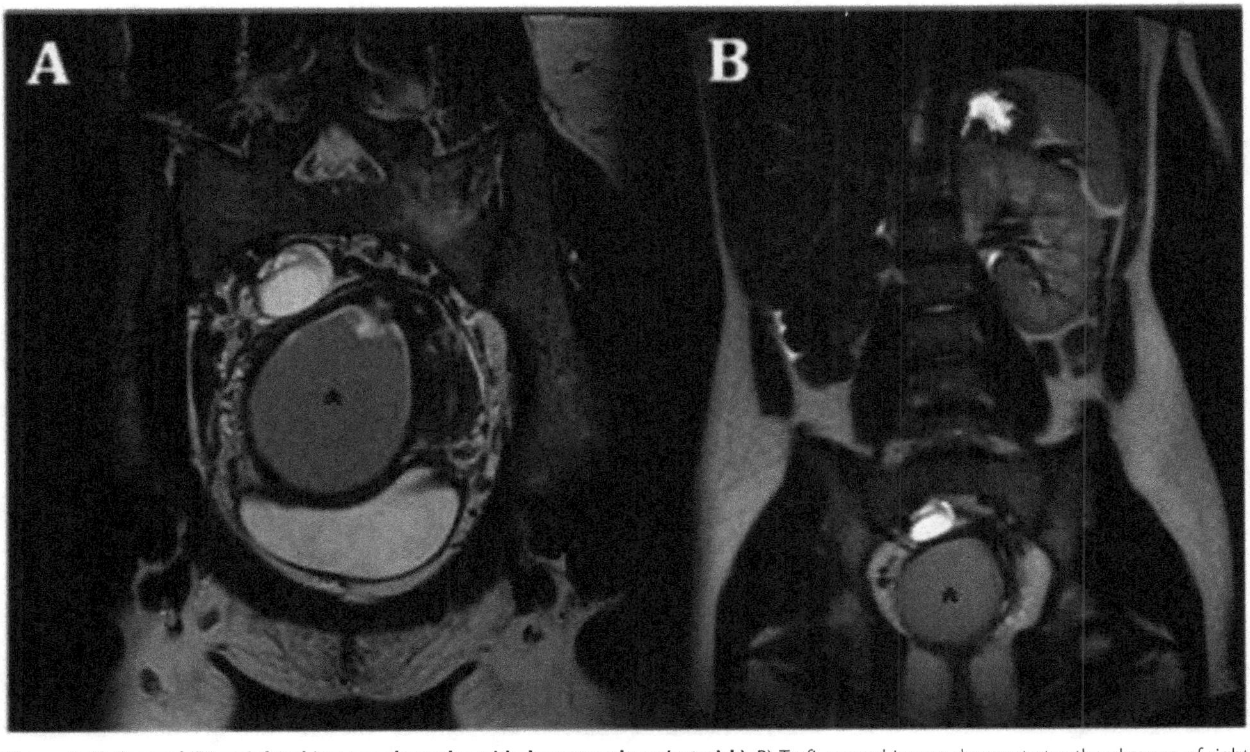

Figure 6 A) Coronal T2 weighted images show the wide hematocolpos (asterisk). B) Trufi coronal image demonstrates the absence of right kidney, omolateral to the pelvic alteration, and a mild compensatory hypertrophy of the left kidney.

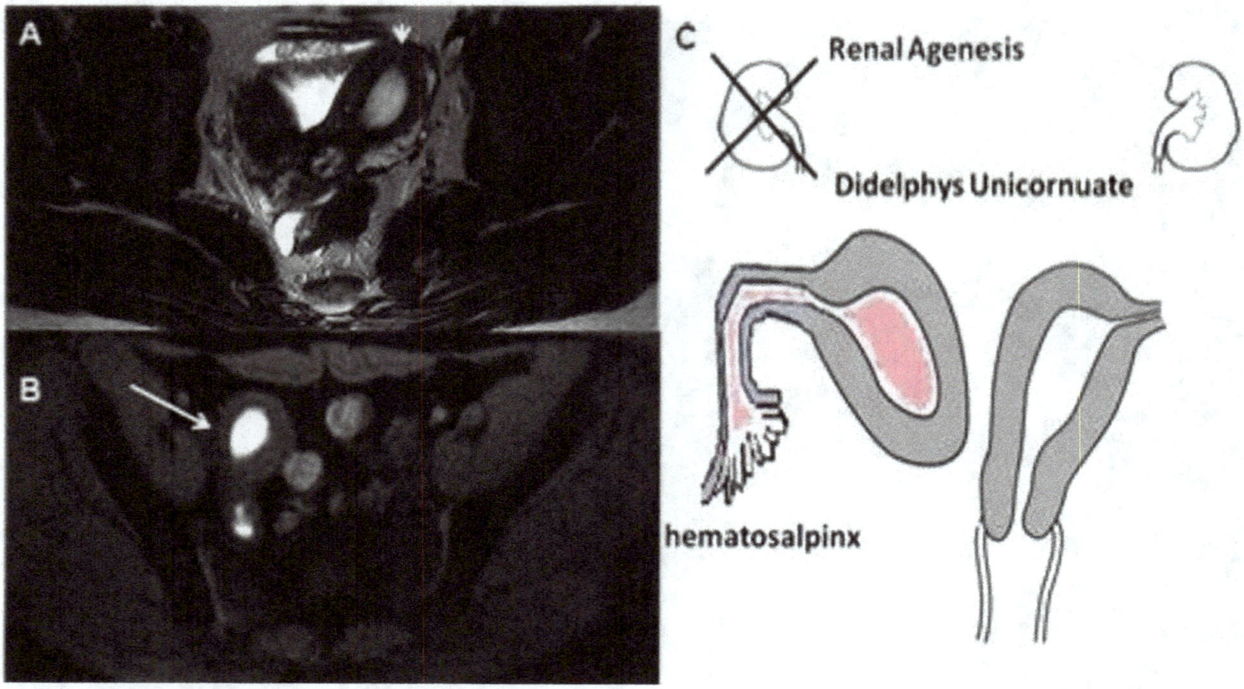

Figure 7 A) TSE axial T2 weighted MR image. B) Axial fat-saturated T1-weighted images. C) Drawing illustrates a 14-year-old girl with an unicornuate uterus and rudimentary right horn with an endometrial cavity that does not communicate with the uterus (class II MDA type) and shows an obstructed functional right uterine horn (long straight arrow) containing blood degradation products and a corresponding high T1fs-signal intensity, exhibiting no communication with the cavity of the normal left uterine horn (short straight arrow).

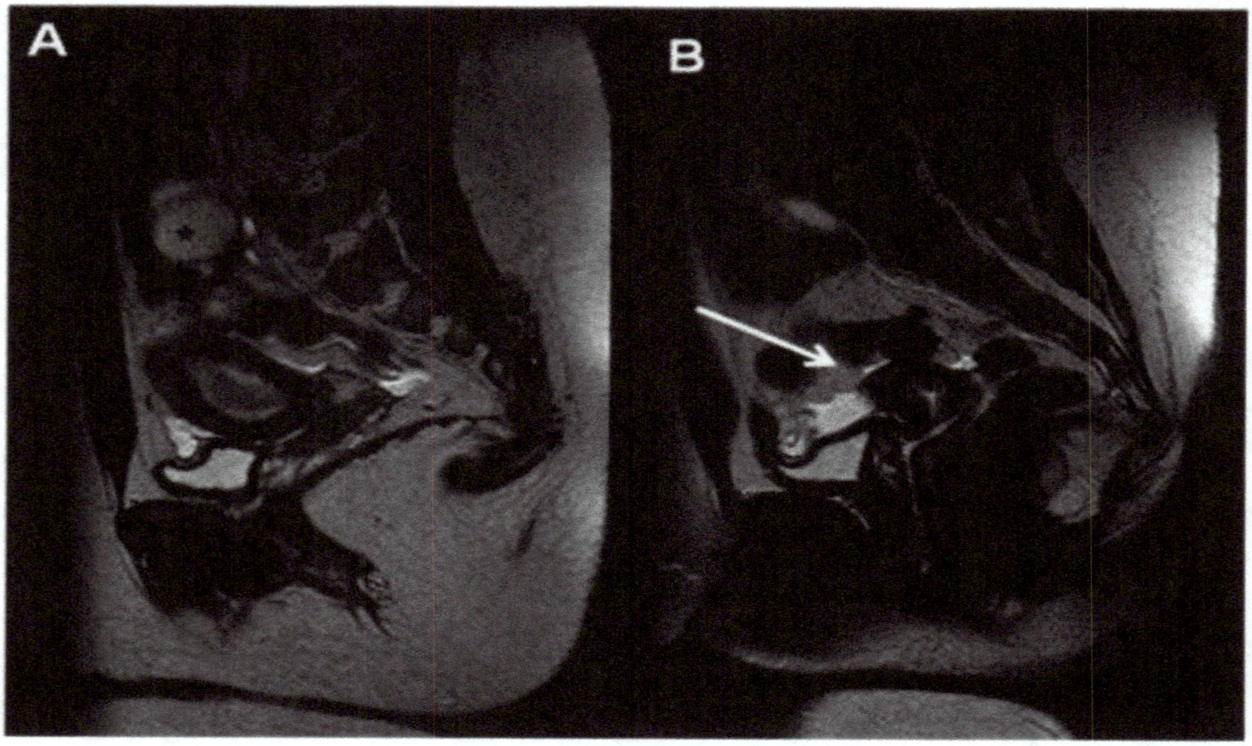

Figure 8 A) Sagittal T2-weighted MR image shows a normal left uterine cavity communicating with a normal cervix (long straight arrow), which in turn communicates with a normal vagina. (B) Right hematosalpinx (asterisk) with a distended non-communicating horn filled with fluid moderately hyperintense on T2 sequences due to haemoglobin degradation products.

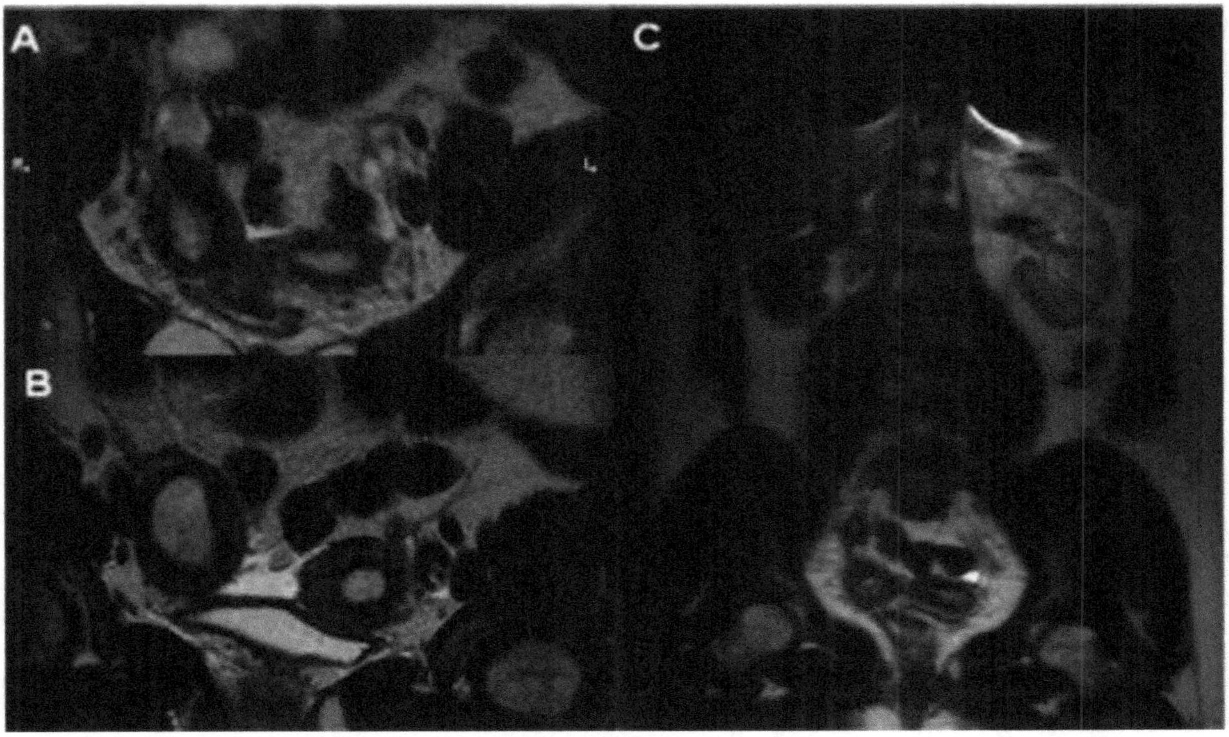

Figure 9 A-B-C) Coronal T2 weighted images demonstrate the absence of right kidney, omolateral to the pelvic alteration.

of endometrial tissue reflux through the fallopian tube, which can result in retrograde endometriosis, is higher, confirming the theory postulated by Sampson [20].

Several reports have confirmed that an association with endometriosis is present in obstructive Müllerian anomalies such as HWW syndrome, but it has not been confirmed to date in non-obstructive malformations. Therefore, it is imperative that MRI technology should be used to evaluate the presence of endometriosis.

Additionally, the presence of associated hematocolpos and hematometra, as well as the presence of an irregularly shaped or sized adnexal structure, or potentially expanding masses inside, need to be detected.

Another kind of obstructive Müllerian anomalies, different from the HWW syndrome, is OHVIRA syndrome, characterized by a variety of associated disorders. Infact, while the classic presentation includes obstructed hemivagina and ipsilateral renal anomaly (OHVIRA), some authors reported other renal anomalies, such as duplicated kidneys, dysplastic kidneys or retrovescical bands [21]. There have been also few reports of varied uterine anatomy; infact, a series of 42 cases of OHVIRA syndrome described, in 22% of cases, a septate uteri [15], but the majorority of cases are duplicated or didelphys uterus, although it has been described a case with two cervices, two uterine cavities and a single uterus [22].

Consent

Written informed consent was obtained from the patient for publication of this case report and accompanying images. A copy of the written consent is available for review by the Editor-in-Chief of this journal.

Abbreviations

HWW syndrome: Herlyn-Werner-Wunderlich syndrome; MDA: Müllerian Duct Anomalies; US: ultrasonography: MR: Magnetic Resonance; MRI: Magnetic Resonance Imaging; ASRM: American Society for Reproductive Medicine; CT: Computed Tomography.

Authors' contributions

SB, VDP, RLC and CP analysed and interpreted the patient data. RDV, IS, RFG and BBZ performed the abdominal magnetic resonance. RDV, SB and VDP were the major contributors in writing the manuscript. All authors read and approved the final manuscript.

Competing interests

The authors declare that they have no competing interests.

References

1. Gholoum S, Puligandla PS, Hui T, Su W, Quiros E, Laberge JM: **Management and outcome of patients with combined vaginal septum, bifid uterus and ipsilateral renal agenesis (Herlin-Werner-Wunderlich syndrome.** *J Pediatr Surg* 2006, 41(5):987-92.
2. Alan JW, Louis RK: **Campbell-Walsh Urology.** Philadelphia: Saunders;, 93270-6.
3. Orazi C, Lucchetti MC, Schingo PM, Marchetti P, Ferro F: **Herlyn-Werner-Wunderlich syndrome: uterus didelphys, blind hemivagina and**

ipsilateral renal agenesis. Sonographic and MR findings in 11 cases. *Pediatr Radiol* 2007, **37**:657-65.

4. Lee BH, Kim JW, Oh SI, *et al*: **3 cases of uterus didelphys with obstructed hemivagina and ipsilateral renal agenesis.** *Korean J Obstet Gynecol* 1997, **40**:1489-95.
5. Heinonen PK: **Clinical implications of the didelphic uterus: long-term follow-up of 49 cases.** *Eur J Obstet Gynecol Reprod Biol* 2000, **91**:183-90.
6. Candiani GB, Fedele L, Candiani M: **Double uterus, blind hemivagina and ipsilateral renal agenesis: 36 cases and long-term follow-up.** *Obstet Gynecol* 1997, **90**:26-32.
7. Park Noh Hyuck, Park Hee Jin, Park Chan Sup, Park Sung Il: **Herlyn-Werner-Wunderlich Syndrome with Unilateral Hemivaginal Obstruction, Ipsilateral Renal Agenesis and Contralateral Renal Thin GBM Disease: A Case Report with Radiological Follow Up.** *J Korean Soc Radiol* 2010, **62**:383-388.
8. Zurawin RK, Dietrich JE, Heard MJ, Edwards CL: **Didelphic uterus and obstructed hemivagina with renal agenesis: case report and review of the literature.** *J Pediatr Adolesc Gynecol* 2004, **17**:137-41.
9. Kim TE, *et al*: **Hysteroscopic resection of the vaginal septum in uterus didelphys with obstructed hemivagina: a case report.** *J Korean Med Sci* 2007, **22**:766-769.
10. Grimbizis GF, *et al*: **Clinical implications of uterine malformations and hysteroscopic treatment results.** *Hum Reprod Update* 2001, **7**:161-174.
11. American Fertility Society: **The American Fertility Society classifications of adnexal adhesions, distal tubal occlusion, tubal occlusion secondary to tubal ligation, tubal pregnancies. Müllerian duct anomalies and intrauterine adhesions.** *Fertil Steril* 1988, **49**:944-55.
12. Rana R, Pasrija S, Puri M: **Herlyn-Werner-Wunderlich syndrome with pregnancy: a rare presentation.** *Congenit Anom* 2008, **48**:142-3.
13. Tanaka YO, Kurosaki Y, Kobayashi T, *et al*: **Uterus didelphys associated with obstructed hemivagina and ipsilateral renal agenesis: MR findings in seven cases.** *Abdom Imaging* 1998, **23(4)**:437-441.
14. Foglia RP, Kim SH, Cleveland RH, Donahoe PK: **Complications of vaginal atresia in association with a duplicated Müllerian duct.** *J Pediatr Surg* 1987, **22(7)**:653-656.
15. Haddad B, Barranger E, Paniel BJ: **Blind hemivagina: long-term follow-up and reproductive performance in 42 cases.** *Hum Reprod* 1999, **14(8)**:1962-1964.
16. Kiechl-Kohlendorfer U, Geley TE, Unsinn KM, Ganer I: **Diagnosing neonatal female genital anomalies using saline-enhanced sonography.** *AJR Am J Roentgenol* 2001, **177**:1041-1044.
17. Burgis J: **Obstructive Müllerian anomalies: Case report, diagnosis, and management.** *Am J Obstet Gynecol* 2001, **185**:338-44.
18. Gruenwald P: **Relation of the growing Müllerian duct to the Wolffian duct and its importance for the genesis of malformation.** *Anat Rec* 1941, **81**:1-20.
19. Park Noh Hyuck, Park Hee Jin, Park Chan Sup, Park Sung Il: **Herlyn-Werner-Wunderlich Syndrome with Unilateral Hemivaginal Obstruction, Ipsilateral Renal Agenesis and Contralateral Renal Thin GBM Disease: A Case Report with Radiological Follow Up.** *J Korean Soc Radiol* 2010, **62**:383-388.
20. Brosens IA, Brosens JJ: **Endometriosis.** *Eur J Obstet Gynecol Reprod Biol* 2000, **90(2)**:159-64.
21. Shavell VI, Montgomery SE, Johnson SC, Diamond MP, Berman JM: **Complete septate uterus, obstructed hemivagina and ipsilateral renal anomaly: pregnancy course complicated by a rare urogenital anomaly.** *Arch Gynecol Obstet* 2009, **280**:449-52.
22. Shah KDivya, Laufer RMarc: **Obstructed hemivagina and ipsilateral renal anomaly (OHVIRA) syndrome with a single uterus.** *Fertility and Sterility* 2011, **96**:e39-e41.

26

MRI to assess chemoprevention in transgenic adenocarcinoma of mouse prostate (TRAMP)

Ali S Arbab[1*], Adarsh Shankar[1], Nadimpalli RS Varma[1], Dorrah Deeb[2], Xiaohua Gao[2], ASM Iskander[1], Branislava Janic[1], Meser M Ali[1] and Subhash C Gautam[2]

Abstract

Background: The current method to determine the efficacy of chemoprevention in TRAMP mouse model of carcinoma of prostate (CaP) is by extracting and weighing the prostate at different time points or by immunohistochemistry analysis. Non-invasive determination of volumes of prostate glands and seminal vesicles before, during and after treatment would be valuable in investigating the efficacy of newer chemopreventive agents in CaP. The purpose of this study was to determine whether *in vivo* magnetic resonance imaging (MRI) using a 3 tesla clinical MRI system can be used to follow the effect of chemoprevention in TRAMP model of mouse CaP.

Methods: Mice were randomized into control and treated groups. The animals in treated group received 10 μmol/kg of CDDO, 5 days a week for 20 weeks. Animals underwent *in vivo* MRI of prostate gland and seminal vesicles by a clinical 3 Tesla MRI system just before (at 5 weeks), during and at the end of treatment, at 25 weeks. T1-weighted and fat saturation (FATSAT) multiecho fast spin echo T2- weighted images (T2WI) were acquired. Volume of the prostate glands and seminal vesicles was determined from MR images. T2 signal intensity changes in the seminal vesicles were determined by subtracting higher echo time (TE) from lower TE T2WI. Following treatments all animals were sacrificed, prostate and seminal vesicles collected, and the tissues prepared for histological staining. All data were expressed as mean ± 1 standard deviation. Two-way or multivariate analysis of variance followed by post-hoc test was applied to determine the significant differences. A p-value of <0.05 was considered significant.

Results: Histological analysis indicated tumor in 100% of control mice, whereas 10% of the treated mice showed tumor in prostate gland. Both MRI and measured prostate weights showed higher volume/weight in control mouse group. MRI showed significantly higher volume of seminal vesicles in control animals and T2 signal intensity changes in seminal vesicles of control mice indicating higher number of tumor foci, which was also proven by histology.

Conclusions: *In vivo* MRI is helpful in determining the efficacy of chemoprevention of prostate cancer in TRAMP mice.

Background

According to American Cancer Society, prostate cancer is the most frequently diagnosed malignant neoplasm among men in America and is the second leading cancer in deaths. The American Cancer Society estimates that there will be 240,890 new cases of prostate cancer diagnosed and 33,720 prostate cancer specific deaths in 2011. To help solve and find a remedy for this illness, investigators in the field of prostate cancer therapy and research are using a mouse model called TRAMP (Transgenic Adenocarcinoma of Mouse Prostate). TRAMP is a transgenic mouse model of carcinoma of prostate (CaP). The mouse model has the ability to develop spontaneous tumors, which have helped study chemopreventive treatment efficacy. This model helps to predict therapeutic responses in different chemopreventive treatment strategies.

Because of the long latency period and slow progression of the preneoplastic lesions to the malignant stage, CaP is ideally suited for developing primary, secondary and tertiary preventive strategies. Thus, intervention with plant-derived polyphenolic compounds or their

* Correspondence: saali@rad.hfh.edu
[1]Department of Radiology, Henry Ford Hospital, 1 Ford Place, 2F, Detroit, MI 48202, USA
Full list of author information is available at the end of the article

synthetic analogs represents a promising approach to preventing/delaying the incidence, progression, recurrence, morbidity and mortality associated with cancer of the prostate. Triterpenes or triterpenoids are members of a larger family of structurally related compounds known as cyclosqualenoids that are widely distributed in the plant kingdom [1]. Oleanolic acid and ursolic acid are naturally occurring triterpenoids that have been used in traditional medicine as anti-cancer and anti-inflammatory agents [2-4]. 2-cyano-3,12-dioxooleana-1,9 (11)-dien-28-oic acid (CDDO) has also shown chemopreventive activity in animal models of liver, breast and lung cancer [5-7], but they have not been investigated for the prevention of prostate cancer.

The current method to determine the efficacy of treatments is by extracting and weighing the prostate at different time points or by immunohistochemistry analysis. Non-invasive determination of prostate glands and seminal vesicles volumes before, during and after treatment will be valuable in investigating the efficacy of different newer chemopreventive agents in prostate cancer. Magnetic resonance imagining (MRI) is often used to analyze therapeutic efficacy in pre-clinical studies [8,9]. Only few investigators have successfully viewed the images of the mouse prostate glands and its tumor by high-resolution magnetic resonance imaging [10-12]. MRI is thought to be one of the best choices among *in vivo* imaging modalities, not only because of its high resolution but also due to its ability to separate tissues based on signal intensities. Unlike human, prostate gland in mouse has different anatomy and does not remain fixed. Mouse prostate is multi-lobed (two anterior, two dorsolateral and one ventral), which surrounds urethra and moves along with urinary bladder. Moreover, tumor in TRAMP model does not remain confined within prostate lobes and spreads in seminal vesicles [11,13,14]. Therefore, lobes of the prostate as well as seminal vesicles should be analyzed by *in vivo* imaging to determine the effects of chemoprevention. The purpose of this paper is to determine whether non-invasive *in vivo* MRI can determine the effects of treatment in TRAMP model of mouse CaP.

Methods

Ethical Statement

Animal experiments described in the manuscript were approved by our animal care and user committee at Henry Ford Health System (protocol number 856) according to the guideline and policies of office of laboratory animal welfare (OLAW) and public health service, National Institutes of Health. All the experiments were performed according to the approved protocol.

Reagents

CDDO was obtained from the National Cancer Institute, Bethesda, MD through the Rapid Access to Intervention Development Program

Mice

TRAMP mice were bred by the Jackson Laboratories (Bar Harbor, ME, USA) through their Speed Expansion Service involving *in vitro* fertilization of C57BL/6 females with C57BL/6-Tg (TRAMP) 8247NG/J males. Mice were genotyped for the transgene (Tag) and delivered to us when 4 weeks old. Mice were maintained in temperature-controlled room (68-72°F) with a 12 h light/dark cycle and provided semi-purified AIN-76A mouse chow and water *ad libitum*. Mice were acclimated for one week before starting the experiment. All animal treatments were according to the protocol approved by the Institutional Animal Care and Use Committee [15].

Treatment protocol

At the age of 5 weeks, 50 male TRAMP mice were weighed and randomized into two groups: Mice in vehicle control group (n = 25) were administered 0.1 ml of vehicle consisting of cremophor-EL:DMSO:PBS (1:1:8), 5 days a week for 20 weeks by p.o. gavage. In the treatment group (n = 25), mice were administered CDDO at a dose of 10 μmol/kg in 0.1 ml of vehicle, 5 days a week for 20 weeks. Body weight of control and CDDO-treated mice was recorded each week and mice were observed for treatment related stress, such as water and food withdrawal, unusual posture, ruffled fur or listlessness. Ten randomly selected animals from each group underwent *in vivo* MRI of prostate glands and seminal vesicles, just before (5 weeks of age), in the middle (at 12 weeks of age) and at the end of treatment. Same selected animals under went MRI at all time points, however, identity of individual animal was not tracked during imaging or at euthanasia due to loss of body markings or ear tags during the long treatment. At the age of 25 wk following MRI, mice from both groups were sacrificed 24 h after the last administration of vehicle or CDDO. After opening the abdomen, mice were visually observed for the presence of tumor mass, enlargement of seminal vesicles, prostate lobes, and pelvic lymph nodes. Urogenital tract and pelvic lymph nodes were removed and weighed. Tissue samples were processed for histological analyses.

In Vivo MRI Studies by 3 Tesla

An appropriate state of anesthesia was obtained with isoflurane (3% for induction, 0.7% to 1.5% for maintenance mixed with O2). MRI was obtained with a 3

Tesla clinical MRI system (Signa Excite, GE health) using 50 mm diameter × 108 mm RF rung length small animal imaging coil (Litzcage small animal imaging system, Doty Scientific Inc, Columbia, SC). After positioning using a triplanar FLASH sequence, T1, and fast spin echo (FSE) fat suppression (FATSAT) T2-weighted images were obtained. T1- weighted images were obtained using following sequence; TR/TE = 300/10 ms, 128 × 128 matrix, 13-15 slices, 0.9 mm thick, 40 mm field of view (FOV), number of excitation (NEX) = 2-4. Fast spin echo T2-weighted images were obtained using standard two-dimensional Fourier transformation (2DFT) multislice (13-15) multiecho (2 echoes) MRI. A series of 2 sets of images (13-15 slices for each set) were obtained using TEs of 11 to 70 msec and a TR of 4000-5000 ms. The images were acquired using 40 mm FOV, 1 mm slice thickness, 128 × 128 matrix, and NEX = 2. We used clinical 3T MRI system due to availability of small animal coil synchronized with 3T MRI and optimized for small animal scanning. Moreover, all the available clinically approved MRI sequences can be used, especially fat suppression during T1 and T2-weighted images. Easy sequence manipulation and shorter acquisition time were also considered as advantages.

Image analysis

All images were analyzed using our home made image analysis software "Eigentool" (http://www.radiologyresearch.org/eigentool.htm). Volume of the prostate glands and seminal vesicles were determined by an investigator blinded to the assignment of animals (treated vs control). The investigators were trained to indentify the prostate glands and the seminal vesicles by going through both axial and coronal images obtained with T1W and T2W sequences. Irregular region of interests (ROIs) were drawn over prostate and seminal vesicles separately and the areas were recorded (Figure 1). All the image sections that contained prostate and seminal vesicles were included in the analysis. Total calculated areas were multiplied by image thickness to determine the volume of prostate and seminal vesicles. The values were expressed in cm^3. The volume of prostate gland calculated from MRI images was compared with the weight of the prostate gland (gm) determined at necropsy. MRI could detect dorsal and anterior/ventral lobes of the prostate gland clearly. However, due to partial volume effect the lateral lobes that continue with coagulating gland could not be separated from surrounding tissues and seminal vesicles. On the other hand, *ex vivo* extracted prostate glands comprised of all the lobes. It is expected that due to differential density between control (due to tumors) and treated animals the volume measured by MRI will not exactly match the weight of the extracted prostate glands and seminal vesicles.

Analysis of signal intensity

According to Dr. Bradley (http://www.e-radiography.net/mrict/fund mr2/fundmri 2.htm) mathematically the intensity (I) of the spin echo signal can be approximated:

$$I = N(H)f(v)(1 - e^{-TR/T1})e^{-TE/T2}$$

where N(H) is the NMR-visible, mobile proton density and f(v) is an unspecified function of flow. This equation indicates that the intensity of the MR signal increases as hydrogen density and T2 increase and as T1 decreases. It should also be noted that T1 and T2 influences are both subject to TR (repetition time) and TE (echo time). Thus, the effect of the T1 and T2 relaxation times of the substance on signal intensity is subject to the specific values of TR and TE selected before the image is acquired. When considered in the most simplistic terms, the spin echo is a two-step process. The first step (longitudinal recovery) determines the starting intensity for the second step (transverse decay). The starting intensity reflects the relationship between T1 and TR and is ultimately limited by the proton density. The subsequent decay from this starting intensity reflects the relationship between T2 and TE. As the TR is prolonged, all substances eventually recover full longitudinal magnetization between repetitions and the pixel intensity becomes dependent only upon proton density and is independent of T1. Substances with longer T2 times will generate stronger signals than substances with shorter T2 times, if both are acquired at the same TE and if proton density and T1 are comparable. Increasing the echo delay time (TE) increases the differences in the T2 decay curves between substances, increasing the T2-weighting. Images obtained with a sufficiently long TR and TE will cause fluid (such as CSF) or edema more intense than solid tissue (such as brain).

It is expected that multiple small tumor foci and associated edema will cause lengthening of T2 values in seminal vesicles of control untreated animals compared to that of treated animals, therefore, signal intensity on T2-weighted images will vary based on the echo delay time (TE). The TR used in image acquisition is long enough to recover full longitudinal magnetization between repetitions and the signal intensity on MR images with different TE will be different between areas of normal seminal vesicle and in areas of tumor growths due to varying T2 values. We expect that tissues with higher T2 will show relatively high signal intensity on images obtained with higher TE and subtraction of the images of higher TE from lower TE will give differential image. To calculate

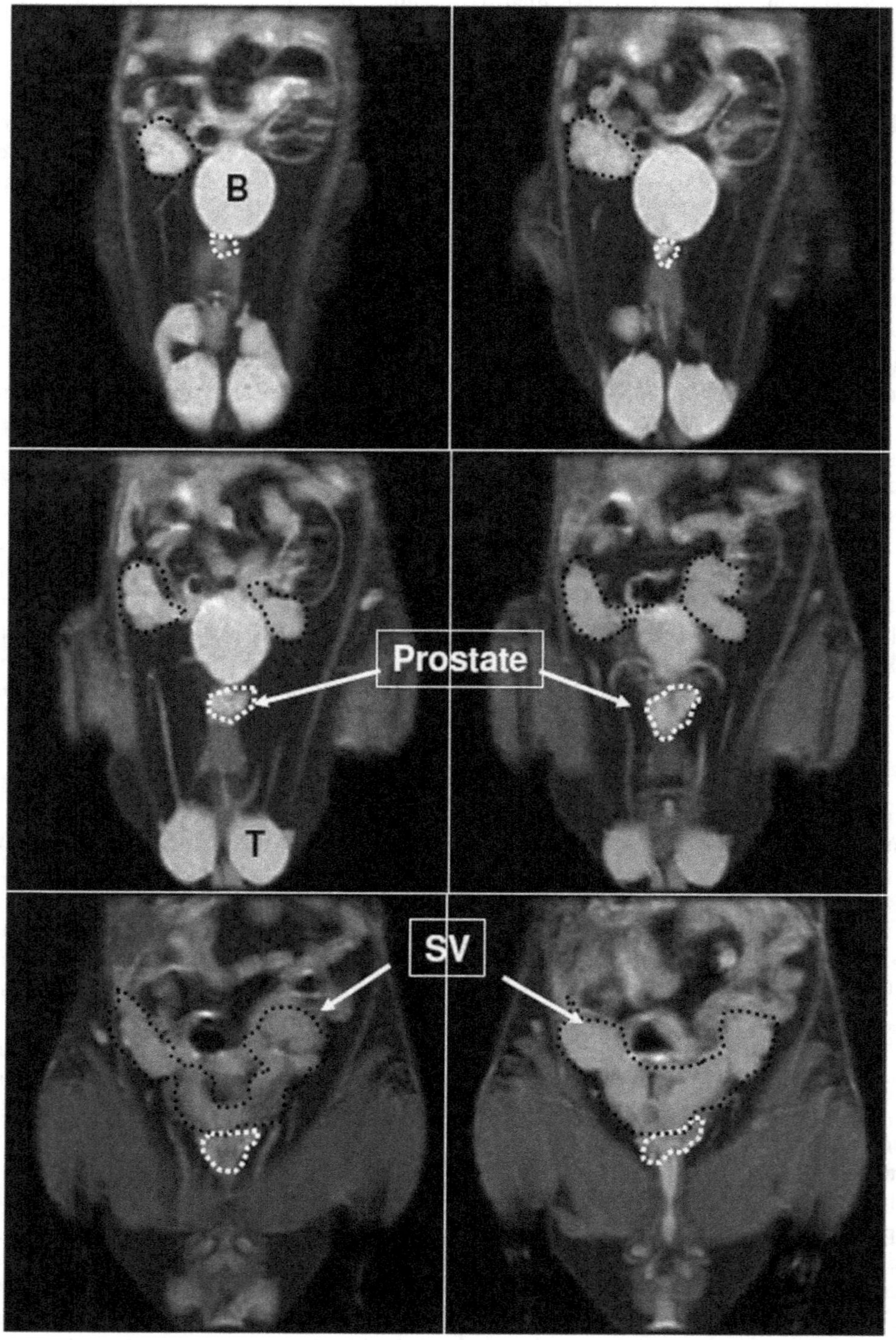

Figure 1 Prostate gland and seminal vesicles on MR images. Identification of prostate gland (areas inside white dots) and seminal vesicles (areas inside black dots) on fat saturation T2-weighted images. Volume of the prostate gland and seminal vesicles was determined by drawing irregular region of interest. B = urinary bladder, T = testes and SV = seminal vesicle.

the changes in signal intensities, images with higher TE (70 ms) were subtracted from corresponding images with lower TE (11 ms) and the resultant images were analyzed. The same investigator blinded to the assignment of animals drew ROIs on the left and right seminal vesicles (to include all areas of seminal vesicles in all sections) and on the skeletal muscles of the corresponding left and right thighs (Figure 2). Average signal intensities of seminal

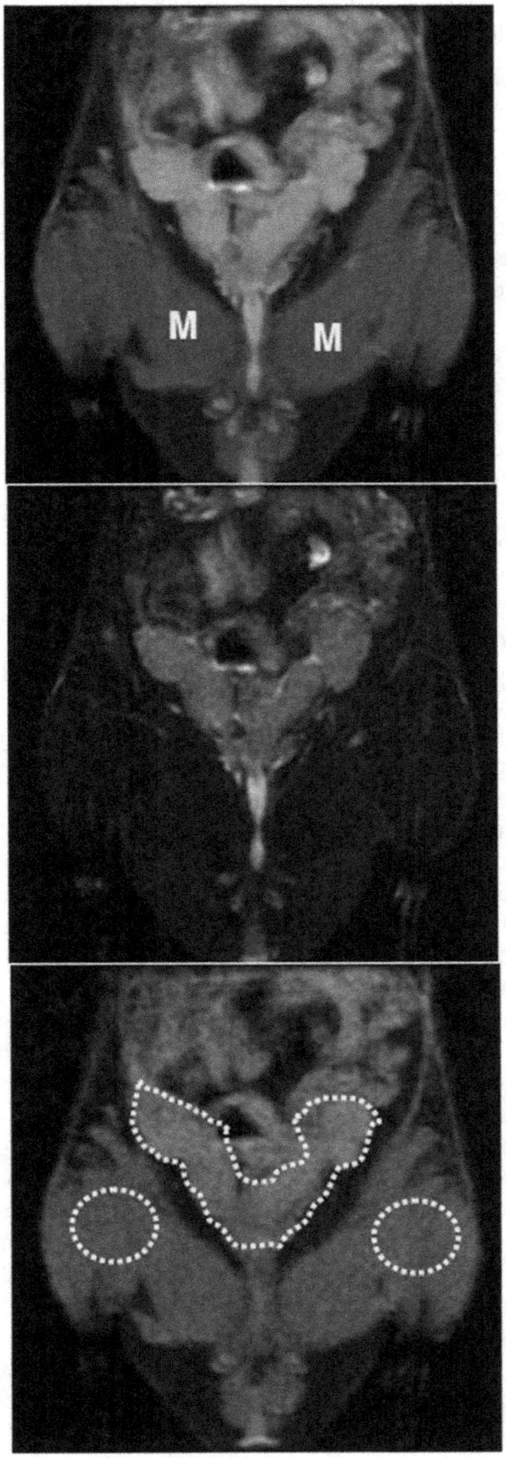

Figure 2 Measurement of signal intensity changes. Representative images of seminal vesicles from a mouse showing signal intensity on FATSAT T2-weighted image with a TE of 11 ms (upper), with a TE of 70 ms (middle) and subtracted image (lower). Note the differential signal intensity among different tissues on higher TE. ROIs on lower image indicate the representative areas from where signal intensity changes were determined. M = muscles.

vesicles were normalized with corresponding average signal intensity of thigh muscles. It is to be cautioned that inflammation or abscess in seminal vesicles may give similar signal intensity changes, however, TRAMP model creates spontaneous small tumor foci in the seminal vesicles, and inflammation or abscess is not expected.

Histological analysis

Tissue specimens of prostate gland and seminal vesicles for all animals that underwent MRI were fixed in 10% neutral buffered formalin for 48 h and then embedded in paraffin. Five to six micrometers thick sections were cut and stained with H&E for routine histology. Tumors were graded according to our published method in prostate glands in all control and treated animals [16] that underwent MRI by using photomicrographs from 5 randomly selected areas. Presence or absence of tumor foci in seminal vesicles was also checked and photomicrographed. For dorso-lateral prostate (DLP), histopathological classification was as follows; normal DLP (ducts lined with single layer of secretory epithelial cells surrounded by 2-3 cell layers of fibromuscular stroma); low-grade prostatic intraepithelial neoplasia (PIN) (epithelial cells with variably elongated nuclei with condensed chromatin); high-grade PIN (epithelial stratification and tufting, presence of micropapillary and cribiform structures); well differentiated (WD) carcinoma (epithelial cells invading fibromuscular stroma) and moderately (MD) to poorly differentiated (PD) adenocarcinoma of the prostate (sheets of neoplastic cells with little or no glandular structures).

Data analysis

All data were expressed as mean ± one standard deviation. Either two way analysis of variance (ANOVA) or multivariate ANOVA followed by post-hoc test Fisher's PLSD was applied to determine the significant differences between treated and control or among different time points (5 weeks, 12 weeks and 25 weeks). A p-value of <0.05 was considered significant.

Results

Treatment with CDDO is well tolerated

Treatment with CDDO for 20 weeks was well tolerated without evidence of any noticeable toxicity with respect to animal appearance, behavior or change in the body weight. Body weight increased as a function of age at the same rate in both the vehicle control and treatment group from 20 ± 0.8 g (control group) and 20.5 ± 0.9 g (treatment group) at 5 weeks of age to 32.7 ± 1.5 g and 31.9 ± 1.9 g, respectively at 25 weeks of age.

Prostate and seminal vesicles by in vivo imaging

MR images were obtained before and after the start of the treatment. The analysis of images showed similar volume of seminal vesicles in control mouse (0.126 ± 0.03 cm^3 at 5 weeks) compared to that of treated (0.143 ± 0.07 cm^3 at 5 weeks) at 5 weeks. However the volume became significantly higher ($p < 0.05$) in control mice (0.596 ± 0.17 cm^3 at 25 weeks) compared to that of treated mice after 20 weeks following the start of the treatment (0.397 ± 0.13 cm^3 at 25 weeks) (Figure 3A). On the other hand, volumes of the prostate glands measured from 10 animals in each group were not different among the control (0.02 ± 0.006 cm^3) and treated (0.02 ± 0.005 cm^3) animals at 5 weeks. Increased volume of prostate gland was observed in control animals (0.044 ± 0.019 cm^3 at 25 weeks) compared to that of treated animals (0.03 ± 0.018 cm^3 at 25 weeks), although significant difference was not achieved ($p = 0.102$) (Figure 3B). Similarly, weights of the prostate glands collected from these same animals that underwent MRI also did not show significant difference ($p = 0.17$) between the control (0.058 ± 0.014 gm at 25 weeks) and treated groups (0.045 ± 0.019 gm at 25 weeks). The measured volume of prostate glands was in agreement with the measured weight determined during collection of tissues following euthanasia (Figure 3C) when compared between controls and treated animals (tendency to increase volume and weight in control group).

Analysis of signal intensity

Similar changes in signal intensity in seminal vesicle were observed in both groups of animals before starting the treatment at the age of week 5. However, when the signal intensity changes in seminal vesicles between the control and treated animals were compared at 25 weeks, significantly ($p < 0.01$) lower changes in signal intensity were observed in treated animals (Figure 4A), indicating less number of tumor foci to the seminal vesicles of treated animals. Control animals showed significantly higher changes in signal intensity in seminal vesicles at 25 weeks when compared with corresponding treated at 25 weeks ($p < 0.001$) and all animals at 5 weeks ($p < 0.01$). The MRI findings were also supported by histology analysis of seminal vesicles from two groups of animals (Figure 4B).

CDDO slows down the progression of prostate carcinoma in TRAMP mice

In mice treated with CDDO for 20 weeks, two of the control mice (out of 25, did not undergo MRI) showed very large tumors originating from the prostate, whereas none of the CDDO treated mice showed these large tumors. In 7 out of 10 control mice (70%) tumor growth was evident in seminal vesicles as opposed to 3 out of 10 CDDO-treated mice (30%). There was no significant difference ($p = 0.17$) in the prostate gland weight when compared between the treated and non-treated animals that underwent MRI (n = 10 in each group). However, significant difference was noticed when all animals (n = 25 in each group) were combined (CDDO = 0.040.9 ± 0.013 gm; Control = 0.073.2 ± 0.014 gm, $p < 0.01$). Histological evaluation of the DLP of control mice (that underwent MRI) showed well-differentiated adenocarcinoma in 8 of the 10 mice (80%), 2 mice showed moderately differentiated CaP (20%), and none showed normal tissue, PIN or high PIN, indicating that 100% of the control mice had cancerous lesions in the DLP (Figure 5). In contrast, 1 CDDO treated mice (10%) had normal DLP, another showed well-differentiated CaP (10%), and 8 mice (80%) had PIN or high PIN lesions (that underwent MRI). These data demonstrated that majority of the treated animals (90%) had noncancerous lesions ranging from normal tissue to preneoplastic PIN and high PIN compared to 100% of the control mice that showed CaP in the DLP. CDDO also inhibited the progression of prostate cancer into the ventral prostate.

Discussion

Although several murine prostate cancer models are available (e.g., LADY transgenic mine, PTEN null, MPAKT etc.), we used TRAMP mouse model in the present study because it is the most well-characterized and extensively used preclinical model of prostate tumorigenesis in chemoprevention studies. Probasin promoter directed expression of SV40 early genes in the prostate epithelium drives the development of prostate cancer in DLP and ventral prostate glands in an age-dependent manner beginning with the emergence of prostatic intraepithelial neoplasia (PIN), a preneoplastic lesion by 6-8 weeks of age followed by high grade PIN (HGPIN) by 10-12 weeks of age. Focal carcinoma develops between 12-18 weeks and poorly differentiated carcinoma is observed by the age of 18-24 weeks [17,18]. Tumor metastasizes to the liver, lungs, bone and pelvic lymph nodes by 24-30 weeks of age [19]. The slow progression of the multistep process of prostatic tumorigenesis over a period of 8-30 weeks renders TRAMP model highly suitable for exploiting the chemopreventive efficacy of novel agents. Indeed, TRAMP mice have been successfully used to evaluate the chemopreventive activity of several natural and synthetic compounds including sulforaphane, green tea polyphenols, garlic constituents, genistein etc. [13,20-23].

Most of the investigations that follow the progression of prostate cancer in chemopreventive treatment strategies use direct measurement of tumor weight/size as well as the weight of total genitourinary system as a measure of tumor progression following euthanasia. However, this method of measuring progression cannot follow the same animals over the span of the treatment duration. *In vivo* imaging modalities could be a great

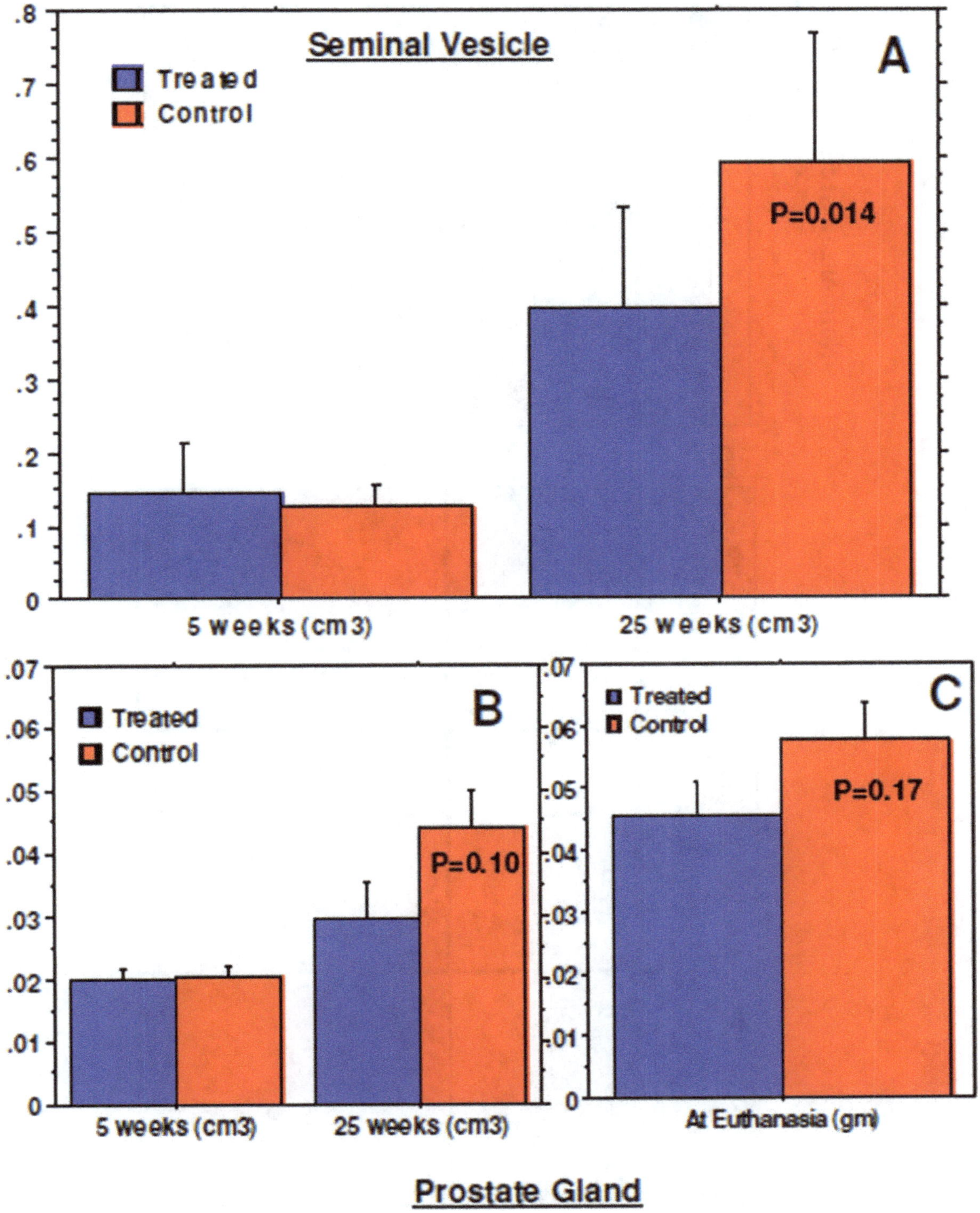

Figure 3 Measurement of seminal vesicles and prostate gland volume by MRI. (A) MR images show significantly increased volume of seminal vesicles by 25 weeks in control animals compared to that of treated animals. Note the similar volume at the beginning of the treatment (at 5 weeks). (B) Similar to seminal vesicles, prostate glands also showed higher volume in control animals on MRI which was also confirmed at necropsy (C, although significant differences were not achieved). Note the similar volume at the beginning of the treatment (at 5 weeks).

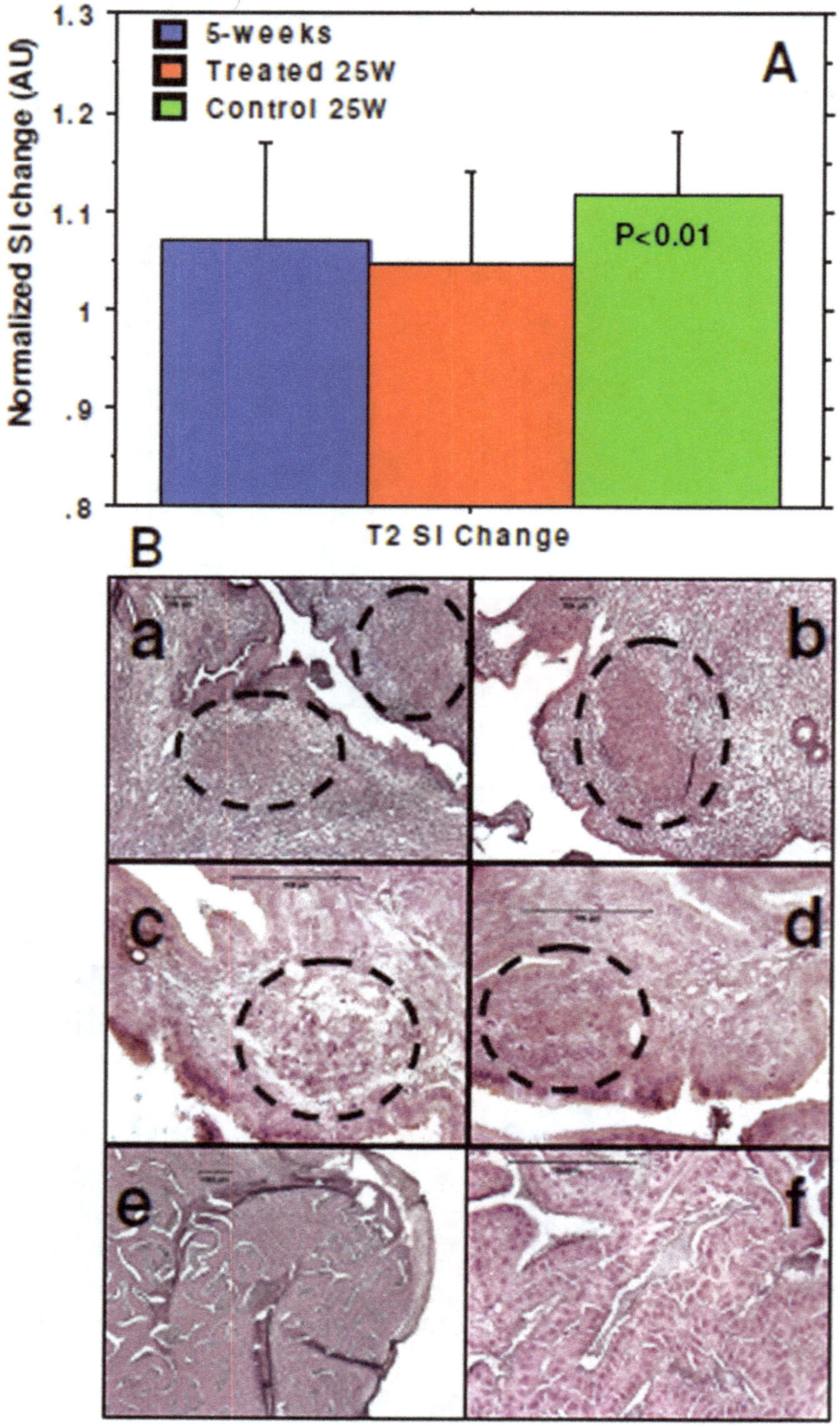

Figure 4 Changes in signal intensity and micro-tumor foci. (A) Changes in T2 signal intensity in seminal vesicles was significantly higher in control animals at 25 weeks, which indicate heterogeneous tissues (involvement of micro-tumor foci) compared to that of treated animals at 25 weeks or of animals at 5 weeks. (B) Multiple tumor foci were observed in seminal vesicles of control animals (a, b, c, d) compared to that of treated animals (e, f). a, b, e are with x10 and c, d, f are with x40 magnifications. Bars in all images represent 100μm.

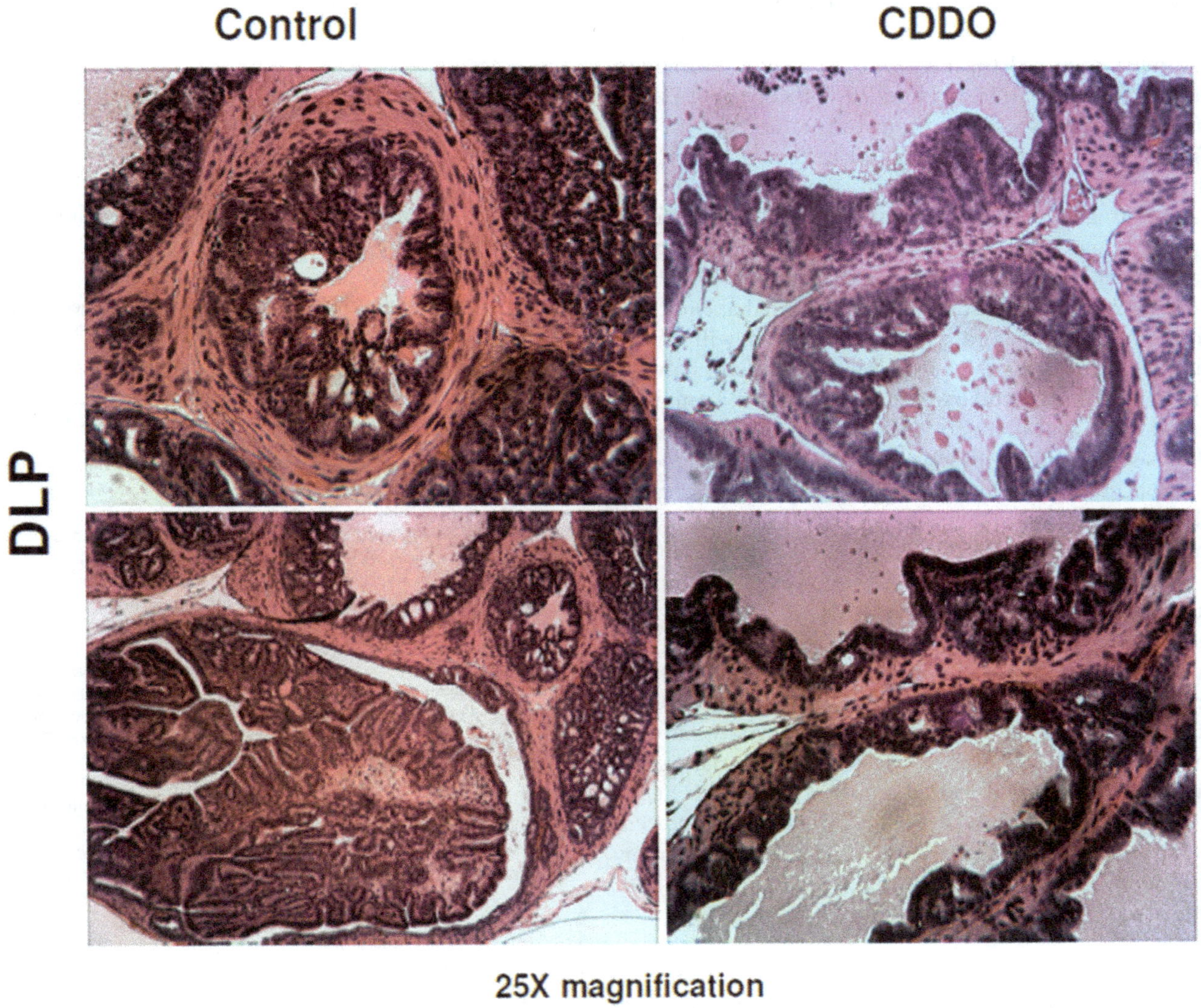

Figure 5 HE staining of prostate gland. H&E-stained sections of DLP from representative cases of 25 week old vehicle control or CDDO-treated TRAMP mouse. Control DLP showing well differentiated carcinoma and CDDO-treated DLP showing low-grade PIN. x25 magnifications.

help to follow the same animals over the span of treatment. In our previous study, we have shown the importance of FATSAT T2-weighted MRI sequence in detecting prostate glands as well as orthotopic implanted prostate cancer [24]. One advantage of MRI is that the images of the prostate gland can be obtained in all planes to identify the glands correctly or MRI can be used to obtain 3D images to reformat later to see the gland in all planes (currently we are optimizing 3D isotropic image sequences). In the current study, we have also used FATSAT sequence to detect the prostate gland, although individual tumor was not detected clearly. Inability to detect the tumor in prostate gland could be due the model itself. TRAMP model produces micro tumors both in prostate and seminal vesicles unless it is in late stages of development. Histopathology also confirmed the size of the tumors in the gland and seminal vesicles. With the current hardware of 3T clinical MRI system, it may not be possible to detect these sub-millimeter size of prostate cancer by *in vivo* imaging. We need to have either high strength dedicated animal MRI system or imaging of animal in an *ex vivo* setting. Other technique would be to use contrast enhancement. We have not tried contrast enhancement in this study, although we think contrast enhancement may not give concrete results, knowing the size of the tumors. However, our *in vivo* imaging method has produced comparable results to that of measured prostate gland weight at necropsy. In that respect, our method of *in vivo* imaging can be used to follow the chemopreventive strategy in TRAMP model of mouse prostate cancer.

Designing an image analysis technique can indirectly show the presence or absence of tumors in any tissues. We have acquired the FATSAT T2-weighted images using two echoes (11 ms and 70 ms). Lower TE T2-weighted images usually indicate total density of the proton in a tissue, which could be almost identical throughout the tissue of interest, whereas high TE images usually produce differential signal intensity from a tissue/organ based on the differential relaxation or T2 parameters [25,26] (http://www.e-radiography.net/mrict/fund mr2/fundmri 2.htm). It is expected that multiple small tumor foci and associated edema will cause lengthening of T2 values in seminal vesicles of control untreated animals compared to that of treated animals, therefore, signal intensity on T2-weighted images will vary based on the echo delay time (TE). The TR used in image acquisition is long enough to recover full longitudinal magnetization between repetitions and the signal intensity on MR images with different TE will be different between areas of normal seminal vesicle and in areas of tumor growths due to varying T2 values. By subtracting high TE images from low TE images, we could have a differential signal intensity patterns which will be different between treated and control groups of animals. Our image analysis proved our hypothesis and there were significant differences in differential signal intensity between the treated and control animals at 25 weeks. Our image analysis findings were also supported by histopathology, where multiple microscopic tumor foci were observed in seminal vesicles of control animals.

Conclusion

In conclusion, our study demonstrated the differences in the volumes of prostate gland and seminal vesicles in TRAMP mice following chemoprevention strategy and these changes can be detected by *in vivo* 3T clinical MRI. *In vivo* MRI is helpful in assessing the chemoprevention of prostate cancer in TRAMP mice.

Acknowledgements

The studies were supported by grants from National Institutes of Health (ASA: R01CA122031, SCG: R01CA130948)

Author details

[1]Department of Radiology, Henry Ford Hospital, 1 Ford Place, 2F, Detroit, MI 48202, USA. [2]Department of Surgery, Henry Ford Hospital, 1 Ford Place, 4D, Detroit, MI 48202, USA.

Authors' contributions

ASA conceived the study and carried out MRI and involved writing the manuscript and trained AS to perform image analysis. AS carried out image analysis and data collection. NRSV helped MRI and histochemistry. DD and XG carried out treatment of the animals, maintenance and collection of tissue following euthanasia. AI maintained animals and prepare the histochemistry samples. BJ helped writing and discussion. MMA helped MRI and data analysis. SCG involved in over all management of the project and critical discussion regarding treatments. All authors read and approved the final manuscript.

Competing interests

The authors declare that they have no competing interests.

References

1. Dzubak P, Hajduch M, Vydra D, Hustova A, Kvasnica M, Biedermann D, Markova L, Urban M, Sarek J: **Pharmacological activities of natural triterpenoids and their therapeutic implications.** *Nat Prod Rep* 2006, **23(3)**:394-411.
2. Huang MT, Ho CT, Wang ZY, Ferraro T, Lou YR, Stauber K, Ma W, Georgiadis C, Laskin JD, Conney AH: **Inhibition of skin tumorigenesis by rosemary and its constituents carnosol and ursolic acid.** *Cancer Res* 1994, **54(3)**:701-708.
3. Nishino H, Nishino A, Takayasu J, Hasegawa T, Iwashima A, Hirabayashi K, Iwata S, Shibata S: **Inhibition of the tumor-promoting action of 12-O-tetradecanoylphorbol-13-acetate by some oleanane-type triterpenoid compounds.** *Cancer Res* 1988, **48(18)**:5210-5215.
4. Ryu SY, Oak MH, Yoon SK, Cho DI, Yoo GS, Kim TS, Kim KM: **Anti-allergic and anti-inflammatory triterpenes from the herb of Prunella vulgaris.** *Planta Med* 2000, **66(4)**:358-360.
5. Yates MS, Kwak MK, Egner PA, Groopman JD, Bodreddigari S, Sutter TR, Baumgartner KJ, Roebuck BD, Liby KT, Yore MM, Honda T, Gribble GW, Sporn MB, Kensler TW: **Potent protection against aflatoxin-induced tumorigenesis through induction of Nrf2-regulated pathways by the triterpenoid 1-[2-cyano-3-,12-dioxooleana-1,9(11)-dien-28-oyl]imidazole.** *Cancer Res* 2006, **66(4)**:2488-2494.
6. Ling X, Konopleva M, Zeng Z, Ruvolo V, Stephens LC, Schober W, McQueen T, Dietrich M, Madden TL, Andreeff M: **The novel triterpenoid C-28 methyl ester of 2-cyano-3, 12-dioxoolen-1, 9-dien-28-oic acid inhibits metastatic murine breast tumor growth through inactivation of STAT3 signaling.** *Cancer Res* 2007, **67(9)**:4210-4218.
7. Liby K, Royce DB, Williams CR, Risingsong R, Yore MM, Honda T, Gribble GW, Dmitrovsky E, Sporn TA, Sporn MB: **The synthetic triterpenoids CDDO-methyl ester and CDDO-ethyl amide prevent lung cancer induced by vinyl carbamate in A/J mice.** *Cancer Res* 2007, **67(6)**:2414-2419.
8. Sarkar SK, Mattingly MA, Kline T, Greig R: **9.4 T imaging studies of human tumor xenografts in nude mice.** *Invest Radiol* 1988, **23(9)**:677-679.
9. Rodriguez O, Fricke S, Chien C, Dettin L, VanMeter J, Shapiro E, Dai HN, Casimiro M, Ileva L, Dagata J, Johnson MD, Lisanti MP, Koretsky A, Albanese C: **Contrast-enhanced in vivo imaging of breast and prostate cancer cells by MRI.** *Cell Cycle* 2006, **5(1)**:113-119.
10. Fricke ST, Rodriguez O, Vanmeter J, Dettin LE, Casimiro M, Chien CD, Newell T, Johnson K, Ileva L, Ojeifo J, Johnson MD, Albanese C: **In vivo magnetic resonance volumetric and spectroscopic analysis of mouse prostate cancer models.** *Prostate* 2006, **66(7)**:708-717.
11. Degrassi A, Russo M, Scanziani E, Giusti A, Ceruti R, Texido G, Pesenti E: **Magnetic resonance imaging and histopathological characterization of prostate tumors in TRAMP mice as model for pre-clinical trials.** *Prostate* 2007, **67(4)**:396-404.
12. Nastiuk KL, Liu H, Hamamura M, Muftuler LT, Nalcioglu O, Krolewski JJ: **In vivo MRI volumetric measurement of prostate regression and growth in mice.** *BMC Urol* 2007, **7**:12.
13. Gupta S, Hastak K, Ahmad N, Lewin JS, Mukhtar H: **Inhibition of prostate carcinogenesis in TRAMP mice by oral infusion of green tea polyphenols.** *Proc Natl Acad Sci USA* 2001, **98(18)**:10350-10355.
14. Gupta S, Ahmad N, Marengo SR, MacLennan GT, Greenberg NM, Mukhtar H: **Chemoprevention of prostate carcinogenesis by alpha-difluoromethylornithine in TRAMP mice.** *Cancer Res* 2000, **60(18)**:5125-5133.
15. Macura KJ, Ouwerkerk R, Jacobs MA, Bluemke DA: **Patterns of enhancement on breast MR images: interpretation and imaging pitfalls.** *Radiographics* 2006, **26(6)**:1719-1734, quiz 1719.
16. Deeb D, Gao X, Liu Y, Jiang D, Divine GW, Arbab AS, Dulchavsky SA, Gautam SC: **Synthetic triterpenoid CDDO prevents the progression and metastasis of prostate cancer in TRAMP mice by inhibiting survival signaling.** *Carcinogenesis* 2011, **32(5)**:757-764.

17. Kaplan-Lefko PJ, Chen TM, Ittmann MM, Barrios RJ, Ayala GE, Huss WJ, Maddison LA, Foster BA, Greenberg NM: **Pathobiology of autochthonous prostate cancer in a pre-clinical transgenic mouse model.** *Prostate* 2003, **55(3)**:219-237.
18. Gingrich JR, Barrios RJ, Foster BA, Greenberg NM: **Pathologic progression of autochthonous prostate cancer in the TRAMP model.** *Prostate Cancer Prostatic Dis* 1999, **2(2)**:70-75.
19. Deeb D, Gao X, Dulchavsky SA, Gautam SC: **CDDO-Me inhibits proliferation, induces apoptosis, down-regulates Akt, mTOR, NF-kappaB and NF-kappaB-regulated antiapoptotic and proangiogenic proteins in TRAMP prostate cancer cells.** *J Exp Ther Oncol* 2008, **7(1)**:31-39.
20. Perkins S, Verschoyle RD, Hill K, Parveen I, Threadgill MD, Sharma RA, Williams ML, Steward WP, Gescher AJ: **Chemopreventive efficacy and pharmacokinetics of curcumin in the min/+ mouse, a model of familial adenomatous polyposis.** *Cancer Epidemiol Biomarkers Prev* 2002, **11(6)**:535-540.
21. Singh SV, Warin R, Xiao D, Powolny AA, Stan SD, Arlotti JA, Zeng Y, Hahm ER, Marynowski SW, Bommareddy A, Desai D, Amin S, Parise RA, Beumer JH, Chambers WH: **Sulforaphane inhibits prostate carcinogenesis and pulmonary metastasis in TRAMP mice in association with increased cytotoxicity of natural killer cells.** *Cancer Res* 2009, **69(5)**:2117-2125.
22. Mentor-Marcel R, Lamartiniere CA, Eltoum IE, Greenberg NM, Elgavish A: **Genistein in the diet reduces the incidence of poorly differentiated prostatic adenocarcinoma in transgenic mice (TRAMP).** *Cancer Res* 2001, **61(18)**:6777-6782.
23. Singh SV, Powolny AA, Stan SD, Xiao D, Arlotti JA, Warin R, Hahm ER, Marynowski SW, Bommareddy A, Potter DM, Dhir R: **Garlic constituent diallyl trisulfide prevents development of poorly differentiated prostate cancer and pulmonary metastasis multiplicity in TRAMP mice.** *Cancer Res* 2008, **68(22)**:9503-9511.
24. Rad AM, Gao X, Deeb D, Gautam SC, Arbab AS: **Imaging Mouse Prostate Gland by 3 Tesla Clinical MRI System.** *Open Magn Reson Rev* 2008, **1**:60-63.
25. Ohtomo K, Itai Y, Furui S, Yashiro N, Yoshikawa K, Iio M: **Hepatic tumors: differentiation by transverse relaxation time (T2) of magnetic resonance imaging.** *Radiology* 1985, **155(2)**:421-423.
26. Arbab AS, Ichikawa T, Sou H, Araki T, Nakajima H, Ishigame K, Yoshikawa T, Kumagai H: **Ferumoxides-enhanced double-echo T2-weighted MR imaging in differentiating metastases from nonsolid benign lesions of the liver.** *Radiology* 2002, **225(1)**:151-158.

27

Volume Tracking: A new method for quantitative assessment and visualization of intracardiac blood flow from three-dimensional, time-resolved, three-component magnetic resonance velocity mapping

Johannes Töger[1,2], Marcus Carlsson[1], Gustaf Söderlind[2], Håkan Arheden[1] and Einar Heiberg[1*]

Abstract

Background: Functional and morphological changes of the heart influence blood flow patterns. Therefore, flow patterns may carry diagnostic and prognostic information. Three-dimensional, time-resolved, three-directional phase contrast cardiovascular magnetic resonance (4D PC-CMR) can image flow patterns with unique detail, and using new flow visualization methods may lead to new insights. The aim of this study is to present and validate a novel visualization method with a quantitative potential for blood flow from 4D PC-CMR, called Volume Tracking, and investigate if Volume Tracking complements particle tracing, the most common visualization method used today.

Methods: Eight healthy volunteers and one patient with a large apical left ventricular aneurysm underwent 4D PC-CMR flow imaging of the whole heart. Volume Tracking and particle tracing visualizations were compared visually side-by-side in a visualization software package. To validate Volume Tracking, the number of particle traces that agreed with the Volume Tracking visualizations was counted and expressed as a percentage of total released particles in mid-diastole and end-diastole respectively. Two independent observers described blood flow patterns in the left ventricle using Volume Tracking visualizations.

Results: Volume Tracking was feasible in all eight healthy volunteers and in the patient. Visually, Volume Tracking and particle tracing are complementary methods, showing different aspects of the flow. When validated against particle tracing, on average 90.5% and 87.8% of the particles agreed with the Volume Tracking surface in mid-diastole and end-diastole respectively. Inflow patterns in the left ventricle varied between the subjects, with excellent agreement between observers. The left ventricular inflow pattern in the patient differed from the healthy subjects.

Conclusion: Volume Tracking is a new visualization method for blood flow measured by 4D PC-CMR. Volume Tracking complements and provides incremental information compared to particle tracing that may lead to a better understanding of blood flow and may improve diagnosis and prognosis of cardiovascular diseases.

* Correspondence: einar.heiberg@med.lu.se
[1]Department of Clinical Physiology, Lund University, Skåne University Hospital Lund, Lund, Sweden
Full list of author information is available at the end of the article

Background

Blood flow patterns are closely linked to the function of valves, vessels and the myocardium, and functional and morphological changes in the heart influence the flow patterns [1-4]. Thus a better understanding of flow patterns may lead to improved diagnosis and prognosis of cardiovascular diseases.

Cardiovascular Magnetic Resonance (CMR) enables the measurement of the full three-dimensional and time-resolved velocity field in the heart and great vessels using four-dimensional Phase Contrast Cardiovascular Magnetic Resonance (4D PC-CMR) [5-7]. Due to the complexity of 4D flow fields, there exists no single natural representation that can show all details of the flow. To handle this abundance of information, flow visualization is often used for discovery, understanding and communication about flow [8]. Visualization is a critical part of the discovery process, as it enables the researcher to interact with the complex data, and by using the powerful pattern recognition systems of the human visual system, new hypotheses about the flow can be formed and then be investigated scientifically. In the case of three-dimensional, time-resolved (4D) flow, visualization is not only beneficial, but a necessity, since it would be an extremely time-consuming and error-prone task to interpret the flow using two-dimensional slices of the velocity volume [9].

Several flow visualization methods have been developed, each showing different aspects of the flow [10,11]. The most commonly used method for visualization of 4D PC-CMR data is particle tracing [9,12], but streamlines, vector plots [13] and vortex cores [14] have also been used. Methods for quantitative analysis have also been presented, including retrospective flow quantification [15], relative pressure mapping [16], turbulence mapping [6], wall shear stress [17], separation of left ventricular flow into components [18] and quantification of helical flow [19].

Visualization plays an important role in generating hypotheses that guide research. The result and performance of flow visualizations has been shown to be heavily influenced by the choice of flow visualization method [20] and even by minor adjustments in the visualization methods themselves [21]. This means that the impression of the flow changes with the visualization method, and therefore also the hypotheses generated and subsequently the studies performed and conclusions drawn. Since a single method may not show all aspects of the flow, research in alternative methods for blood flow visualization is motivated.

We have therefore developed a new visualization method, called Volume Tracking. Volume Tracking is similar to particle tracing in that it displays the path taken by the blood through the circulation, but follows and displays volumes and surfaces instead of points, changing the visual representation of the flow. Additionally, Volume Tracking adds a quantitative component to the visualizations. The purposes of this article are *1.* To present and validate a newly developed flow visualization method, Volume Tracking, and *2.* To investigate if Volume Tracking complements particle tracing and provides incremental information.

Methods

Study population and CMR protocol

Eight healthy volunteers were included in the study. All volunteers had normal blood pressure, normal ECG and no history of cardiovascular disease. One patient was also included to investigate if Volume Tracking was feasible in patients. This patient was hypertensive and had an apical aneurysm that developed after a major anterior infarction, resulting in an LV ejection fraction of 15%. A standard CMR examination consisting of Cine images in the 2-chamber, 3-chamber, 4-chamber and short-axis views was performed on all subjects. An experienced observer verified normal anatomy, myocardial function and valve function in the healthy volunteers. The study was approved by the Regional Ethical Review Board in Lund, Sweden. Written informed consent was obtained from all subjects. Subject characteristics are summarized in Table 1.

Three-dimensional, time-resolved, three-component velocity mapping (4D PC-CMR) was performed over the whole heart on all subjects using a three-dimensional Turbo Field Echo (TFE) Phase Contrast sequence [6] on a Philips Achieva 3T CMR scanner. The 4D flow and cine images were acquired in the same imaging session, so that the cine images could be used as spatial orientation when visualizing the 4D flow data. For the 4D flow measurements, the following parameters were used:

Table 1 Subject characteristics

	Subject	Age (years)	Gender	Weight (kg)	Height (cm)
Normals:	1	52	F	57	160
	2	23	M	89	194
	3	28	M	64	173
	4	36	F	70	177
	5	29	M	83	185
	6	63	M	70	170
	7	24	M	85	188
	8	25	F	67	165
	n = 8	23 - 63	5M, 3F	57 - 89	160 - 194
Patient:	AA	74	M	83	180

Characteristics for the subjects included in the study. AA = Apical Aneurysm.

Spatial resolution 3 × 3 × 3 mm, flip angle 8°, TE 3.7 ms, TR 6.2 ms, velocity encoding (VENC) 100 cm/s, and temporal resolution typically 50 ms. Parallel imaging (SENSE) was used with a factor of 2, and the turbo factor was 2. Respiratory gating to the end-expiratory phase was performed with a navigator beam for the diaphragm. Synchronization to the cardiac cycle was performed using retrospective ECG triggering, covering the whole R-R interval. All imaging was performed with the subjects at rest. Scan time for the flow measurement was typically 35 minutes. The flow measurement and standard CMR examination were performed in the same session, bringing the total scan time to about 50 minutes.

Volume Tracking

This section presents an overview of the Volume Tracking theory and implementation. The full mathematical formulation and technical details of Volume Tracking, necessary to reproduce and analyze the method, are given in Additional File 1: VT-Appendix.pdf.

Volume Tracking is based on the concept of a *flow map* $\phi_{t_0}^{t_1}(\bar{x})$, which is a function that maps the location $\bar{x}$ of a particle at one time t_0 to its position at another time t_1, thereby answering the question "Where will this particle go?" or "Where did this particle come from?". Using the flow map, the evolution of any volume in the flow can be defined: If the volume at the starting time t_0 is V_0, and the volume at another time t is $V(t)$, we define $V(t)$ as the image of V_0 under the flow map as

$$V(t) = \phi_{t_0}^{t}(V_0).$$

To compute the flow map, an auxiliary function $\psi(\bar{x}, t) = \phi_t^{t_0}(\bar{x})$ is introduced, mapping particles from their current position to their positions at time t_0, the *starting time*. Denoting the velocity field by $\bar{v}$, and decomposing ψ into its cartesian components (ψ^x, ψ^y, ψ^z), and decomposing $\bar{x} = (x, y, z)$, the advection equations

$$\begin{aligned} \partial_t \psi^x + \bar{v} \cdot \nabla \psi^x &= 0 \\ \partial_t \psi^y + \bar{v} \cdot \nabla \psi^y &= 0 \\ \partial_t \psi^z + \bar{v} \cdot \nabla \psi^z &= 0 \end{aligned} \qquad (1)$$

then describe the motion of volumes in the flow. The initial conditions at $t = t_0$ are

$$\begin{aligned} \psi^x(\bar{x}, t_0) &= x \\ \psi^y(\bar{x}, t_0) &= y \\ \psi^z(\bar{x}, t_0) &= z. \end{aligned}$$

These equations can be efficiently solved using a finite volume method, further described Additional File 1: VT-Appendix.pdf.

A starting volume V_0 is specified using a *volume function f*:

$$V_0 = \{\bar{x} \in \Omega | f(\bar{x}) \leq C\},$$

and the evolution of a volume can then be computed as

$$V(t) = \{\bar{x} \in \Omega | f(\phi_t^{t_0}(\bar{x})) \leq C\}. \qquad (2)$$

The solution to the Volume Tracking equations can be pre-computed, and the evolution of any volume is encoded in the flow map. Blood volumes of different shape, such as spheres and planes, can then be followed forward or backward in time interactively. Using the current implementation of Volume Tracking, the pre-computation step typically lasts 10-15 minutes per starting time. However, the pre-computation step can be performed offline without human interaction once the starting times have been chosen. Once the pre-computation has been completed, the flow map can be used to select volumes of several shapes and any position, and the movement and deformation of this volume can be displayed instantaneously.

The full mathematical formulation and technical details of Volume Tracking, necessary to reproduce and analyze the method, are given in Additional File 1: VT-Appendix.pdf.

Volume Tracking was implemented in MATLAB (The Mathworks, USA), using the freely available Finite Volume solver CLAWPACK [22-24] for the numerical calculations. User interaction, image display and animation were performed in the visualization software package Ensight (CEI, USA).

Software

To correct for eddy currents and other phase background effects, a first-order polynomial was fitted to velocities in stationary tissue and subtracted from the acquired velocity field [25]. Additionally, automatic phase unwrapping was performed to correct for phase aliasing effects [26]. Concomitant gradient effects were compensated by the CMR scanner software. Correction of background effects and phase unwrapping of the velocity data was implemented as a plugin to Segment [27], a freely available software for cardiovascular image analysis based on MATLAB (The Mathworks, USA). The visualization software package Ensight 9.1 (CEI, USA) was used to display Volume Tracking surfaces, compute particle traces and to create images and animations. Particle traces were computed using Ensight's default fourth-order Runge-Kutta integration algorithm [28], which uses linear interpolation between timesteps and grid points. The implementation of Volume Tracking is described in Additional File 1: VT-Appendix.pdf.

Evaluation and validation of Volume Tracking

Particle tracing and Volume Tracking both display the path taken by blood through the cardiovascular system, although giving different visual impressions of the flow. Therefore, to evaluate the visualization aspects of Volume Tracking, Volume Tracking and particle trace visualizations were generated in the visualization software package Ensight (CEI, USA) and compared side-by-side. Side-by-side visualizations were generated for diastolic inflow in left ventricle and right ventricle in a healthy volunteer, and diastolic inflow in the left ventricle in the ischemic cardiomyopathy patient. In the visualizations of left ventricular flow, the Volume Tracking surface shows the boundary between inflowing blood and blood already in the ventricle from the previous heartbeat.

To validate Volume Tracking against particle tracing, combined visualizations were generated of LV inflow in all subjects, with Volume Tracking and particle tracing displayed superimposed in the same image (see Figure 1 and Additional File 2: VT-PT-Combination.mpg). Since both Volume Tracking and particle tracing compute and display the motion of blood through the heart, no particles should cross the Volume Tracking surface if the methods display the exact same blood motion. Therefore, a particle was defined as fulfilling the validation criterion if it was located on the same side of the Volume Tracking plane as it was released on. The agreement between Volume Tracking and particle tracing at mid-diastole and end-diastole was calculated as the number of particles fulfilling the validation criterion, divided by the number of particles released up to that timepoint, and expressed as a percentage. At least 1000 particles were released in each subject. To ensure that this validation methodology was not sensitive to the number of released particles, the number of particles was varied between 1000 and 8000 in subject 7.

Analysis of LV inflow patterns

To demonstrate one of the possible applications of Volume Tracking, Volume Tracking visualizations were used to describe blood flow patterns in the left ventricle (LV). Using a Volume Tracking plane, as shown in Figure 2, panels D-E, the boundary between blood flowing into the ventricle and blood already in the ventricle was determined for the whole diastolic period. To map the location of the inflow blood, the LV lumen was divided into segments according to Figure 3. The LV lumen was divided into Apical, Mid-ventricular and Basal parts

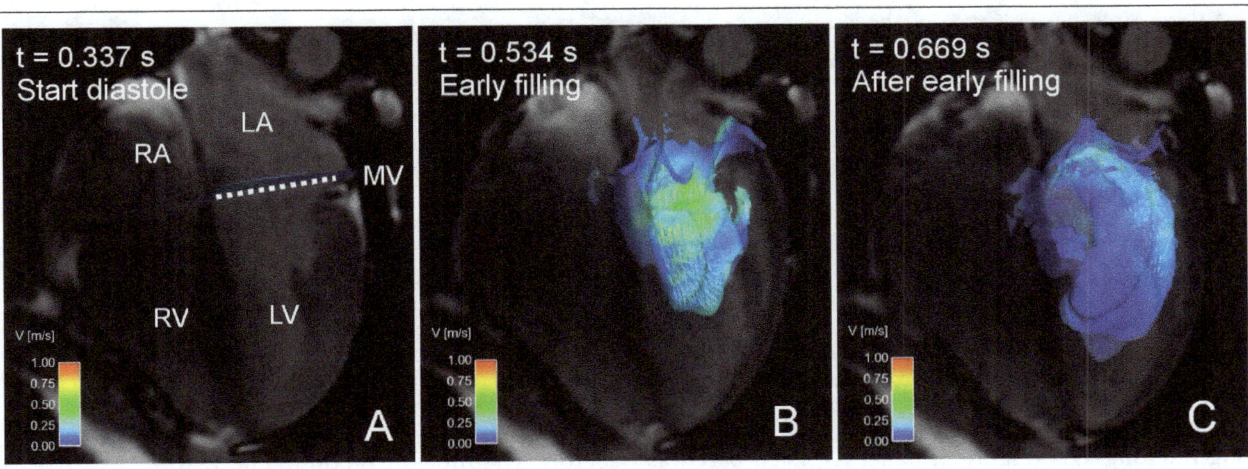

Figure 1 Composite visualization using both Volume Tracking and particle tracing. Combined particle tracing and Volume Tracking visualization of LV filling in volunteer 7. See Additional File 2: VT-PT-Combination.mpg for an animated version. In each image, an anatomical 4-chamber Cine image is shown for orientation. The 4-chamber image is transparent to show flow behind the plane. Time is counted from the start of systole. Panel A shows the heart at the start of diastole. A Volume Tracking plane is visible near the mitral valve, and a collection of particles is located above the plane. Particles are released in this position every 20 milliseconds during LV filling. Panel B shows the early filling wave. The Volume Tracking surface shows the inflowing blood volume. Particles have been released in the atrium and have flowed into the ventricle. The particles are visible through the transparent Volume Tracking surface. Panel C shows the flow in early diastasis. The Volume Tracking surface shows how the blood has flowed further into the ventricle. The particles have also moved further into the ventricle. Note that the particles are released on the basal side of the Volume Tracking plane. This means that all particles belong to the blood flowing into the ventricle. Since the Volume Tracking surface shows the inflowing blood, the particles should stay on the inflow side of the surface if the methods agree. Panels B and C show that very few particles have passed through the surface. This shows the correspondence between Volume Tracking and particle tracing, and that the theory and implementation of Volume Tracking are reliable. *LV = left ventricle, RV = right ventricle, LA = left atrium, RA = right atrium, MV = mitral valve, dashed line = approximate location of mitral valve, color = velocity from 0 (blue) to 1 m/s (red).*

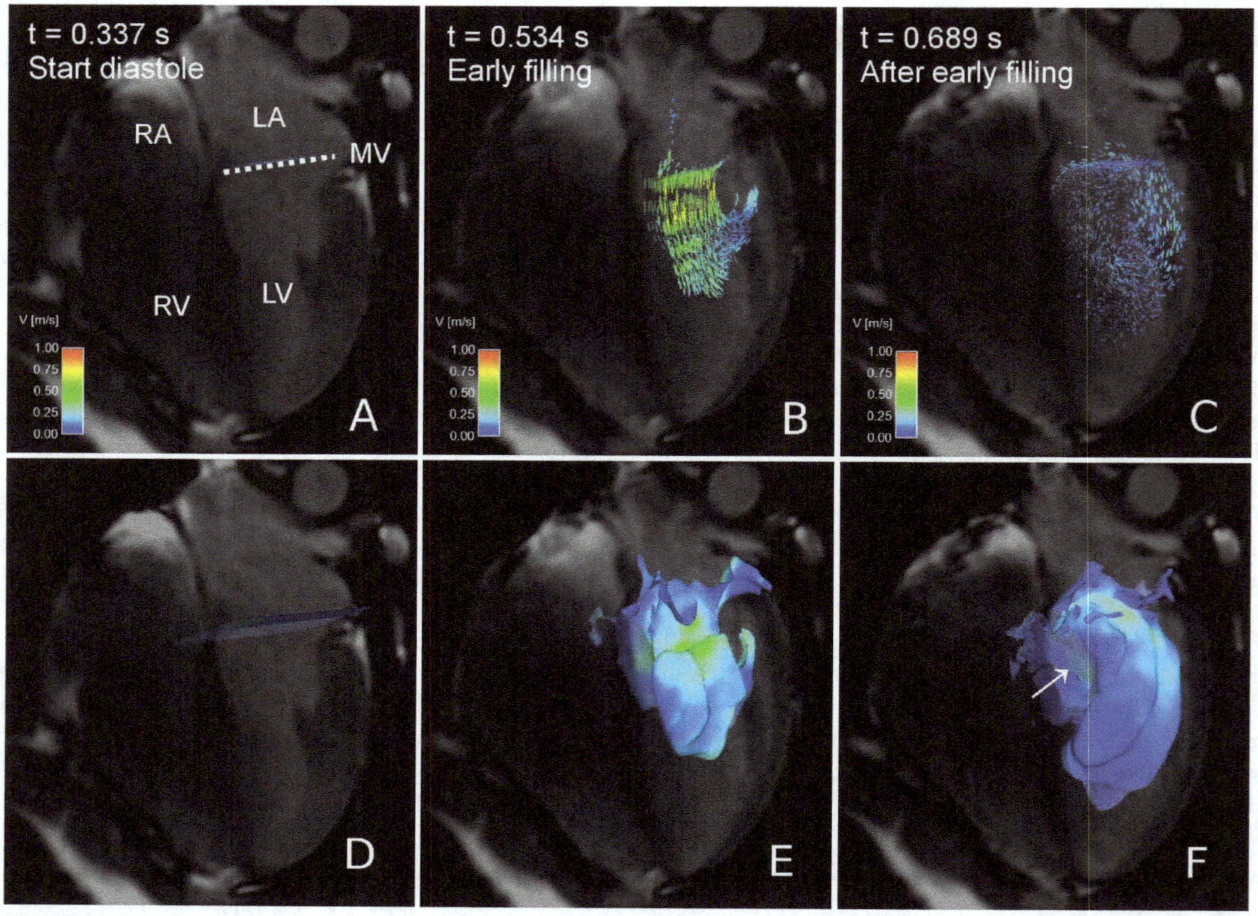

Figure 2 Particle tracing and Volume Tracking visualizations of LV filling. Particle tracing (A-C) and Volume Tracking (D-F) visualizations of LV filling in volunteer 7. See Additional File 3: VT-Comparison.mpg for an animated version. In each image, an anatomical 4-chamber Cine image is shown for orientation. The 4-chamber image is transparent to show flow behind the plane. Time is counted from the start of ventricular systole. Panels A-C show the particle tracing visualization. Particles are released every 20 milliseconds at the level of the white dotted line (MV). In panel A, at the start of diastole, particles can be seen at their starting position just above the dotted white line. In panel B, during the early phase of the filling, the particle traces flow from the atrium into the ventricle. In panel C, during diastasis, the particles have decelerated and dispersed in the ventricle. Panels D-F show the Volume Tracking visualization corresponding to panels A-C. Panel D shows a plane at the level of the mitral valve just before ventricular diastole. In panel E, Volume Tracking shows the volume of blood flowing into the ventricle. In panel F, the blood has flowed further into the ventricle. Panels E and F show how the Volume Tracking plane is deformed as if it were an in finitely stretchable, flexible sheet, i.e. the Volume Tracking visualization shows the boundary between blood flowing into the ventricle and blood already in the ventricle. Panel F clearly shows an absence of filling blood in an area near the basal parts of the septum (white arrow), something which is not easily seen in the corresponding particle trace image (panel C). *LV = left ventricle, RV = right ventricle, LA = left atrium, RA = right atrium, MV = mitral valve, dotted line = approximate location of mitral valve, color = velocity from 0 (blue) to 1 m/s (red).*

along the long-axis (Figure 3, panel A). Each part was then divided into seven segments (Figure 3, panel B) adjusted from the AHA model [29]. The intersection between the Volume Tracking surface and short-axis slices at the Apical, Mid-ventricular and Basal levels was then visualized (Figure 3, panel C). Two independent observers estimated whether each segment contained more or less than 25% blood. The location of the inflow blood was determined in this way at two times during diastole: at mid-diastole, defined as halfway between peak flow during the E-wave and peak flow during the A-wave, and at end-diastole, defined as the time just before systolic contraction. The E-wave and A-wave were measured in the mitral annulus in the 4D PC-CMR flow data and used for timing reference only. Agreement between the observers was measured using the kappa coefficient [30].

Results

Volume Tracking

When using Volume Tracking, a starting volume of blood is first chosen. In Figure 2, Panel D the blood in the left atrium has been chosen, and the surface of this volume is displayed. As the blood flows, the volume will

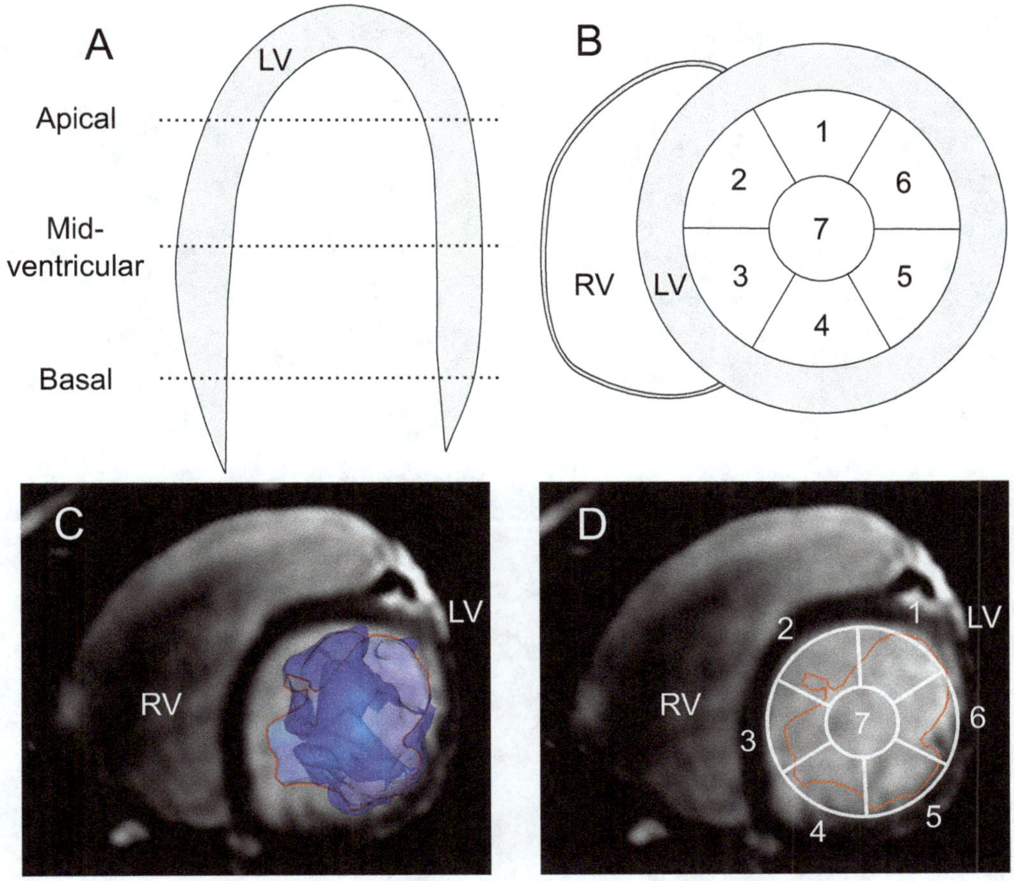

Figure 3 Division of the LV lumen into segments. In panel A the LV lumen is divided into apical, mid-ventricular and basal parts along the long-axis. Panel B shows how each short-axis part is divided into seven segments, where six (labels 1-6) are located along the endocardial border adjusted from the AHA standard [29], and the seventh (label 7) in the center of the lumen. Panel C shows a representative slice and Volume Tracking surface (blue transparent surface). The intersection of the Volume Tracking surface with the short-axis slice is shown as a red line. Panel D shows the intersection in red and the segment model from panel B in white. *LV = left ventricle, RV = right ventricle, 1-7 = segment numbers.*

move and deform with the flow as if the volume's surface was infinitely flexible and stretchable, as seen in Figure 2, panel D-F, and Additional File 3: VT-Comparison.mpg. The Volume Tracking surface shows the boundary between inflowing blood and blood already in the ventricle from the previous heartbeat.

Although only one shape is used in this example, a wide variety of sizes and shapes can be used. Planes are used in Figures 1, 2 and 4, and Figure 5 shows a sphere as initial volume. A more detailed discussion of the possible shapes can be found in Additional File 1: VT-Appendix.pdf. The formulation of the method allows the volume selection to be performed interactively using a point-and-click user interface.

Evaluation and validation of Volume Tracking

In Figure 2 a comparison of visualizations of LV inflow using Volume Tracking and particle tracing is shown. Additional File 3: VT-Comparison.mpg shows an animated version of Figure 2, showing the effect of animation on Volume Tracking. Particle tracing shows an intricate pattern of swirling flows during diastolic filling, especially apparent in the animation (Additional File 3: VT-Comparison.mpg). Volume Tracking, in contrast, shows the boundary between the inflowing blood and the blood already in the ventricle. Additionally, Volume Tracking reveals an area close to the basal parts of the septum with no filling blood in subject 7 (Figure 2, lower right panel). This area was not observed when studying the particle trace visualization alone. Particle tracing shows a dynamic, complex scene, while Volume Tracking shows the combined movement of the whole inflow volume.

Figure 4 and Additional File 4: VT-Patient.mpg shows inflow into the left ventricle (LV) in a patient with a LV apical aneurysm, visualized using Volume Tracking and

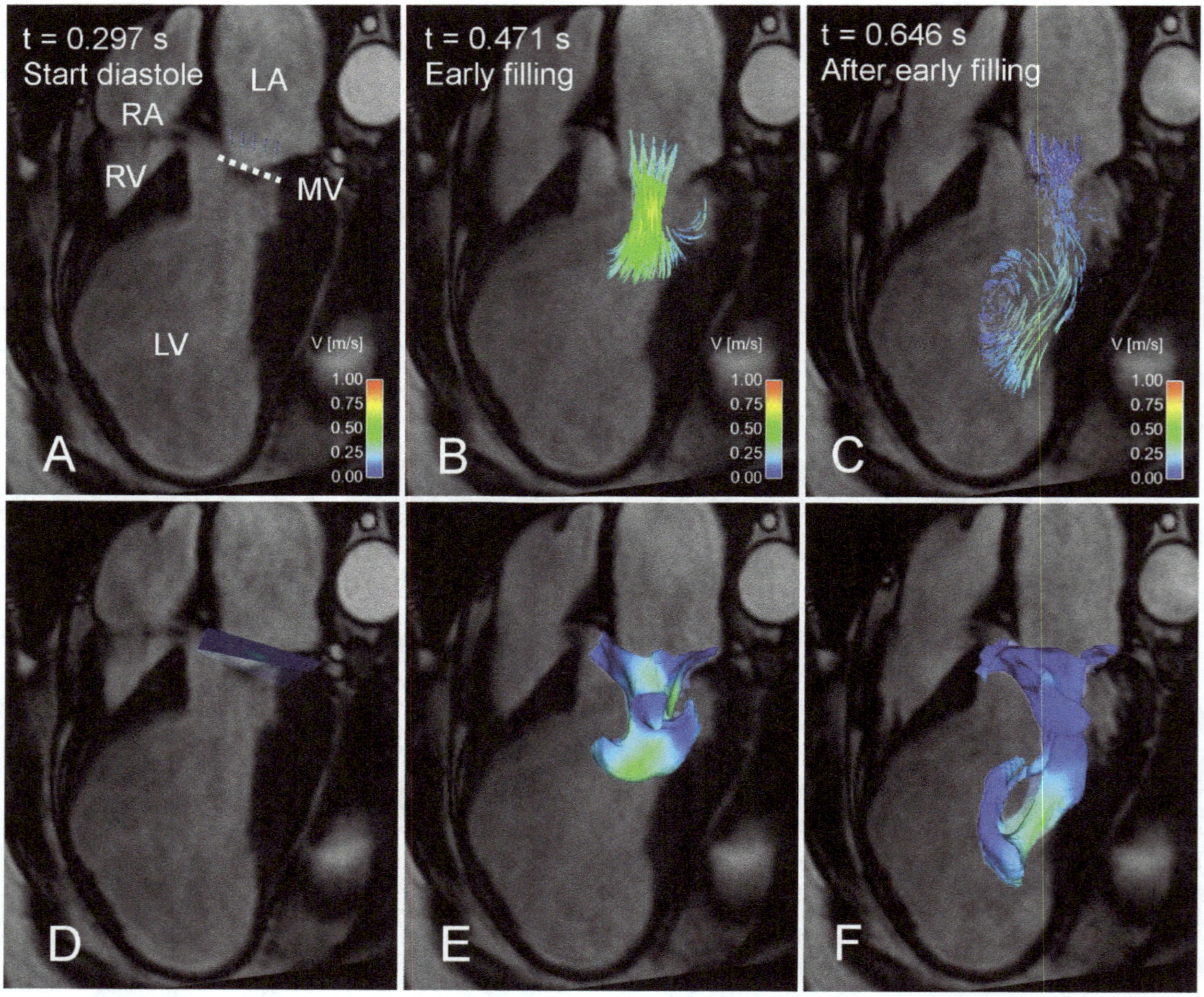

Figure 4 Particle tracing and Volume Tracking visualizations of LV filling in a patient with apical aneurysm. Particle tracing (A-C) and Volume Tracking (D-F) visualizations of LV filling in a patient with a large LV apical aneurysm, which appeared after a major anterior infarction. See Additional File 4: VT-Patient.mpg for an animated version. In each image, an anatomical 4-chamber Cine image is shown for orientation. The 4-chamber image is transparent to show flow behind the plane. Time is counted from the start of ventricular systole. In the particle trace images in panels A-C, particles are released every 20 milliseconds at the level of the white, dotted line (MV). In panel A, at the start of diastole, particles are shown at their starting position just above the dotted white line. In panel B, during early filling, the traces show the flow from the atrium into the ventricle. In panel C, at mid-diastole, the particles have moved further into the ventricle and entered a twisting pattern. Panels D-F show a Volume Tracking visualization corresponding to the particle trace visualization in panels A-C. In panel D, at the start of diastole, a Volume Tracking plane can be seen at the level of the mitral valve just before ventricular diastole. In panel E, during early filling, the plane has deformed and shows the blood flowing into the ventricle. In panel F, in mid-diastole, the blood has moved further into the ventricle. The inflow pattern is distinctly different from the pattern observed in the healthy volunteer in Figure 2. *LV = left ventricle, RV = right ventricle, LA = left atrium, RA = right atrium, MV = mitral valve, dotted line = approximate location of mitral valve, color = velocity from 0 (blue) to 1 m/s (red).*

particle tracing. As in Figure 2, the visual impression of the LV inflow is different for the two methods. The inflow is distinctly different from the flow pattern in the healthy volunteer in Figure 2.

Figure 5 shows particle trace and Volume Tracking visualizations of inflow in the right ventricle (RV). Additional File 5: VT-RV.mpg shows an animated version of Figure 5. To demonstrate that Volume Tracking can be used with many different shapes, a sphere of blood in the right atrium (panel D) is used instead of a plane. The particle tracing visualization shows a vortex or helix motion of particles into the ventricle, and the particles coming to rest in the RV. Volume Tracking shows the initial volume deforming and moving into the right ventricle, but the vortex motion is not clearly visible. As the blood comes to rest in the RV during diastasis, it spreads out in a complex pattern. This complex pattern is not apparent in the particle tracing visualization.

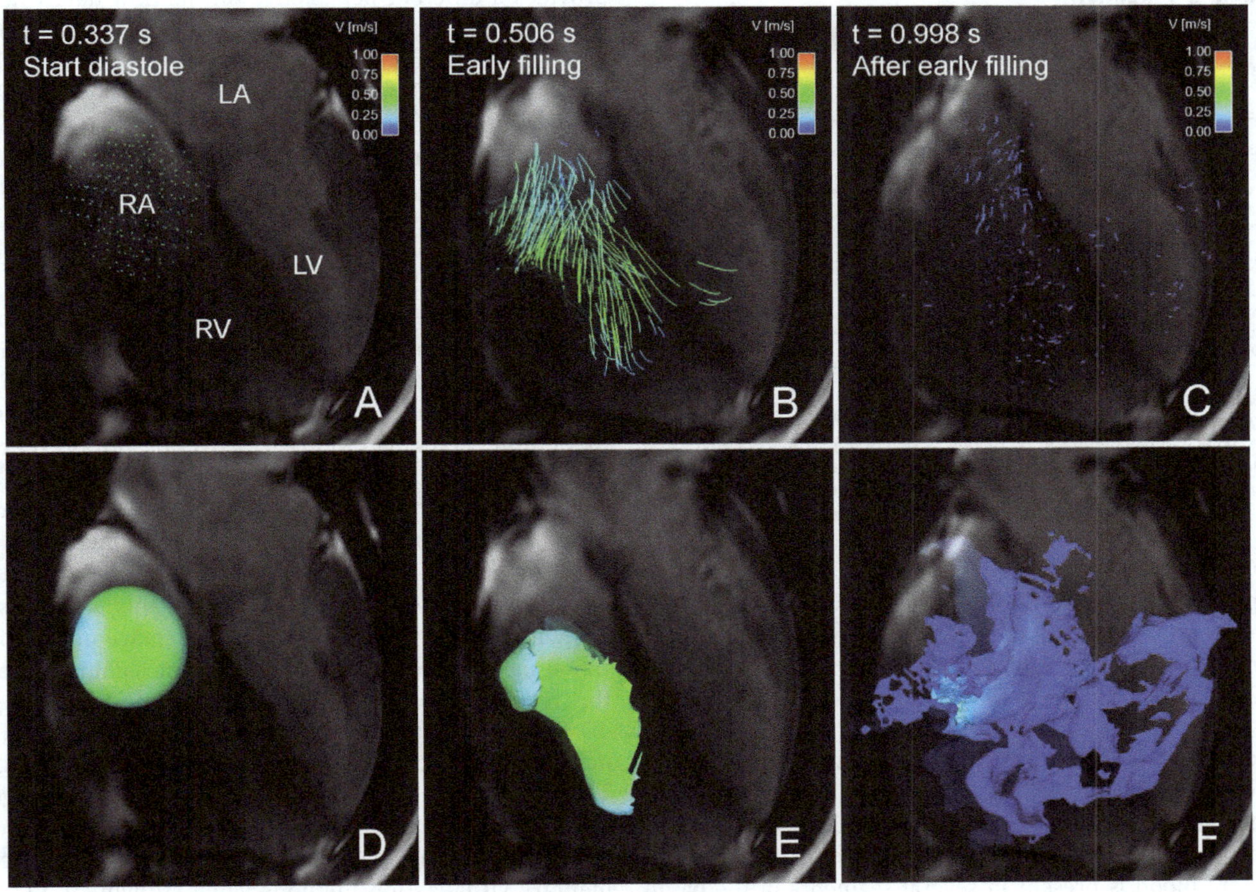

Figure 5 Particle tracing and Volume Tracking visualizations of right ventricular filling flow. Particle tracing (panels A-C) and Volume Tracking (panels D-F) visualizations of RV filling in volunteer 7. See Additional File 5: VT-RV.mpg for an animated version. In each image, an anatomical 4-chamber cine image is shown. The 4-chamber image is transparent to show flow behind the plane. The scene has been rotated in comparison to Figures 1, 2 and 4, to better show the visualizations. Due to the rotation, the RV is in the foreground, with the LV behind. Time is counted from the start of systole. Panels A-C show particle tracing. In panel A, at the start of diastole, a collection of particles has been placed in the right atrium. In panel B, during early filling, the particle traces move in a vortex pattern from the atrium into the ventricle. In panel C, at end-diastole, the particles have slowed down and spread in the right ventricle. Panels D-F show a Volume Tracking visualization corresponding to the particle tracing in panels A-C. Panel D, at the start of diastole, shows a spherical volume of blood in the right atrium. In Panel E, during early filling, the blood volume has deformed and flowed into the right ventricle. In Panel F, at end-diastole, the volume has been deformed further and has spread in the right ventricle. Comparing panels B and E, the vortex flow pattern is more apparent in the particle trace visualization in panel B. Comparing panels C and F, the Volume Tracking visualization in panel F shows how blood has spread in a complex pattern in the right ventricle. This is not apparent in the particle tracing visualization in panel C. *LV = left ventricle, RV = right ventricle, LA = left atrium, RA = right atrium, MV = mitral valve, color = velocity from 0 (blue) to 1 m/s (red).*

Additional File 5: VT-RV.mpg clearly shows the breakdown of ordered, vortical inflow to the complex deformation in late diastole.

Figure 1 shows the superposition of Volume Tracking and particle tracing visualizations of LV filling in a healthy volunteer. Additional File 2: VT-PT-Combination.mpg shows an animated version of Figure 1. Notice that very few particles pass through the plane. Table 2 shows the agreement between Volume Tracking and particle tracing, i.e. the fraction of particles that stay on the inflow side of the Volume Tracking surface. Mean agreement for all 9 subjects was 90.5% in mid-diastole and 87.8% in end-diastole. When varying the number of particles in subject 7 between 1000 and 8000, the standard deviation in the mid-diastolic agreement was 0.30% and in the end-diastolic agreement 0.17%.

Analysis of LV inflow patterns

Semi-quantitative analysis of the inflow patterns was feasible in all subjects. The results of the flow pattern analysis are given in Tables 3 and 4 for Observer 1, and in Additional File 6: Distribution of LV inflow blood.xls. Agreement between the observers was excellent with a kappa coefficient of $\kappa = 0.91$. In seven out of eight

Table 2 Validation

	Subject	MD %	ED %
Normals:	1	90.0	88.4
	2	82.1	71.4
	3	96.4	95.5
	4	96.6	92.2
	5	90.3	88.8
	6	90.8	90.1
	7	90.6	89.7
	8	87.1	90.1
Patient:	AA	90.2	84.1
Mean ± SD:		90.5 ± 4.4	87.8 ± 6.8

Agreement between Volume Tracking and particle tracing, calculated as the percentage of released traces on the inflow side of the Volume Tracking surface (see Figure 1) at mid-diastole (MD) and end-diastole (ED). The mean agreement was 90.5% in mid-diastole and 87.8% in end-diastole.

volunteers an in the patient, blood did not reach the apical level by mid-diastole. In end-diastole, blood has reached the apical level in the majority of healthy subjects (observer 1: 6 of 8, observer 2: 8 of 8). In the patient, the inflowing blood did not reach the apical level at all. There was a large variability inflow patterns between the healthy volunteers. In the patient with ischemic cardiomyopathy, the inflow blood is only present in segments 4, 5, 6 and 7 in the basal third of the ventricle. This is notably different from the normals, where blood is present in several segments in the basal and mid-ventricular thirds.

Discussion

In this article, a new method for visualization and analysis of 4D PC-CMR data, called Volume Tracking, is presented for the first time. Visually, Volume Tracking provides a different perspective on the flow data when compared to particle tracing. Volume Tracking and particle tracing have a mean agreement of 90.5% in mid-diastole and 87.8% in end-diastole. In the analysis of LV inflow patterns, observer agreement was excellent. The flow patterns varied between the normals, and in the ischemic cardiomyopathy patient, the inflow was notably different from the normals.

Evaluation and validation of Volume Tracking

Three examples demonstrate that Volume Tracking provides incremental value to particle tracing: a) Volume Tracking shows the surface of the blood volume flowing into the left ventricle rather than the detailed dynamics; b) Volume Tracking emphasizes overall motion more than particle tracing; and c) Volume Tracking shows a complex flow pattern in RV filling not visible using particle tracing. This is in line with previous studies, where the visualization method influences the results of the visualization process [20,21]. However, this is the first study investigating the influence of the choice of visualization method for 4D PC-CMR data. The significance of this result may be that when visualizing and analyzing 4D PC-CMR data, researchers can extract more information from a given dataset using Volume Tracking. This may lead to new insights and additional knowledge about blood flow and cardiac pumping.

In general, it may be beneficial to use several complementary visualization methods when studying 4D PC-CMR data, since it may reveal more aspects of the flow. One example of this is that the vortex in the right ventricular inflow was less apparent with Volume Tracking than with particle tracing. To detect this type of flow patterns, vortex detection methods [14] and quantitative indices of helix flow [19,31] may be effective

Table 3 Distribution of left ventricular inflow blood for observer 1 at mid-diastole

	Segment Apical							Mid-ventricular							Basal						
Subject	1	2	3	4	5	6	7	1	2	3	4	5	6	7	1	2	3	4	5	6	7
1								X	X	X	X	X	X	X	X	X	X	X	X	X	X
2								X	X	X	X	X			X			X	X		
3							X	X	X	X	X			X	X			X			
4								X	X		X	X		X					X	X	X
5								X	X	X	X			X		X	X	X	X	X	X
6									X	X		X	X	X	X	X	X	X	X	X	X
7								X	X		X	X		X	X		X	X	X		X
8								X	X			X	X	X	X	X	X	X	X	X	X
AA																			X		

This table shows the distribution of the blood flowing into the left ventricle in the volunteers (1-8) and the patient (AA) at mid-diastole for observer 1. Observer 1 at end-diastole can be seen in Table 4. The results from both observers can be seen in Additional file 6: Distribution of LV inflow blood.xls. Inflow blood locations were determined using Volume Tracking visualizations of LV filling (see Figure 2) and the segment model described in Figure 3. This table shows observer 1 at mid-diastole. Each row in the table shows one of the subjects included in the study. Columns correspond to segments in the segment model in Figure 3. Each segment was marked with an 'X' if the inflow blood occupied 25% or more of the area of the segment.

Table 4 Distribution of left ventricular inflow blood for observer 1 at end-diastole

	Segment Apical							Mid-ventricular							Basal						
Subject	**1**	**2**	**3**	**4**	**5**	**6**	**7**	**1**	**2**	**3**	**4**	**5**	**6**	**7**	**1**	**2**	**3**	**4**	**5**	**6**	**7**
1						X	X	X	X	X			X		X	X	X	X	X	X	X
2							X				X	X	X	X	X			X	X	X	X
3								X	X	X				X			X	X	X		X
4	X								X	X	X	X		X	X		X	X	X	X	X
5							X	X	X	X	X			X	X	X	X	X	X	X	X
6	X						X	X	X	X	X	X		X	X	X	X	X	X	X	X
7							X	X		X	X	X		X	X		X	X	X	X	X
8								X	X		X	X	X	X	X	X	X	X	X	X	X
AA																		X	X	X	X

This table shows the distribution of the blood flowing into the left ventricle in the volunteers (1-8) and the patient (AA) at end-diastole for observer 1. Observer 1 at end-diastole can be seen in Table 4. The results from both observers can be seen in Additional file 6: Distribution of LV inflow blood.xls. Inflow blood locations were determined using Volume Tracking visualizations of LV filling (see Figure 2) and the segment model described in Figure 3. Each row in the table shows one of the subjects included in the study. Columns correspond to segments in the segment model in Figure 3. Each segment was marked with an 'X' if the inflow blood occupied 25% or more of the area of the segment.

complements to Volume Tracking. Complementary to the large-scale flow dynamics shown by Volume Tracking, the flow dynamics in vessel wall boundary layers can be quantified using wall shear stress (WSS) [17] analysis. Simultaneous use of WSS analysis and Volume Tracking may provide a link between WSS and large-scale flow. Furthermore, the visual impression of the flow gained by Volume Tracking can be quantified by classifying particle traces according to origin and destination of flow [18,32].

The high agreement between Volume Tracking and particle tracing shows that Volume Tracking displays the same blood motion as the particle traces, which in this study were computed using a numerical algorithm independent from Volume Tracking and known to be accurate [28]. This suggests that the Volume Tracking numerical algorithm performs well in the presence of noise, acceleration and vortices in the 4D PC-CMR datasets used in this study. Additionally, the agreement between Volume Tracking and particle tracing shows that the differences in interpretation of the flow is not due to differences in blood transport calculations. The differences in interpretation of the flow may instead be explained by the differences in visual representation (surfaces instead of particles and lines). The low variation in agreement when changing the number of particles suggests that the agreement is not dependent on the number of particles.

In this study, only ventricular inflow has been studied. However, Volume Tracking is a general method, which may be used to study flow in all parts of the cardiovascular system. One example where Volume Tracking may also provide incremental value is the human aorta, where flow patterns may be influential in plaque formation and rupture.

Analysis of LV inflow patterns

The physiological significance of the present findings may be an increased understanding of the complex, and clinically intangible, hemodynamics that may help clarify normal cardiac pumping. The different filling patterns in the healthy volunteers suggest that normal hemodynamics may display additional degrees of freedom that could explain differences in normal physiology.

The pathophysiological significance of the present findings may be that the transition from normal to pathological LV hemodynamics which may take several years to develop can be better understood and discovered at an earlier sub-clinical stage. These gradual changes over time may also be coupled to early morphological and physiological changes. In line with previous studies [33], we agree that flow patterns may be a sensitive measure of LV function and may be able to detect early stages of dysfunction.

Limitations

Errors in the velocity measurements accumulate in particle paths and Volume Tracking surfaces over time [9]. This problem is minimized in this study by limiting the tracking to diastole.

Blood flow patterns may be influenced by factors which were not measured in the present experimental setting, such as changes in blood viscosity and hematocrit.

Long 4D PC-CMR acquisition times lead to averaging over several heartbeats, obscuring small flow details so that the resulting flow data describes large-scale flow features that are present in the majority of heartbeats. The 4D PC-CMR technique is also limited in spatial resolution, does not provide absolute pressure levels, and is not feasible during exercise. Noise in the 4D PC-

CMR measurements and the complicated flow patterns in the human heart may also influence the Volume Tracking calcuations. The high agreement between particle tracing and Volume Tracking suggests that accuracy in the Volume Tracking algorithm is a minor problem for the present application.

Volume Tracking shows how a certain volume is deformed in the flow. This means that flow inside the volume is only seen indirectly. To overcome this limitation, Volume Tracking and particle tracing can be used simultaneously, as in Figure 1.

Ensight uses linear interpolation of the velocity fields in space and time to compute particle traces, which may introduce errors into the calculation. Since Ensight does not allow the user to choose interpolation method, the influence of the interpolation could not be checked. The authors are not aware of any studies of the effects of interpolation strategies in particle tracing, but the effects are probably small in relation to the smoothing, noise, low resolution and phase background effects of the 4D PC-CMR technique.

The evaluation of the visualization aspects of Volume Tracking was performed by visual comparison to particle tracing. An independent, quantitative evaluation for both methods would be desirable. However, the state of the art in evaluation methods for flow visualization has not yet been extended to treat time-resolved flow [20,21] and may not adress the hypothesis-generating aspects of visualization.

Conclusion

In this study Volume Tracking, a new method for visualization of blood flow from 4D PC-CMR, is presented. Compared to particle tracing, Volume Tracking can provide incremental information that may lead to a better understanding of blood flow and may improve diagnosis and prognosis of cardiovascular diseases. The diastolic inflow pattern in the patient is notably different from the volunteers, suggesting that blood flow patterns may be used as a measure of LV function and as an early indicator of disease.

Additional material

Additional file 1: Appendix: Theory and implementation. Appendix: Document describing the mathematical theory and technical details of the implementation of Volume Tracking.

Additional file 2: Animation: Composite visualization of LV filling using both Volume Tracking and particle tracing. Composite particle trace and Volume Tracking visualization of LV filling in volunteer 7, also shown in Figure 1. Anatomical four-chamber Cine images are displayed in the background for orientation. See Figure 1 for a description of the anatomy. The image is semi-transparent to show flow behind the four-chamber plane. Time is counted from the start of ventricular systole. At the beginning of the movie a Volume Tracking plane is visible at the level of the mitral valve, and a collection of particles are visible just above the plane. Particles are released every 20 milliseconds in the same location. The Volume Tracking plane can be seen as an infinitely flexible and stretchable sheet, deformed effortlessly with the flow. Between t = 0.337 s and t = 0.5 s, the Volume Tracking plane is deformed as blood flows into the ventricle. The particles show an ordered inflow. The Volume Tracking plane shows that the front of inflowing blood moves quickly towards the apex. After t = 0.5 s the particle traces show a complex arrangement of vortices, which slows down almost to a standstill around t = 0.8 s. The Volume Tracking surface keeps on deforming slowly even after t = 0.8s, when the particles seem to have stopped moving. Notice the correspondence between the two methods. Specifically, very few particles cross through the Volume Tracking plane. This is due to the fact that all particles are released in the inflowing blood and that the Volume Tracking plane separates the inflowing blood from the blood already in the ventricle.

Additional file 3: Animation: Comparison between particle tracing and Volume Tracking. Visualization of LV filling in volunteer 7, also shown in Figure 2. Left: particle tracing. Right: Volume Tracking. The left and right panels differ only in the visualization method used. Anatomical four-chamber Cine images are displayed in the background for orientation. See Figure 2 for a description of the anatomy. The four-chamber plane image is semi-transparent to show flow behind the plane. The color scale indicates velocities between 0 and 1.0 meters per second. Time is counted from the start of ventricular systole. The video starts just before the opening of the mitral valve. In the left panel, particles are released every 20 milliseconds. In the right panel, a plane is placed near the mitral valve. The plane is infinitely flexible and stretchable and deforms effortlessly with the flow, showing the boundary between inflow blood and blood already in the ventricle. Between t = 0.337 s and t = 0.5 s, particle tracing shows an ordered inflow, and Volume Tracking shows the inflow blood progressing quickly into the ventricle. After t = 0.5 s, particle tracing shows a complex arrangement of vortices decelerating almost to standstill around t = 0.8 s. In contrast, Volume Tracking clearly shows a clockwise rotation and further deformation in the apical region after t = 0.8s. Additionally, Volume Tracking shows that inflow blood is located closer to the lateral wall of the LV in this subject. A region near the basal parts of the septum contains no filling blood (see Figure 2, white arrow), something which is not clearly visible using particle trace visualization.

Additional file 4: Animation: Particle trace and Volume Tracking visualizations of LV inflow in patient with apical aneurysm. Particle tracing (left) and Volume Tracking (right) visualizations of LV inflow in a patient diagnosed with a large LV apical aneurysm. Anatomical four-chamber Cine images are displayed in the background for orientation. See Figure 4 for a description of the anatomy. The four-chamber image is transparent to show flow behind the four-chamber plane. The color scale in the lower left corner indicates velocities between zero and 1.0 meters per second (m/s). Time is counted from the start of ventricular systole. At the start of the movie, just before the filling of the LV begins, the starting location of the particles is visible just above the mitral valve (left). A Volume Tracking plane is visible at the level of the mitral valve (right). As the movie plays, the particles flow into the ventricle. The plane deforms to show the boundary between inflowing blood and blood already in the ventricle.

Additional file 5: Animation: Particle trace and Volume Tracking visualizations of right ventricular inflow. Particle tracing (left) and Volume Tracking (right) visualizations of RV diastolic inflow. Anatomical four-chamber Cine images are displayed in the background for orientation. See Figure 5 for a description of the anatomy. The four-chamber image is transparent to show flow behind the four-chamber plane, and the scene has been rotated in comparison to Figures 1, 2 and 4. Due to the rotation, the RV is in the foreground, with the LV behind. The color scale in the lower left corner indicates velocities between zero and 1.0 meters per second (m/s). Time is counted from the start of ventricular systole. The animation starts at the beginning of RV filling. After this the animation can be divided into two parts. First an organized inflow into the right ventricle is shown between t = 0.337 s and t = 0.63 s. Particle tracing (left) shows a distinct swirling vortex of flow into the right ventricle. Volume Tracking does not show the vortex clearly. During the remaining time, from t = 0.63 s to t = 1.00 s, the flow decelerates during diastasis. Particle tracing shows the blood coming to rest in an uncomplicated manner. However, Volume Tracking shows the blood volume becoming stretched and twisted, finally occupying most of the right ventricle in a complex structure. The volume is spread out in three dimensions, outside the image plane, but is still completely within the RA and RV.

Additional file 6: Distribution of left ventricular inflow blood. This file shows the distribution of left ventricular inflow blood as assessed by the two independent observers. Observer 1 is also shown in Tables 3 and 4.

Acknowledgements
The authors would like to thank the Cardiovascular MR Research Group at Linköping University, Linköping, Sweden for help and support in our work on intracardiac blood flow.
Ann-Helen Arvidsson, Christel Carlander and Martin Ugander at the Cardiac MR Group, Department of Clinical Physiology, Lund University Hospital, Lund, Sweden assisted in data collection.
Freddy Ståhlberg and Anders Nilsson at the Department of Medical Radiation Physics, Lund University Hospital, Lund, Sweden and Karin Markenroth-Bloch at Philips Medical Systems, Best, the Netherlands provided expertise in MRI physics and data acquisition.
This study was supported by Swedish Research Council grants VR 621-2005-3129, VR 621-2008-2949 and VR K2009-65X-14599-07-3, National Visualization Program and Knowledge Foundation grant 2009-0080, the Medical Faculty at Lund University, Sweden, the Region of Scania, Sweden and the Swedish Heart-Lung Foundation.

Author details
[1]Department of Clinical Physiology, Lund University, Skåne University Hospital Lund, Lund, Sweden. [2]Department of Numerical Analysis, Centre for Mathematical Sciences, Lund University, Lund, Sweden.

Authors' contributions
JT developed the details of the method and implemented it in software, wrote the manuscript, created all figures and animations, performed analysis of LV inflow patterns and merged feedback from the other authors. MC collected data, supplied expertise in cardiac physiology and revised the manuscript for intellectual content. GS contributed to the design and development of the numerical method. HA supplied expertise in cardiac physiology and revised the manuscript for intellectual content. EH conceived the method, performed analysis of LV inflow patterns, contributed to the method design and revised the manuscript for intellectual content. All authors have read and approved the final manuscript.

Competing interests
The authors declare that they have no competing interests.

References

1. Beppu S, Izumi S, Miyatake K, Nagata S, Park Y, Sakakibara H, Nimura Y: **Abnormal blood pathways in left ventricular cavity in acute myocardial infarction. Experimental observations with special reference to regional wall motion abnormality and hemostasis.** *Circulation* 1988, **78(1)**:157.
2. Reiter G, Reiter U, Kovacs G, Kainz B, Schmidt K, Maier R, Olschewski H, Rienmueller R: **Magnetic Resonance-Derived 3-Dimensional Blood Flow Patterns in the Main Pulmonary Artery as a Marker of Pulmonary Hypertension and a Measure of Elevated Mean Pulmonary Arterial Pressure.** *Circulation: Cardiovascular Imaging* 2008, **1(1)**:23.
3. Thanigaraj S, Chugh R, Schechtman K, Lee L, Wade R, Pérez J: **Defining left ventricular segmental and global function by echocardiographic intraventricular contrast flow patterns.** *The American journal of cardiology* 2000, **85(1)**:65-68.
4. Garcia M, Smedira N, Greenberg N, Main M, Firstenberg M, Odabashian J, Thomas J: **Color M-mode Doppler flow propagation velocity is a preload insensitive index of left ventricular relaxation: animal and human validation.** *Journal of the American College of Cardiology* 2000, **35(1)**:201-208.
5. Wigström L, Sjövist L, Wranne B: **Temporally resolved 3D phase-contrast imaging.** *Magn Reson Med* 1996, **36(5)**:800-3.
6. Dyverfeldt P, Kvitting J, Sigfridsson A, Engvall J, Bolger A, Ebbers T: **Assessment of fluctuating velocities in disturbed cardiovascular blood flow: In vivo feasibility of generalized phase-contrast MRI.** *Journal of Magnetic Resonance Imaging* 2008, **28(3)**:655-663.
7. Markl M, Kilner P, Ebbers T: **Comprehensive 4D velocity mapping of the heart and great vessels by cardiovascular magnetic resonance.** *Journal of Cardiovascular Magnetic Resonance* 2011, **13**:7.
8. DeFanti T, Brown M, McCormick B: **Visualization: Expanding Scientific and Engineering Research Opportunities.** *Computer* 1989, **22(8)**:12-25.
9. Napel S, Lee D, Frayne R, Rutt B: **Visualizing three-dimensional flow with simulated streamlines and three-dimensional phase-contrast MR imaging.** *J Magn Reson Imaging* 1992, **2(2)**:143-153.
10. McLoughlin T, Laramee R, Peikert R, Post F, Chen M: **Over two decades of integration-based, geometric flow visualization.** *Computer Graphics Forum* 2010, **29(6)**:1807-1829.
11. Post FH, Vrolijk B, Hauser H, Laramee RS, Doleisch H: **Feature Extraction and Visualisation of Flow Fields.** In *Proceedings of the Eurographics Conference 2002.* Edited by: Fellner D, Scopigno R. Saarbrücken, Germany: Eurographics Association; 2002:.
12. Wigström L, Ebbers T, Fyrenius A, Karlsson M, Engvall J, Wranne B, Bolger A: **Particle Trace Visualization of Intracardiac Flow Using Time-Resolved 3D Phase Contrast MRI.** *Magnetic Resonance in Medicine* 1999, **41(4)**:793-799.
13. Buonocore M: **Visualizing blood flow patterns using streamlines, arrows, and particle paths.** *Magnetic resonance in medicine* 1998, **40(2)**:210-226.
14. Heiberg E, Ebbers T, Wigstrom L, Karlsson M: **Three-dimensional flow characterization using vector pattern matching.** *Visualization and Computer Graphics, IEEE Transactions on* 2003, **9(3)**:313-319.
15. Westenberg J, Roes S, Ajmone Marsan N, Binnendijk N, Doornbos J, Bax J, Reiber J, de Roos A, van der Geest R: **Mitral Valve and Tricuspid Valve Blood Flow: Accurate Quantification with 3D Velocity-encoded MR Imaging with Retrospective Valve Tracking.** *Radiology* 2008, **249(3)**:792.
16. Ebbers T, Wigström L, Bolger A, Wranne B, Karlsson M: **Noninvasive Measurement of Time-Varying Three-Dimensional Relative Pressure Fields Within the Human Heart.** *Journal of Biomechanical Engineering* 2002, **124(3)**:288.
17. Stalder A, Russe M, Frydrychowicz A, Bock J, Hennig J, Markl M: **Quantitative 2D and 3D phase contrast MRI: optimized analysis of blood flow and vessel wall parameters.** *Magnetic Resonance in Medicine* 2008, **60(5)**:1218-1231.
18. Eriksson J, Carlhäll C, Dyverfeldt P, Engvall J, Bolger A, Ebbers T: **Semi-automatic quantification of 4 D left ventricular blood flow.** *Journal of Cardiovascular Magnetic Resonance* 2010, **12**:9.
19. Morbiducci U, Ponzini R, Rizzo G, Cadioli M, Esposito A, De Cobelli F, Del Maschio A, Montevecchi F, Redaelli A: **In vivo quantification of helical blood flow in human aorta by time-resolved three-dimensional cine phase contrast magnetic resonance imaging.** *Annals of biomedical engineering* 2009, **37(3)**:516-531.
20. Laidlaw D, Kirby R, Jackson C, Davidson J, Miller T, Da Silva M, Warren W, Tarr M: **Comparing 2D vector field visualization methods: A user study.** *IEEE Transactions on Visualization and Computer Graphics* 2005, **11(1)**:59-70.
21. Forsberg A, Chen J, Laidlaw D: **Comparing 3D Vector Field Visualization Methods: A User Study.** *IEEE Transactions on Visualization and Computer Graphics* 2009, **15(6)**:1219-1226.
22. LeVeque R, Berger M: **CLAWPACK Software 4.3.** [http://www.clawpack.org/], [Accessed 2009-10-23].
23. LeVeque R: **High-Resolution Conservative Algorithms for Advection in Incompressible Flow.** *SIAM Journal on Numerical Analysis* 1996, **33(2)**:627-665.
24. Langseth J, LeVeque R: **A Wave Propagation Method for Three-Dimensional Hyperbolic Conservation Laws.** *Journal of Computational Physics* 2000, **165(1)**:126-166.
25. Ebbers T, Haraldsson H, Dyverfeldt P, Sigfridsson A, Warntjes M, Wigström L: **Higher order weighted least-squares phase offset correction for improved accuracy in phase-contrast MRI.** *Proceedings of the International Society for Magnetic Resonance in Medicine* 2008, **16**:1367.
26. Xiang Q: **Temporal phase unwrapping for CINE velocity imaging.** *J Magn Reson Imaging* 1995, **5(5)**:529-34.

27. Heiberg E, Sjögren J, Ugander M, Carlsson M, Engblom H, Arheden H: **Design and validation of Segment-available software for cardiovascular image analysis.** *BMC Medical Imaging* 2010, **10**:1.
28. Darmofal D, Haimes R: **An Analysis of 3D Particle Path Integration Algorithms.** *Journal of Computational Physics* 1996, **123(1)**:182-195.
29. Cerqueira M, Weissman N, Dilsizian V, Jacobs A, Kaul S, Laskey W, Pennell D, Rumberger J, Ryan T, Verani M: **Standardized myocardial segmentation and nomenclature for tomographic imaging of the heart: a statement for healthcare professionals from the Cardiac Imaging Committee of the Council on Clinical Cardiology of the American Heart Association.** *Circulation* 2002, **105(4)**:539-542.
30. Cohen J: **A coefficient of agreement for nominal scales.** *Educational and psychological measurement* 1960, **20(1)**:37.
31. Morbiducci U, Ponzini R, Rizzo G, Cadioli M, Esposito A, Montevecchi F, Redaelli A: **Mechanistic insight into the physiological relevance of helical blood flow in the human aorta: an in vivo study.** *Biomechanics and Modeling in Mechanobiology* .
32. Bolger A, Heiberg E, Karlsson M, Wigstrom L, Engvall J, Sigfridsson A, Ebbers T, Kvitting J, Carlhall C, Wranne B: **Transit of Blood Flow Through the Human Left Ventricle Mapped by Cardiovascular Magnetic Resonance.** *Journal of Cardiovascular Magnetic Resonance* 2007, **9(5)**:741-747.
33. Hong G, Pedrizzetti G, Tonti G, Li P, Wei Z, Kim J, Baweja A, Liu S, Chung N, Houle H, *et al*: **Characterization and quantification of vortex flow in the human left ventricle by contrast echocardiography using vector particle image velocimetry.** *JACC: Cardiovascular Imaging* 2008, **1(6)**:705-717.

Permissions

All chapters in this book were first published in MI, by BioMed Central; hereby published with permission under the Creative Commons Attribution License or equivalent. Every chapter published in this book has been scrutinized by our experts. Their significance has been extensively debated. The topics covered herein carry significant findings which will fuel the growth of the discipline. They may even be implemented as practical applications or may be referred to as a beginning point for another development.

The contributors of this book come from diverse backgrounds, making this book a truly international effort. This book will bring forth new frontiers with its revolutionizing research information and detailed analysis of the nascent developments around the world.

We would like to thank all the contributing authors for lending their expertise to make the book truly unique. They have played a crucial role in the development of this book. Without their invaluable contributions this book wouldn't have been possible. They have made vital efforts to compile up to date information on the varied aspects of this subject to make this book a valuable addition to the collection of many professionals and students.

This book was conceptualized with the vision of imparting up-to-date information and advanced data in this field. To ensure the same, a matchless editorial board was set up. Every individual on the board went through rigorous rounds of assessment to prove their worth. After which they invested a large part of their time researching and compiling the most relevant data for our readers.

The editorial board has been involved in producing this book since its inception. They have spent rigorous hours researching and exploring the diverse topics which have resulted in the successful publishing of this book. They have passed on their knowledge of decades through this book. To expedite this challenging task, the publisher supported the team at every step. A small team of assistant editors was also appointed to further simplify the editing procedure and attain best results for the readers.

Apart from the editorial board, the designing team has also invested a significant amount of their time in understanding the subject and creating the most relevant covers. They scrutinized every image to scout for the most suitable representation of the subject and create an appropriate cover for the book.

The publishing team has been an ardent support to the editorial, designing and production team. Their endless efforts to recruit the best for this project, has resulted in the accomplishment of this book. They are a veteran in the field of academics and their pool of knowledge is as vast as their experience in printing. Their expertise and guidance has proved useful at every step. Their uncompromising quality standards have made this book an exceptional effort. Their encouragement from time to time has been an inspiration for everyone.

The publisher and the editorial board hope that this book will prove to be a valuable piece of knowledge for researchers, students, practitioners and scholars across the globe.

List of Contributors

Paola Di Carlo, Marcello Trizzino, Lucina Titone, Giuseppina Capra and Daniela Pistoia
Dipartimento di Scienze per la Promozione della Salute, Università di Palermo, Italy

Giovanni Mazzola and Piero Colletti
Dipartimento di Medicina Clinica e delle Patologie Emergenti, Azienda Ospedaliera Universitaria Policlinico "Paolo Giaccone" di Palermo, Palermo, Italy

Caterina Sarno
Dipartimento di Scienze Radiologiche, Azienda Ospedaliera Universitaria Policlinico "Paolo Giaccone" di Palermo, Palermo, Italy

Mikael Montelius
Department of Radiation Physics, Institute of Clinical Sciences, Sahlgrenska Cancer Centre, Sahlgrenska Academy, University of Gothenburg, Sahlgrenska University Hospital, Gothenburg SE-413 45, Sweden

Maria Ljungberg and Eva Forssell-Aronsson
Division of Medical Physics and Medical Engineering, Sahlgrenska University Hospital, Gothenburg SE-413 45, Sweden
Department of Radiation Physics, Institute of Clinical Sciences, Sahlgrenska Cancer Centre, Sahlgrenska Academy, University of Gothenburg, Sahlgrenska University Hospital, Gothenburg SE-413 45, Sweden

Michael Horn
Department of Radiology, University of Würzburg, Würzburg, Germany
Department of Radiation Physics, Institute of Clinical Sciences, Sahlgrenska Cancer Centre, Sahlgrenska Academy, University of Gothenburg, Sahlgrenska University Hospital, Gothenburg SE-413 45, Sweden

Chevrefils Claudia
Ecole Polytechnique de Montreal, Biomedical Engineering Institute, Montreal, QC H3C 3A7, Canada

Grimard Guy and Miron Marie-Claude
Sainte-Justine University Hospital Center, Montreal, QC H3T 1C5, Canada

Cheriet Farida
Department of Computer Engineering and Software, Ecole Polytechnique de Montreal, Montreal, QC H3C 3A7, Canada
Sainte-Justine University Hospital Center, Montreal, QC H3T 1C5, Canada
Department of Mechanical Engineering, Ecole Polytechnique de Montreal, Montreal, QC H3C 3A7, Canada

Aubin Carl-Eric
Department of Mechanical Engineering, Ecole Polytechnique de Montreal, Montreal, QC H3C 3A7, Canada
Sainte-Justine University Hospital Center, Montreal, QC H3T 1C5, Canada

Sima Chalavi and A A T Simone Reinders
Department of Neuroscience, University Medical Center Groningen, and BCN Neuroimaging Center, University of Groningen, Groningen, The Netherlands
King's College London, Institute of Psychiatry, Department of Psychosis Studies, London, UK

Gareth J Barker
King's College London, Institute of Psychiatry, Department of Neuroimaging, London, UK
Centre for Neurodegeneration Research, King's College London, London, UK

Andrew Simmons
Biomedical Research Centre for Mental Health at South London and Maudsley NHS Foundation Trust and Institute of Psychiatry, King's College London, London, UK
King's College London, Institute of Psychiatry, Department of Neuroimaging, London, UK
Centre for Neurodegeneration Research, King's College London, London, UK

Hildebrand Dijkstra
Department of Radiology, University Medical Center Groningen, University of Groningen, Groningen, The Netherlands

Jacob Lønborg
Department of Cardiology, Rigshospitalet, Copenhagen, Denmark
North Shore Heart Research Group, Kolling Institute of Medical Research, University of Sydney, Sydney, Australia

Gemma A Figtree
Department of Cardiology, Royal North Shore Hospital, St Leonards, NSW 2065, Australia
North Shore Heart Research Group, Kolling Institute of Medical Research, University of Sydney, Sydney, Australia

Michael Ward
Department of Cardiology, Royal North Shore Hospital, St Leonards, NSW 2065, Australia
North Shore Heart Research Group, Kolling Institute of Medical Research, University of Sydney, Sydney, Australia

Stuart M Grieve
Department of Radiology, Royal Prince Alfred Hospital, Sydney, Australia
North Shore Heart Research Group, Kolling Institute of Medical Research, University of Sydney, Sydney, Australia

Anthony Gill
Department of Pathology, Royal North Shore Hospital, Sydney, Australia

Kristina I Ringe
Department of Diagnostic and Interventional Radiology, Hannover Medical School, Carl-Neuberg Str. 1, 30625 Hannover, Germany

Daniel T Boll, Daniela B Husarik, Mustafa R Bashir and Rajan T Gupta
Department of Radiology, Duke University Medical Center, Durham, North Carolina 27710, USA

Elmar M Merkle
University Hospital Basel, Radiology and Nuclear Medicine, Petersgraben 4, CH-4031 Basel, Switzerland
Department of Radiology, Duke University Medical Center, Durham, North Carolina 27710, USA

Hiroyuki Tokue, Ayako Taketomi-Takahashi, Azusa Tokue and Yoshito Tsushima
TDepartment of Diagnostic and Interventional Radiology, Gunma University Hospital, 3-39-22 Showa-machi, Maebashi, Gunma 371-8511, Japan

Junjie Li, Jan Bogaert, Raymond Oyen and Yicheng Ni
Radiology Section, Department of Imaging and Pathology, University Hospitals, KU Leuven, Belgium

Yuanbo Feng, Feng Chen, Huaijun Wang, Marlein Miranda Cona, Junjie Li and Jie Yu
Radiology Section, Department of Imaging and Pathology, University Hospitals, KU Leuven, Belgium
Molecular Small Animal Imaging Center (MoSAIC), Biomedical Sciences Group, University Hospitals, KU Leuven, Belgium

Yi Xie
Departments of Electronics and Information System (ELIS), Ghent University, Ghent, Belgium

Stefan Janssens
Department of Cardiovascular Diseases, University Hospitals, KU, Leuven, Belgium

Barbara Blasiak, Tadeusz Foniok, David Rushforth, Garnette R Sutherland and Boguslaw Tomanek
3330 Hospital Dr NW, Calgary, Alberta T2N 4N1, Canada

Wladyslaw P Weglarz
Polish Academy of Sciences, Institute of Nuclear Physics, Krakow,152 Radzikowskiego, Krakow, Malopolska 31-342, Poland

Boguslaw Tomanek
Thunder Bay Regional Research Institute, 980 Oliver Road, Thunder Bay, Ontario P7B 6V4, Canada
Polish Academy of Sciences, Institute of Nuclear Physics, Krakow,152 Radzikowskiego, Krakow, Malopolska 31-342, Poland

Andre Obenaus and Samuel Barnes
Departments of Radiation Medicine, Radiology, Pediatrics, Loma Linda University Chan Shun Pavilion, Room A101011175 Campus Street, Loma Linda, California 92354, USA

Dragana Ponjevic and John Matyas
Faculty of Veterinary Medicine, University of Calgary, 3330 Hospital Dr NW, Calgary, Alberta T2N 4N1, Canada

Abedelnasser Abulrob
Department of Cellular and Molecular Medicine, Faculty of Medicine, University of Ottawa, 451 Smyth Road, Ottawa, Ontario K1H 8M5, Canada
Human Health Therapeutics Portfolio, National Research Council of Canada, Ottawa K1A 0R6, Ontario, Canada

Umar Iqbal
Human Health Therapeutics Portfolio, National Research Council of Canada, Ottawa K1A 0R6, Ontario, Canada

Randy Tyson
Alberta Innovates - Technology Futures, 3608 33 Street NW, Calgary T2L 2A6, Alberta, Canada

Michael Haimerl, Max Wächtler, Rene Müller-Wille, Christoph Niessen, Patrick Hoffstetter Andreas Georg Schreyer, Christian Stroszczynski and Philipp Wiggermann
Department of Radiology, University Medical Center Regensburg, Regensburg 93042, Germany

Ivan Platzek
Department of Radiology, University Hospital Carl Gustav Carus Dresden, Dresden, Germany
Institute for Biomedical Engineering, University and ETH Zurich, Zurich, Switzerland

Cosima Jahnke and Rolf Gebker
Department of Cardiology, University Hospital Zurich, Rämistrasse 100, 8091, Zurich, Switzerland

Robert Manka
Institute of Diagnostic and Interventional Radiology, University Hospital Zurich, Zurich, Switzerland
Department of Cardiology, University Hospital Zurich, Rämistrasse 100, 8091, Zurich, Switzerland

Ingo Paetsch
Department of Cardiology, University Hospital RWTH Aachen, Aachen, Germany

Kristof Graf, Thomas Hucko and Thore Dietrich
Department of Cardiology, German Heart Institute Berlin, Berlin, Germany

Bernhard Schnackenburg
Philips Healthcare, Hamburg, Germany

Rasheed Zakaria and Michael D Jenkinson
Department of Neurosurgery, The Walton Centre NHS Foundation Trust, Liverpool, UK

Philip R Rudland and Rasheed Zakaria
Institute of Integrative Biology, University of Liverpool, Liverpool, UK

Kumar Das, Mark Radon and Maneesh Bhojak
Department of Neuroradiology, The Walton Centre NHS Foundation Trust, Liverpool, UK

Vanessa Sluming
Magnetic resonance and image analysis research centre (MARIARC), University of Liverpool, Liverpool, UK

Michael D Jenkinson
Institute of Translational Medicine, University of Liverpool, Liverpool, UK

Rasheed Zakaria
Neurosciences Research Centre, The Walton Centre NHS Foundation Trust, Liverpool L9 7LJ, UK

Niklas Klasson, Erik Olsson, Carl Eckerström, Helge Malmgren and Anders Wallin
Institute of Psychiatry and Neurochemistry, Department of Neuroscience and physiology, The Sahlgrenska Academy, University of Gothenburg, SE-405 30 Göteborg, Sweden

Mats Rudemo
Department of Mathematical Sciences, Chalmers University of Technology and University of Gothenburg, SE-412 96 Göteborg, Sweden

Helge Malmgren
Department of Philosophy, Linguistics and Theory of Science, University of Gothenburg, SE-405 30 Göteborg, Sweden

Christos Xanthis
Department of Computer Science and Biomedical informatics, University of Thessaly, Lamia, Greece

Karin Markenroth Bloch
Philips Healthcare, Lund, Sweden

Einar Heiberg
Department of Biomedical Engineering, Faculty of Engineering, Lund University, Lund, Sweden
Department of Clinical Physiology, Lund University, Lund University Hospital, Lund, Sweden
Center for Mathematics, Faculty of Engineering, Lund University, Lund, Sweden

Ann-Christin Ostwaldt, Christian H. Nolte, Kersten Villringer and Jochen B. Fiebach
Center for Stroke Research Berlin (CSB), Charité Universitätsmedizin Berlin, Hindenburgdamm 30, 12200 Berlin, Germany

Tatiana Usnich and Christian H. Nolte
Department of Neurology, Charité Universitätsmedizin Berlin, Hindenburgdamm 30, 12200 Berlin, Germany

Sayaka Kodaira, Takahito Nakajima, Ryosuke Takahashi, Shingo Moriya, Hidenori Ohtake and Yoshito Tsushima
Department of Diagnostic Radiology and Nuclear Medicine, 3-39-22, Showa, Maebashi, Gunma, Japan

Tomoyuki Nakagawa
Zenshukai Hospital, 1381, Ninomiya, Maebashi, Gunma, Japan

Tomas Lapinskas and Remigijus Zaliunas
Department of Cardiology, Medical Academy, Lithuanian University of Health Sciences, Eiveniu Street 2, LT-50161 Kaunas, Lithuania

Burkert Pieske, Heike Meyborg, Daniel Messroghli Rolf Gebker and Seyedeh Mahsa Zamani
Department of Internal Medicine / Cardiology, Deutsches Herzzentrum Berlin, Augustenburger Platz 1, 13353 Berlin, Germany

Ulrich Kintscher
Center for Cardiovascular Research, Institute of Pharmacology, Charité-Universitätsmedizin Berlin, Berlin, Germany

Jana Grune
Center for Cardiovascular Research, Institute of Pharmacology, Charité-Universitätsmedizin Berlin, Berlin, Germany
Department of Internal Medicine / Cardiology, Deutsches Herzzentrum Berlin, Augustenburger Platz 1, 13353 Berlin, Germany
DZHK (German Centre for Cardiovascular Research), Partner Site Berlin, Berlin, Germany

Sarah Jeuthe
Department of Internal Medicine / Cardiology, Charité-Universitätsmedizin Berlin, Berlin, Germany

Sebastian Kelle and Philipp Stawowy
DZHK (German Centre for Cardiovascular Research), Partner Site Berlin, Berlin, Germany
Department of Internal Medicine / Cardiology, Deutsches Herzzentrum Berlin, Augustenburger Platz 1, 13353 Berlin, Germany

Ulrich Kintscher
DZHK (German Centre for Cardiovascular Research), Partner Site Berlin, Berlin, Germany

Yanguang Shen, Yan Zhong, Haiyi Wang, Lu Ma, Yingwei Wang, Jinjin Pan and Huiyi Ye
Department of Radiology, Chinese PLA General Hospital, Fuxing Road NO.28, Beijing, China

Zhonghua Sun
Department of Medical Radiation Sciences, Curtin University, Perth 6102, Australia

Matthieu Dumont, Luc Tremblay and Martin Lepage
Centre d'Imagerie Moléculaire de Sherbrooke, CHUS - Hôpital Fleurimont, Sherbrooke, Canada

Benoit Tricot
Center for Systems Biology, Massachusetts General Hospital and Harvard Medical School, Boston, USA
Centre d'Imagerie Moléculaire de Sherbrooke, CHUS - Hôpital Fleurimont, Sherbrooke, Canada

Maxime Descoteaux
Département d'Informatique, Université de Sherbrooke, Sherbrooke, Canada
Centre d'Imagerie Moléculaire de Sherbrooke, CHUS - Hôpital Fleurimont, Sherbrooke, Canada

Frederic Chagnon
Soins Intensifs Médicaux, CHUS - Hôpital Fleurimont, Sherbrooke, Canada

Olivier Lesur
Soins Intensifs Médicaux, CHUS - Hôpital Fleurimont, Sherbrooke, Canada
Centre d'Imagerie Moléculaire de Sherbrooke, CHUS - Hôpital Fleurimont, Sherbrooke, Canada

André Carpentier
Département de Médecine, CHUS - Hôpital Fleurimont, Sherbrooke, Canada

Alain Lalande
Le2I, Faculté de Médecine, Université Bourgogne Franche-Comté, 7 Bld Jeanne d'Arc, 21079 Dijon Cedex, BP 87900, France

Bo Hu, Jin Zhang, Ying Yu, Qian Sun, Lin-Feng Yan, Yu-Chuan Hu, Hai-Yan Nan, Yang Yang, Guang-Bin Cui and Wen Wang
Department of Radiology & Functional and Molecular Imaging Key Lab of Shaanxi Province, Tangdu Hospital, Fourth Military Medical University (Air Force Medical University), 569 Xinsi Road, Xi'an 710038, Shaanxi, China

Xu Wang and Jie-bing He
Student Brigade, Fourth Military Medical University (Air Force Medical University), 169 West Changle Road, Xi'an 710032, Shaanxi Province, China

Yu-jie Dai
Department of Clinical Nutrition, Xijing Hospital, The Fourth Military Medical University, Xi'an, China

Alan D. Kaye
Departments of Anesthesiology and Pharmacology, Louisiana State University School of Medicine, New Orleans, Louisiana, USA

B. G. Sibinga Mulder, K. Visser, A. L. Vahrmeijer, R. J. Swijnenburg, H. H. Hartgrink and J. S. D. Mieog
Department of Surgery, Leiden University Medical Center, Leiden 2300 RC, The Netherlands

R. van den Boom, M. C. Burgmans and S. Feshtali
Department of Radiology, Leiden University Medical Center, Leiden 2300 RC, The Netherlands

Jacob A. Macdonald
Department of Medical Physics, University of Wisconsin, 1111 Highland Avenue, Room 1005, Madison, WI 53705, USA

Christopher J. François
Department of Radiology, University of Wisconsin, Madison, USA

Oliver Wieben
Department of Radiology, University of Wisconsin, Madison, USA
Department of Biomedical Engineering, University of Wisconsin, Madison, USA
Department of Medical Physics, University of Wisconsin, 1111 Highland Avenue, Room 1005, Madison, WI 53705, USA

Omid Forouzan and Naomi C. Chesler
Department of Biomedical Engineering, University of Wisconsin, Madison, USA

Katarina Kindberg
Department of Management and Engineering, Linköping University, SE-581 83 Linköping, Sweden
Center for Medical Image Science and Visualization (CMIV), Linköping University, SE-581 85 Linköping, Sweden

Henrik Haraldsson
Department of Management and Engineering, Linköping University, SE-581 83 Linköping, Sweden
Center for Medical Image Science and Visualization (CMIV), Linköping University, SE-581 85 Linköping, Sweden
Department of Medical and Health Sciences, Linköping University, SE-581 85 Linköping, Sweden

Matts Karlsson
Department of Management and Engineering, Linköping University, SE-581 83 Linköping, Sweden
Center for Medical Image Science and Visualization (CMIV), Linköping University, SE-581 85 Linköping, Sweden

Andreas Sigfridsson
Center for Medical Image Science and Visualization (CMIV), Linköping University, SE-581 85 Linköping, Sweden
Department of Medical and Health Sciences, Linköping University, SE-581 85 Linköping, Sweden

Jan Engvall
Department of Medical and Health Sciences, Linköping University, SE-581 85 Linköping, Sweden

Neil B Ingels Jr
Department of Cardiothoracic Surgery, School of Medicine, Stanford University, Stanford, CA 94305, USA
Research Institute of the Palo Alto Medical Foundation, Palo Alto, CA 94305, USA

Tino Ebbers
Department of Science and Technology, Linköping University, SE-581 83 Linköping, Sweden
Department of Management and Engineering, Linköping University, SE-581 83 Linköping, Sweden
Center for Medical Image Science and Visualization (CMIV), Linköping University, SE-581 85 Linköping, Sweden
Department of Medical and Health Sciences, Linköping University, SE-581 85 Linköping, Sweden

Zikuan Chen
The Mind Research Network and LBERI, Albuquerque 87106, NM, USA

Vince Calhoun
Department of Electrical and Computer Engineering, Albuquerque 87131, NM, USA
The Mind Research Network and LBERI, Albuquerque 87106, NM, USA

Riccardo Del Vescovo, Sofia Battisti, Valerio Di Paola, Claudia L Piccolo, Roberto L Cazzato, Ilaria Sansoni, Rosario F Grasso and Bruno Beomonte Zobel
Department of Radiology, Campus Bio-Medico Univeristy of Rome, Italy

Ali S Arbab, Adarsh Shankar, Nadimpalli RS Varma, Xiaohua Gao, ASM Iskander, Branislava Janic and Meser M Ali
Department of Radiology, Henry Ford Hospital, 1 Ford Place, 2F, Detroit, MI 48202, USA

Subhash C Gautam and Dorrah Deeb
Department of Surgery, Henry Ford Hospital, 1 Ford Place, 4D, Detroit, MI 48202, USA

Mikael Kanski, Katarina Steding-Ehrenborg, Marcus Carlsson, Håkan Arheden and Einar Heiberg
Department of Clinical Physiology, Lund University, Skåne University Hospital Lund, Lund, Sweden

Gustaf Söderlind
Department of Numerical Analysis, Centre for Mathematical Sciences, Lund University, Lund, Sweden

Johannes Töger
Department of Numerical Analysis, Centre for Mathematical Sciences, Lund University, Lund, Sweden
Department of Clinical Physiology, Lund University, Skåne University Hospital Lund, Lund, Sweden

Index

www.ingramcontent.com/pod-product-compliance
Lightning Source LLC
LaVergne TN
LVHW080911210926
848485LV00004B/630